THE NUTRI~~

CARBOHYDRATES CALORIES & FAT

IN YOUR FOOD

DR. ART ULENE

Avery Publishing Group

Garden City Park, New York

The information in this book is based upon the latest data made available by government agencies, food manufacturers, and trade associations. It is important to note that all nutrient breakdowns for processed foods are subject to change by manufacturers without notice and may therefore vary from printing to printing.

ISBN 0-89529-632-2

Printed in the United States of America

10   9   8   7   6   5

CONTENTS

INTRODUCTION

Throughout history, people have recognized the connection between the food we eat and the state of our health. But only recently have we begun to appreciate just how important this connection is. Researchers have now proven a strong relationship between excess fat consumption and obesity, high blood pressure, and stroke; between excess fat and coronary heart disease; between excess calorie consumption and premature death. The list goes on and on.

But not all of the associations are negative. Research has also shown that by changing the quantity and quality of the fats and carbohydrates you consume, you can have a positive effect on your health. For instance, by reducing your intake of fat and cholesterol, you can lower blood cholesterol levels. By changing the carbohydrates you consume, you can reduce your risk of colon cancer and lower your blood cholesterol. And if you have diabetes, by consuming complex carbohydrates, you can more easily maintain blood sugars within the normal range.

Some people are surprised to learn that carbohydrates can be a useful part of a weight-loss program. Years ago, dieters were often advised to shun carbohydrates in favor of protein-rich foods like steak and cheese. This advice was given because pasta, potatoes, and breads were thought to be a major cause of excess weight gain. Now we know that the real culprit usually isn't the pasta; it's the fat-rich sauces that go on top. In fact, carbohydrates provide dieters with a feeling of satisfaction and fullness, as well as a continuing source of energy. Better yet, on an ounce-for-ounce basis, carbohydrates have less than half the calories of fat. (More on this later.)

This book was designed to help you make wiser choices when you buy food and when you dine out. It will help you interpret nutritional stories in the media so you can distinguish useful information from nonsense. It will give you the control you need over your personal nutrition.

Many people refer to books of this sort as "counter" books because of the nutritional numbers that fill the pages. But this is not a book about counting. This is a book about control and choices. Use this book to learn more about the foods you should consume or avoid. Don't be intimidated by the huge number of choices listed or by the impossible-to-memorize nutritional value numbers. It is not necessary to memorize these numbers. Instead, just try to familiarize yourself with the foods and food categories that are best suited to your needs.

Begin by looking up the foods that you eat most often or in the largest quantities. If these foods are not providing you with the nutrients you need, use the book to find better alternatives that are just as tasty. Once you are familiar with the nutritional content of your most common food choices, gradually look up the remainder of the foods in your diet. You'll be surpised by how easy it is to learn about these foods and to make any necessary changes.

The following section will explain some of the basics about fats, carbohydrates, and calories. After that, you will learn how to use this book to locate the information you need to improve your diet.

UNDERSTANDING CARBOHYDRATES

Carbohydrates supply the body with the energy it needs to function. Carbohydrates are metabolized, or "burned," by the body, providing 4 calories—4 units of energy—per gram. (There are 454 grams in one pound.) Carbohydrates are found almost exclusively in plant foods, such as fruits, vegetables, grains, peas, and beans. Milk is the only food derived from animals that contains a significant amount of carbohydrates.

Carbohydrates are divided into two groups—simple carbohydrates and complex carbohydrates. *Simple carbohydrates,* sometimes called simple sugars, include fructose (fruit sugar), sucrose (table sugar), and lactose (milk sugar), as well as several other sugars. Fruits are one of the richest sources of simple carbohydrates. Complex carbohydrates are also made up of sugars, but the sugar molecules are strung together to form longer, more complex chains. Complex carbohydrates include fiber and starches. Foods rich in complex carbohydrates include vegetables, whole grains, peas, and beans.

Carbohydrates are the main source of blood glucose, which is a major fuel for all of our cells, and the only source of energy for the brain and red blood cells. Except for fiber, which cannot be digested, both simple and complex carbohydrates are converted into glucose, which is either used directly to provide energy for the body, or stored in the liver for future use. When a person consumes more calories than the body is using, a portion of the carbohydrates consumed may also be stored in the body as fat.

When choosing carbohydrate-rich foods for your diet, it is a good idea to select unrefined foods, such as fruits, vegetables, peas, beans, and whole-grain products, as opposed to refined, processed foods such as soft drinks, candy, and sugar. Refined foods offer few, if any, of the vitamins and minerals that are important to your health. Also, be cautious in your use of any carbohydrate-rich foods that are combined with large quantities of fat in their preparation. These foods, which include

astries and snack foods, are usually loaded with calories far out of proportion to
heir overall nutrient value.

UNDERSTANDING FATS

Recently, much attention has been focused on the need to reduce dietary fat.
Nevertheless, the body does need fats—but only the right fats, and only in the
appropriate quantities. Fats are essential for growth and development, and for the
maintenance of healthy skin, hair, and nails. And, as one of the four nutrients, fat
provides the body with the energy it needs to carry on all functions. Most of us know,
though, that there are several kinds of dietary fat, and that some fats are more likely
than others to contribute to high blood pressure and coronary heart disease. A basic
understanding of the different types of fat is important for anyone who wants to
maximize health through wise dietary choices.

Fats have been classified into three major categories—saturated fats, polyunsaturated fats, and monounsaturated fats. This classification is based on the
number of hydrogen atoms each has in its chemical structure.

Saturated fats, which are usually solid at room temperature, are found primarily
in animal products, including fatty meats like beef, veal, lamb, pork, and ham; and
in dairy items, such as whole milk, cream, ice cream, and cheese. For example, the
marbleized fat you can see in beef is saturated. Some types of vegetable products—including coconut oil, palm kernel oil, and vegetable shortening—are also
high in saturates.

The liver uses saturated fats to manufacture cholesterol. Therefore, excessive
dietary intake of saturated fats can significantly raise the blood cholesterol level,
especially in people who have inherited a tendency toward high blood cholesterol.
Guidelines issued by the National Cholesterol Education Program (NCEP), and
widely supported by most experts, recommend that your intake of saturated fats
should be kept below 10 percent of your total calorie intake. However, for people
who have severe problems with high blood cholesterol, even that level may be too
high.

Polyunsaturated fats are found in greatest abundance in corn, soybean, saf-
flower, and sunflower oils. Certain fish oils, particularly the omega-3 fatty acids, are
also high in polyunsaturates. Unlike the saturated fats, polyunsaturates may actually
lower your total blood cholesterol level. In doing so, however, large amounts of
polyunsaturates also have a tendency to reduce your HDLS—the "good" cholesterol
that helps lower blood cholesterol levels. For this reason—and because, like all fats,
polyunsaturates are high in calories for their weight and volume—the NCEP
guidelines state that your intake of polyunsaturated fats should not exceed 10
percent of your total calorie intake.

Monounsaturated fats are found mostly in vegetable and nut oils such as olive peanut, and canola. These fats appear to reduce blood levels of LDL cholesterol—the "bad" cholesterol that contributes to coronary heart disease—without affecting HDLs in any way. However, this positive impact upon LDL cholesterol is relatively modest. The NCEP guidelines recommend that your intake of monounsaturated fats be kept between 10 and 15 percent of your total calorie intake.

Although most foods—including some plant-derived foods—contain a combination of all three types of fats, one of the types usually predominates. Thus, a food is considered "saturated" or "high in saturates" when it is composed primarily of saturated fatty acids. Similarly, a food composed mostly of polyunsaturated fatty acids is called "polyunsaturated," while a food composed mostly of monounsaturated fatty acids is called "monounsaturated."

One other element, trans-fatty acids, might also play a role in blood cholesterol levels. Trans-fatty acids occur when polyunsaturated oils are altered through hydrogenation, a process used to harden liquid vegetable oils into solid foods like margarine and shortening. One recent study found that trans-monounsaturated fatty acids raise LDL cholesterol levels, behaving much like saturated fats. Simultaneously, these trans-fatty acids reduced HDL cholesterol readings. Much more research is necessary, since some studies have not produced clear-cut conclusions about these substances. But your dietary choices could become less matter-of-fact than they now appear. For now, however, it is clear that when your goal is to lower cholesterol, polyunsaturated and monounsaturated fats are much more desirable than saturated fats.

UNDERSTANDING CALORIES

When we talk about foods, we often mention the number of calories a certain food has. Yet calories are not nutrients, like carbohydrates and fat. What, then, are calories?

A calorie is an energy unit. As already mentioned, carbohydrates and fats—as well as protein, still another nutrient—provide the body with the energy it needs to function. This energy is measured in calories. There are 4 calories in every gram of protein, 4 calories in every gram of carbohydrate, and 9 calories in every gram of fat. So on a gram-for-gram basis, fat is more than twice as fattening than carbohydrates or protein. It is no wonder, then, that when people try to lose weight, it is important that they cut down on fatty foods.

In addition to fat's having more calories than protein or carbohydrates, fat is metabolized differently by the body. Therefore, the excess fat in your diet is more likely to be stored as fat in your body than is excess carbohydrate or protein. That's because dietary fat is similar in chemical composition to body fat, so it takes less energy to convert it to body fat. In fact, it takes only 3 percent of the calories in the fat you eat to turn that food into body fat, while it takes at least 25 percent of the carbohydrate and protein calories you eat to convert them into body fat.

THE FOOD GUIDE PYRAMID

Over the years, the United States Department of Agriculture (USDA) has tried to insure adequate nutrition by encouraging Americans to eat a "well-balanced diet"—a concept that has changed dramatically over the years. Most of us still remember the four food groups that the USDA once promoted. These food groups—fruits and vegetables; breads and cereals; meat, poultry, fish and eggs; and dairy products— were developed to encourage a balanced diet that was rich in meat, poultry, and dairy products. Clearly, we now have a greater understanding of how such a diet affects our health, and the government now recommends a diet high in complex carbohydrates and low in fat. With this in mind, in May 1992, the government abandoned the four food groups in favor of the Food Guide Pyramid, which has dramatically changed the recommended amounts of foods in each group.

At the base of the Food Guide Pyramid is the bread, cereal, rice, and pasta group. Six to eleven servings from this group are recommended daily—more servings than from any other food group. The next level of the pyramid is occupied by the vegetable group, with three to five servings recommended daily, and the fruit group, with two to four servings recommended daily. Moving upward, the next pyramid level is shared by the milk, yogurt, and cheese group, and the meat, poultry, fish, dry beans, eggs, and nuts group, with two to three servings recommended daily from each group. Finally, at the peak of the pyramid—and occupying the smallest area—are fats, oils, and sweets, a group of foods that is to be eaten only sparingly.

Government health officials recommend that no more than 30 percent of your calories should come from fat. Others, myself included, believe that levels of 20 to 25 percent would be even healthier. In contrast, it is recommended that about 60 percent of your calories come from complex carbodrates—those foods found in the two largest levels of the pyramid.

How Americans Measure Up

How many Americans are now following the government's lead and using the Food Guide Pyramid as their model? Unfortunately, most Americans—97 percent, by some estimates—are not eating a balanced diet by any definition. What are Americans eating? The Standard American Diet, appropriately nicknamed SAD, now gets about 36 percent of its calories from fat. This is significantly higher than

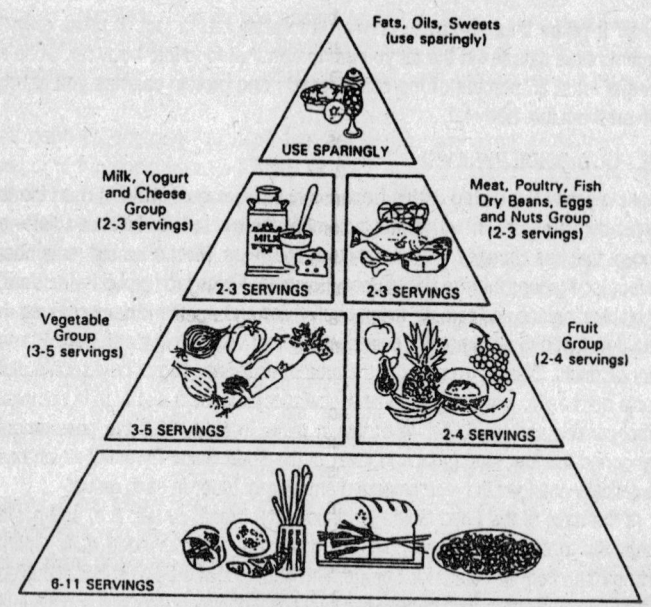

Bread, Cereal, Rice, and Pasta Group (6–11 servings)

The Food Guide Pyramid

the government recommendation of 30 percent, and far above the 20- to 25-percent target that many physicians think is healthier.

Are Americans getting adequate amounts of carbohydates? Recent studies show that Americans get only about 45 percent of their calories from carbohydrates, rather than the 60 percent now recommended. Even worse, about half of these calories come from refined foods—soft drinks, cakes, candies, and other low-nutrient foods—rather than from unrefined foods that contain a variety of other nutrients.

GUIDELINES FOR HEALTHY EATING

The remainder of this book will help you choose foods that are low in health-compromising fat, and high in nutrient-rich carbohydrates. But as the Food Guide Pyramid illustrates, to maximize your health, you must eat adequate servings from each of the pyramid's first three levels. The following guidelines should help:

■ When eating foods from the bread, cereal, rice, and pasta group, always choose whole-grain, high-fiber, low-fat breads and cereals—preferably without added sugar, coloring, or unnecessary preservatives. Choose brown rice over white rice, and whole-wheat or other whole-grain pastas over pastas made from white flour.

■ When eating fruits and vegetables, eat fresh raw produce as often as possible. Water-soluble vitamins, such as vitamin C, may leach out of foods during cooking, be damaged by overprocessing, or be destroyed when foods are overcooked. Even fat-soluble vitamins, which are fairly stable during low-temperature cooking, can be affected by frying. For this reason, it is best to steam or microwave vegetables rather than boiling or frying them. And, unless the produce was grown organically, be sure to peel or thoroughly wash it to eliminate pesticide residues and waxes.

■ When choosing foods from the milk, yogurt, and cheese group, select low-fat and nonfat brands, which provide the most nutrients and the least amount of fat. When eating meat, poultry, and fish, choose the leanest cuts available, trim off any excess fat, and bake or broil the foods instead of frying them.

■ Select as few foods as possible from the fats, oils, and sweets group. When you do use fats and oils, though, choose monounsaturated and polyunsaturated fats instead of saturated fats. Limit your intake of sweets, choosing fresh fruits instead of cakes, cookies, and other high-fat desserts.

THE NEW FOOD LABELING

For many years, consumers complained about the confusing nature of food labels. For instance, the word "light" might mean light in calories when used by one manufacturer, and light in taste or color when used by another. Serving sizes, too, varied greatly, making it nearly impossible to compare the nutrient values of one product with those of another.

Because of this confusion, as of 1994, new food labels were required on all processed foods regulated by the Food and Drug Administration (FDA) and on all processed meat products regulated by the U.S. Department of Agriculture (USDA). Let's take a look at the most significant features of the new food label.

Nutrition Facts

One of the new label's features is a revamped nutrition panel, identified by its "Nutrition Facts" heading. The new nutrition panel features more consistent serving sizes, in both household and metric measures, and states how many servings are found in each container. In addition, the panel lists the following dietary components:

- Total calories
- Sugars
- Saturated fat
- Protein
- Total carbohydrates

- Dietary fiber
- Total fat
- Calories from fat
- Sodium
- Cholesterol

- Vitamin A
- Vitamin C
- Calcium
- Iron

For the last four nutrients listed above—vitamin A, vitamin C, calcium, and iron—the amount is expressed only as a percentage of its Daily Value, a recommended daily amount based on a 2,000-calorie diet. For most of the other nutrients listed, the amount is expressed both in grams or milligrams and as a percentage of its Daily Value. To educate the consumer, reference values are provided at the bottom of the label to show how much total fat, saturated fat, cholesterol, sodium, total carbohydrates, and dietary fiber should be included in both a 2,000-calorie and a 2,500-calorie diet.

Nutrient Content Descriptions

On the new food label, terms once used inconsistently, and often misleadingly, now must be applied uniformly to insure that such terms mean the same on each product on which they appear. Following are definitions of some of the most frequently used terms.

■ **Free.** The product contains no amount of, or only "physiologically inconsequential" amounts of one or more of these components: fat, saturated fat, cholesterol, sodium, sugars, and calories. For instance, "calorie free" means that there are fewer than 5 calories per serving, and "sugar free" and "fat free" indicate that there are less than 0.5 grams per serving.

■ **Low.** This food could be eaten frequently without exceeding dietary guidelines for one or more of the following components: fat, saturated fat, cholesterol, sodium, and calories. Thus, the following terms are used:

    ■ **Low fat.** 3 grams or less per serving.

    ■ **Low saturated fat.** 1 gram or less per serving.

    ■ **Low sodium.** Less than 140 milligrams per serving.

    ■ **Very low sodium.** Less than 35 milligrams per serving.

    ■ **Low cholesterol.** Less than 20 milligrams per serving.

    ■ **Low calorie.** 40 calories or less per serving.

■ **Lean and extra lean.** The following terms can be used to describe the fat content of meat, poultry, seafood, and game meats:

■ **Lean.** Less than 10 grams of fat, less than 4 grams of saturated fat, and less than 95 milligrams of cholesterol per serving and per 100 grams.

■ **Extra lean.** Less than 5 grams of fat, less than 2 grams of saturated fat, and less than 95 milligrams of cholesterol per serving and per 100 grams.

■ **High.** One serving of the food contains 20 percent or more of the Daily Value for a particular nutrient.

■ **Good source.** One serving of the food contains 10 to 19 percent of the Daily Value for a particular nutrient.

■ **Reduced.** A nutritionally altered product that contains 25 percent less of a nutrient or of calories than the regular, or reference, product.

■ **Less.** A food, whether altered or not, that contains 25 percent less of a nutrient or of calories than the reference food.

■ **Light.** A nutritionally altered product that contains one-third fewer calories or half of the fat of the reference food, or the sodium content of a low-calorie, low-fat food has been reduced by 50 percent.

■ **More.** One serving of the food, altered or not, contains a nutrient in a quantity that is at least 10 percent of the Daily Value more than the reference food.

The following section should provide you with the details you need to better access and understand the data contained in this volume. I hope this book inspires you to learn more about your unique nutritional needs and the foods you are using to meet those needs. You will enjoy the sense of control this knowledge gives you. More important, you will make better food choices and take a major step toward better health. I wish you good health always.

Arthur Ulene, MD

How to Use This Book

This book was designed to provide nutritional information on a wide range of foods, both generic and brand name, raw and prepared. The information provided here was gleaned from a number of government agencies, from hundreds of manufacturers, and from food trade associations. This information was compiled and later supplemented through countless hours of follow-up that involved hundreds of additional sources. Because scientific techniques are constantly being improved and nutritional theory continues to advance, this book will be continuously updated to reflect the most current nutritional data available.

FINDING THE LISTING YOU WANT

This easy-to-use guide is an A-to-Z reference to the calorie, carbohydrate, and fat contents of foods. All of the foods in this reference have been listed alphabetically. For instance, if you were looking for the nutrient values of ground beef, you would turn to the *B's* and look under *Beef*. For convenience, similar foods have been grouped together in categories such as *Baby Foods, Breads, Candies, Cereals, Cheese, Cookies, Pasta,* and *Sauces*. Therefore, if the food you are looking for is not listed individually by its own name, you should try looking it up under a logical category.

Some foods are known by two or more names. In most cases, the food is listed under just one name, and cross-references have been provided to guide you to the proper listing. For instance, garbanzo beans are also called chick peas and ceci beans. In this book, you will find the nutrient information under *Garbanzo beans,* with cross-references under *Ceci beans* and *Chick peas*.

If you are unable to find a particular food, look for the listing of a similar food. The nutritional data should be close, if not exact, for any product not listed. When doing this, make sure you are comparing weight measure against weight measure and volume measure against volume measure.

After you locate the listing of the food you are interested in, you may find that abbreviations have been used to provide you with the information you need. Refer to page xvii for a complete key to the abbreviations used throughout this book.

UNDERSTANDING FISH, MEAT, AND VEGETABLE LISTINGS

When examining the nutrient values of *cooked* fish, meat, poultry, and vegetables, keep in mind that unless otherwise noted, no additional ingredients have been added. Also be aware that unless otherwise noted, the food values for fish, meats, and poultry are for meat only, and do not include skin or bones.

We hope that you will find *The Nutribase Guide to Carbohydrates, Calories, and Fat in Your Food* a valuable companion that provides the information you need to take control of your eating habits. Should you have any comments about this book, feel free to write to the following address: Nutribase Comments, c/o Avery Publishing Group, 120 Old Broadway, Garden City Park, NY 11040.

CODES AND ABBREVIATIONS

>	greater than
<	less than
%	percentage
approx	approximately
cal	calories
carbs	carbohydrates
diam	diameter
fl	fluid
gm	gram
lb	pound
mcg	microgram(s)
med	medium-sized
mgs	milligrams

(mq)	may contain a measurable quantity
na	not available
pkg	package
prep	prepared according to directions
tbsp	tablespoon
tr	trace
(tr)	may contain a trace amount
tsp	teaspoon
w/	with
w/o	without
wt	weight

A

Food Name	Serv. Size	Total Cal.	Carbs GMS	Fat GMS
ABALONE, MIXED SPECIES, raw	3 oz	89	5.1	0.7
ABALONE MUSHROOM. See MUSHROOM, OYSTER.				
ACEROLA CHERRY/Barbados cherry				
trimmed	1 cup	31	7.5	0.3
trimmed	1 oz	9	2.2	0.1
trimmed	1 fruit	2	0.4	0.0
untrimmed	1 lb	114	27.9	1.1
ACEROLA CHERRY JUICE/Barbados cherry juice				
	1 cup	51	11.6	0.7
	1 oz	6	1.5	0.1
ACORN				
dried	1 oz	145	15.2	8.9
dried, in shell	1 lb	1432	150.9	88.3
raw, in shell	1 lb	1037	114.6	67.1
raw, shelled	1 oz	105	11.6	6.8
ACORN FLOUR, full fat	1 oz	142	15.5	8.6
ACORN SQUASH. See SQUASH, ACORN.				
ADZUKI BEAN				
boiled, mature seeds	1/2 cup	147	28.5	0.1
raw	1 oz	93	17.8	0.2
raw *(Arrowhead Mills)*	2 oz	190	35.0	1.0
raw, mature seeds	1/2 cup	322	61.6	0.5
yokan, mature seeds, 1/4-inch slice	1 slice	36	8.5	0.0
ADZUKI BEAN, CANNED				
mature seeds, sweetened	1/2 cup	351	81.4	0.0
organic, no salt added *(Eden Foods)*	1/2 cup	80	18.0	<1.0
organic, w/liquid *(Eden Foods)*	1/2 cup	100	17.0	<1.0
AGAR				
dried	100 gm	306	80.9	0.3
raw	1 lb	116	30.6	0.1
raw	100 gm	26	6.8	0.0
raw	1 oz	7	1.9	tr
AHI. See TUNA, YELLOWFIN.				
AKU. See TUNA, SKIPJACK.				
ALBACORE. See TUNA, CANNED; TUNA, FROZEN.				
ALCOHOL-FREE BEVERAGES				
BEER				
(Cutter)	12 oz	76	19.6	0.0
(Kaliber)	12 oz	71	10.6	0.0
(Sharp's)	12 oz	86	9.5	0.0

Food Name	Serv. Size	Total Cal.	Carbs GMS	Fat GMS
MIXED-DRINK MIXERS				
Banana Daiquiri, frozen, diluted w/water *(Bacardi)*	7 oz	150	35.0	1.0
Bloody Mary				
bottled *(Mr. & Mrs. T)*	4.5 oz	20	4.0	0.0
bottled, rich & spicy *(Mr. & Mrs. T)*	4.5 oz	30	6.0	0.0
bottled 'Smooth N' Spicy' *(Holland House)*	1 oz	3	<1.0	0.0
Daiquiri				
bottled *(Holland House)*	1 oz	36	9.0	0.0
instant, dry *(Holland House)*	.56 oz	65	16.0	0.0
Grenadine				
syrup *(Roses)*	1 oz	65	16.0	0.0
syrup *(Roses)*	.5 oz	32	8.0	<1.0
Lime Daiquiri, shelf stable, w/water *(Bacardi)*	7 oz	130	33.0	0.0
Mai Tai				
bottled *(Holland House)*	1 oz	32	8.0	0.0
instant, dry *(Holland House)*	.56 oz	64	16.0	0.0
Manhattan, bottled *(Holland House)*	1 oz	28	7.0	0.0
Margarita				
bottled *(Holland House)*	1 oz	27	6.0	0.0
bottled *(Mr. & Mrs. T)*	3 oz	80	20.0	<1.0
frozen, diluted w/water *(Bacardi)*	7 oz	90	24.0	0.0
instant, dry *(Holland House)*	.5 oz	57	14.0	0.0
shelf stable, w/water *(Bacardi)*	7 oz	130	33.0	0.0
Old Fashioned, bottled *(Holland House)*	1 oz	33	8.0	0.0
Peach Daiquiri, frozen, diluted w/water *(Bacardi)*	7 oz	130	33.0	0.0
Piña Colada				
bottled *(Holland House)*	1 oz	33	8.0	0.0
bottled *(Mr. & Mrs. T)*	4 oz	150	39.0	<1.0
frozen, diluted w/water *(Bacardi)*	7 oz	200	37.0	6.0
instant, dry *(Holland House)*	.56 oz	82	12.0	<3.0
shelf stable, w/water *(Bacardi)*	7 oz	170	36.0	2.0
Raspberry Daiquiri, bottled *(Holland House)*	1 oz	30	7.0	0.0
Rum Runner, shelf stable, w/water *(Bacardi)*	7 oz	140	33.0	0.0
Strawberry Colada, shelf stable, w/water *(Bacardi)*	7 oz	150	34.0	1.0
Strawberry Daiquiri				
bottled *(Holland House)*	1 oz	31	7.0	0.0
frozen, diluted w/water *(Bacardi)*	7 oz	140	34.0	0.0
shelf stable, w/water *(Bacardi)*	7 oz	130	31.0	0.0
Strawberry Margarita				
bottled *(Holland House)*	1 oz	31	7.0	0.0
bottled *(Mr. & Mrs. T)*	3.5 oz	100	24.0	<1.0
instant, dry *(Holland House)*	.56 oz	66	16.0	0.0

Food Name	Serv. Size	Total Cal.	Carbs GMS	Fat GMS
Sweet and Sour				
bottled *(Mr. & Mrs. T)*	3 oz	70	17.0	<1.0
liquid *(Holland House)*	1 oz	34	8.0	0.0
Tom Collins				
bottled *(Holland House)*	1 oz	47	11.0	0.0
instant, dry *(Holland House)*	.56 oz	65	16.0	0.0
Whiskey Sour				
bottled *(Holland House)*	1 oz	37	9.0	0.0
instant, dry *(Holland House)*	.56 oz	64	16.0	0.0
ALCOHOLIC BEVERAGES. See also ALCOHOL-FREE BEVERAGES.				
BEER, ALE, and MALT LIQUOR				
(Anheuser Marzen)	12 oz	168	15.2	0.0
(Beck's)	12 oz	148	10.0	0.0
(Budweiser)	12 oz	144	11.3	0.0
(Budweiser) 'Bud Light'	12 oz	110	6.9	0.0
(Busch)	12 oz	144	11.9	0.0
(Carlsberg)	12 oz	149	11.9	0.0
(Carlsberg) 'Light'	12 oz	110	6.5	0.0
(Coors)	12 oz	137	11.6	<0.0
(Coors) 'Dry'	12 oz	119	6.0	<0.0
(Coors) 'Dry' 3.2%	12 oz	101	5.3	<0.0
(Coors) 'Extra Gold'	12 oz	151	12.5	<0.0
(Coors) 'Extra Gold' 3.2%	12 oz	121	10.2	<0.0
(Coors) 'Light'	12 oz	103	4.7	<0.0
(Coors) 'Light' 3.2%	12 oz	98	4.7	<0.0
(Coors) 3.2%	12 oz	119	9.7	<0.0
(Coqui)	12 oz	208	9.8	0.0
(Dribeck's)	12 oz	94	7.0	0.0
(Elephant)	12 oz	208	16.9	0.0
(Keystone)	12 oz	121	6.8	<0.0
(Keystone) 'Dry'	12 oz	121	6.4	<0.0
(Keystone) 'Light'	12 oz	100	4.4	<0.0
(Keystone) 'Light' 3.2%	12 oz	99	5.0	<0.0
(Keystone) 3.2%	12 oz	104	6.1	<0.0
(Killian's)	12 oz	161	15.0	<0.0
(Killian's) 3.2%	12 oz	128	11.4	<0.0
(King Cobra)	12 oz	182	15.2	0.0
(Knickerbocker)	12 oz	140	12.3	0.0
(LA) light alcohol	12 oz	114	16.4	0.0
(Lite) 'Genuine Draft'	12 oz	98	3.5	0.0
(Lite) 'Lite'	12 oz	96	2.8	0.0
(Lowenbräu) 'Dark Special'	12 oz	158	14.3	0.0
(Lowenbräu) 'Special'	12 oz	158	14.3	0.0

Food Name	Serv. Size	Total Cal.	Carbs GMS	Fat GMS
(McSorley's)	12 oz	166	14.7	0.0
(Meister Brau)	12 oz	141	12.8	0.0
(Meister Brau) 'Light'	12 oz	98	3.5	0.0
(Michelob)	12 oz	156	13.6	0.0
(Michelob) 'Classic Dark'	12 oz	158	14.4	0.0
(Michelob) 'Dry'	12 oz	133	7.8	0.0
(Michelob) 'Light'	12 oz	134	11.9	0.0
(Miller) 'Genuine Draft'	12 oz	147	13.1	0.0
(Miller) 'High Life'	12 oz	147	13.1	0.0
(Miller) 'Magnum'	12 oz	162	10.2	0.0
(Milwaukee) 'Milwaukee's Best'	12 oz	133	11.4	0.0
(Milwaukee) 'Milwaukee's Best Light'	12 oz	98	3.5	0.0
(Natural Light)	12 oz	110	6.6	0.0
(Ortlieb's)	12 oz	140	12.3	0.0
(Prior) 'Double Dark'	12 oz	171	15.4	0.0
(Rheingold)	12 oz	148	12.9	0.0
(Rheingold) 'Light'	12 oz	96	2.8	0.0
(Rolling Rock) 'Light'	12 oz	104	8.0	0.0
(Rolling Rock) 'Premium'	12 oz	145	10.0	0.0
(Schmidt's)	12 oz	148	12.9	0.0
(Schmidt's) 'Classic'	12 oz	144	12.8	0.0
(Schmidt's) 'Light'	12 oz	96	2.8	0.0
(Tiger Head)	12 oz	166	14.7	0.0
(Zima)	12 oz	148	14.0	na
CHAMPAGNE				
brut *(Jacques Bonet)*	4 oz	92	2.1	0.0
brut *(Lejon)*	4 oz	92	3.4	0.0
extra dry *(Jacques Bonet)*	4 oz	97	3.4	0.0
extra dry *(Lejon)*	4 oz	97	2.1	0.0
pink *(Jacques Bonet)*	4 oz	98	3.7	0.0
pink *(Lejon)*	4 oz	98	3.7	0.0
LIQUOR AND LIQUEUR				
Bourbon				
80 proof, distilled	1 oz	65	tr	0.0
86 proof, distilled	1 oz	70	tr	0.0
90 proof, distilled	1 oz	74	tr	0.0
94 proof, distilled	1 oz	77	tr	0.0
100 proof, distilled	1 oz	83	tr	0.0
Brandy				
80 proof, distilled	1 oz	65	tr	0.0
86 proof, distilled	1 oz	70	tr	0.0
90 proof, distilled	1 oz	74	tr	0.0
94 proof, distilled	1 oz	77	tr	0.0

Food Name	Serv. Size	Total Cal.	Carbs GMS	Fat GMS
100 proof, distilled	1 oz	83	tr	0.0
Coffee Liqueur				
53 proof	1 oz	117	16.3	0.1
63 proof	1 oz	107	11.2	0.1
Creme de Menthe, 72 proof	1 oz	125	14.0	0.1
Gin				
80 proof, distilled	1 oz	64	0.0	0.0
86 proof, distilled	1 oz	69	0.0	0.0
90 proof, distilled	1 oz	73	0.0	0.0
94 proof, distilled	1 oz	76	0.0	0.0
100 proof, distilled	1 oz	82	0.0	0.0
Rum				
80 proof, distilled	1 oz	64	0.0	0.0
86 proof, distilled	1 oz	69	0.0	0.0
90 proof, distilled	1 oz	73	0.0	0.0
94 proof, distilled	1 oz	76	0.0	0.0
100 proof, distilled	1 oz	82	0.0	0.0
Rye Whiskey				
80 proof, distilled	1 oz	65	tr	0.0
86 proof, distilled	1 oz	70	tr	0.0
90 proof, distilled	1 oz	74	tr	0.0
94 proof, distilled	1 oz	77	tr	0.0
100 proof, distilled	1 oz	83	tr	0.0
Scotch				
80 proof, distilled	1 oz	65	tr	0.0
86 proof, distilled	1 oz	70	tr	0.0
90 proof, distilled	1 oz	74	tr	0.0
94 proof, distilled	1 oz	77	tr	0.0
100 proof, distilled	1 oz	83	tr	0.0
Tequila				
80 proof, distilled	1 oz	65	tr	0.0
86 proof, distilled	1 oz	70	tr	0.0
90 proof, distilled	1 oz	74	tr	0.0
94 proof, distilled	1 oz	77	tr	0.0
100 proof, distilled	1 oz	83	tr	0.0
Vodka				
80 proof, distilled	1 oz	64	0.0	0.0
86 proof, distilled	1 oz	69	0.0	0.0
90 proof, distilled	1 oz	73	0.0	0.0
94 proof, distilled	1 oz	76	0.0	0.0
100 proof, distilled	1 oz	82	0.0	0.0
Whiskey				
80 proof, distilled	1 oz	64	0.0	0.0

Food Name	Serv. Size	Total Cal.	Carbs GMS	Fat GMS
86 proof, distilled	1 oz	69	0.0	0.0
90 proof, distilled	1 oz	73	0.0	0.0
94 proof, distilled	1 oz	76	0.0	0.0
100 proof, distilled	1 oz	82	0.0	0.0

MIXED DRINKS. See also ALCOHOL-FREE BEVERAGES, MIXED-DRINK MIXERS.

Food Name	Serv. Size	Total Cal.	Carbs GMS	Fat GMS
Banana Daiquiri				
frozen, prepared w/1/2-can rum, diluted as directed (Bacardi)	7 oz	210	35.0	1.0
Bloody Mary, prepared from recipe	5 oz	115	4.9	0.2
Bourbon and Soda, prepared from recipe	4 oz	104	0.0	0.0
Daiquiri				
instant, prepared as directed (Bar-Tender's)	3.5 oz	177	18.0	0.0
prepared from recipe	1 oz	56	2.0	0.0
Gin and Tonic, prepared from recipe	1 oz	23	2.1	0.0
Lime Daiquiri, mix, shelf stable, prepared w/1/2-can rum (Bacardi)	7 oz	210	33.0	0.0
Manhattan, prepared from recipe	1 oz	64	0.9	0.0
Margarita				
frozen, prepared w/1/2-can rum, diluted as directed (Bacardi)	7 oz	160	24.0	0.0
shelf stable, prepared w/1/2-can rum (Bacardi)	7 oz	210	33.0	0.0
Martini, prepared from recipe	1 oz	63	0.1	0.0
Peach Daiquiri				
frozen, prepared w/1/2-can rum, diluted as directed (Bacardi)	7 oz	200	33.0	0.0
Piña Colada				
frozen, prepared w/1/2-can rum, diluted as directed (Bacardi)	7 oz	260	37.0	6.0
mix, shelf stable, prepared w/1/2-can rum (Bacardi)	7 oz	240	36.0	2.0
prepared from recipe	1 oz	58	8.9	0.6
Rum Runner, shelf stable, prepared w/1/2-can rum (Bacardi)	7 oz	210	33.0	0.0
Screwdriver, prepared from recipe	1 oz	25	2.6	0.0
Strawberry Colada				
mix, shelf stable, prepared w/1/2-can rum (Bacardi)	7 oz	230	34.0	1.0
Strawberry Daiquiri				
frozen, prepared w/1/2-can rum, diluted as directed (Bacardi)	7 oz	200	34.0	0.0
mix, shelf stable, prepared w/1/2-can rum (Bacardi)	7 oz	200	31.0	0.0
Tequila Sunrise, prepared from recipe	1 oz	34	2.7	0.0
Tom Collins, prepared from recipe	1 oz	16	0.4	0.0
Whiskey Sour				
mix, powder, instant, prepared w/whiskey (Bar-Tender's)	3.5 oz	177	18.0	0.0

Food Name	Serv. Size	Total Cal.	Carbs GMS	Fat GMS
prepared from recipe	1 oz	41	1.7	0.0
WINE. See also WINE, COOKING.				
'Arriba' *(Mission Bell)*	2 oz	95	6.8	0.0
'Diamond Red' *(Mission Bell)*	2 oz	95	6.8	0.0
'Silver Satin' *(Mission Bell)*	2 oz	83	5.4	0.0
'Silver Satin Bitter Lemon' *(Mission Bell)*	2 oz	83	5.5	0.0
'Swiss Up' *(Mission Bell)*	2 oz	84	5.6	0.0
Barbera, white *(Colony)*	4 oz	91	3.5	0.0
Burgundy				
(Bravo)	4 oz	91	1.7	0.0
(Carlo Rossi)	4 oz	92	1.6	0.0
(Colony) 'Classic'	4 oz	90	1.2	0.0
(Gallo)	4 oz	88	0.8	0.0
(Gallo) 'Hearty'	4 oz	92	1.6	0.0
(Gambarelli & Davitto) 'Parma'	4 oz	91	1.7	0.0
(Petri)	4 oz	91	1.7	0.0
Cabernet Sauvignon				
(Colony)	4 oz	88	0.7	0.0
(Gallo)	4 oz	88	0.0	0.0
Carbonated				
(Carlo Rossi) 'Paisano'	4 oz	92	1.6	0.0
(Jacques Bonet) almond	4 oz	104	7.7	0.0
(Jacques Bonet) apricot	4 oz	111	9.5	0.0
(Jacques Bonet) cherry	4 oz	106	8.3	0.0
(Jacques Bonet) peach	4 oz	111	9.5	0.0
(Jacques Bonet) raspberry	4 oz	106	8.3	0.0
Chablis				
(Bravo)	4 oz	86	1.7	0.0
(Carlo Rossi)	4 oz	84	2.0	0.0
(Carlo Rossi) pink	4 oz	92	3.6	0.0
(Colony)	4 oz	98	4.5	0.0
(Colony) 'Classic'	4 oz	84	1.8	0.0
(Colony) emerald	4 oz	102	5.3	0.0
(Colony) gold	4 oz	97	4.3	0.0
(Colony) ruby	4 oz	104	5.9	0.0
(Gallo)	4 oz	80	4.0	0.0
(Gallo) 'Blanc'	4 oz	80	0.6	0.0
(Gambarelli & Davitto) 'Parma'	4 oz	86	1.7	0.0
(Petri)	4 oz	98	4.5	0.0
(Petri) 'Blanc'	4 oz	86	1.7	0.0
Chardonnay *(Gallo)*	4 oz	88	na	0.0
Chenin Blanc				
(Colony)	4 oz	86	2.4	0.0

Food Name	Serv. Size	Total Cal.	Carbs GMS	Fat GMS
(Gallo)	4 oz	88	1.6	0.0
Chianti				
(Carlo Rossi) 'Light'	4 oz	92	2.4	0.0
(Petri)	4 oz	91	1.7	0.0
Cold duck				
(Jacques Bonet)	4 oz	108	5.9	0.0
(Lejon)	4 oz	108	5.9	0.0
French colombard				
(Colony)	4 oz	84	1.8	0.0
(Gallo)	4 oz	88	2.0	0.0
Gewurztraminer *(Gallo)*	4 oz	88	1.6	0.0
Marsala *(Gambarelli & Davitto)*	4 oz	77	4.0	0.0
Moselle *(Colony)* 'Rhineskeller'	4 oz	97	4.3	0.0
Muscatel *(Italian Swiss Colony)*	2 oz	122	5.9	0.0
Pastoso *(Petri)*	4 oz	92	1.8	0.0
Port				
(Gallo)	2 oz	64	2.0	0.0
(Gallo) white	2 oz	86	5.6	0.0
(Italian Swiss Colony)	2 oz	85	5.7	0.0
(Italian Swiss Colony) white	2 oz	86	6.3	0.0
(Livingston Cellars) tawny	2 oz	86	6.4	0.0
Rhine				
(Bravo)	4 oz	97	4.3	0.0
(Carlo Rossi)	4 oz	84	4.4	0.0
(Colony) 'Classic'	4 oz	89	3.8	0.0
(Gallo)	4 oz	80	4.0	0.0
(Gambarelli & Davitto) 'Parma'	4 oz	92	1.2	0.0
(Petri)	4 oz	97	4.3	0.0
Reisling *(Gallo)* 'Johannisberg'	4 oz	84	1.6	0.0
Rosé				
(Bravo)	4 oz	92	3.1	0.0
(Carlo Rossi) 'Vin Rosé'	4 oz	88	2.8	0.0
(Colony) 'Classic'	4 oz	89	3.0	0.0
(Gallo) 'Grenache'	4 oz	88	2.4	0.0
(Gallo) 'Red Rosé'	4 oz	112	6.4	0.0
(Gallo) 'Vin Rosé'	4 oz	88	2.8	0.0
(Gambarelli & Davitto) 'Parma'	4 oz	92	3.1	0.0
(Petri)	4 oz	92	3.1	0.0
Sauvignon Blanc *(Gallo)*	4 oz	80	0.8	0.0
Sherry				
(Gallo)	2 oz	64	2.0	0.0
(Italian Swiss Colony) cream	2 oz	85	6.8	0.0
(Italian Swiss Colony) dry	2 oz	63	1.2	0.0

Food Name	Serv. Size	Total Cal.	Carbs GMS	Fat GMS
(Livingston Cellars) cream	2 oz	78	5.6	0.0
(Livingston Cellars) 'Very Dry'	2 oz	60	1.0	0.0
Tokay *(Italian Swiss Colony)*	2 oz	82	5.1	0.0
Vermouth				
(Gallo) dry	2 oz	56	0.8	0.0
(Gallo) sweet	2 oz	90	9.4	0.0
(Gambarelli & Davitto) dry	2 oz	64	1.5	0.0
(Gambarelli & Davitto) sweet	2 oz	77	8.4	0.0
(Lejon) dry	2 oz	64	1.5	0.0
(Lejon) sweet	2 oz	77	8.4	0.0
Zinfandel				
(Colony)	4 oz	91	0.7	0.0
(Colony) white	4 oz	82	2.7	0.0
(Gallo)	4 oz	92	0.0	0.0
WINE COOLERS				
(Bartles & Jaymes) Berry Cooler 'Light'	12 oz	150	32.0	0.0
(Bartles & Jaymes) Black Cherry Cooler 'Light'	12 oz	139	30.0	0.0
(Bartles & Jaymes) Citrus Cooler 'Light'	6 oz	67	12.0	<1.0
(Bartles & Jaymes) Tropical Cooler 'Light'	12 oz	151	32.0	0.0
ALE. See ALCOHOLIC BEVERAGES.				
ALFALFA SEEDS				
(Arrowhead Mills)	1 cup	40	4.0	1.0
sprouted, raw	1 lb	132	17.1	3.1
sprouted, raw	1/2 cup	5	0.6	0.1
sprouted, raw	1 tbsp	1	0.1	0.0
sprouted, raw	1 oz	8	1.1	0.2
ALLIGATOR	1 oz	41	na	0.8
ALLSPICE				
ground	1 oz	75	20.4	2.5
ground	1 tbsp	16	4.3	0.5
ground	1 tsp	5	1.4	0.2
ground *(Durkee)*	1 tsp	7	0.0	tr
ground *(Laurel Leaf)*	1 tsp	7	0.0	tr
ground *(Spice Islands)*	1 tsp	6	1.3	tr
ALMOND				
(Beer Nuts)	1 oz	180	7.0	14.4
(Dole)	1 oz	170	12.0	14.0
(Fisher)	1 oz	170	3.0	15.0
chopped	1 cup	766	26.5	67.9
in shell	1 lb	1069	37.0	94.7
sliced	1 cup	554	19.2	49.1
slivered, tightly packed	1 cup	795	27.5	70.5
whole kernels	1 cup	836	29.0	74.1

Food Name	Serv. Size	Total Cal.	Carbs GMS	Fat GMS
whole kernels, approx 24	1 oz	167	5.8	14.8
Blanched				
sliced	1 cup	615	19.5	55.2
whole kernels	1 cup	850	26.9	76.2
whole kernels	1 oz	166	5.3	14.9
Dry-roasted				
(Planters)	1 oz	170	6.0	15.0
whole kernels	1 cup	810	33.4	71.2
whole kernels	1 oz	167	6.9	14.7
Honey-roasted				
(Planters)	1 oz	170	9.0	13.0
whole kernels	1 cup	855	40.2	71.9
whole kernels	1 oz	168	7.9	14.1
Oil-roasted				
whole kernels	1 cup	970	24.9	90.5
whole kernels, approx 22	1 oz	176	4.5	16.4
Oil-roasted and blanched				
approx 24 whole kernels	1 oz	174	5.1	16.1
toasted	1 cup	870	25.6	80.3
toasted	1 oz	167	6.5	14.4
Raw				
blanched (Planters)	1 oz	170	6.0	15.0
sliced (Planters)	1 oz	170	6.0	15.0
slivered (Planters)	1 oz	170	6.0	15.0
whole (Planters)	1 oz	170	6.0	15.0
Toasted				
(Dole)	1 oz	170	5.0	14.0
unblanched	1 oz	167	6.5	14.4
ALMOND BUTTER				
Plain				
	1/2 cup	791	26.5	73.9
	1 oz	179	6.0	16.8
blanched, toasted (Hain)	2 tbsp	220	3.0	19.0
gourmet (Roaster Fresh)	1 oz	184	6.0	16.0
no salt, crunchy 'Natural' (Westbrae)	2 tbsp	190	7.0	17.0
no salt, smooth 'Natural' (Westbrae)	2 tbsp	190	7.0	17.0
raw 'Natural' (Hain)	2 tbsp	190	3.0	18.0
raw, organic (Maranatha Natural)	2 tbsp	190	8.0	15.0
roasted (Maranatha Natural)	2 tbsp	190	8.0	15.0
salted	1 cup	791	26.5	73.9
salted	1 oz	179	6.0	16.8
salted	1 tbsp	101	3.4	9.5

Food Name	Serv. Size	Total Cal.	Carbs GMS	Fat GMS
Honey and cinnamon				
. . . .	1/2 cup	753	33.7	65.3
. . . .	1 oz	171	7.6	14.8
salted	1/2 cup	753	33.7	65.3
salted	1 oz	171	7.6	14.8
ALMOND MEAL				
partially defatted	4 oz	463	32.8	20.8
partially defatted, salted	4 oz	463	32.8	20.8
ALMOND OIL				
. . . .	1/2 cup	964	0.0	109.0
. . . .	1 oz	251	0.0	28.4
. . . .	1 tbsp	120	0.0	13.6
(Hain)	1 tbsp	120	0.0	14.0
(Spectrum Naturals)	1 tbsp	120	0.0	14.0
ALMOND PASTE				
. . . .	4 oz	506	49.4	30.8
. . . .	1 oz	127	12.4	7.7
firmly packed	1 cup	1012	98.9	61.7
ALMOND POWDER				
full-fat	1 oz	168	6.3	14.7
full-fat, not packed	1 cup	385	14.5	33.6
partially defatted	1 oz	112	9.0	4.5
partially defatted, not packed	1 cup	255	20.7	10.4
ALOE VERA JUICE				
sodium free, certified 100% juice *(Sunburst)*	2 oz	5	1.0	0.0
ALPINE SPICED CIDER *(Krusteaz)*	8 oz	80	21.0	0.0
AMARANTH				
boiled, drained	1/2 cup	14	2.7	0.1
raw	1 cup	7	1.1	0.1
AMARANTH DINNER, CANNED				
w/garden vegetables 'Fast Menu' fat-free *(Health Valley)*	7.5 oz	120	16.0	3.0
w/garden vegetables 'Fast Menu' fat-free *(Health Valley)*	5 oz	70	11.0	0.0
AMARANTH FLOUR *(Arrowhead Mills)*	2 oz	200	35.0	<3.0
AMARANTH SEED *(Arrowhead Mills)*	2 oz	200	35.0	3.0
AMBERJACK				
raw	1 lb	386	0.0	4.1
raw	1 oz	24	0.0	0.3
AMBROSIA SALAD *(Sunfresh)* in light syrup	2/3 cup	70	18.0	0.0
AMBROSIA JUICE *(Knudsen & Sons)*	8 oz	110	27.0	0.0
ANASAZI BEAN raw *(Arrowhead Mills)*	2 oz	200	35.0	1.0
ANCHOVY, European, meat only, raw	1 oz	37	0.0	1.4
ANCHOVY, CANNED				
in olive oil, drained	1 oz	60	0.0	2.8

Food Name	Serv. Size	Total Cal.	Carbs GMS	Fo GM
in olive oil, drained, 5 medium	.7 oz	42	0.0	1.
in olive oil, drained, yield from 2-oz can	1.6 oz	94	0.0	4.
ANGLER FISH. See MONKFISH.				
ANISE SEED				
whole	1 oz	95	14.2	4.
whole	1 tbsp	23	3.3	1.
whole	1 tsp	7	1.0	0.
ANTELOPE				
raw	1 oz	32	0.0	0.
roasted	3 oz	127	0.0	2.
roasted, diced	1 cup	210	0.0	3.
APPLE				
boiled, peeled slices	1/2 cup	60	15.5	0.
boiled, unpeeled slices	1/2 cup	46	11.7	0.
microwaved, peeled slices	1/2 cup	64	16.3	0.
microwaved, unpeeled slices	1/2 cup	48	12.3	0.
raw, peeled	1 oz	16	4.2	0.
raw, peeled slices	1 cup	63	16.3	0.
raw, peeled whole fruit, approx 3 per lb	1 med	73	19.0	0.
raw, unpeeled	1 oz	17	4.3	0.
raw, unpeeled slices	1 cup	65	16.8	0.
raw, unpeeled whole fruit, approx 3 per lb	1 med	81	21.0	0.
raw, unpeeled whole fruit	1 lb	244	63.7	1.
APPLE, CANNED				
Chipped				
(Lucky Leaf)	4 oz	50	12.0	0.
(Musselman's)	4 oz	50	12.0	0.0
(White House) in water	4 oz	50	12.0	0.
Diced				
(Lucky Leaf)	4 oz	50	12.0	0.0
(Musselman's)	4 oz	50	12.0	0.0
Rings, spiced				
(Lucky Leaf) green	4 oz	100	24.0	0.0
(Lucky Leaf) red	4 oz	100	24.0	0.0
(Musselman's) green	4 oz	100	24.0	0.0
(Musselman's) red	4 oz	100	24.0	0.0
(White House)	3.5 oz	180	44.0	0.0
Sliced				
(Lucky Leaf) dessert	4 oz	70	16.0	0.0
(Lucky Leaf) sweetened, in syrup	4 oz	50	13.0	0.0
(Lucky Leaf) sweetened, in water	4 oz	50	12.0	0.0
(Lucky Leaf) sweetened, unpeeled	4 oz	90	22.0	0.0
(Musselman's) dessert	4 oz	70	16.0	0.0

Food Name	Serv. Size	Total Cal.	Carbs GMS	Fat GMS
(Musselman's) sweetened, in syrup	4 oz	50	13.0	0.0
(Musselman's) sweetened, in water	4 oz	50	12.0	0.0
(Musselman's) sweetened, unpeeled	4 oz	90	22.0	0.0
(White House) sweetened	4 oz	54	14.0	0.0
(White House) sweetened, in water	4 oz	40	12.0	0.0
Whole				
(Lucky Leaf) baked	1 apple	110	28.0	0.0
(Lucky Leaf) sweetened, peeled, cored	1 apple	90	21.0	0.0
(Musselman's) baked	1 apple	110	28.0	0.0
(Musselman's) sweetened, peeled, cored	1 apple	90	21.0	0.0
(White House) baked	3.5 oz	118	29.0	0.0
APPLE, DEHYDRATED/SULFURED				
chips *(Weight Watchers)*	.75 oz	70	19.0	0.0
cooked	4 oz	84	22.6	0.1
stewed, low-moisture	1/2 cup	72	19.3	0.1
uncooked	4 oz	392	111.7	0.7
uncooked, low-moisture	1/2 cup	104	28.1	0.2
APPLE, DRIED				
chunks *(Sun•Maid)*	2 oz	150	42.0	0.0
chunks *(SunSweet)*	2 oz	150	42.0	0.0
sliced, uncooked *(Del Monte)*	2 oz	140	37.0	0.0
sulfured, stewed	1/2 cup	73	19.6	0.1
sulfured, uncooked	4 oz	276	74.7	0.4
sulfured, uncooked	1 cup	209	56.7	0.3
sulfured, uncooked, approx 2.3 oz	10 rings	155	42.2	0.2
APPLE, FROZEN				
escalloped *(Stouffer's)*	4 oz	130	27.0	2.0
glazed, in raspberry sauce 'Side Dish' *(Budget Gourmet)*	5 oz	110	22.0	3.0
unsweetened	4 oz	54	14.0	0.4
unsweetened, heated	4 oz	53	13.6	0.4
unsweetened, heated, sliced	1/2 cup	48	12.4	0.3
unsweetened, sliced	1/2 cup	41	10.6	0.3
APPLE APRICOT JUICE *(Knudsen & Sons)*	8 oz	120	29.0	0.0
APPLE BANANA JUICE *(Knudsen & Sons)*	8 oz	85	21.0	0.0
APPLE BLACKBERRY JUICE				
(Knudsen & Sons)	8 oz	100	24.0	0.0
(Santa Cruz Natural) organic	8 oz	120	29.0	1.0
APPLE BOYSENBERRY JUICE				
(Knudsen & Sons)	8 oz	110	28.0	0.0
(Santa Cruz Natural) organic	8 oz	120	29.0	1.0
APPLE BUTTER				
	1 cup	519	134.5	0.9
	1 tbsp	33	8.6	0.1

Food Name	Serv. Size	Total Cal.	Carbs GMS	Fat GMS
APPLE CHERRY BERRY DRINK (Veryfine)	8 oz	130	33.0	0.0
APPLE CHERRY CIDER				
(Indian Summer)	6 oz	100	25.0	<1.0
(McCain) 100%-juice 'Junior'	4.2 oz	50	13.0	0.0
(Musselman's) 'Breakfast Cocktail'	6 oz	100	26.0	0.0
(Red Cheek) 'Naturally 100%'	6 oz	113	28.0	0.0
APPLE CIDER				
(Indian Summer) can or bottle	6 oz	80	20.0	<1.0
(Indian Summer) can or bottle, cinnamon	6 oz	90	21.0	<1.0
(Lucky Leaf) can or bottle	6 oz	90	21.0	0.0
(Lucky Leaf) can or bottle, sparkling	6 oz	80	18.0	0.0
(Musselman's) can or bottle	6 oz	90	21.0	0.0
(S. Martinelli) 'Sparkling'	6 oz	100	25.0	0.0
(Tree Top) canned or frozen, diluted as directed	6 oz	90	22.0	0.0
APPLE CIDER MIX (Swiss Miss)	.776 oz	84	20.3	0.3
APPLE CITRUS JUICE (Tree Top) canned or frozen	6 oz	90	22.0	0.0
APPLE CRANBERRY CIDER (Indian Summer)	6 oz	100	24.0	<1.0
APPLE CRANBERRY DRINK				
(Mott's)	10 oz	176	44.0	0.0
(Mott's)	9.5 oz	167	42.0	0.0
(Tropicana)	6 oz	110	27.0	<1.0
(Tropicana) 'Single Serve'	10 oz	175	43.0	0.0
APPLE CRANBERRY JUICE				
(Apple & Eve)	6 oz	80	19.0	0.0
(Knudsen & Sons)	8 oz	110	28.0	0.0
(Lucky Leaf)	6 oz	130	32.0	0.0
(Mott's)	9.5 oz	147	38.0	0.0
(Mott's)	6 oz	83	24.0	0.0
(Mott's) aseptic box	8.45 oz	136	34.0	0.0
(Santa Cruz Natural) organic	8 oz	115	28.0	<1.0
(Smucker's) 'Naturally 100%'	8 oz	120	32.0	0.0
(Tree Top) canned	6 oz	100	25.0	0.0
(Tree Top) frozen	6 oz	100	25.0	0.0
(Veryfine) cocktail	8 oz	130	33.0	0.0
APPLE DRINK				
(Hi-C) 'Candy Apple Cooler'	8.45 oz	132	32.6	<.1
(Hi-C) 'Candy Apple Cooler'	6 oz	94	23.1	<.1
(Hi-C) 'Jamin' Apple Drink,' aseptic box	6 oz	90	23.0	0.0
(10-K)	8 oz	60	15.0	0.0
APPLE DUMPLING, frozen (Pepperidge Farm)	3 oz	260	33.0	13.0
APPLE GRAPE CHERRY JUICE				
(Welch's) 'Orchard Cocktail'	6 oz	110	27.0	0.0
(Welch's) 'Orchard Cocktail-in-a-Box'	8.45 oz	150	38.0	0.0

Food Name	Serv. Size	Total Cal.	Carbs GMS	Fat GMS
(Welch's) 'Orchard Cocktail' frozen	6 oz	90	22.0	0.0
APPLE GRAPE JUICE				
(Juicy Juice)	6 oz	90	22.0	0.0
(Juicy Juice) box	8.45 oz	120	29.0	0.0
(Mott's)	9.5 oz	139	37.0	0.0
(Mott's)	6 oz	86	23.0	0.0
(Mott's) aseptic box	8.45 oz	128	32.0	0.0
(Musselman's) 'Breakfast Cocktail'	6 oz	110	28.0	0.0
(Red Cheek)	6 oz	109	27.0	0.0
(Tree Top) canned	6 oz	100	25.0	0.0
(Tree Top) frozen	6 oz	100	25.0	0.0
(Welch's) 'Orchard Cocktail'	6 oz	110	27.0	0.0
(Welch's) 'Orchard Cocktail,' frozen	6 oz	110	27.0	0.0
(Welch's) 'Orchard Cocktail,' frozen, w/raspberry	6 oz	90	22.0	0.0
(Welch's) 'Orchard Cocktail-in-a Box' w/raspberry	8.45 oz	140	35.0	0.0
APPLE JUICE				
Can, bottle, or box				
(Heinz) strained, 'Saver Size'	4.2 oz	70	17.0	0.0
(IGA) 'Unsweetened'	6 oz	74	18.0	0.0
(Indian Summer)	6 oz	90	21.0	<1.0
(J. Hungerford)	9.03 oz	128	32.2	0.0
(J. Hungerford) 50%-juice	9.03 oz	119	29.9	0.0
(J. Hungerford) 100%-juice	9.03 oz	112	28.0	0.0
(Juicy Juice)	6 oz	90	21.0	0.0
(Knudsen & Sons) Gravenstein	8 oz	110	28.0	0.0
(Knudsen & Sons) 'Natural'	8 oz	85	21.0	0.0
(Kraft) 'Pure 100%'	6 oz	80	20.0	0.0
(Lucky Leaf) 'Individual Portion Control'	3.8 oz	60	14.0	0.0
(Lucky Leaf) 100% vitamin-C enriched	6 oz	90	21.0	0.0
(Lucky Leaf) regular	6 oz	90	21.0	0.0
(McCain) 100%-juice 'Junior'	4.2 oz	50	13.0	0.0
(Minute Maid) aseptic box	6 oz	80	21.0	0.0
(Minute Maid) 'Juices to Go'	6 oz	80	21.0	0.0
(Mott's)	10 oz	148	37.0	0.0
(Mott's)	9.5 oz	141	35.0	0.0
(Mott's)	8.45 oz	124	31.0	0.0
(Mott's)	6 oz	88	22.0	0.0
(Mott's) natural style	6 oz	76	19.0	0.0
(Musselman's) 'Individual Portion Control'	3.8 oz	60	14.0	0.0
(Musselman's) 100% vitamin-C enriched	6 oz	90	21.0	0.0
(Musselman's) regular	6 oz	90	21.0	0.0
(Ocean Spray)	6 oz	90	23.0	0.0
(Red Cheek) 'Natural'	6 oz	97	24.0	0.0

Food Name	Serv. Size	Total Cal.	Carbs GMS	Fat GMS
(Red Cheek) '100%-Pure'	6 oz	97	24.0	0.0
(S&W) '100% Pure Unsweetened'	6 oz	85	20.0	0.0
(S. Martinelli)	6 oz	100	25.0	0.0
(S. Martinelli) 'Sparkling'	6 oz	100	25.0	0.0
(Sippin' Pak) 100%-pure, from concentrate	8.45 oz	110	28.0	0.0
(Snapple) 'Apple Crisp'	8 oz	140	36.0	0.0
(Tree Top)	6 oz	90	22.0	0.0
(TreeSweet)	6 oz	90	22.0	0.0
(Tropicana) '100%-Pure'	8 oz	116	28.5	0.0
(Tropicana) 100%-pure	6 oz	80	20.0	<1.0
(Veryfine) '100%'	8 oz	107	27.0	0.0
(Welch's) sparkling	6 oz	100	24.0	0.0
(White House)	6 oz	87	22.0	0.0
Chilled or frozen				
(A&P) diluted as directed	6 oz	90	22.0	<1.0
(Knudsen & Sons) clear	8 oz	90	22.0	0.0
(Minute Maid) diluted as directed	6 oz	80	21.0	0.0
(Sunkist) diluted as directed	8 oz	79	19.4	0.2
(Tree Top) diluted as directed	6 oz	90	22.0	0.0
(Welch's) 'Orchard Cocktail'	10 oz	170	42.0	0.0
APPLE KIT				
Candy *(Concord)* microwaveable	1 apple	50	14.0	0.0
Caramel *(Concord)* microwaveable	1 apple	150	27.0	3.0
APPLE ORANGE PINEAPPLE COCKTAIL				
(Welch's) 'Orchard Tropical Cocktails'	8.45 oz	140	35.0	0.0
(Welch's) 'Orchard Tropical Cocktails'	6 oz	100	25.0	0.0
APPLE PASTRY				
Fresh				
(Entenmann's) 'Apple Puffs'	1 puff	280	39.0	13.0
(Tastykake) pocket	3 oz	323	38.3	17.6
Frozen				
(Hormel) 'Apple Dulcita'	4 oz	290	44.0	10.0
(Mrs. Paul's) 'Apple Fritter'	2 pieces	240	35.0	9.0
(Pepperidge Farm) 'Apple Dumpling'	3 oz	260	33.0	13.0
(Pepperidge Farm) apple fruit square	1 piece	220	27.0	12.0
(Pepperidge Farm) 'Berkshire' apple crisps	1 ramekin	250	43.0	8.0
(Weight Watchers) 'Sweet Celebrations' apple crisps	3.5 oz	190	40.0	5.0
APPLE PEACH JUICE *(Knudsen & Sons)*	8 oz	140	34.0	0.0
APPLE PEAR JUICE *(Tree Top)* frozen	6 oz	90	22.0	0.0
APPLE PIE. See PIE.				
APPLE PIE FILLING. See PIE FILLING.				
APPLE PIE SPICE *(Tone's)*	1 tsp	9	2.4	0.2

Food Name	Serv. Size	Total Cal.	Carbs GMS	Fat GMS
APPLE PUNCH				
(Minute Maid) chilled	6 oz	90	23.0	0.0
(Minute Maid) frozen concentrate	6 oz	90	23.0	0.0
APPLE PUNCH DRINK (Red Cheek)	6 oz	113	28.0	0.0
APPLE RASPBERRY DRINK				
(Mott's)	10 oz	158	40.0	0.0
(Mott's)	9.5 oz	150	38.0	0.0
APPLE RASPBERRY JUICE				
(Knudsen & Sons)	8 oz	110	28.0	0.0
(Mott's)	9.5 oz	134	35.0	0.0
(Mott's)	6 oz	83	22.0	0.0
(Mott's) aseptic box	8.45 oz	124	31.0	0.0
(Red Cheek)	6 oz	113	28.0	0.0
(Santa Cruz Natural) organic	8 oz	120	29.0	1.0
(Tree Top) canned or frozen	6 oz	80	21.0	0.0
(Veryfine) cocktail	8 oz	110	27.0	0.0
APPLE STICKS, frozen, breaded, fried (Farm Rich)	4 oz	260	44.0	8.0
APPLE STRAWBERRY JUICE				
(Knudsen & Sons)	8 oz	110	28.0	0.0
(Santa Cruz Natural) organic	8 oz	120	29.0	<1.0
APPLE STRAWBERRY NECTAR (Kern's) can or bottle	6 oz	110	26.0	0.0
APPLE STRUDEL				
(Aunt Fanny's) individual	3 oz	330	38.0	18.0
(Entenmann's) old fashioned	1.5 oz	120	17.0	5.0
APPLE SYRUP (Knudsen & Sons)	1 oz	75	15.0	<1.0
APPLE-WHITE GRAPE JUICE				
(Welch's) 'No Sugar Added' frozen cocktail	6 oz	40	10.0	0.0
APPLESAUCE				
(A&P)				
regular	1/2 cup	110	25.0	<1.0
unsweetened	1/2 cup	50	10.0	<1.0
(Del Monte)				
'Lite'	1/2 cup	50	13.0	0.0
regular	1/2 cup	90	24.0	0.0
(Featherweight)	1/2 cup	50	12.0	0.0
(Finast)				
regular	1/2 cup	105	25.0	0.0
unsweetened	1/2 cup	56	15.0	0.2
(Lucky Leaf)				
chunky	4 oz	80	20.0	0.0
'Juice Pack'	4 oz	50	12.0	0.0
'Natural' individual portion control	4 oz	50	13.0	0.0
regular	4 oz	80	20.0	0.0

Food Name	Serv. Size	Total Cal.	Carbs GMS	Fa GM
'Regular' individual portion control	4 oz	80	20.0	0.0
unsweetened	4 oz	50	12.0	0.0
(Mott's)				
chunky	6 oz	86	21.0	0.0
cinnamon	6 oz	152	36.0	<0.0
'Natural'	6 oz	80	20.0	0.0
'Natural Single Serve'	4 oz	53	13.0	0.0
regular	6 oz	150	36.0	<0.0
'Single Serve'	4 oz	100	24.0	<0.0
'Single Serve' cinnamon	4 oz	101	24.0	<0.0
(Musselman's)				
chunky	4 oz	80	20.0	0.0
'Juice Pack'	4 oz	50	12.0	0.0
'Natural' individual portion control	4 oz	50	13.0	0.0
regular	4 oz	80	20.0	0.0
'Regular' individual portion control	4 oz	80	20.0	0.0
unsweetened	4 oz	50	12.0	0.0
(S&W)				
regular	1/2 cup	90	24.0	0.0
unsweetened	1/2 cup	55	14.0	0.0
(S&W Nutradiet)	1/2 cup	55	14.0	0.0
(Stokely)				
regular	1/2 cup	90	23.0	0.0
unsweetened	1/2 cup	45	12.0	0.0
(Tree Top) 'Original'	1/2 cup	80	21.0	0.0
(White House)				
chunky	4 oz	80	22.0	0.0
in apple juice	4 oz	50	13.0	0.0
'Regular'	4 oz	80	22.0	0.0
unsweetened	4 oz	50	12.0	0.0
APRICOT				
candied	100 gm	338	86.5	0.2
pitted	1 oz	14	3.2	<0.1
raw, halves	1 cup	74	17.2	0.6
untrimmed	1 lb	202	46.9	1.7
APRICOT, CANNED				
In extra heavy syrup				
peeled	4 oz	109	28.2	<.1
peeled, whole	1/2 cup	118	30.6	0.1
In extra light syrup				
unpeeled	4 oz	56	14.2	0.1
unpeeled, halves	1/2 cup	61	15.4	0.1

Food Name	Serv. Size	Total Cal.	Carbs GMS	Fat GMS
In heavy syrup				
peeled	4 oz	94	24.3	0.1
peeled, halves	1 cup	214	55.4	0.2
peeled, whole	1/2 cup	107	27.7	0.1
peeled, whole (S&W)	1/2 cup	100	26.0	0.0
unpeeled	4 oz	94	24.3	0.1
unpeeled (A&P)	1/2 cup	110	28.0	1.0
unpeeled, halves	1/2 cup	107	27.7	0.1
unpeeled, halves (IGA)	1 cup	220	56.0	0.0
unpeeled, halves (S&W)	1/2 cup	110	28.0	0.0
In juice				
peeled (Featherweight)	1/2 cup	50	12.0	0.0
unpeeled	4 oz	54	14.0	<.1
unpeeled, halves	1/2 cup	60	15.3	<.1
unpeeled, 'Lite' (Libby's)	1/2 cup	60	17.0	0.0
In light syrup				
unpeeled	4 oz	71	18.7	0.1
unpeeled, halves	1/2 cup	80	20.9	0.1
unpeeled, halves 'No Frills' (Pathmark)	1/2 cup	80	20.0	0.0
In water				
peeled	1/2 cup	25	6.2	<.1
peeled, whole (S&W Nutradiet)	1/2 cup	28	7.0	0.0
unpeeled	4 oz	31	7.2	0.2
unpeeled, halves	1/2 cup	33	7.8	0.2
unpeeled, halves (S&W)	1/2 cup	35	9.0	0.0
unpeeled, halves (S&W Nutradiet)	1/2 cup	35	9.0	0.0
APRICOT, DEHYDRATED/SULFURED				
cooked	4 oz	143	37.0	0.3
stewed, low-moisture	1/2 cup	156	40.4	0.3
uncooked	4 oz	363	94.0	0.7
uncooked, low-moisture	1/2 cup	192	49.7	0.4
APRICOT, DRIED				
sulfured, cooked	4 oz	96	24.8	0.2
sulfured, stewed, halves	1/2 cup	106	27.4	0.2
sulfured, uncooked	4 oz	270	70.0	0.5
sulfured, uncooked, approx 1.2 oz	10 halves	83	21.6	0.2
sulfured, uncooked, halves	1 cup	309	80.3	0.6
(Del Monte)	2 oz	140	35.0	0.0
(Mariani) California, sun-dried, premium	1/4 cup	140	35.0	0.0
(Mariani) Mediterranean, sun-dried, premium	1/4 cup	140	35.0	0.0
(Sun•Maid)	2 oz	140	35.0	0.0
(SunSweet)	2 oz	140	35.0	0.0

Food Name	Serv. Size	Total Cal.	Carbs GMS	Fat GMS
APRICOT, FROZEN				
sweetened	4 oz	111	28.5	0.1
sweetened, unthawed	1 cup	237	60.7	0.2
APRICOT KERNEL OIL				
	1/2 cup	964	0.0	109.0
	1 oz	251	0.0	28.4
	1 tbsp	120	0.0	13.6
(Hain)	1 tbsp	120	0.0	14.0
(Spectrum Naturals)	1 tbsp	120	0.0	14.0
APRICOT NECTAR				
(Del Monte)	6 oz	100	26.0	0.0
(Kern's)	6 oz	110	27.0	0.0
(Knudsen & Sons)	8 oz	105	24.0	0.0
(Libby's)	6 oz	110	26.0	0.0
(S&W)	6 oz	100	26.0	0.0
APRICOT PIE FILLING. See PIE FILLING.				
APRICOT PINEAPPLE NECTAR				
(Kern's)	6 oz	110	27.0	0.0
(S&W Nutradiet)	4 oz	35	12.0	0.0
ARCTIC BONITO. See TUNA, SKIPJACK.				
ARROWHEAD				
boiled, drained	4 oz	88	18.3	0.1
boiled, drained	1 med	9	1.9	0.0
raw	1 large	25	5.1	0.1
raw	1 med	12	2.4	0.0
raw, trimmed	1 oz	28	5.7	0.1
raw, untrimmed	1 lb	337	68.8	1.0
ARROWROOT, powdered (Tone's)	1 tsp	10	2.3	0.0
ARROWROOT FLOUR				
	1/3 cup	154	37.9	(mq)
	1 oz	101	25.0	(mq)
ARTICHOKE HEARTS				
boiled, drained	4 oz	57	12.7	0.2
boiled, drained	1/2 cup	42	9.4	0.1
canned, marinated (S&W)	3.5 oz	225	6.0	26.0
frozen, boiled, drained	4 oz	51	10.4	0.6
frozen, 'Deluxe' (Birds Eye)	3 oz	30	7.0	0.0
frozen (Seabrook)	3 oz	25	4.0	0.0
ARTICHOKES, FRENCH				
boiled, drained	1 med	60	13.4	0.2
boiled, drained, hearts	1/2 cup	42	9.4	0.1
frozen, boiled, drained	3 oz	36	7.3	0.4
raw	1 large	76	17.0	0.2

Food Name	Serv. Size	Total Cal.	Carbs GMS	Fat GMS
raw	1 med	60	13.4	0.2
ARTICHOKES, GLOBE				
boiled, drained	1 med	60	13.4	0.2
boiled, drained, hearts	1/2 cup	42	9.4	0.1
boiled, drained, trimmed	4 oz	57	12.7	0.2
boiled, drained, untrimmed	4 oz	23	5.1	0.1
fresh (Dole)	1 large	23	5.0	0.1
frozen, boiled, drained	3 oz	36	7.3	0.4
frozen, unprepared	9 oz	97	19.8	1.1
raw	1 large	76	17.0	0.2
raw	1 med	60	13.4	0.2
raw, untrimmed	1 lb	85	19.1	0.3
ARTICHOKES, JERUSALEM				
raw, slices	1/2 cup	57	13.1	0.0
trimmed	1 oz	22	4.9	tr
untrimmed	1 lb	238	54.6	<.1
ARUGULA/rocket/roquette/ruculo/rugula				
raw	1 leaf	1	0.1	0.0
raw	1/2 cup	3	0.4	0.1
(Frieda's)	1 lb	104	17.7	1.4
(Frieda's)	1 oz	7	1.1	<.1
ASPARAGUS				
boiled, drained	1/2 cup	22	3.8	0.3
boiled, drained, cuts and spears	4 oz	28	5.0	0.4
fresh (Dole)	5 spears	18	2.0	0.0
raw, cuts and spears	1/2 cup	15	2.5	0.2
raw, trimmed	1 oz	6	1.0	0.1
raw, untrimmed	1 lb	54	8.9	0.5
ASPARAGUS, CANNED				
Cuts and tips (Finast)	1 cup	35	6.0	0.0
Points, all green (S&W Nutradiet)	1/2 cup	17	3.0	0.0
Spears				
and tips, all green (Del Monte)	1/2 cup	20	3.0	0.0
colossal, all green 'Fancy' (S&W)	1/2 cup	20	4.0	0.0
cut (Green Giant)	1/2 cup	18	3.0	0.0
cut, 50% less salt (Green Giant)	1/2 cup	18	3.0	0.0
cut, green (Pathmark)	1/2 cup	20	2.0	0.0
cut, green 'No Salt Added' (Pathmark)	1/2 cup	20	2.0	0.0
green (Stokely)	1/2 cup	20	3.0	0.0
green 'Fancy' (S&W)	1/2 cup	18	3.0	0.0
green, w/liquid (Green Giant)	1/2 cup	20	3.0	0.0
'No Salt or Sugar Added' (Stokely)	1/2 cup	20	3.0	0.0
white (Green Giant)	1/2 cup	16	3.0	0.0

Food Name	Serv. Size	Total Cal.	Carbs GMS	Fat GMS
white, w/liquid *(Green Giant)*	1/2 cup	16	3.0	0.0
w/liquid, 50% less salt *(Green Giant)*	1/2 cup	20	3.0	0.0
w/liquid, green, tipped *(Del Monte)*	1/2 cup	20	3.0	0.0
ASPARAGUS, FROZEN				
boiled, drained	10-oz pkg	82	14.3	1.2
boiled, drained, cuts and spears	4 oz	32	5.5	0.5
cuts *(Birds Eye)*	3.3 oz	25	4.0	0.0
cuts *(Seabrook)*	3.3 oz	25	4.0	0.0
cuts 'Harvest Fresh' *(Green Giant)*	1/2 cup	25	4.0	0.0
cuts and spears *(Frosty Acres)*	3.3 oz	25	4.0	0.0
spears *(Birds Eye)*	3.3 oz	25	4.0	0.0
spears *(Finast)*	3.3 oz	25	4.0	0.0
spears *(Frosty Acres)*	3.3 oz	25	4.0	0.0
spears *(Seabrook)*	3.3 oz	25	4.0	0.0
spears *(Southern)*	3.5 oz	27	4.1	0.2
unprepared	10-oz pkg	68	11.6	0.7
ASPARAGUS BEAN. See YARDLONG BEAN.				
AUBERGINE. See EGGPLANT.				
AU JUS. See GRAVY.				
AVOCADO				
All commercial varieties				
puréed	1/2 cup	185	8.5	17.6
trimmed	1 oz	46	2.1	4.3
untrimmed	1 lb	540	24.8	51.4
California				
puréed	1/2 cup	204	8.0	19.9
trimmed	1 oz	50	2.0	4.9
untrimmed	1 lb	610	23.8	59.8
Florida				
puréed	1/2 cup	129	10.3	10.2
trimmed	1 oz	32	2.5	2.5
untrimmed	1 lb	339	27.1	26.9
AVOCADO OIL				
	1/2 cup	964	0.0	109.0
	1 oz	251	0.0	28.4
	1 tbsp	124	0.0	14.0
(Hain)	1 tbsp	120	0.0	14.0
(Spectrum Naturals)	1 tbsp	120	0.0	14.0
AWA/milkfish				
dry-heat cooked	3 oz	161	0.0	7.3
raw	1 lb	673	0.0	30.5
raw	1 oz	42	0.0	1.9

B

Food Name	Serv. Size	Total Cal.	Carbs GMS	Fat GMS
BABASSU OIL. See PALM KERNEL OIL.				
BABY FOOD				
CEREAL				
Barley				
dry	1 tbsp	9	9.0	2.3
dry	.5 oz	52	10.7	0.5
instant, dry, '1st Foods' (Gerber)	.5 oz	60	11.0	1.0
instant, dry, 'Stage 1' (Beech-Nut)	.5 oz	60	12.0	0.0
instant, .5 oz cereal prepared w/2.4 oz formula, 'Stage 1' (Beech-Nut)	1 serving	120	18.0	4.0
instant, .5 oz cereal prepared w/2.4 oz whole milk (Gerber)	1 serving	100	14.0	4.0
instant, .5 oz cereal prepared w/2.4 oz formula	1 serving	110	16.0	4.0
instant (Heinz)	3.5 oz	370	78.5	3.7
prepared w/whole milk	3.5 oz	111	16.3	3.3
Cereal w/applesauce and bananas, '3rd Foods' (Gerber)	7 tbsp	82	17.9	0.6
Cereal w/egg yolks				
junior	7.5 oz	111	15.1	3.8
junior	1 oz	15	2.0	0.5
strained	1 oz	14	2.0	0.5
w/bacon, junior	4.5 oz	101	7.9	6.4
w/bacon, junior	1 oz	22	1.8	1.4
w/bacon, strained	7.5 oz	179	15.1	11.1
w/bacon, strained	1 oz	24	2.0	1.5
Cereal w/eggs				
strained	4.5 oz	74	10.2	1.9
strained	1 oz	16	2.3	0.4
Corn				
instant, dry, 'Tropical Foods' (Gerber)	.5 oz	60	12.0	1.0
instant, dry, 'Tropical Foods' (Gerber)	3.5 oz	390	80.8	4.6
instant, prepared w/milk, 'Tropical Foods' (Gerber)	2.4 oz	110	15.0	4.0
Grits and egg yolks				
strained	4.5 oz	73	9.5	2.9
strained	1 oz	16	2.1	0.7
High-protein				
instant, dry	1 tbsp	9	1.1	0.1
instant, dry	.5 oz	51	6.6	0.8
instant, 1 oz cereal prepared w/whole milk	1 serving	31	3.3	1.1
instant, w/apple and orange, dry	1 tbsp	9	1.4	0.2
instant, w/apple and orange, dry	.5 oz	53	8.2	0.9

Food Name	Serv. Size	Total Cal.	Carbs GMS	Fat GMS
instant, w/apple and orange, 1 oz cereal				
prepared w/whole milk	1 serving	32	3.8	1.1
Mixed				
dry	1 tbsp	9	1.8	0.1
dry	.5 oz	54	10.4	0.6
instant, dry *(Earth's Best)*	.5 oz	60	11.0	0.0
instant, dry, '2nd Foods' *(Gerber)*	.5 oz	60	11.0	1.0
instant, dry, 'Stages 2' *(Beech-Nut)*	.5 oz	60	12.0	0.0
instant, .5 oz cereal prepared w/2.4 oz formula, 'Stages 2' *(Beech-Nut)*	1 serving	120	17.0	4.0
instant, .5 oz cereal prepared w/2.5 oz formula *(Earth's Best)*	1 serving	110	16.0	3.0
instant, .5 oz cereal prepared w/2.4 oz whole milk, 'Stages 2' *(Beech-Nut)*	1 serving	100	14.0	3.0
instant *(Heinz)*	3.5 oz	373	71.9	4.9
instant, prepared w/apple juice, '2nd Foods' *(Gerber)*	2.4 oz	90	20.0	1.0
1 oz cereal prepared w/whole milk	1 serving	32	4.5	1.0
w/apples and bananas, 'Stages 2' *(Beech-Nut)*	4.5 oz	90	19.0	1.0
w/apples and bananas, strained *(Heinz)*	3.5 oz	70	15.7	0.3
w/applesauce and bananas, junior	7.75 oz	183	40.5	0.9
w/applesauce and bananas, junior	1 oz	24	5.2	0.1
w/applesauce and bananas, '2nd Foods' *(Gerber)*	4 oz	90	20.0	1.0
w/applesauce and bananas, '2nd Foods' *(Gerber)*	7 tbsp	81	17.8	0.6
w/applesauce and bananas, strained	4.75 oz	111	24.2	0.7
w/applesauce and bananas, strained	1 oz	23	5.1	0.1
w/applesauce and bananas, '3rd Foods' *(Gerber)*	7 tbsp	82	18.9	0.6
w/bananas, dry	1 tbsp	9	1.9	0.1
w/bananas, dry	.5 oz	56	10.9	0.7
w/bananas, instant, dry, '2nd Foods' *(Gerber)*	.5 oz	60	11.0	1.0
w/bananas, 1 oz cereal prepared w/whole milk	1 serving	33	4.7	1.0
w/fruit and nuts, no sugar added, 1-4 yr., dry *(Familia)*	1.5 oz	170	31.0	3.0
w/fruit and nuts, no sugar added, 1-4 yr., 1.5 oz cereal prepared w/whole milk *(Familia)*	1 serving	270	38.0	8.0
w/fruit and nuts, 1-4 yr., 1.5 oz cereal prepared w/2/3 cup milk *(Familia)*	1 serving	270	39.0	8.0
w/fruit and nuts, 100%-natural, 1-4 yr., dry *(Familia)*	1.5 oz	170	32.0	3.0
w/honey, dry	1 tbsp	9	1.8	0.1
w/honey, dry	.5 oz	56	10.4	0.7
w/honey, 1 oz cereal prepared w/whole milk	1 serving	33	4.5	1.0
Oatmeal				
instant, dry	1 tbsp	10	1.7	0.2
instant, dry	.5 oz	57	9.8	1.1
prepared w/whole milk	1 oz	33	4.3	1.2

Food Name	Serv. Size	Total Cal.	Carbs GMS	Fat GMS
w/apples and bananas, 'Stages 2' (Beech-Nut)	4.5 oz	90	17.0	1.0
w/apples and bananas, strained (Heinz)	3.5 oz	76	16.1	0.6
w/apples and cinnamon, instant, '3rd Foods' (Gerber)	1 pkt	90	16.0	2.0
w/applesauce and bananas, '2nd Foods' (Gerber)	4 oz	90	20.0	1.0
w/applesauce and bananas, '2nd Foods' (Gerber)	7 tbsp	83	17.6	0.8
w/applesauce and bananas, '3rd Foods' (Gerber)	7 tbsp	80	17.0	0.8
w/applesauce and bananas, junior	7.75 oz	165	34.5	1.5
w/applesauce and bananas, junior	1 oz	21	4.4	0.2
w/applesauce and bananas, strained	4.75 oz	99	20.8	0.9
w/applesauce and bananas, strained	1 oz	21	4.4	0.2
w/bananas, dry	1 tbsp	9	1.8	0.1
w/bananas, dry	.5 oz	56	10.4	0.9
w/bananas, instant, '3rd Foods' (Gerber)	1 pkt	90	16.0	2.0
w/bananas, prepared w/whole milk	1 oz	33	4.5	1.1
w/bananas, prepared w/whole milk	3.5 oz	116	16.0	3.8
w/bananas, 100%-natural, organic, dry (Healthy Times)	.5 oz	60	12.0	0.0
w/bananas, organic, .5 oz cereal prepared w/2.4 oz formula (Healthy Times)	.5 oz	100	17.0	3.0
w/honey, dry	1 tbsp	9	1.7	0.2
w/honey, dry	.5 oz	56	9.8	1.0
w/honey, prepared w/whole milk	1 oz	33	4.3	1.1
Rice				
dry	1 tbsp	9	1.9	0.1
dry	.5 oz	56	11.0	0.7
dry (Earth's Best)	.5 oz	60	12.0	0.0
dry (Health Valley)	1 tbsp	60	10.0	1.0
dry, .5 oz cereal prepared w/2.5 oz formula (Earth's Best)	3 oz	110	17.0	3.0
dry, prepared w/whole milk	1 oz	33	4.7	1.0
instant, dry, '1st Foods' (Gerber)	.5 oz	60	11.0	1.0
instant, dry, '1st Foods' (Gerber)	3.5 oz	380	79.3	3.3
instant, dry, 'Stages 1' (Beech-Nut)	.5 oz	60	12.0	0.0
instant, .5 oz cereal prepared w/2.4 oz formula (Beech-Nut)	.5 oz	120	18.0	4.0
instant, .5 oz cereal prepared w/2.4 oz whole milk (Beech-Nut)	2.9 oz	110	17.0	3.0
instant (Heinz)	3.5 oz	376	78.0	4.1
sprouted (Health Valley)	1 tbsp	60	10.0	1.0
w/apples, instant, dry, 'Stages 2' (Beech-Nut)	.5 oz	60	13.0	0.0
w/apples, instant, .5 oz cereal prepared w/2.4 oz formula (Beech-Nut)	.5 oz	120	19.0	4.0
w/apples, instant, .5 oz cereal prepared w/2.4 oz whole milk (Beech-Nut)	2.9 oz	110	17.0	3.0
w/apples and bananas, 'Stages 2' (Beech-Nut)	4.5 oz	100	24.0	0.0

Food Name	Serv. Size	Total Cal.	Carbs GMS	Fat GMS
w/apples and bananas, strained *(Heinz)*	3.5 oz	70	16.2	0.2
w/applesauce and bananas, '2nd Foods' *(Gerber)*	4 oz	90	21.0	0.0
w/applesauce and bananas, '2nd Foods' *(Gerber)*	7 tbsp	79	18.2	0.2
w/applesauce and bananas, strained	4.75 oz	107	23.1	0.5
w/applesauce and bananas, strained	1 oz	22	4.8	0.1
w/bananas, dry	1 tbsp	10	1.9	0.1
w/bananas, dry	.5 oz	57	11.4	0.6
w/bananas, instant, dry, '2nd Foods' *(Gerber)*	.5 oz	60	11.0	1.0
w/bananas, instant, dry, 'Stages 2' *(Beech-Nut)*	.5 oz	60	13.0	0.0
w/bananas, instant, .5 oz cereal prepared w/2.4 oz formula *(Beech-Nut)*	.5 oz	120	19.0	4.0
w/bananas, instant, .5 oz cereal prepared w/2.4 oz whole milk *(Beech-Nut)*	2.9 oz	100	17.0	3.0
w/bananas, prepared w/whole milk	1 oz	33	4.8	1.0
w/formula, instant, '1st Foods' *(Gerber)*	2.4 oz	110	16.0	4.0
w/honey, dry	1 tbsp	9	1.9	0.1
w/honey, dry	.5 oz	56	11.5	0.4
w/honey, prepared w/whole milk	1 oz	33	4.8	0.9
w/mango, instant, dry, 'Tropical Foods' *(Gerber)*	3.5 oz	386	84.3	2.6
w/mango, instant, prepared w/milk, 'Tropical Foods' *(Gerber)*	2.4 oz	100	15.0	3.0
w/mixed fruit, junior	7.75 oz	185	41.1	0.4
w/mixed fruit, junior	1 oz	24	5.3	0.1
w/mixed fruit, junior *(Gerber)*	6 oz	140	31.0	1.0
w/mixed fruit, '3rd Foods' *(Gerber)*	7 tbsp	79	18.3	0.2
DESSERTS AND SNACKS				
Apple betty				
junior	7.75 oz	154	41.8	0.0
junior	1 oz	20	5.4	0.0
strained	4.75 oz	97	26.5	0.0
strained	1 oz	20	5.6	0.0
Apple Juice Dessert, w/yogurt, '2nd Foods' *(Gerber)*	4 oz	100	18.0	2.0
Apple yogurt				
apple yogurt dessert, 'Stages 2' *(Beech-Nut)*	4.5 oz	120	25.0	2.0
'Breakfast' *(Earth's Best)*	4.5 oz	100	17.0	2.0
Banana yogurt				
'2nd Foods' *(Gerber)*	7 tbsp	74	16.4	0.4
'Stages 2' *(Beech-Nut)*	4.5 oz	120	26.0	2.0
strained *(Heinz)*	3.5 oz	83	18.7	0.5
Banana-apple dessert, '2nd Foods' *(Gerber)*	7 tbsp	68	16.4	0.1
Banana-pineapple dessert, 'Stages 2' *(Beech-Nut)*	4.5 oz	110	27.0	0.0
Banana-vanilla dessert, 'Tropical Foods' *(Gerber)*	7 tbsp	85	18.7	0.9
Blueberry yogurt, 'Breakfast' *(Earth's Best)*	4.5 oz	100	16.0	2.0

Food Name	Serv. Size	Total Cal.	Carbs GMS	Fat GMS
Cereal snack				
apple-banana finger snacks, 'Graduates' (Gerber)	3.2 oz	405	82.6	4.8
apple-cinnamon finger snacks, 'Graduates' (Gerber)	3.2 oz	407	82.6	5.0
Cherry vanilla dessert				
junior	7.75 oz	152	40.5	0.4
junior	1 oz	20	5.2	0.1
strained	4.75 oz	92	24.0	0.4
strained	1 oz	19	5.1	0.1
Cookies and crackers				
animal-shaped, baked, chunky (Gerber)	3.5 oz	443	74.8	13.1
apple, organic, 'Hugga Bears' (Healthy Times)	1 oz	120	17.0	3.0
arrowroot	1 oz	125	20.2	4.1
arrowroot, baked finger snacks, 'Graduates' (Gerber)	3.5 oz	452	70.3	15.3
arrowroot, w/maple, wheat-free (Healthy Times)	1 cookie	120	17.0	3.0
baked, chunky, 'Biter Biscuit' (Gerber)	1 biscuit	50	9.0	1.0
cinnamon animal crackers, baked, 'Graduates' (Gerber)	3.5 oz	449	78.7	12.3
pretzel	1 oz	113	23.3	0.6
pretzel, baked, finger snacks, 'Graduates' (Gerber)	3.5 oz	403	83.0	3.3
strawberry, organic, 'Hugga Bears' (Healthy Times)	1 oz	120	17.0	3.0
teething biscuit	1 biscuit	43	8.4	0.5
teething biscuit	1 oz	111	21.7	1.2
zwieback, baked, chunky (Gerber)	3.5 oz	432	69.4	11.5
Cottage cheese w/pineapple				
junior	7.75 oz	172	35.0	1.5
junior	1 oz	22	4.5	0.2
strained	4.75 oz	93	17.8	1.1
strained	1 oz	20	3.7	0.2
'Stages 2' (Beech-Nut)	4.5 oz	130	26.0	1.0
'Stages 3' (Beech-Nut)	6 oz	170	36.0	2.0
Custard/pudding				
banana pudding, 'Stages 2' (Beech-Nut)	4.5 oz	100	25.0	0.0
banana pudding, strained (Heinz)	3.5 oz	74	16.8	0.5
caramel pudding, junior	7.75 oz	168	36.2	1.9
caramel pudding, junior	1 oz	22	4.8	0.3
caramel pudding, strained	4.75 oz	104	23.2	0.9
caramel pudding, strained	1 oz	22	4.9	0.2
cherry vanilla pudding, '2nd Foods' (Gerber)	7 tbsp	69	16.6	0.2
cherry vanilla pudding, strained (Gerber)	4.5 oz	90	21.0	1.0
chocolate custard, junior	7.75 oz	196	38.3	3.5
chocolate custard, junior	1 oz	25	4.9	0.5
chocolate custard, junior (Heinz)	3.5 oz	75	14.0	1.2
chocolate custard, strained	4.75 oz	108	20.6	2.2
chocolate custard, strained	1 oz	24	4.6	0.5

Food Name	Serv. Size	Total Cal.	Carbs GMS	Fat GMS
orange pudding, strained	4.75 oz	108	23.9	1.2
orange pudding, strained	1 oz	23	5.0	0.3
pineapple pudding, junior	7.75 oz	191	47.5	0.9
pineapple pudding, junior	1 oz	25	6.1	0.1
pineapple pudding, strained	4.75 oz	104	26.0	0.4
pineapple pudding, strained	1 oz	23	5.8	0.1
vanilla custard, junior	7.75 oz	196	35.6	5.1
vanilla custard, junior	1 oz	25	4.6	0.7
vanilla custard, junior *(Gerber)*	6 oz	150	31.0	2.0
vanilla custard, '2nd Foods' *(Gerber)*	7 tbsp	88	18.2	0.9
vanilla custard, 'Stages 2' *(Beech-Nut)*	4.5 oz	140	24.0	4.0
vanilla custard, 'Stages 3' *(Beech-Nut)*	6 oz	180	30.0	5.0
vanilla custard, strained	4.75 oz	109	20.6	2.6
vanilla custard, strained	1 oz	24	4.6	0.6
vanilla custard, strained *(Gerber)*	4.5 oz	100	22.0	1.0
vanilla custard, '3rd Foods' *(Gerber)*	7 tbsp	89	18.4	0.9
vanilla custard, strained *(Heinz)*	3.5 oz	75	14.0	1.2
Dutch apple dessert				
junior	7.75 oz	152	37.0	2.2
junior	1 oz	20	4.8	0.3
junior *(Heinz)*	3.5 oz	69	16.3	0.4
'2nd Foods' *(Gerber)*	7 tbsp	79	17.4	1.0
'Stages 2' *(Beech-Nut)*	4.5 oz	100	24.0	0.0
strained	4.75 oz	92	22.5	1.2
strained	1 oz	19	4.7	0.3
strained *(Heinz)*	3.5 oz	69	16.3	0.4
'3rd Foods' *(Gerber)*	7 tbsp	77	16.9	0.9
Fruit dessert				
junior *(Gerber)*	6 oz	130	30.0	1.0
junior *(Heinz)*	3.5 oz	65	15.7	0.2
'2nd Foods' *(Gerber)*	7 tbsp	82	19.7	0.2
'Stages 2' *(Beech-Nut)*	4.5 oz	80	20.0	0.0
'Stages 3' *(Beech-Nut)*	6 oz	120	28.0	0.0
strained *(Gerber)*	4.5 oz	100	24.0	1.0
strained *(Heinz)*	3.5 oz	66	15.8	0.2
'3rd Foods' *(Gerber)*	7 tbsp	73	17.6	0.2
w/o ascorbic acid, junior	7.75 oz	139	37.8	0.0
w/o ascorbic acid, junior	1 oz	18	4.9	0.0
w/o ascorbic acid, strained	4.75 oz	80	21.6	0.0
w/o ascorbic acid, strained	1 oz	17	4.5	0.0
Guava dessert, w/tapioca, 'Tropical Foods' *(Gerber)*	7 tbsp	69	16.8	0.1
Hawaiian dessert				
junior *(Gerber)*	6 oz	150	33.0	1.0

Food Name	Serv. Size	Total Cal.	Carbs GMS	Fat GMS
'2nd Foods' (Gerber)	7 tbsp	86	19.7	0.2
'3rd Foods' (Gerber)	7 tbsp	87	20.2	0.1
strained (Gerber)	4.5 oz	120	25.0	1.0
Mango dessert, w/tapioca 'Tropical Foods' (Gerber)	7 tbsp	75	18.2	0.2
Mango-banana dessert, w/passion fruit, 'Tropical Foods' (Gerber)	7 tbsp	73	17.7	0.1
Mixed fruit yogurt, '2nd Foods' (Gerber)	7 tbsp	79	18.0	0.3
Papaya dessert, w/tapioca, 'Tropical Foods' (Gerber)	7 tbsp	62	15.1	0.2
Papaya-pineapple dessert, 'Tropical Foods' (Gerber)	7 tbsp	76	18.6	0.0
Peach cobbler				
junior	7.75 oz	147	40.3	0.0
junior	1 oz	19	5.2	0.0
'2nd Foods' (Gerber)	7 tbsp	77	18.2	0.2
strained	4.75 oz	88	24.0	0.0
strained	1 oz	18	5.1	0.0
strained (Heinz)	3.5 oz	72	16.9	0.3
'3rd Foods' (Gerber)	7 tbsp	77	18.4	0.1
Peach melba				
junior	7.75 oz	132	36.1	0.0
junior	1 oz	17	4.7	0.0
strained	4.75 oz	81	22.3	0.0
strained	1 oz	17	4.7	0.0
Peach yogurt				
'2nd Foods' (Gerber)	7 tbsp	76	17.2	0.4
'Stages 2' (Beech-Nut)	4.5 oz	120	25.0	2.0
Peach-mango dessert, 'Tropical Foods' (Gerber)	7 tbsp	60	16.8	0.2
Pear yogurt				
'Stages 2' (Beech-Nut)	4.5 oz	130	29.0	2.0
strained (Heinz)	3.5 oz	80	18.1	0.4
Pineapple-banana dessert, 'Tropical Foods' (Gerber)	7 tbsp	79	19.3	0.1
Pineapple-orange dessert				
strained	4.75 oz	90	24.4	0.0
strained	1 oz	20	5.4	0.0
Tropical fruit dessert				
junior	7.75 oz	132	36.1	0.0
junior	1 oz	17	4.7	0.0
medley, 'Tropical Foods' (Gerber)	7 tbsp	64	15.4	0.1
w/tapioca, strained	4.5 oz	80	20.0	0.0
Tropical yogurt, 'Breakfast' (Earth's Best)	4.5 oz	110	19.0	2.0
Tutti frutti dessert, junior (Heinz)	3.5 oz	67	15.7	0.4
DINNERS AND MAIN DISHES				
Apples and chicken dinner, 'Simple Recipe' '2nd Foods' (Gerber)	7 tbsp	66	11.0	1.4

Food Name	Serv. Size	Total Cal.	Carbs GMS	Fat GMS
Apples and ham dinner, 'Simple Recipe'				
'2nd Foods' (Gerber)	7 tbsp	67	12.2	0.8
Apples and turkey dinner				
'Simple Recipe,' '2nd Foods' (Gerber)	4 oz	80	13.0	2.0
'Simple Recipe,' '2nd Foods' (Gerber)	7 tbsp	67	11.3	1.2
Beans and rice dinner				
'Tropical Foods' (Gerber)	7 tbsp	52	7.4	1.5
w/green beans (Earth's Best)	4.5 oz	70	14.0	0.0
Beef and egg noodle dinner				
'2nd Foods' (Gerber)	7 tbsp	62	8.3	2.0
'3rd Foods' (Gerber)	7 tbsp	64	8.9	1.9
strained (Heinz)	3.5 oz	49	6.3	1.8
Beef and rice dinner				
toddler	6.25 oz	145	15.6	5.1
toddler	1 oz	23	2.5	0.8
Beef dinner				
junior (Gerber)	2.5 oz	80	1.0	4.0
'Stages 1' (Beech-Nut)	2.8 oz	90	0.0	5.0
'Stages 3' (Beech-Nut)	6 oz	150	14.0	8.0
supreme, 'Stages 2' (Beech-Nut)	4.5 oz	120	13.0	6.0
'3rd Foods' (Gerber)	7 tbsp	103	0.2	4.6
w/vegetables, lean meat, junior (Gerber)	4.5 oz	100	10.0	3.0
w/vegetables, lean meat, strained (Gerber)	4.5 oz	90	9.0	3.0
Beef lasagna dinner				
toddler	6.25 oz	136	17.7	3.7
toddler	1 oz	22	2.8	0.6
Beef noodle dinner				
junior	7.5 oz	121	15.8	4.1
junior	1 oz	16	2.1	0.5
strained	4.5 oz	68	9.0	2.2
strained	1 oz	15	2.0	0.5
Beef stew				
'Stages Table Time' (Beech-Nut)	6 oz	150	16.0	6.0
toddler	6.25 oz	90	9.7	2.1
toddler	1 oz	14	1.6	0.3
Beef vegetable dinner				
high-meat, junior	4.5 oz	109	6.8	5.9
high-meat, junior	1 oz	24	1.5	1.3
high-meat, strained	4.5 oz	96	5.4	5.4
high-meat, strained	1 oz	21	1.2	1.2
Beef vegetable entrée				
'Stages 2' (Beech-Nut)	4.5 oz	90	10.0	4.0
'Stages 3' (Beech-Nut)	6 oz	160	16.0	7.0

Food Name	Serv. Size	Total Cal.	Carbs GMS	Fat GMS
Broccoli-chicken dinner, 'Simple Recipe'				
'2nd Foods' *(Gerber)*	7 tbsp	42	3.4	1.5
Carrots and beef dinner, 'Simple Recipe'				
'2nd Foods' *(Gerber)*	7 tbsp	59	5.7	2.5
Chicken dinner				
junior *(Gerber)*	2.5 oz	110	1.0	7.0
'3rd Foods' *(Gerber)*	7 tbsp	132	0.2	7.9
vegetable entrée, 'Stages 2' *(Beech-Nut)*	4.5 oz	90	14.0	3.0
vegetable entrée, 'Stages 3' *(Beech-Nut)*	6 oz	90	13.0	2.0
w/vegetables, lean meat, junior *(Gerber)*	4.5 oz	90	10.0	3.0
w/vegetables, lean meat, strained *(Gerber)*	4.5 oz	90	8.0	3.0
Chicken noodle dinner				
junior	7.5 oz	109	16.0	3.0
junior	1 oz	14	2.1	0.4
'2nd Foods' *(Gerber)*	7 tbsp	55	8.6	1.2
strained	4.5 oz	67	9.6	1.9
strained	1 oz	15	2.1	0.4
'3rd Foods' *(Gerber)*	7 tbsp	56	8.6	1.3
Chicken rice dinner				
'Stages 2' *(Beech-Nut)*	4.5 oz	80	11.0	3.0
'Tropical Foods' *(Gerber)*	7 tbsp	48	6.9	1.3
Chicken stew dinner				
toddler	6 oz	133	10.9	6.3
toddler	1 oz	22	1.8	1.0
w/noodles, 'Graduates'	3.2 oz	69	8.5	2.0
Chicken vegetable dinner				
high-meat, junior	4.5 oz	118	5.4	7.0
high-meat, junior	1 oz	26	1.2	1.6
high-meat, strained	4.5 oz	100	7.6	4.6
high-meat, strained	1 oz	22	1.7	1.0
Green bean dinner, w/turkey, 'Simple Recipe,'				
'2nd Foods' *(Gerber)*	7 tbsp	55	6.5	1.5
Ham dinner				
ham and vegetable entrée, 'Stages 2' *(Beech-Nut)*	4.5 oz	80	12.0	3.0
w/vegetables, lean meat, junior *(Gerber)*	4.5 oz	110	11.0	4.0
w/vegetables, lean meat, strained *(Gerber)*	4.5 oz	100	10.0	4.0
Ham vegetable dinner				
high-meat, junior	4.5 oz	99	7.8	4.2
high-meat, junior	1 oz	22	1.7	0.9
high-meat, strained	4.5 oz	97	7.0	4.5
high-meat, strained	1 oz	22	1.6	1.0
Lamb and vegetable entrée, 'Stages 2' *(Beech-Nut)*	4.5 oz	90	13.0	4.0

Food Name	Serv. Size	Total Cal.	Carbs GMS	Fat GMS
Lamb noodle dinner				
junior	7.5 oz	138	18.5	4.7
junior	1 oz	18	2.5	0.6
Macaroni dinner				
tomato beef, '2nd Foods' (Gerber)	7 tbsp	57	9.1	1.1
tomato beef, '3rd Foods' (Gerber)	7 tbsp	60	10.2	0.9
tomatoes and beef, junior (Heinz)	3.5 oz	52	8.2	1.2
w/bacon, junior	7.5 oz	160	18.3	7.0
w/bacon, junior	1 oz	21	2.4	0.9
w/beef, 'Stages 2' (Beech-Nut)	4.5 oz	90	13.0	4.0
w/beef, 'Stages 3' (Beech-Nut)	6 oz	160	17.0	8.0
w/cheese (Earth's Best)	4.5 oz	100	12.0	4.0
w/cheese, junior	7.5 oz	130	17.5	4.3
w/cheese, junior	1 oz	17	2.3	0.6
w/cheese, strained	4.5 oz	76	9.6	2.7
w/cheese, strained	1 oz	17	2.1	0.6
w/cheese, '2nd Foods' (Gerber)	7 tbsp	63	8.6	2.0
Macaroni main dish				
alphabets w/beef and tomato sauce, chunky (Gerber)	7 tbsp	80	11.4	2.0
w/beef, in sauce, 'Graduates' (Gerber)	3.2 oz	78	11.1	1.7
w/ham, junior	7.5 oz	128	18.1	3.0
w/ham, junior	1 oz	17	2.4	0.4
w/tomato and beef, junior	7.5 oz	126	20.0	2.3
w/tomato and beef, junior	1 oz	17	2.7	0.3
w/tomato and beef, strained	4.5 oz	70	11.3	1.4
w/tomato and beef, strained	1 oz	16	2.5	0.3
Mixed vegetable dinner				
junior	7.5 oz	70	16.8	0.0
junior	1 oz	9	2.2	0.0
strained	4.5 oz	52	12.2	0.1
strained	1 oz	12	2.7	0.0
Noodle main dish				
w/beef, chunky, 'Homestyle' (Gerber)	7 tbsp	88	9.8	3.5
w/chicken, carrots, and peas, chunky (Gerber)	7 tbsp	65	8.8	1.5
Pasta dinner (Earth's Best)	4.5 oz	90	13.0	3.0
Potato dinner, w/green beans (Earth's Best)	4.5 oz	100	13.0	3.0
Ravioli				
beef, w/tomato sauce, 'Graduates' (Gerber)	3.2 oz	97	16.3	2.0
beef, w/tomato sauce, 'Graduates' micro cup (Gerber)	6 oz	170	28.0	4.0
cheese, w/tomato sauce, 'Graduates' (Gerber)	3.2 oz	99	16.3	2.2
cheese, w/tomato sauce, 'Graduates' micro cup (Gerber)	6 oz	170	28.0	4.0
Rice and lentil dinner, (Earth's Best)	4.5 oz	80	13.0	2.0

Food Name	Serv. Size	Total Cal.	Carbs GMS	Fat GMS
Rice main dish				
saucy, w/chicken, chunky *(Gerber)*	7 tbsp	67	10.1	1.5
w/beef and tomato sauce, chunky *(Gerber)*	7 tbsp	79	11.7	1.9
Spaghetti				
rings, in meat sauce, 'Stages Table Time' *(Beech-Nut)*	6 oz	160	22.0	4.0
w/beef, 'Stages 3' *(Beech-Nut)*	6 oz	170	17.0	8.0
w/mini meatballs and sauce,'Graduates' *(Gerber)*	6 oz	160	21.0	5.0
w/mini meatballs and sauce, 'Graduates' *(Gerber)*	3.2 oz	91	12.0	2.8
w/tomato and meat, junior	7.5 oz	134	21.5	2.8
w/tomato and meat, junior	1 oz	18	2.9	0.4
w/tomato and meat, toddler	6.25 oz	133	19.1	1.8
w/tomato and meat, toddler	1 oz	21	3.1	0.3
w/tomato sauce and beef, chunky *(Gerber)*	7 tbsp	85	12.5	1.9
w/tomato sauce and beef, junior *(Gerber)*	6 oz	120	19.0	3.0
w/tomato sauce and beef, '3rd Foods' *(Gerber)*	7 tbsp	64	10.6	1.2
w/tomato sauce and meat, junior *(Heinz)*	3.5 oz	58	9.6	1.3
Split pea and ham dinner				
junior	7.5 oz	151	24.1	2.8
junior	1 oz	20	3.2	0.4
Sweet potato dinner, w/chicken *(Earth's Best)*	4.5 oz	90	13.0	2.0
Turkey dinner				
junior *(Gerber)*	2.5 oz	100	1.0	6.0
supreme, 'Stages 2' *(Beech-Nut)*	4.5 oz	120	11.0	6.0
Turkey rice dinner				
junior	7.5 oz	104	15.3	3.0
junior	1 oz	14	2.0	0.4
junior *(Gerber)*	6 oz	110	14.0	4.0
'2nd Foods' *(Gerber)*	7 tbsp	55	7.5	1.5
'Stages 2' *(Beech-Nut)*	4.5 oz	70	12.0	2.0
'Stages 3' *(Beech-Nut)*	6 oz	110	14.0	4.0
strained	4.5 oz	63	9.3	1.7
strained	1 oz	14	2.1	0.4
strained *(Gerber)*	4.5 oz	80	10.0	3.0
'3rd Foods' *(Gerber)*	7 tbsp	55	7.8	1.4
w/vegetables, junior *(Heinz)*	3.5 oz	42	7.9	0.6
w/vegetables, strained *(Heinz)*	3.5 oz	47	8.2	1.1
Turkey stew main dish, w/rice, 'Graduates' *(Gerber)*	3.2 oz	59	7.6	1.0
Turkey-vegetable dinner				
high-meat, junior	4.5 oz	115	7.6	6.4
high-meat, junior	1 oz	26	1.7	1.4
high-meat, strained	4.5 oz	111	7.7	6.1
high-meat, strained	1 oz	25	1.7	1.4
lean meat, junior *(Gerber)*	4.5 oz	100	10.0	4.0

Food Name	Serv. Size	Total Cal.	Carbs GMS	Fat GMS
lean meat, strained *(Gerber)*	4.5 oz	100	9.0	4.0
Veal-vegetable dinner				
high-meat, junior	4.5 oz	93	7.4	4.0
high-meat, junior	1 oz	21	1.6	0.9
high-meat, strained	4.5 oz	88	7.8	3.5
high-meat, strained	1 oz	20	1.7	0.8
Vegetable-bacon dinner				
junior	7.5 oz	151	16.2	8.3
junior	1 oz	20	2.2	1.1
'2nd Foods' *(Gerber)*	7 tbsp	73	8.8	3.3
strained	4.5 oz	88	11.0	4.2
'3rd Foods' *(Gerber)*	7 tbsp	77	9.3	3.4
Vegetable-beef dinner				
(Earth's Best)	4.5 oz	90	11.0	3.0
junior	7.5 oz	113	15.8	3.6
junior	1 oz	15	2.1	0.5
'2nd Foods' *(Gerber)*	7 tbsp	65	8.5	2.4
strained	4.5 oz	68	9.0	2.6
strained	1 oz	15	2.0	0.6
'3rd Foods' *(Gerber)*	7 tbsp	62	9.2	1.6
Vegetable-chicken dinner				
junior	7.5 oz	107	18.1	2.3
junior	1 oz	14	2.4	0.3
'2nd Foods' *(Gerber)*	7 tbsp	58	9.4	1.3
strained	4.5 oz	55	8.4	1.4
strained	1 oz	12	1.9	0.3
'3rd Foods' *(Gerber)*	7 tbsp	51	8.1	1.1
vegetable dinner, 'Summer' *(Earth's Best)*	4.5 oz	90	12.0	3.0
Vegetable-dumpling dinner				
w/beef, junior	7.5 oz	102	17.0	1.7
w/beef, junior	1 oz	14	2.3	0.2
w/beef, junior *(Heinz)*	3.5 oz	47	7.2	1.2
w/beef, strained	4.5 oz	61	9.9	1.1
w/beef, strained	1 oz	14	2.2	0.3
w/beef, strained *(Heinz)*	3.5 oz	49	8.6	1.3
Vegetable-ham dinner				
junior	7.5 oz	111	14.9	3.6
junior	1 oz	15	2.0	0.5
'2nd Foods' *(Gerber)*	7 tbsp	59	8.6	1.9
strained	4.5 oz	61	8.8	2.2
strained	1 oz	14	2.0	0.5
'3rd Foods' *(Gerber)*	7 tbsp	61	9.2	1.8
toddler	6.25 oz	127	14.0	5.3

Food Name	Serv. Size	Total Cal.	Carbs GMS	Fat GMS
toddler	1 oz	20	2.2	0.9
Vegetable-lamb dinner				
junior	7.5 oz	109	15.1	3.6
junior	1 oz	14	2.0	0.5
strained	4.5 oz	67	8.8	2.6
strained	1 oz	15	2.0	0.6
Vegetable-liver dinner				
junior	7.5 oz	94	17.5	1.3
junior	1 oz	12	2.3	0.2
strained	4.5 oz	50	8.8	0.5
strained	1 oz	11	2.0	0.1
Vegetable main dish				
w/beef, chunky *(Gerber)*	7 tbsp	70	9.2	2.0
w/chicken, chunky *(Gerber)*	7 tbsp	66	9.5	1.4
w/ham, chunky *(Gerber)*	7 tbsp	70	8.7	2.3
w/turkey, chunky *(Gerber)*	7 tbsp	61	8.4	4.4
Vegetable-noodle dinner				
w/chicken, junior	7.5 oz	136	19.4	4.7
w/chicken, junior	1 oz	18	2.6	0.6
w/chicken, junior *(Heinz)*	3.5 oz	57	8.7	1.8
w/chicken, strained	4.5 oz	81	10.1	3.2
w/chicken, strained	1 oz	18	2.2	0.7
w/chicken, strained *(Heinz)*	3.5 oz	54	7.5	1.7
w/turkey, junior	7.5 oz	111	16.2	3.2
w/turkey, junior	1 oz	15	2.2	0.4
w/turkey, junior *(Heinz)*	3.5 oz	48	6.4	2.0
w/turkey, strained	4.5 oz	56	8.7	1.5
w/turkey, strained	1 oz	12	1.9	0.3
w/turkey, strained *(Heinz)*	3.5 oz	47	6.7	1.6
Vegetable stew				
w/beef, 'Graduates' *(Gerber)*	3.2 oz	71	8.8	1.4
w/beef, 'Graduates' micro cup *(Gerber)*	6 oz	130	15.0	3.0
w/chicken, 'Stages Table Time' *(Beech-Nut)*	6 oz	190	23.0	8.0
Vegetable-turkey dinner				
(Earth's Best)	4.5 oz	60	11.0	1.0
junior	7.5 oz	100	16.4	2.6
junior	1 oz	13	2.2	0.3
'2nd Foods' *(Gerber)*	7 tbsp	49	7.5	1.2
'3rd Foods' *(Gerber)*	7 tbsp	53	8.7	1.0
strained	4.5 oz	54	8.4	1.5
strained	1 oz	12	1.9	0.3
toddler	6.25 oz	142	14.2	6.0
toddler	1 oz	23	2.3	1.0

Food Name	Serv. Size	Total Cal.	Carbs GMS	Fat GMS
EGG YOLK				
'2nd Foods' (Gerber)	7 tbsp	193	1.0	16.8
strained	3.3 oz	191	0.9	16.3
strained	1 oz	58	0.3	4.9
FRUIT				
Apple (Earth's Best)	4.5 oz	60	14.0	1.0
Apple, peach, and strawberry, 'Stages 2' (Beech-Nut)	4.5 oz	100	24.0	0.0
Apple, pear, and banana, 'Stages 2' (Beech-Nut)	4.5 oz	100	24.0	0.0
Apple and apricot				
(Earth's Best)	4.5 oz	70	15.0	1.0
strained (Heinz)	3.5 oz	55	12.9	0.3
Apple and banana				
(Earth's Best)	4.5 oz	80	18.0	1.0
'2nd Foods' (Gerber)	4 oz	60	15.0	0.0
Apple and blueberry				
(Earth's Best)	4.5 oz	60	14.0	1.0
junior	7.75 oz	136	36.5	0.4
junior	1 oz	18	4.7	0.1
junior (Gerber)	6 oz	80	19.0	1.0
'2nd Foods' (Gerber)	7 tbsp	51	12.1	0.2
strained	4.75 oz	82	22.0	0.3
strained	1 oz	17	4.6	0.1
strained (Gerber)	4.5 oz	60	14.0	1.0
'3rd Foods' (Gerber)	7 tbsp	50	11.8	0.2
Apple and cranberry, w/tapioca, strained (Heinz)	3.5 oz	66	15.9	0.3
Apple and pear				
(Heinz)	3.5 oz	56	13.4	0.2
junior	3.5 oz	57	12.9	0.2
Apple and plum (Earth's Best)	4.5 oz	70	16.0	1.0
Apple and raspberry				
w/sugar, junior	7.75 oz	128	34.1	0.4
w/sugar, junior	1 oz	16	4.4	0.1
w/sugar, strained	4.75 oz	78	21.2	0.3
w/sugar, strained	1 oz	16	4.4	0.1
Applesauce				
'Beginner Foods' (Heinz)	3.5 oz	73	18.0	0.1
'1st Foods' (Gerber)	2.5 oz	35	9.0	0.0
'1st Foods' (Gerber)	7 tbsp	56	13.2	0.2
golden delicious, 'Baby's First' (Beech-Nut)	2.5 oz	50	11.0	0.0
golden delicious, 'Stages 1' (Beech-Nut)	4.5 oz	70	17.0	0.0
golden delicious, 'Stages 1' (Beech-Nut)	2.8 oz	50	13.0	0.0
junior	7.5 oz	79	21.9	0.0
junior	1 oz	10	2.9	0.0

Food Name	Serv. Size	Total Cal.	Carbs GMS	Fat GMS
junior (Gerber)	6 oz	90	20.0	1.0
junior (Heinz)	3.5 oz	53	12.4	0.2
'2nd Foods' (Gerber)	7 tbsp	52	12.3	0.2
'Stages 3' (Beech-Nut)	6 oz	90	22.0	0.0
strained	4.5 oz	52	14.0	0.3
strained	1 oz	12	3.1	0.1
strained (Gerber)	4.5 oz	60	14.0	1.0
strained (Heinz)	3.5 oz	53	12.4	0.2
'3rd Foods' (Gerber)	7 tbsp	51	12.1	0.2
w/apricot, junior	7.75 oz	103	27.3	0.4
w/apricot, junior	1 oz	13	3.5	0.1
w/apricot, '2nd Foods' (Gerber)	7 tbsp	53	12.5	0.2
w/apricot, 'Stages 2' (Beech-Nut)	4.5 oz	80	19.0	0.0
w/apricot, strained	4.75 oz	61	15.7	0.3
w/apricot, strained	1 oz	13	3.3	0.1
w/apricot, strained (Gerber)	4.5 oz	70	15.0	1.0
w/banana, 'Stages 2' (Beech-Nut)	4.5 oz	80	18.0	0.0
w/banana, 'Stages 3' (Beech-Nut)	6 oz	100	25.0	0.0
w/cherry, junior	7.75 oz	106	29.0	0.0
w/cherry, junior	1 oz	14	3.7	0.0
w/cherry, 'Stages 2' (Beech-Nut)	4.5 oz	70	18.0	0.0
w/cherry, 'Stages 3' (Beech-Nut)	6 oz	100	24.0	0.0
w/cherry, strained	4.75 oz	65	17.7	0.0
w/cherry, strained	1 oz	14	3.7	0.0
w/pineapple, junior	7.5 oz	83	22.4	0.2
w/pineapple, junior	1 oz	11	3.0	0.0
w/pineapple, strained	4.5 oz	47	12.9	0.1
w/pineapple, strained	1 oz	10	2.9	0.0
Apricot				
w/pear, 'Stages 3' (Beech-Nut)	6 oz	120	27.0	0.0
w/pear and applesauce, 'Stages 2' (Beech-Nut)	4.5 oz	90	21.0	0.0
w/tapioca, junior	7.75 oz	139	38.1	0.0
w/tapioca, junior	1 oz	18	4.9	0.0
w/tapioca, junior (Gerber)	6 oz	130	29.0	1.0
w/tapioca, junior (Heinz)	3.5 oz	66	15.9	0.2
w/tapioca, '2nd Foods' (Gerber)	7 tbsp	67	16.2	0.2
w/tapioca, strained	4.75 oz	81	22.0	0.0
w/tapioca, strained	1 oz	17	4.6	0.0
w/tapioca, strained (Gerber)	4.5 oz	90	20.0	1.0
w/tapioca, strained (Heinz)	3.5 oz	64	15.3	0.2
w/tapioca, '3rd Foods' (Gerber)	7 tbsp	71	17.1	0.2
Banana				
'Beginner Foods' (Heinz)	3.5 oz	107	25.0	0.2

Food Name	Serv. Size	Total Cal.	Carbs GMS	Fat GMS
Chiquita, 'Baby's First' (Beech-Nut)	2.5 oz	70	16.0	0.0
Chiquita, 'Stages 1' (Beech-Nut)	4.5 oz	110	26.0	0.0
Chiquita, 'Stages 1' (Beech-Nut)	2.8 oz	70	16.0	0.0
(Earth's Best)	4.5 oz	100	22.0	0.0
'1st Foods' (Gerber)	2.5 oz	70	17.0	0.0
'1st Foods' (Gerber)	7 tbsp	100	23.3	0.3
w/pineapple and tapioca, '2nd Foods' (Gerber)	7 tbsp	52	12.3	0.1
w/pineapple and tapioca,'3rd Foods' (Gerber)	7 tbsp	52	12.3	0.1
w/tapioca, junior	7.75 oz	147	39.2	0.4
w/tapioca, junior	1 oz	19	5.1	0.1
w/tapioca, junior (Gerber)	6 oz	140	31.0	1.0
w/tapioca, junior (Heinz)	3.5 oz	73	17.6	0.2
w/tapioca, '2nd Foods' (Gerber)	7 tbsp	78	18.5	0.2
w/tapioca, '3rd Foods' (Gerber)	7 tbsp	77	18.4	0.2
w/tapioca, strained	4.75 oz	77	20.7	0.1
w/tapioca, strained	1 oz	16	4.3	0.0
w/tapioca, strained (Gerber)	4.5 oz	110	24.0	1.0
w/tapioca, strained (Heinz)	3.5 oz	73	17.6	0.2
Banana and apple, strained (Gerber)	4.5 oz	90	20.0	1.0
Banana and pear, w/applesauce, 'Stages 2' (Beech-Nut)	4.5 oz	100	24.0	0.0
Banana and pineapple				
'Stages 2' (Beech-Nut)	4.5 oz	110	27.0	0.0
w/tapioca, junior	4.75 oz	92	24.8	0.1
w/tapioca, junior	1 oz	19	5.2	0.0
w/tapioca, junior (Gerber)	6 oz	90	20.0	1.0
w/tapioca, strained	7.75 oz	143	39.2	0.0
w/tapioca, strained	1 oz	18	5.1	0.0
w/tapioca, strained (Gerber)	4.5 oz	60	15.0	0.0
w/tapioca, strained (Heinz)	3.5 oz	64	15.3	0.2
Guava				
w/tapioca, strained	4.5 oz	86	23.4	0.0
w/tapioca, strained	1 oz	19	5.2	0.0
w/tapioca, strained (Gerber)	4.5 oz	90	20.0	1.0
w/tapioca, strained, 'Stages 2' (Beech-Nut)	4.5 oz	100	24.0	0.0
Guava and papaya				
w/tapioca, strained	4.5 oz	81	21.8	0.1
w/tapioca, strained	1 oz	18	4.8	0.0
Mango				
tropical fruit dessert, 'Stages 2' (Beech-Nut)	4.5 oz	100	25.0	0.0
w/tapioca, strained	4.75 oz	108	29.2	0.3
w/tapioca, strained	1 oz	23	6.1	0.1
w/tapioca, strained (Gerber)	4.5 oz	90	21.0	1.0

Food Name	Serv. Size	Total Cal.	Carbs GMS	Fat GMS
Mango and banana, w/passion fruit and tapioca, strained *(Gerber)*	4.5 oz	100	25.0	0.0
Papaya				
'Stages 2' *(Beech-Nut)*	4.5 oz	100	24.0	0.0
w/tapioca, strained *(Gerber)*	4.5 oz	80	19.0	1.0
Papaya and applesauce				
w/tapioca, strained	4.5 oz	90	24.2	0.1
w/tapioca, strained	1 oz	20	5.4	0.0
Peach				
'Beginner Foods' *(Heinz)*	3.5 oz	80	18.3	0.2
'1st Foods' *(Gerber)*	2.5 oz	30	7.0	0.0
'1st Foods' *(Gerber)*	7 tbsp	43	9.6	0.2
junior *(Gerber)*	6 oz	110	25.0	1.0
junior *(Heinz)*	3.5 oz	68	15.4	0.3
'2nd Foods' *(Gerber)*	7 tbsp	66	15.3	0.2
'Stages 3' *(Beech-Nut)*	6 oz	90	22.0	0.0
strained *(Gerber)*	4.5 oz	90	19.0	1.0
strained *(Heinz)*	3.5 oz	68	15.4	0.3
'3rd Foods' *(Gerber)*	7 tbsp	65	15.1	0.2
w/mango and tapioca, strained *(Gerber)*	4.5 oz	100	24.0	1.0
w/oatmeal and banana *(Earth's Best)*	4.5 oz	70	15.0	1.0
w/sugar, junior	7.75 oz	156	41.6	0.4
w/sugar, junior	1 oz	20	5.4	0.1
w/sugar, strained	4.75 oz	96	25.5	0.3
w/sugar, strained	1 oz	20	5.4	0.1
w/yogurt, 'Stages 2' *(Beech-Nut)*	4.5 oz	120	25.0	2.0
yellow cling, 'Baby's First' *(Beech-Nut)*	2.5 oz	45	10.0	0.0
yellow cling, 'Stages 1' *(Beech-Nut)*	4.5 oz	70	15.0	0.0
yellow cling, 'Stages 1' *(Beech-Nut)*	2.8 oz	50	12.0	0.0
Pear				
Bartlett, 'Baby's First' *(Beech-Nut)*	2.5 oz	50	12.0	0.0
Bartlett, 'Stages 1' *(Beech-Nut)*	4.5 oz	70	18.0	0.0
Bartlett, 'Stages 1' *(Beech-Nut)*	2.8 oz	50	13.0	0.0
Bartlett, 'Stages 3' *(Beech-Nut)*	6 oz	100	24.0	0.0
Bartlett, w/applesauce, 'Stages 2' *(Beech-Nut)*	4.5 oz	80	20.0	0.0
Bartlett, w/pineapple, 'Stages 2' *(Beech-Nut)*	4.5 oz	90	21.0	0.0
'Beginner Foods' *(Heinz)*	3.5 oz	76	18.0	0.2
(Earth's Best)	4.5 oz	60	14.0	0.2
'1st Foods' *(Gerber)*	2.5 oz	40	11.0	0.0
'1st Foods' *(Gerber)*	7 tbsp	57	13.2	0.3
junior	7.5 oz	92	24.7	0.2
junior	1 oz	12	3.3	0.0
junior *(Gerber)*	6 oz	100	21.0	1.0

Food Name	Serv. Size	Total Cal.	Carbs GMS	Fat GMS
junior *(Heinz)*	3.5 oz	60	14.1	0.2
'2nd Foods' *(Gerber)*	7 tbsp	55	12.9	0.2
strained	4.5 oz	52	13.8	0.3
strained	1 oz	12	3.1	0.1
strained *(Gerber)*	4.5 oz	80	16.0	1.0
strained *(Heinz)*	3.5 oz	60	14.1	0.2
'3rd Foods' *(Gerber)*	7 tbsp	55	12.9	0.2
Pear and pineapple				
junior	7.5 oz	94	24.3	0.4
junior	1 oz	12	3.2	0.1
junior *(Gerber)*	6 oz	100	21.0	1.0
'2nd Foods' *(Gerber)*	7 tbsp	55	12.8	0.2
strained	4.5 oz	52	14.0	0.1
strained	1 oz	12	3.1	0.0
strained *(Gerber)*	4.5 oz	80	16.0	1.0
'3rd Foods' *(Gerber)*	7 tbsp	54	12.7	0.2
Pears and raspberries, *(Earth's Best)*	4.5 oz	60	15.0	
Plum				
w/banana and rice *(Earth's Best)*	4.5 oz	90	19.0	0.0
w/rice, 'Stages 2' *(Beech-Nut)*	4.5 oz	150	34.0	0.0
w/tapioca, junior *(Gerber)*	6 oz	130	30.0	1.0
w/tapioca, '2nd Foods' *(Gerber)*	7 tbsp	74	17.7	0.2
w/tapioca, strained *(Gerber)*	4.5 oz	90	22.0	0.0
w/tapioca, strained *(Heinz)*	3.5 oz	67	16.2	0.2
w/tapioca, '3rd Foods' *(Gerber)*	7 tbsp	75	18.1	0.2
w/tapioca, w/o ascorbic acid, junior	7.75 oz	163	44.9	0.0
w/tapioca, w/o ascorbic acid, junior	1 oz	21	5.8	0.0
w/tapioca, w/o ascorbic acid, strained	4.75 oz	96	26.6	0.0
w/tapioca, w/o ascorbic acid, strained	1 oz	20	5.6	0.0
Prune				
'1st Foods' *(Gerber)*	2.5 oz	70	17.0	0.0
'1st Foods' *(Gerber)*	7 tbsp	101	23.8	0.2
w/oatmeal *(Earth's Best)*	4.5 oz	100	24.0	0.0
w/pear, 'Stages 2' *(Beech-Nut)*	4.5 oz	90	22.0	0.0
w/tapioca, '2nd Foods' *(Gerber)*	7 tbsp	77	18.1	0.2
w/tapioca, strained *(Gerber)*	4.5 oz	100	22.0	1.0
w/tapioca, strained *(Heinz)*	3.5 oz	90	21.5	0.2
w/tapioca, w/o ascorbic acid, junior	7.75 oz	154	41.1	0.2
w/tapioca, w/o ascorbic acid, junior	1 oz	20	5.3	0.0
w/tapioca, w/o ascorbic acid, strained	4.75 oz	94	25.0	0.1
w/tapioca, w/o ascorbic acid, strained	1 oz	20	5.2	0.0

Food Name	Serv. Size	Total Cal.	Carbs GMS	Fat. GMS
INFANT FORMULA				
Mix				
liquid, iron-fortified, prepared, 'Follow-Up' (Carnation)	5 oz	100	13.2	4.1
liquid, iron-fortified, prepared, 'Good Start' (Carnation)	5 oz	100	11.0	5.1
liquid, low-iron, prepared (Enfamil)	5 oz	100	10.3	5.6
liquid, low-iron, prepared (Gerber)	5 oz	100	10.0	5.3
liquid, low-iron, prepared (Similac)	5 oz	100	10.7	5.4
liquid, soy, iron-fortified, milk-free (Nursoy)	5 oz	100	10.2	5.3
liquid, soy, iron-fortified, milk-free, prepared (Gerber)	5 oz	100	10.0	5.3
liquid, soy, iron-fortified, milk-free, prepared (ProSobee)	5 oz	100	10.0	5.3
liquid, soy, w/iron, milk-free, prepared (Isomil)	5 oz	100	10.3	5.4
liquid, w/iron, prepared (Enfamil)	5 oz	100	10.3	5.6
liquid, w/iron, prepared (Gerber)	5 oz	100	10.7	5.4
liquid, w/iron, prepared (Similac)	5 oz	100	10.7	5.4
powder, iron-fortified, prepared, 'Follow-Up' (Carnation)	5 oz	100	13.2	4.1
powder, iron-fortified, prepared, 'Good Start' (Carnation)	5 oz	100	11.0	5.1
powder, low-iron, prepared (Enfamil)	5 oz	100	10.3	5.6
powder, low-iron, prepared (Gerber)	5 oz	100	10.0	5.3
powder, low-iron, prepared (Similac)	5 oz	100	10.7	5.4
powder, soy, iron-fortified, milk-free, prepared (Gerber)	5 oz	100	10.0	5.3
powder, soy, iron-fortified, milk-free, prepared (ProSobee)	5 oz	100	10.0	5.3
powder, soy, w/iron, milk-free, prepared (Isomil)	5 oz	100	10.3	5.5
powder, w/iron, prepared (Enfamil)	5 oz	100	10.3	5.6
powder, w/iron, prepared (Gerber)	5 oz	100	10.7	5.4
powder, w/iron, prepared (Similac)	5 oz	100	10.7	5.4
Ready to use				
iron-fortified, 'Follow-Up' (Carnation)	5 oz	100	13.2	4.1
iron-fortified, 'Good Start' (Carnation)	5 oz	100	11.0	5.1
low-iron (Enfamil)	5 oz	100	10.3	5.6
low-iron (Gerber)	5 oz	100	10.0	5.3
low-iron (Similac)	5 oz	100	10.7	5.4
soy, iron-fortified, milk-free (Gerber)	5 oz	100	10.0	5.3
soy, iron-fortified, milk-free (ProSobee)	5 oz	100	10.0	5.3
soy, w/iron, milk-free (Isomil)	5 oz	100	10.3	5.4
w/iron (Enfamil)	5 oz	100	10.3	5.6
w/iron (Gerber)	5 oz	100	10.7	5.4
w/iron (Similac)	5 oz	100	10.7	5.4
JUICE				
Apple				
	4.2 oz	61	15.2	0.1
	1 oz	15	3.6	0.0
(Earth's Best)	4.2 oz	60	14.0	0.0
'Graduates' (Gerber)	6 oz	80	21.0	0.0

Food Name	Serv. Size	Total Cal.	Carbs GMS	Fat GMS
'Graduates' (Gerber)	3.2 oz	48	11.7	0.1
100%-juice, 'Junior' (McCain)	4.2 oz	50	13.0	0.0
'Stages 1' (Beech-Nut)	4.2 oz	60	14.0	0.0
strained, '1st Foods' (Gerber)	4 oz	60	14.0	0.0
strained, '1st Foods' (Gerber)	3.2 oz	46	11.0	0.1
strained (Heinz)	3.5 oz	48	11.7	0.2
strained, 'Saver Size' (Heinz)	4.2 oz	70	17.0	0.0
w/yogurt, 2nd Foods' (Gerber)	3.2 oz	73	14.2	0.9
Apple-apricot, strained (Heinz)	3.5 oz	47	11.2	0.2
Apple-banana				
(Earth's Best)	4.2 oz	60	14.0	0.0
'Graduates' (Gerber)	6 oz	90	23.0	0.0
'Graduates' (Gerber)	3.2 oz	51	12.5	0.1
'2nd Foods' (Gerber)	3.2 oz	51	12.3	0.1
strained (Heinz)	3.5 oz	52	12.5	0.2
Apple-carrot				
'3rd Foods' (Gerber)	4 oz	50	12.0	0.0
'3rd Foods' (Gerber)	3.2 oz	42	10.0	0.1
Apple-cherry				
	4.2 oz	53	12.9	0.3
	1 oz	13	3.1	0.1
'Graduates' (Gerber)	6 oz	80	21.0	0.0
'Graduates' (Gerber)	3.2 oz	51	12.4	0.1
100%-juice, 'Junior' (McCain)	4.2 oz	50	13.0	0.0
'2nd Foods' (Gerber)	4 oz	60	14.0	0.0
'2nd Foods' (Gerber)	3.2 oz	48	11.5	0.1
'Stages 2' (Beech-Nut)	4 oz	60	14.0	0.0
strained (Heinz)	3.5 oz	45	10.7	0.2
Apple-cranberry				
'Stages 2' (Beech-Nut)	4 oz	60	14.0	0.0
strained (Heinz)	3.5 oz	48	11.5	0.2
Apple-grape				
	4.2 oz	60	14.8	0.3
	1 oz	14	3.5	0.1
(Earth's Best)	4.2 oz	60	14.0	0.0
'Graduates' (Gerber)	6 oz	90	22.0	0.0
'Graduates' (Gerber)	3.2 oz	51	12.4	0.1
'2nd Foods' (Gerber)	4 oz	60	15.0	0.0
'2nd Foods' (Gerber)	3.2 oz	48	11.7	0.1
'Stages 2' (Beech-Nut)	4 oz	70	16.0	0.0
strained (Heinz)	3.5 oz	47	11.3	0.2
Apple-peach				
	4.2 oz	55	13.6	0.1

Food Name	Serv. Size	Total Cal.	Carbs GMS	Fat GMS
....	1 oz	13	3.3	0.0
'2nd Foods' *(Gerber)*	3.2 oz	47	11.3	0.1
'2nd Foods' *(Gerber)*	4 oz	60	14.0	0.0
strained *(Heinz)*	3.5 oz	44	10.4	0.2
Apple-pineapple, strained *(Heinz)*	3.5 oz	47	11.1	0.2
Apple-plum				
....	4.2 oz	64	16.0	0.0
....	1 oz	15	3.8	0.0
'2nd Foods' *(Gerber)*	4 oz	60	15.0	0.0
'2nd Foods' *(Gerber)*	3.2 oz	48	11.7	0.1
Apple-prune				
....	4.2 oz	95	23.4	0.1
....	1 oz	23	5.6	0.0
'2nd Foods' *(Gerber)*	4 oz	60	16.0	0.0
'2nd Foods' *(Gerber)*	3.2 oz	53	12.8	0.1
strained *(Heinz)*	3.5 oz	50	11.9	0.2
Apple-sweet potato, '3rd Foods' *(Gerber)*	3.2 oz	48	11.4	0.1
Banana				
w/yogurt, '2nd Foods' *(Gerber)*	4 oz	110	21.0	2.0
w/yogurt, '2nd Foods' *(Gerber)*	3.2 oz	84	16.5	1.0
Grape				
'Juice Plus,' 'Stages 2' *(Beech-Nut)*	4 oz	90	22.0	0.0
red, '1st Foods' *(Gerber)*	4 oz	80	20.0	0.0
red, '1st Foods' *(Gerber)*	3.2 oz	65	15.4	0.1
white, '1st Foods' *(Gerber)*	4 oz	80	19.0	0.0
white, '1st Foods' *(Gerber)*	3.2 oz	65	15.6	0.1
white, 'Stages 1' *(Beech-Nut)*	4.2 oz	80	20.0	0.0
white, strained *(Heinz)*	3.5 oz	58	13.8	0.2
Guava, w/mixed fruit, 'Tropical Foods' *(Gerber)* ...	3.2 oz	58	13.8	0.1
Mango, w/mixed fruit 'Tropical Foods' *(Gerber)* ...	3.2 oz	59	14.2	0.1
Mango nectar, w/grape and pear juice				
'Stages 2' *(Beech-Nut)*	4 oz	80	19.0	0.0
Mixed fruit				
....	4.2 oz	61	15.1	0.1
....	1 oz	15	3.6	0.0
100% juice, 'Junior' *(McCain)*	4.2 oz	60	15.0	0.0
'2nd Foods' *(Gerber)*	4 oz	60	14.0	0.0
'2nd Foods' *(Gerber)*	3.2 oz	49	11.8	0.1
'Stages 2' *(Beech-Nut)*	4 oz	70	16.0	0.0
strained *(Heinz)*	3.5 oz	50	11.7	0.2
w/yogurt, '2nd Foods' *(Gerber)*	4 oz	100	18.0	2.0
w/yogurt, '2nd Foods' *(Gerber)*	3.2 oz	75	14.4	0.9

Food Name	Serv. Size	Total Cal.	Carbs GMS	Fat GMS
Orange				
.... 4.2 oz	4.2 oz	57	13.3	0.4
.... 1 oz	1 oz	14	3.2	0.1
'2nd Foods' (Gerber) .... 4 oz	4 oz	60	13.0	0.0
'2nd Foods' (Gerber) .... 3.2 oz	3.2 oz	46	10.3	0.3
'Stages 3' (Beech-Nut) .... 4 oz	4 oz	60	14.0	0.0
strained (Heinz) .... 3.5 oz	3.5 oz	48	10.7	0.3
Orange-apple				
.... 4.2 oz	4.2 oz	56	13.1	0.3
.... 1 oz	1 oz	13	3.1	0.1
strained (Heinz) .... 3.5 oz	3.5 oz	50	11.4	0.3
w/banana .... 4.2 oz	4.2 oz	61	14.9	0.1
w/banana .... 1 oz	1 oz	15	3.6	0.0
Orange-apricot				
.... 4.2 oz	4.2 oz	60	14.2	0.1
.... 1 oz	1 oz	14	3.4	0.0
Orange-banana				
.... 4.2 oz	4.2 oz	65	15.5	0.1
.... 1 oz	1 oz	15	3.7	0.0
Orange-carrot, '3rd Foods' (Gerber) .... 3.2 oz	3.2 oz	43	9.9	0.1
Orange-pineapple				
.... 4.2 oz	4.2 oz	62	15.2	0.1
.... 1 oz	1 oz	15	3.6	0.0
Papaya, w/mixed fruit, 'Tropical Foods' (Gerber) .... 3.2 oz	3.2 oz	57	13.5	0.2
Papaya nectar, w/pear and grape juice, 'Stages 2' (Beech-Nut) .... 4 oz	4 oz	70	17.0	0.0
Peach nectar, w/pear and grape juice, 'Stages 2' (Beech-Nut) .... 4 oz	4 oz	70	17.0	0.0
Pear				
(Earth's Best) .... 4.2 oz	4.2 oz	60	15.0	0.0
'Stages 1' (Beech-Nut) .... 4 oz	4 oz	60	15.0	0.0
strained (Heinz) .... 3.5 oz	3.5 oz	49	11.7	0.2
strained, '1st Foods' (Gerber) .... 4 oz	4 oz	60	14.0	0.0
strained, '1st Foods' (Gerber) .... 3.2 oz	3.2 oz	46	11.1	0.1
strained, 'Saver Size' (Heinz) .... 4.2 oz	4.2 oz	70	15.0	1.0
Pear-grape, strained (Heinz) .... 3.5 oz	3.5 oz	43	10.5	0.1
Pear-peach				
w/yogurt, '2nd Foods' (Gerber) .... 4 oz	4 oz	90	18.0	1.0
w/yogurt, '2nd Foods' (Gerber) .... 3.2 oz	3.2 oz	72	14.0	0.9
Pineapple-carrot				
'3rd Foods' (Gerber) .... 4 oz	4 oz	60	13.0	0.0
'3rd Foods' (Gerber) .... 3.2 oz	3.2 oz	47	11.0	0.1

Food Name	Serv. Size	Total Cal.	Carbs GMS	Fat GMS
Prune-orange				
....	4.2 oz	91	21.8	0.4
....	1 oz	22	5.2	0.1
Tropical blend, 'Stages 2' (Beech-Nut)	4 oz	70	17.0	0.0
Tropical blend nectar, 'Stages 2' (Beech-Nut)	4 oz	90	21.0	0.0
MEAT				
Beef				
junior	3.5 oz	105	0.0	4.8
junior	1 oz	30	0.0	1.4
'2nd Foods' (Gerber)	7 tbsp	100	0.1	4.7
strained	3.5 oz	106	0.0	5.3
strained	1 oz	30	0.0	1.5
'3rd Foods' (Gerber)	7 tbsp	103	0.2	4.6
w/beef heart, strained	3.5 oz	93	0.0	4.4
w/beef heart, strained	1 oz	27	0.0	1.3
w/broth, junior (Heinz)	3.5 oz	123	0.3	7.2
w/broth, 'Stages 1' (Beech-Nut)	2.5 oz	80	0.0	5.0
w/broth, strained (Heinz)	3.5 oz	123	0.3	7.2
w/egg yolks, strained (Gerber)	2.5 oz	80	0.0	4.0
Chicken				
junior	3.5 oz	148	0.0	9.5
junior	1 oz	42	0.0	2.7
'2nd Foods' (Gerber)	7 tbsp	128	0.0	7.9
'Stages 1' (Beech-Nut)	2.8 oz	80	0.0	4.0
strained	3.5 oz	129	0.1	7.8
strained	1 oz	37	0.0	2.2
'3rd Foods' (Gerber)	7 tbsp	132	0.2	7.9
w/broth, junior (Heinz)	3.5 oz	143	0.7	9.7
w/broth, 'Stages 1' (Beech-Nut)	2.5 oz	70	0.0	4.0
w/broth, strained (Heinz)	3.5 oz	143	0.7	9.7
Chicken sticks				
finger snacks, 'Graduates' (Gerber)	10 sticks	143	1.6	8.3
junior	1 stick	19	0.1	1.4
Ham				
junior	3.5 oz	124	0.0	6.6
junior	1 oz	35	0.0	1.9
junior (Gerber)	2.5 oz	90	0.0	5.0
'2nd Foods' (Gerber)	7 tbsp	120	0.2	7.1
strained	3.5 oz	110	0.0	5.7
strained	1 oz	31	0.0	1.6
'3rd Foods' (Gerber)	7 tbsp	123	0.1	7.2
w/egg yolks, strained (Gerber)	2.5 oz	90	1.0	5.0

Food Name	Serv. Size	Total Cal.	Carbs GMS	Fat GMS
Lamb				
junior	3.5 oz	111	0.0	5.2
junior	1 oz	32	0.0	1.5
'2nd Foods' (Gerber)	7 tbsp	104	0.0	4.8
'Stages 1' (Beech-Nut)	2.8 oz	70	0.0	3.0
strained	3.5 oz	102	0.1	4.7
strained	1 oz	29	0.0	1.3
w/broth, 'Stages 1' (Beech-Nut)	2.5 oz	60	0.0	3.0
w/broth, strained (Heinz)	3.5 oz	129	0.2	7.6
w/egg yolks, strained (Gerber)	2.5 oz	70	1.0	3.0
Liver				
strained	3.5 oz	100	1.4	3.8
strained	1 oz	29	0.4	1.1
w/liver broth, strained (Heinz)	3.5 oz	100	3.6	3.2
Meat sticks				
finger snacks, 'Graduates' (Gerber)	10 sticks	150	1.5	9.6
junior	1 stick	18	0.1	1.5
Pork				
strained	3.5 oz	123	0.0	7.0
strained	1 oz	35	0.0	2.0
Turkey				
junior	3.5 oz	128	0.0	7.0
junior	1 oz	37	0.0	2.0
'2nd Foods' (Gerber)	7 tbsp	109	0.2	5.9
'Stages 1' (Beech-Nut)	2.8 oz	100	0.0	6.0
strained	3.5 oz	113	0.1	5.7
strained	1 oz	32	0.0	1.6
'3rd Foods' (Gerber)	7 tbsp	115	0.1	6.1
w/broth, 'Stages 1' (Beech-Nut)	2.5 oz	90	0.0	6.0
w/broth, strained (Heinz)	3.5 oz	137	0.4	8.6
w/egg yolks, strained (Gerber)	2.5 oz	100	1.0	6.0
Turkey sticks				
finger snacks, 'Graduates' (Gerber)	10 sticks	141	1.5	8.5
junior	1 stick	18	0.1	1.4
Veal				
junior	3.5 oz	109	0.0	4.9
junior	1 oz	31	0.0	1.4
junior (Gerber)	2.5 oz	80	0.0	4.0
'2nd Foods' (Gerber)	7 tbsp	102	0.1	5.1
'Stages 1' (Beech-Nut)	2.8 oz	60	0.0	2.0
strained	3.5 oz	100	0.0	4.8
strained	1 oz	29	0.0	1.4
'3rd Foods' (Gerber)	7 tbsp	108	0.0	5.0

Food Name	Serv. Size	Total Cal.	Carbs GMS	Fat GMS
w/broth, 'Stages 1' *(Beech-Nut)*	2.5 oz	70	0.0	3.0
w/broth, strained *(Heinz)*	3.5 oz	130	0.2	7.9
w/egg yolks, strained *(Gerber)*	2.5 oz	80	1.0	4.0
Veal and beef				
junior *(Gerber)*	6 oz	110	16.0	3.0
strained *(Gerber)*	4.5 oz	90	11.0	4.0
Veal and ham				
junior *(Gerber)*	6 oz	120	17.0	4.0
strained *(Gerber)*	4.5 oz	80	11.0	3.0
Veal and turkey				
junior *(Gerber)*	6 oz	100	15.0	3.0
strained *(Gerber)*	4.5 oz	70	10.0	2.0
SOUP				
Chicken				
hearty, w/stars, 'Stages Table Time' *(Beech-Nut)*	6 oz	180	20.0	9.0
strained	4.5 oz	64	9.2	2.2
strained	1 oz	14	2.0	0.5
strained *(Heinz)*	3.5 oz	49	7.2	1.7
Cream of broccoli, '3rd Foods' *(Gerber)*	3.2 oz	26	2.7	1.1
Cream of chicken				
strained	4.5 oz	74	10.8	2.0
strained	1 oz	16	2.4	0.5
Cream of potato, '3rd Foods' *(Gerber)*	3.2 oz	33	5.2	0.8
Cream of tomato, '3rd Foods' *(Gerber)*	3.2 oz	41	7.3	0.7
Cream of vegetable, '3rd Foods' *(Gerber)*	3.2 oz	29	4.4	0.8
VEGETABLES				
Beet				
'2nd Foods' *(Gerber)*	7 tbsp	39	8.1	0.2
strained	4.5 oz	44	9.9	0.1
strained	1 oz	10	2.2	0.0
strained *(Gerber)*	4.5 oz	60	11.0	1.0
strained *(Heinz)*	3.5 oz	40	8.3	0.2
Broccoli, carrot, and cheese, '3rd Foods' *(Gerber)*	7 tbsp	44	7.2	1.0
Carrot				
(Earth's Best)	4.5 oz	40	7.0	1.0
'Beginner Foods' *(Heinz)*	3.5 oz	30	6.1	0.3
buttered, junior	7.5 oz	70	14.3	1.3
buttered, junior	1 oz	9	1.9	0.2
buttered, strained	4.5 oz	46	9.5	0.8
buttered, strained	1 oz	10	2.1	0.2
diced, 'Graduates' *(Gerber)*	3.2 oz	22	4.7	0.1
'1st Foods' *(Gerber)*	2.5 oz	25	5.0	0.0
'1st Foods' *(Gerber)*	7 tbsp	34	6.9	0.3

Food Name	Serv. Size	Total Cal.	Carbs GMS	Fat GMS
junior	7.5 oz	68	15.3	0.4
junior	1 oz	9	2.0	0.1
junior *(Gerber)*	6 oz	80	16.0	1.0
junior *(Heinz)*	3.5 oz	23	4.9	0.2
'Regal Imperial,' 'Baby's First' *(Beech-Nut)*	2.5 oz	25	6.0	0.0
'Regal Imperial,' 'Stages 1' *(Beech-Nut)*	4.5 oz	40	9.0	0.0
'Regal Imperial,' 'Stages 1' *(Beech-Nut)*	2.8 oz	30	7.0	0.0
'2nd Foods' *(Gerber)*	7 tbsp	30	6.1	0.2
'Stages 3' *(Beech-Nut)*	6 oz	60	13.0	0.0
strained	4.5 oz	35	7.7	0.1
strained	1 oz	8	1.7	0.0
strained *(Gerber)*	4.5 oz	35	8.0	0.0
strained *(Heinz)*	3.5 oz	23	4.9	0.2
'3rd Foods' *(Gerber)*	7 tbsp	29	6.0	0.2
Carrot and parsnip *(Earth's Best)*	4.5 oz	60	14.0	0.0
Corn, creamed				
junior	7.5 oz	138	34.7	0.9
junior	1 oz	18	4.6	0.1
junior *(Heinz)*	3.5 oz	65	14.1	0.5
'2nd Foods' *(Gerber)*	7 tbsp	62	12.7	0.5
'Stages 2' *(Beech-Nut)*	4.5 oz	100	20.0	1.0
strained	4.5 oz	73	18.0	0.5
strained	1 oz	16	4.0	0.1
strained *(Gerber)*	4.5 oz	80	16.0	1.0
strained *(Heinz)*	3.5 oz	63	14.0	0.4
Garden vegetable				
(Earth's Best)	4.5 oz	70	15.0	0.0
'2nd Foods' *(Gerber)*	7 tbsp	39	6.4	0.4
'Stages 2' *(Beech-Nut)*	4.5 oz	60	11.0	0.0
strained	4.5 oz	47	8.7	0.3
strained	1 oz	10	1.9	0.1
strained *(Gerber)*	4.5 oz	50	8.0	1.0
Green bean				
'Beginner Foods' *(Heinz)*	3.5 oz	30	5.9	0.3
buttered, junior	7.25 oz	66	12.6	1.9
buttered, junior	1 oz	9	1.7	0.3
buttered, strained	4.5 oz	42	8.4	1.0
buttered, strained	1 oz	9	1.9	0.2
creamed, junior	7.5 oz	68	15.3	0.9
creamed, junior	1 oz	9	2.0	0.1
creamed, junior *(Gerber)*	6 oz	80	16.0	1.0
creamed, junior *(Heinz)*	3.5 oz	41	6.6	1.0
creamed, '3rd Foods' *(Gerber)*	7 tbsp	45	9.1	0.2

Food Name	Serv. Size	Total Cal.	Carbs GMS	Fat GMS
diced, 'Graduates' (Gerber)	3.2 oz	21	4.2	0.1
'1st Foods' (Gerber)	2.5 oz	25	5.0	0.0
'1st Foods' (Gerber)	7 tbsp	32	6.2	0.2
junior	7.25 oz	52	11.7	0.2
junior	1 oz	7	1.6	0.0
'2nd Foods' (Gerber)	7 tbsp	30	5.8	0.2
'Stages 3' (Beech-Nut)	6 oz	45	10.0	0.0
'Stages 1' (Beech-Nut)	4.5 oz	35	8.0	0.0
strained	4.5 oz	32	7.6	0.1
strained	1 oz	7	1.7	0.0
strained (Heinz)	3.5 oz	25	4.9	0.2
Mixed				
junior	7.5 oz	87	17.5	0.9
junior	1 oz	12	2.3	0.1
junior (Gerber)	6 oz	70	14.0	1.0
'2nd Foods' (Gerber)	7 tbsp	42	8.4	0.4
'Stages 2' (Beech-Nut)	4.5 oz	50	12.0	0.0
strained	4.5 oz	52	10.2	0.6
strained	1 oz	12	2.3	0.1
strained (Gerber)	4.5 oz	60	11.0	1.0
strained (Heinz)	3.5 oz	44	8.8	0.4
'3rd Foods' (Gerber)	7 tbsp	39	8.0	0.2
Peas				
'Beginner Foods' (Heinz)	3.5 oz	55	9.5	0.5
buttered, junior	7.25 oz	124	23.3	2.7
buttered, junior	1 oz	17	3.2	0.4
buttered, strained	4.5 oz	72	13.6	1.4
buttered, strained	1 oz	16	3.0	0.3
buttered, tender, sweet, 'Stages 1' (Beech-Nut)	4.5 oz	60	10.0	0.0
buttered, tender, sweet, 'Stages 1' (Beech-Nut)	2.8 oz	40	6.0	0.0
creamed, strained	4.5 oz	68	11.4	2.4
creamed, strained	1 oz	15	2.5	0.5
creamed, strained (Heinz)	3.5 oz	52	7.6	1.5
diced, 'Graduates' (Gerber)	3.2 oz	44	8.4	0.1
'1st Foods' (Gerber)	2.5 oz	30	6.0	0.0
'1st Foods' (Gerber)	7 tbsp	47	7.7	0.4
junior (Gerber)	6 oz	90	16.0	1.0
'2nd Foods' (Gerber)	7 tbsp	47	7.7	0.5
strained	4.5 oz	51	10.4	0.4
strained	1 oz	11	2.3	0.1
strained (Gerber)	4.5 oz	60	10.0	1.0
tender, sweet, 'Baby's First' (Beech-Nut)	2.5 oz	40	7.0	0.0
'3rd Foods' (Gerber)	7 tbsp	47	7.8	0.4

Food Name	Serv. Size	Total Cal.	Carbs GMS	Fat GMS
Peas and brown rice *(Earth's Best)*	4.5 oz	80	16.0	0.0
Peas and carrots, 'Stages 2' *(Beech-Nut)*	4.5 oz	60	11.0	0.0
Potato, diced, 'Graduates' *(Gerber)*	3.2 oz	38	8.5	0.1
Spinach, creamed				
junior	7.5 oz	89	13.6	3.0
junior	1 oz	12	1.8	0.4
'2nd Foods' *(Gerber)*	7 tbsp	47	7.3	0.6
strained	4.5 oz	47	7.3	1.7
strained	1 oz	10	1.6	0.4
strained *(Gerber)*	4.5 oz	60	9.0	1.0
Spinach and potato *(Earth's Best)*	4.5 oz	60	8.0	2.0
Squash				
'Beginner Foods' *(Heinz)*	3.5 oz	36	7.3	0.2
buttered, junior	7.5 oz	64	13.6	1.3
buttered, junior	1 oz	9	1.8	0.2
buttered, strained	4.5 oz	37	8.8	0.4
buttered, strained	1 oz	8	2.0	0.1
butternut, 'Baby's First' *(Beech-Nut)*	2.5 oz	30	7.0	0.2
butternut, 'Stages 1' *(Beech-Nut)*	4.5 oz	50	11.0	0.0
butternut, 'Stages 1' *(Beech-Nut)*	2.8 oz	30	7.0	0.0
'1st Foods' *(Gerber)*	2.5 oz	25	5.0	0.0
'1st Foods' *(Gerber)*	7 tbsp	33	7.0	0.3
junior	7.5 oz	51	11.9	0.4
junior	1 oz	7	1.6	0.1
junior *(Gerber)*	6 oz	60	11.0	1.0
'2nd Foods' *(Gerber)*	7 tbsp	32	6.8	0.2
strained	4.5 oz	31	7.2	0.3
strained	1 oz	7	1.6	0.1
strained *(Gerber)*	4.5 oz	35	8.0	0.0
strained *(Heinz)*	3.5 oz	32	6.6	0.3
'3rd Foods' *(Gerber)*	7 tbsp	33	6.8	0.2
winter *(Earth's Best)*	4.5 oz	50	12.0	0.0
Sweet potato				
(Earth's Best)	4.5 oz	60	12.0	1.0
'Baby's First' *(Beech-Nut)*	2.5 oz	50	11.0	0.0
'Beginner Foods' *(Heinz)*	3.5 oz	69	15.7	0.2
buttered, junior	7.75 oz	125	26.8	1.5
buttered, junior	1 oz	16	3.5	0.2
buttered, strained	4.75 oz	76	15.9	0.9
buttered, strained	1 oz	16	3.3	0.2
'1st Foods' *(Gerber)*	2.5 oz	45	10.0	0.0
'1st Foods' *(Gerber)*	7 tbsp	67	15.0	0.2
junior	7.75 oz	132	30.6	0.2

Food Name	Serv. Size	Total Cal.	Carbs GMS	Fat GMS
junior	1 oz	17	3.9	0.0
junior *(Gerber)*	6 oz	110	24.0	1.0
junior *(Heinz)*	3.5 oz	69	15.6	0.3
'2nd Foods' *(Gerber)*	7 tbsp	62	14.1	0.2
'Stages 1' *(Beech-Nut)*	2.8 oz	60	14.0	0.0
'Stages 1' *(Beech-Nut)*	4.5 oz	90	20.0	0.0
'Stages 3' *(Beech-Nut)*	6 oz	110	26.0	0.0
strained	4.75 oz	77	17.8	0.1
strained	1 oz	16	3.7	0.0
strained *(Gerber)*	4.5 oz	80	18.0	1.0
strained *(Heinz)*	3.5 oz	69	15.6	0.3
'3rd Foods' *(Gerber)*	7 tbsp	63	14.2	0.2
WATER, w/fluoride, sodium-free *(Beech-Nut)*	4 oz	0	0.0	0.0
BACON				
cooked, yield from 1 lb raw	4.5 oz	732	0.8	62.5
cured, approx 20 slices per lb, cooked	3 slices	109	0.1	9.4
cured, breakfast strips, cooked	3 slices	156	0.4	12.5
cured, broiled	4.5 oz	732	0.8	62.5
cured, broiled	3 med slices	109	0.1	9.4
cured, canned	100 gm	685	1.0	71.5
cured, pan-fried	4.5 oz	732	0.8	62.5
cured, pan-fried	3 med slices	109	0.1	9.4
cured, roasted	4.5 oz	732	0.8	62.5
cured, roasted	3 med slices	109	0.1	9.4
cured, strips, cooked	6 oz	780	1.8	62.4
cured, 12 slices per lb, raw	1 slice	211	0.0	21.9
cured, strips, 15 slices per 12 oz, raw	3 slices	264	0.5	25.3
raw	1 oz	158	<.1	16.3
(Hormel)				
'Black Label' cooked	1 oz	142	2.0	14.0
'Black Label' low-salt, cooked	1.76 oz	250	2.0	25.0
'Black Label' sliced, cooked	2 slices	60	0.0	5.0
'Range' thick sliced, cooked	1 oz	152	2.0	16.0
(JM)				
cooked	2 slices	100	1.0	9.0
'Lower Sodium' cooked	2 slices	100	1.0	9.0
'Lower Sodium' raw	2 slices	290	1.0	30.0
raw	2 slices	280	1.0	29.0
(Jones Dairy Farm), raw	1 slice	165	tr	17.0
(Kahn's), 'American Beauty,' cooked	2 slices	100	na	9.0
(Oscar Mayer)				
'Center Cut' cooked, approx .2-oz slices	1 slice	25	0.1	1.8
'Center Cut' cooked, yield from 1 lb raw	6 oz	852	3.5	62.5

Food Name	Serv. Size	Total Cal.	Carbs GMS	Fat GMS
cooked, approx .2-oz slices	1 slice	33	0.1	2.8
cooked, yield from 16-oz pkg raw	5 oz	784	3.0	64.9
'Lower Salt' cooked, approx .2-oz slices	1 slice	33	0.1	2.6
'Lower Salt,' cooked, yield from 1 lb raw	5.6 oz	870	2.3	70.3
thick-sliced, cooked, approx .4-oz slices	1 slice	58	0.1	4.8
thick-sliced, cooked, yield from 1 lb raw	5 oz	811	1.1	67.1
(Range Brand) 'Sliced,' cooked	2 slices	110	0.0	9.0
(Red Label) cooked	3 slices	110	0.0	10.0
BACON, ALTERNATIVE				
BEEF				
heated (JM)	2 slices	100	1.0	7.0
heated (Sizzlean)	2 strips	70	0.0	5.0
heated, yield from 12-oz pkg	6 oz	764	2.4	58.5
raw	1 oz	115	0.2	11.0
raw (JM)	2 slices	200	1.0	18.0
unheated	1 oz	115	0.2	11.0
PORK				
80%-fat-free (Louis Rich)	1 slice	35	<1.0	2.0
heated (Sizzlean)	2 strips	90	0.0	8.0
heated, brown-sugar-cured (Sizzlean)	2 strips	110	2.0	9.0
heated, yield from 12-oz pkg	6 oz	780	1.8	62.4
raw	1 oz	110	0.2	10.5
TURKEY, heated (Louis Rich)	1 slice	32	0.3	2.4
VEGETARIAN				
	1 cup	446	9.1	42.5
	1 oz	88	1.8	8.4
(Morningstar Farms) 'Breakfast Strips' frozen	3 strips	80	4.0	6.0
(White Wave SoyFood) 'Healthy'	1 oz	27	4.0	1.0
(Worthington) 'Stripples' frozen	4 strips	120	6.0	9.0
Canadian style				
(Heartline)	2 oz	176	9.0	7.0
(Heartline) 'Canadian Bacon Style' lite	.5 oz	22	1.0	0.0
BACON, CANADIAN-STYLE				
cured, grilled	2 slices	86	0.6	3.9
cured, grilled, yield from 6 oz raw	4.9 oz	257	1.9	11.7
cured, packed 6 slices per 6 oz, unheated	2 slices	89	1.0	4.0
cured, unheated	6 oz	267	2.9	11.9
unheated	1 oz	45	0.5	2.0
(Hormel) 'Sliced'	1 oz	45	0.0	2.0
(Jones Dairy Farm) unheated	1 slice	25	tr	1.0
(Light & Lean)	2 slices	35	0.0	1.0
(Oscar Mayer)	.8 oz	28	0.1	1.0

Food Name	Serv. Size	Total Cal.	Carbs GMS	Fat GMS
BACON BITS				
(Hormel)	1 oz	117	1.0	7.0
(Hormel)	1 tbsp	30	0.0	2.0
(Libby's) 'Bacon Crumbles'	1 tbsp	25	2.0	1.0
(Oscar Mayer)	3 oz	248	2.5	12.4
(Oscar Mayer)	1 tbsp	20	0.2	1.0
BACON BITS, ALTERNATIVE				
(Bac•Os)	2 tsp	25	2.0	1.0
(McCormick) 'Bac'N Pieces' no cholesterol	1 1/2 tbsp	30	2.0	1.0
(Schilling) 'Bac'N Pieces'	1 tsp	26	2.0	0.4
BACON PIECES (Hormel)	1 oz	94	2.0	5.0
BAGEL				
BLUEBERRY				
(Earth Grains) 3 oz	1 bagel	245	48.0	0.0
(Western Bagel)	1 bagel	240	43.0	4.0
CINNAMON-RAISIN				
(Dunkin' Donuts)	1 bagel	250	49.0	2.0
(Earth Grains) 3 oz	1 bagel	245	48.0	0.0
(Thomas') 'Deli Style'	1 bagel	170	33.0	2.0
(Western Bagel)	1 bagel	230	40.0	4.0
EGG				
	1 oz	79	15.0	0.6
(Dunkin' Donuts)	1 bagel	250	47.0	2.0
(Lender's) 'Bagel Shop'	1 bagel	230	41.0	2.5
(Lender's) 'Bakery Style'	1 bagel	210	41.0	2.0
HONEY WHEAT (Earth Grains) 3 oz	1 bagel	240	45.0	0.0
ONION				
enriched, 3.5-inch diam	1 bagel	195	37.9	1.1
enriched, w/calcium proprianate, 3.5-inch diam	1 bagel	195	37.9	1.1
enriched, w/calcium proprianate, toasted	1 oz	84	16.3	0.5
unenriched, 3.5-inch diam	1 bagel	195	37.9	1.1
unenriched, w/calcium proprianate, 3.5-inch diam	1 bagel	195	37.9	1.1
(Dunkin' Donuts)	1 bagel	230	46.0	1.0
(Earth Grains) 3 oz	1 bagel	240	45.0	0.0
(Lender's) 'Bagel Shop'	1 bagel	220	40.0	2.0
(Western Bagel)	1 bagel	220	39.0	4.0
PLAIN				
enriched, 3.5-inch diam	1 bagel	195	37.9	1.1
enriched, w/calcium proprianate, 3.5-inch diam	1 bagel	195	37.9	1.1
unenriched, 3.5-inch diam	1 bagel	195	37.9	1.1
unenriched, w/calcium proprianate, 3.5-inch diam	1 bagel	195	37.9	1.1
(Dunkin' Donuts)	1 bagel	240	47.0	1.0
(Earth Grains) 3 oz	1 bagel	240	45.0	0.0

Food Name	Serv. Size	Total Cal.	Carbs GMS	Fat GMS
(Lender's) 'Bagel Shop'	1 bagel	210	40.0	1.5
(Lender's) 'Bakery Style'	1 bagel	210	42.0	2.0
POPPY SEED				
enriched, 3.5 inch diam	1 bagel	195	37.9	1.1
enriched, w/calcium proprianate, 3.5-inch diam	1 bagel	195	37.9	1.1
enriched, w/calcium proprianate, toasted	1 oz	84	16.3	0.5
unenriched, 3.5-inch diam	1 bagel	195	37.9	1.1
unenriched, w/calcium proprianate, 3.5-inch diam	1 bagel	195	37.9	1.1
RAISIN				
(Lender's) 'Bagel Shop'	1 bagel	240	44.0	3.0
(Lender's) 'Bakery Style'	1 bagel	220	44.0	2.0
RAISIN-HONEY CINNAMON *(Finast)* 2.5 oz	1 bagel	200	40.0	1.0
SESAME				
enriched, 3.5-inch diam	1 bagel	195	37.9	1.1
enriched, w/calcium proprianate, 3.5-inch diam	1 bagel	195	37.9	1.1
enriched, w/calcium proprianate, toasted	1 oz	84	16.3	0.5
unenriched, 3.5-inch diam	1 bagel	195	37.9	1.1
unenriched, w/calcium proprianate, 3.5-inch diam	1 bagel	195	37.9	1.1
WATER *(Western Bagel)*	1 bagel	230	41.0	4.0
BAGEL, FROZEN				
BLUEBERRY *(Lender's)* 2.5 oz	1 bagel	190	38.0	1.0
CINNAMON-RAISIN				
(Lender's) 'Big'n Crusty' 3 1/8 oz	1 bagel	250	49.0	2.0
(Sara Lee) 3.1 oz	1 bagel	240	48.0	2.0
(Sara Lee) 2.5 oz	1 bagel	200	39.0	2.0
EGG				
(Lender's) 2 oz	1 bagel	150	29.0	1.0
(Lender's) 'Big'n Crusty' 3 1/8 oz	1 bagel	250	47.0	2.0
(Sara Lee) 3.1 oz	1 bagel	250	48.0	2.0
(Sara Lee) 2.5 oz	1 bagel	200	38.0	2.0
GARLIC				
(Lender's) 2 oz	1 bagel	160	32.0	1.0
(Lender's) 'Big'n Crusty' 3 1/8 oz	1 bagel	250	50.0	1.0
OAT BRAN				
(Lender's) 2.5 oz	1 bagel	170	36.0	2.0
(Sara Lee) 3 oz	1 bagel	220	47.0	1.0
(Sara Lee) 2.5 oz	1 bagel	180	38.0	1.0
ONION				
(Lender's) 2 oz	1 bagel	160	31.0	1.0
(Lender's) 'Bagelettes' .9 oz	1 bagel	70	14.0	<1.0
(Lender's) 'Big'n Crusty' 3 1/8 oz	1 bagel	230	46.0	1.0
(Sara Lee) 3.1 oz	1 bagel	230	45.0	1.0
(Sara Lee) 2.5 oz	1 bagel	190	37.0	1.0

Food Name	Serv. Size	Total Cal.	Carbs GMS	Fat GMS
PLAIN				
(Lender's) 2 oz	1 bagel	150	30.0	1.0
(Lender's) 'Bagelettes' .9 oz	1 bagel	70	13.0	<1.0
(Lender's) 'Big'n Crusty'	1 bagel	240	47.0	1.0
(Lender's) soft, 2.5 oz	1 bagel	210	36.0	3.0
(Sara Lee) 3.1 oz	1 bagel	230	46.0	1.0
(Sara Lee) 2.5 oz	1 bagel	190	38.0	1.0
POPPY SEED				
(Lender's) 2 oz	1 bagel	160	29.0	1.0
(Sara Lee) 3.1 oz	1 bagel	230	46.0	1.0
(Sara Lee) 2.5 oz	1 bagel	190	37.0	1.0
PUMPERNICKEL (Lender's) 2 oz	1 bagel	160	31.0	1.0
RAISIN (Lender's) 'Bagelettes' .9 oz	1 bagel	70	14.0	<1.0
RAISIN-HONEY (Lender's) 2.5 oz	1 bagel	200	40.0	1.0
RYE (Lender's) 2 oz	1 bagel	150	30.0	1.0
SESAME				
(Lender's) 2 oz	1 bagel	160	31.0	1.0
(Sara Lee) 3.1 oz	1 bagel	240	46.0	2.0
(Sara Lee) 2.5 oz	1 bagel	190	37.0	1.0
WHEAT-RAISIN (Lender's) 2.5 oz	1 bagel	190	39.0	1.0
BAGEL CHIP				
(Burns & Ricker) cinnamon raisin 'Original Bagel Crisps'	1 oz	130	20.0	4.0
(Burns & Ricker) garlic 'Original Bagel Crisps'	1 oz	130	20.0	4.0
BAKED BEANS, CANNED. See also BEANS, CANNED.				
(Allens)	1/2 cup	170	21.0	6.0
(Grandma Brown's)	1 cup	301	53.9	3.0
(Green Giant)	1/2 cup	150	28.0	2.0
(Open Range)	4.656 oz	152	30.5	2.3
(Van Camp's)	1 cup	260	52.0	2.0
bacon and brown sugar, 'Premium' (Van Camp's)	6 oz	170	36.0	2.0
barbecue (B&M)	8 oz	260	48.0	6.0
barbecue (Campbell's)	7 7/8 oz	210	43.0	4.0
Boston (Health Valley)	4 oz	213	43.0	1.0
Boston, 'No Salt Added' (Health Valley)	4 oz	213	43.0	1.0
Boston, w/ham 'Homestyle' (Hunt's)	9.03 oz	248	41.8	1.9
'Brick Oven' (S&W)	1/2 cup	160	28.0	2.0
brown sugar (Van Camp's)	1 cup	290	51.0	5.1
'Deluxe' (Van Camp's)	1 cup	320	57.0	4.0
'Dry Beans in Sauce' (Green Giant)	1/2 cup	130	30.0	1.0
'Dry Beans in Sauce' (Joan of Arc)	1/2 cup	130	30.0	1.0
'Home Style' (Campbell's)	8 oz	220	48.0	4.0
honey (B&M)	8 oz	240	50.0	2.0
hot 'n spicy (B&M)	8 oz	240	50.0	3.0

Food Name	Serv. Size	Total Cal.	Carbs GMS	Fat GMS
in homestyle sauce *(Bush's Best)*	4 oz	110	25.0	1.0
in molasses, brown sugar, 'Old Fashioned' *(Campbell's)*	8 oz	230	49.0	3.0
in tomato sauce *(B&M)*	8 oz	230	48.0	3.0
in tomato sauce *(Campbell's)*	8 oz	200	43.0	3.0
in tomato sauce *(Pathmark)*	1/2 cup	150	23.0	2.0
in tomato sauce, 40-oz can *(Finast)*	1/2 cup	120	21.0	1.0
in tomato sauce, 'No Frills' *(Pathmark)*	1/2 cup	160	28.0	2.0
in tomato sauce, 16-oz can *(Finast)*	1 cup	270	50.0	3.0
maple *(B&M)*	8 oz	240	52.0	2.0
maple *(Friends)*	8 oz	240	52.0	2.0
no salt added, fat-free *(Health Valley)*	7.5 oz	190	41.0	0.0
pea beans *(B&M)*	8 oz	270	50.0	6.0
pea, small *(Friends)*	8 oz	360	62.0	4.0
pea, small, w/pork *(Friends)*	8 oz	260	53.0	5.0
pork and beans, 'Deluxe' *(Bush's Best)*	4 oz	110	25.0	1.0
pork and beans, 'Showboat' *(Bush's Best)*	4 oz	80	19.0	<1.0
regular, fat-free *(Health Valley)*	7.5 oz	190	41.0	0.0
'Saucepan' *(Grandma Brown's)*	1 cup	307	52.3	4.8
vegetarian	1/2 cup	118	26.0	0.6
vegetarian *(A&P)*	1/2 cup	130	25.0	<1.0
vegetarian *(Allens)*	1/2 cup	110	19.0	1.0
vegetarian *(B&M)*	8 oz	230	50.0	3.0
vegetarian *(Campbell's)*	7.75 oz	170	40.0	1.0
vegetarian 'Vegetarian Style' *(Van Camp's)*	1 cup	206	42.0	0.6
vegetarian, w/miso 'Vegetarian' *(Health Valley)*	4 oz	90	19.0	1.0
w/beef	1/2 cup	161	22.5	4.6
w/franks	1/2 cup	182	19.7	8.4
w/franks, 'Beanee Weenee' *(Van Camp's)*	1 cup	326	31.7	15.4
w/onions, approx 1/2 cup *(Bush's Best)*	4 oz	110	27.0	1.0
w/pork	1/2 cup	134	25.2	2.0
w/pork *(A&P)*	1/2 cup	150	25.0	2.0
w/pork *(Hunt's)*	4 oz	140	26.0	1.0
w/pork *(S&W)*	1/2 cup	130	22.0	2.0
w/pork *(Van Camp's)*	1 cup	216	41.0	1.9
w/pork 'Extra Fancy' *(Allens)*	1/2 cup	125	24.0	1.0
w/pork, 'Extra Standard' *(Allens)*	1/2 cup	90	15.0	1.0
w/pork,'Fancy' *(Allens)*	1/2 cup	110	18.0	1.0
w/pork, 'Micro-Cup' *(Hormel)*	7.5 oz	254	41.0	5.0
w/pork and sweet sauce	1/2 cup	140	26.5	1.8
w/pork and tomato sauce	1/2 cup	123	24.4	1.3
w/pork and tomato sauce *(Green Giant)*	1/2 cup	90	21.0	1.0
w/pork and tomato sauce *(Joan of Arc)*	1/2 cup	90	21.0	1.0

Food Name	Serv. Size	Total Cal.	Carbs GMS	Fat GMS
BAKING POWDER				
....	1 tbsp	11	2.6	0.0
....	1 tsp	3	0.7	0.0
commercial	3 1/2 oz	109	26.5	0.0
commercial *(Calumet)*	1/4 tsp	0	0.0	0.0
cream of tartar, w/tartaric acid	1 tbsp	7	1.8	0.0
double-acting, sodium aluminum sulfate ...	1 tsp	2	1.3	0.0
double-acting, straight phosphate	1 tsp	2	1.1	0.0
'Low Salt' *(Featherweight)*	1 tsp	8	2.0	0.0
low-sodium	1 tsp	5	2.3	0.0
low-sodium, commercial	1 tbsp	23	5.6	0.0
low-sodium, commercial	1 tsp	7	1.8	0.0
low-sodium, non-commercial	1 tsp	2	0.6	0.0
w/monohydrate	1 tbsp	14	3.4	0.0
w/monohydrate	1 tsp	4	0.9	0.0
w/straight phosphate	1 tbsp	15	3.7	0.0
w/straight phosphate	1 tsp	5	1.1	0.0
BAKING SODA				
....	1 tsp	0	0.0	0.0
(Arm & Hammer)	1/2 tsp	0	0.0	0.0
BALSAM PEAR/bitter melon				
Leafy tips				
boiled, drained	4 oz	40	7.7	0.2
boiled, drained	1/2 cup	10	2.0	0.1
raw	1/2 cup	7	0.8	0.2
raw, trimmed	1 oz	9	0.9	0.2
raw, untrimmed	1 lb	52	5.7	1.2
Pods				
boiled, drained	4 oz	22	4.9	0.2
boiled, drained, 1/2-inch pieces	1/2 cup	12	2.7	0.1
raw	1 pear	21	4.6	0.2
raw, approx 9 3/8 inch x 1 1/2 inch, 5.3 oz each	1 pod	21	4.6	0.2
raw, 1/2-inch pieces	1 cup	16	3.4	0.2
raw, trimmed	1 oz	5	1.1	0.1
raw, untrimmed	1 lb	64	13.9	0.6
BAMBOO SHOOTS				
boiled, drained	4 oz	14	2.2	0.2
boiled, drained, 1/2-inch slices	1 cup	14	2.3	0.3
canned *(LaChoy)*	1.5 oz	8	1.4	0.2
canned *(LaChoy)*	2 tbsp	3	0.7	0.1
canned, drained solids, 1/8-inch slices ...	1 cup	25	4.2	0.5
raw, 1/2-inch slices	1 cup	41	7.8	0.5
raw, trimmed	1 oz	8	1.5	0.1

Food Name	Serv. Size	Total Cal.	Carbs GMS	Fat GMS
raw, w/sheath	1 lb	36	6.8	0.4
BANANA				
fresh *(Dole)*	1 fruit	120	28.0	1.0
mashed	1/2 cup	104	26.4	0.5
peeled	1 oz	26	6.6	<0.1
powdered	1 oz	98	25.0	0.5
powdered	1/4 cup	87	22.1	0.5
powdered	1 tbsp	21	5.5	0.1
raw, w/o skin and seeds	1 fruit	105	26.7	0.6
unpeeled	1 lb	271	69.1	1.4
BANANA, COOKING. See PLANTAIN.				
BANANA, DEHYDRATED				
	1 oz	98	25.0	0.5
	1/4 cup	87	22.1	0.5
BANANA, RED				
raw	100 gm	90	23.4	0.2
raw, approx 7.25 inch x 1.5 inch	1 med	118	30.7	0.3
raw, sliced	1/2 cup	68	17.6	0.2
BANANA BERRY DRINK				
'Stompin' Banana Berry Drink' *(Hi-C)*	6 oz	90	22.0	0.0
BANANA BREAD. See BREAD, QUICK.				
BANANA CHIPS				
	1 oz	147	16.6	9.5
freeze-dried *(Mountain House)*	1/2 cup	248	15.0	8.0
premium *(Mariani)*	1 oz	150	17.0	<9.0
BANANA NECTAR *(Libby's)*	6 oz	110	26.0	0.0
BANANA PEPPER. See PEPPER, BANANA.				
BANANA PINEAPPLE NECTAR *(Kern's)*	6 oz	110	27.0	0.0
BANANA SQUASH. See SQUASH, BANANA.				
BANNER BEAN SEED, whole, dried	1 oz	95	17.4	0.3
BARBADOS CHERRY. See ACEROLA CHERRY.				
BARBADOS CHERRY JUICE. See ACEROLA CHERRY JUICE.				
BARBECUE SAUCE				
(Bull's Eye)	.5 oz	22	5.0	0.0
(Cattleman's) mild	1 tbsp	25	5.0	0.0
(Enrico's) 'Original'	1 tbsp	18	3.0	1.0
(Healthy Choice) original	1.1 oz	25	5.7	0.2
(Heinz) 'Old Fashioned'	1 tbsp	18	4.1	0.1
(Heinz) 'Select'	1 oz	40	9.0	0.0
(Heinz) 'Thick and Rich' old fashioned	1 oz	35	8.0	0.0
(Heinz) 'Thick and Rich' original	1 oz	35	8.0	0.0
(Hunt's) 'Bold' original	1.2 oz	46	10.8	0.3
(Hunt's) 'Light' original	1.1 oz	26	6.1	0.1

Food Name	Serv. Size	Total Cal.	Carbs GMS	Fat GMS
(Hunt's) original	1.2 oz	40	9.4	0.3
(Kraft)	2 tbsp	45	10.0	1.0
(Kraft) 'Thick 'n Spicy' original	2 tbsp	50	12.0	1.0
(Open Range) original	1.2 oz	38	9.0	0.2
(Ott's)	1 tbsp	14	3.2	0.1
(Skipper's)	1 tbsp	25	5.0	1.0
CAJUN STYLE				
(Golden Dipt)	1 oz	90	5.0	8.0
(Heinz)	1 tbsp	15	3.4	0.1
(Heinz) 'Thick and Rich'	1 oz	35	8.0	0.0
CHUNKY				
(Heinz) 'Thick and Rich'	1 oz	30	6.0	0.0
(Kraft) 'Thick 'n Spicy'	2 tbsp	60	13.0	1.0
COUNTRY STYLE				
(Hunt's)	1.2 oz	39	8.8	0.3
(Hunt's)	1 tbsp	20	5.0	<1.0
DIJON AND HONEY				
(Estee)	1 tbsp	18	3.0	<1.0
(Lawry's)	1/2 cup	203	27.0	1.2
GARLIC (Kraft)	2 tbsp	40	9.0	0.0
HAWAIIAN STYLE				
(Heinz)	1 tbsp	19	4.4	0.1
(Heinz) 'Thick and Rich'	1 oz	40	10.0	0.0
HICKORY				
(Healthy Choice)	1.1 oz	26	5.6	0.2
(Heinz) 'Select'	1 oz	35	8.0	0.0
(Hunt's)	1 tbsp	20	5.0	<1.0
(Hunt's) bold	1.2 oz	46	10.6	0.4
(Hunt's) 'Light'	1.1 oz	27	6.2	0.2
(Open Range)	1.2 oz	37	8.6	0.2
HICKORY SMOKE				
(Heinz)	1 tbsp	19	4.4	0.1
(Heinz) 'Thick and Rich'	1 oz	35	8.0	0.0
(Heinz) 'Thick and Rich'	1 tbsp	20	5.0	0.0
(Kraft)	2 tbsp	45	10.0	1.0
(Kraft) 'Thick 'n Spicy'	2 tbsp	50	12.0	1.0
(Kraft) w/onion bits	2 tbsp	50	11.0	1.0
HOMESTYLE (Hunt's)	1.2 oz	41	9.8	0.1
HONEY				
(Hain)	1 tbsp	14	1.0	1.0
(Kraft) 'Thick 'n Spicy'	2 tbsp	60	13.0	1.0
HONEY MUSTARD (Hunt's)	1.2 oz	48	11.5	0.2

Food Name	Serv. Size	Total Cal.	Carbs GMS	Fat GMS
HOT				
(Healthy Choice) and spicy	1.1 oz	25	5.7	0.2
(Heinz) 'Thick and Rich'	1 tbsp	20	5.0	0.0
(Hunt's) and spicy	1.2 oz	48	11.5	0.2
(Kraft)	2 tbsp	45	9.0	1.0
(Kraft) hickory smoke	2 tbsp	45	9.0	1.0
ITALIAN SEASONING (Kraft)	2 tbsp	50	10.0	1.0
KANSAS CITY STYLE				
(Hunt's)	1.2 oz	43	10.0	0.2
(Kraft)	2 tbsp	50	11.0	1.0
(Kraft) 'Thick 'n Spicy'	2 tbsp	60	13.0	1.0
MESQUITE SMOKE				
(Enrico's)	1 tbsp	18	3.0	1.0
(Heinz) 'Thick and Rich'	1 oz	30	7.0	0.0
(Hunt's)	2 tbsp	40	9.0	0.0
(Kraft)	2 tbsp	45	10.0	1.0
(Kraft) 'Thick 'n Spicy'	2 tbsp	50	12.0	1.0
MUSHROOM				
(Heinz)	1 tbsp	14	3.2	0.1
(Heinz) 'Thick and Rich'	1 oz	30	6.0	0.0
NEW ORLEANS STYLE (Hunt's)	1.2 oz	41	9.4	0.2
ONION				
(Heinz)	1 tbsp	15	3.4	0.1
(Heinz) 'Thick and Rich'	1 oz	30	7.0	0.0
(Kraft) w/onion bits	2 tbsp	50	11.0	1.0
ORANGE JUICE, 'California Grill' (Lawry's)	1/4 cup	34	3.4	0.7
ORIENTAL (LaChoy)	1 tbsp	16	3.8	<.1
SALSA STYLE (Kraft)	2 tbsp	45	9.0	0.0
SLOPPY JOE, w/beef (Libby's)	1/3 cup	110	7.0	7.0
SMOKY				
(Cattleman's)	1 tbsp	25	5.0	0.0
(Maull's)	1 tbsp	20	4.0	<1.0
(Ott's)	1 tbsp	14	3.3	0.1
SOUTHERN STYLE (Hunt's)	1 tbsp	20	5.0	<1.0
TEXAS STYLE				
(Heinz) hot 'Thick and Rich'	1 oz	30	7.0	0.0
(Hunt's)	1 tbsp	25	6.0	<1.0
WESTERN STYLE (Hunt's)	1 tbsp	20	5.0	<1.0
BARBECUE SPICE (Tone's)	1 tsp	9	1.4	0.4
BARLEY				
	1 cup	651	135.2	4.2
flakes (Arrowhead Mills)	2 oz	200	45.0	1.0
pearled, cooked	1 cup	193	44.3	0.7

Food Name	Serv. Size	Total Cal.	Carbs GMS	Fat GMS
pearled, cooked	4 oz	139	32.0	0.5
pearled, raw	1 cup	704	155.4	2.3
pearled, raw	1 oz	100	22.0	0.3
pearled, raw *(Arrowhead Mills)*	2 oz	200	45.0	1.0
pearled, raw, medium 'Scotch Brand' 1.7 oz *(Quaker)*	1/4 cup	172	36.3	0.5
pearled, raw, quick 'Scotch Brand' *(Quaker)*	1/3 cup	172	36.3	0.5
raw	1 oz	100	20.8	0.7
BARLEY FLOUR *(Arrowhead Mills)*	2 oz	200	35.0	1.0
BARRACUDA, PACIFIC				
raw	1 lb	426	0.0	5.0
raw	100 gm	113	0.0	2.6
raw	1 oz	27	0.0	0.3
BASELLA. See VINE SPINACH.				
BASIL				
dried *(Golden Dipt)*	2 grams	8	1.0	0.0
dried, crumbled	1 oz	71	17.3	1.1
dried, crumbled	1 tbsp	11	2.7	0.2
dried, crumbled *(Spice Islands)*	1 tsp	3	0.7	<.1
dried, ground *(Durkee)*	1 tsp	5	0.0	tr
dried, ground *(Laurel Leaf)*	1 tsp	5	0.0	tr
fresh	2 tbsp	1	0.2	0.0
fresh	5 leaves	1	0.1	0.0
BASS, FRESHWATER, MIXED SPECIES				
dry-heat cooked	3 oz	124	0.0	4.0
raw	1 lb	516	0.0	16.7
raw	3 oz	97	0.0	3.1
raw	1 oz	32	0.0	1.0
BASS, SEA, MIXED SPECIES				
baked	4 oz	141	0.0	2.9
broiled	4 oz	141	0.0	2.9
dry-heat cooked	3 oz	105	0.0	2.2
microwaved	4 oz	141	0.0	2.9
raw	1 lb	439	0.0	9.1
raw	3 oz	82	0.0	1.7
raw	1 oz	27	0.0	0.6
BASS, STRIPED				
dry-heat cooked	3 oz	105	0.0	2.5
raw	1 lb	439	0.0	10.6
raw	3 oz	82	0.0	2.0
raw	1 oz	27	0.0	0.7
BATTER MIX				
beer, dry mix *(Golden Dipt)*	1 oz	100	22.0	0.0
corn dog, dry mix *(Golden Dipt)*	1 oz	100	22.0	0.0

Food Name	Serv. Size	Total Cal.	Carbs GMS	Fat GMS
fish and chips, dry mix *(Golden Dipt)*	1.25 oz	120	27.0	0.0
onion ring, dry mix *(Golden Dipt)*	1 oz	100	22.0	0.0
original, dry mix *(Golden Dipt)*	1 oz	100	21.0	0.0
tempura, dry mix *(Golden Dipt)*	1 oz	100	22.0	0.0
BAY LEAF				
dried, crumbled	1 oz	89	21.3	2.4
dried, crumbled	1 tbsp	6	1.4	0.2
dried, crumbled	1 tsp	2	0.5	0.1
dried, crumbled *(Durkee)*	1 tsp	2	0.0	tr
dried, crumbled *(Laurel Leaf)*	1 tsp	2	0.0	tr
dried, crumbled *(Spice Islands)*	1 tsp	5	0.3	<0.1
BEAN. See individual listings.				
BEAN DINNER, W/FRANKFURTERS, FROZEN				
(Banquet)	10 oz	520	57.0	25.0
(Morton)	10 oz	350	46.0	13.0
(Swanson)	10.5 oz	440	53.0	19.0
BEAN ENTRÉE, MICROWAVE				
w/frankfurters, in sauce, 'Diner' micro cup *(Libby's)*	7.75 oz	330	38.0	15.0
w/wieners, microwave cup *(Kid's Kitchen)*	7.5 oz	310	36.0	13.0
BEAN MIX				
Cajun, w/sauce, dry *(Lipton)*	1/4 pkg	130	28.0	<1.0
Cajun, w/sauce, prepared *(Lipton)*	1/2 cup	160	28.0	3.0
chicken and sauce, dry *(Lipton)*	1/4 pkg	120	26.0	1.0
chicken and sauce, prepared *(Lipton)*	1/2 cup	150	26.0	4.0
'Kettle Creations' bean medley with pasta, dry *(Lipton)*	1/4 cup	130	23.0	1.5
BEAN SALAD, CANNED				
four-bean *(Joan of Arc)*	1/2 cup	100	23.0	1.0
four-bean *(Read)*	1/2 cup	100	23.0	1.0
green bean, German-style *(Joan of Arc)*	1 cup	180	27.0	7.0
green bean, German-style *(Read)*	1 cup	180	27.0	7.0
three-bean *(Joan of Arc)*	1/2 cup	90	22.0	0.0
three-bean *(Read)*	1/2 cup	90	22.0	0.0
'Three Bean Salad' *(Green Giant)*	1/2 cup	70	18.0	<1.0
BEAN SPROUTS, CANNED				
(LaChoy)	2 oz	6	1.4	0.1
(LaChoy)	2.928 oz	12	2.2	0.1
BEANS, BAKED. See BAKED BEANS, CANNED.				
BEANS, CANNED. See also BAKED BEANS, CANNED; BEAN SPROUTS, CANNED; BEAN SALAD, CANNED; and individual listings.				
barbecue *(Open Range)*	4.75 oz	185	36.4	3.3
'Beans 'N' Fixins' *(Big John's)*	4.7 oz	127	22.6	3.5
'Big John's Beans 'n Fixin's' *(Hunt's)*	4 oz	170	26.0	6.0
'Mexe-Beans' *(Old El Paso)*	1/2 cup	163	31.0	1.0

Food Name	Serv. Size	Total Cal.	Carbs GMS	Fat GMS
'Mix and Serve' (Hunt's)	4.75 oz	125	30.3	2.8
mixed (Bush's Best)	1/2 cup	70	17.0	0.0
'Pork and Beans' (Hunt's)	4.5 oz	130	27.5	1.2
'Pork and Beans' (Open Range)	4.6 oz	157	26.8	4.8
ranch (Open Ranch)	4.7 oz	124	22.7	3.2
spiced (Gebhardt)	4.5 oz	100	19.3	1.6
vegetarian, 'Deluxe' (Bush's Best)	4 oz	110	25.0	0.0
'Vegetarian Style' (Van Camp's)	1 cup	206	42.0	0.6
w/beef, 'Homestyle' (Hunt's)	9 oz	246	30.6	6.5
w/franks, 'Homestyle' (Hunt's)	9 oz	319	41.0	9.9
w/sausage, 'Homestyle' (Hunt's)	9 oz	306	35.7	9.8

BEAR

raw	1 lb	730	0.0	37.7
raw	1 oz	45	0.0	2.3
simmered	3 oz	220	0.0	11.4
simmered, diced	1 cup	363	0.0	18.7

BEARNAISE. See SAUCE.

BEAVER

raw	1 lb	662	0.0	21.8
raw	1 oz	41	0.0	1.3
roasted	3 oz	180	0.0	5.9
roasted, diced	1 cup	232	0.0	7.6

BEECHNUT, DRIED

in shell	1 lb	1595	92.7	138.4
shelled	1 oz	164	9.5	14.2

BEEF

(NOTE: TRIMMED = Lean; separable fat removed after cooking. UNTRIMMED = Separable fat not removed.)

BRAIN

pan-fried	3 oz	167	0.0	13.5
raw	4 oz	142	0.0	10.5
simmered	4 oz	181	0.0	14.2

BRISKET, FLAT HALF

Trimmed

all grades, 0-inch fat, braised	4 oz	217	0.0	7.0
all grades, 0-inch fat, braised	3 oz	162	0.0	5.3
all grades, 1/4-inch fat, braised	3 oz	189	0.0	8.2
all grades, 1/2-inch fat, braised	3 oz	180	0.0	7.3

Untrimmed

all grades, 0-inch fat, braised	4 oz	244	0.0	10.7
all grades, 1/4-inch fat, braised	11.5 oz	1189	0.0	93.1
all grades, 1/4-inch fat, braised	3 oz	309	0.0	24.2
all grades, 1/4-inch fat, raw	4 oz	328	0.0	26.7

Food Name	Serv. Size	Total Cal.	Carbs GMS	Fat GMS
all grades, 1/2-inch fat, braised	3 oz	311	0.0	24.6
all grades, 1/2-inch fat, raw	1 lb	1338	0.0	110.7
all grades, 1/2-inch fat, raw	1 oz	84	0.0	6.9
BRISKET, POINT HALF				
Trimmed				
all grades, 0-inch fat, braised	4 oz	277	0.0	15.6
all grades, 0-inch fat, braised	3 oz	207	0.0	11.7
all grades, 1/4-inch fat, braised	3 oz	222	0.0	13.3
all grades, 1/2-inch fat, braised	3 oz	224	0.0	13.5
all grades, 1-inch fat, braised	4 oz	296	0.0	17.8
Untrimmed				
all grades, 0-inch fat, braised	3 oz	304	0.0	24.2
all grades, 1/4-inch fat, braised	3 oz	343	0.0	29.1
all grades, 1/4-inch fat, raw	1 lb	1501	0.0	131.9
all grades, 1/4-inch fat, raw	1 oz	94	0.0	8.3
all grades, 1/2-inch fat, braised	3 oz	347	0.0	29.6
all grades, 1/2-inch fat, raw	1 lb	1601	0.0	143.5
all grades, 1/2-inch fat, raw	1 oz	100	0.0	9.0
BRISKET, WHOLE				
Trimmed				
all grades, 0-inch fat, braised	4 oz	247	0.0	11.4
all grades, 0-inch fat, braised	3 oz	185	0.0	8.6
all grades, 1/4-inch fat, braised	4 oz	274	0.0	14.5
all grades, 1/4-inch fat, braised	3 oz	206	0.0	10.9
all grades, 1/2-inch fat, braised	3 oz	205	0.0	10.9
Untrimmed				
all grades, 0-inch fat, braised	3 oz	247	0.0	16.6
all grades, 1/4-inch fat, braised	3 oz	327	0.0	26.8
all grades, 1/4-inch fat, raw	1 lb	1415	0.0	120.4
all grades, 1/4-inch fat, raw	1 oz	88	0.0	7.5
all grades, 1/2-inch fat, braised	3 oz	332	0.0	27.6
all grades, 1/2-inch fat, raw	1 lb	1474	0.0	127.7
all grades, 1/2-inch fat, raw	1 oz	92	0.0	8.0
CHUCK, ARM POT ROAST				
Trimmed				
all grades, 0-inch fat, braised	3 oz	178	0.0	6.5
all grades, 1/4-inch fat, braised	3 oz	184	0.0	7.1
all grades, 1/2-inch fat, braised	3 oz	196	0.0	8.5
choice, 0-inch fat, braised	3 oz	186	0.0	7.4
choice, 1/4-inch fat, braised	3 oz	191	0.0	7.9
choice, 1/2-inch fat, braised	3 oz	199	0.0	8.8
prime, 1/2-inch fat, braised	3 oz	222	0.0	11.4
prime, 1/2-inch fat, raw	1 lb	699	0.0	31.6

Food Name	Serv. Size	Total Cal.	Carbs GMS	Fat GMS
prime, 1/2-inch, raw	1 oz	44	0.0	2.0
select, 0-inch fat, braised	3 oz	168	0.0	5.3
select, 1/4-inch fat, braised	3 oz	175	0.0	6.1
select, 1/2-inch fat, braised	3 oz	189	0.0	7.6
Untrimmed				
all grades, 0-inch fat, braised	3 oz	238	0.0	14.5
all grades, 1/4-inch fat, braised	3 oz	282	0.0	20.2
all grades, 1/4-inch fat, raw	1 lb	1111	0.0	83.3
all grades, 1/4-inch fat, raw	1 oz	69	0.0	5.2
all grades, 1/2-inch fat, braised	3 oz	297	0.0	22.1
all grades, 1/2-inch fat, raw	1 lb	1166	0.0	89.8
all grades, 1/2-inch fat, raw	1 oz	73	0.0	5.6
choice, 0-inch fat, braised	3 oz	249	0.0	15.8
choice, 1/4-inch fat, braised	3 oz	296	0.0	21.9
choice, 1/4-inch fat, raw	1 lb	1157	0.0	88.8
choice, 1/4-inch fat, raw	1 oz	72	0.0	5.6
choice, 1/2-inch fat, braised	3 oz	301	0.0	22.5
choice, 1/2-inch fat, raw	1 lb	1188	0.0	92.9
choice, 1/2-inch fat, raw	1 oz	74	0.0	5.8
prime, 1/2-inch fat, braised	3 oz	332	0.0	26.3
prime, 1/2-inch fat, raw	1 lb	1334	0.0	109.6
prime, 1/2-inch fat, raw	1 oz	83	0.0	6.8
select, 0-inch fat, braised	3 oz	221	0.0	12.4
select, 1/4-inch fat, braised	3 oz	268	0.0	18.5
select, 1/4-inch fat, raw	1 lb	1061	0.0	77.4
select, 1/4-inch fat, raw	1 oz	66	0.0	4.8
select, 1/2-inch fat, braised	3 oz	286	0.0	20.8
select, 1/2-inch fat, raw	1 lb	1075	0.0	79.2
select, 1/2-inch fat, raw	1 oz	67	0.0	4.9
CHUCK, BLADE ROAST				
Trimmed				
all grades, 0-inch fat, braised	3 oz	215	0.0	11.3
all grades, 1/4-inch fat, braised	3 oz	213	0.0	11.1
all grades, 1/2-inch fat, braised	3 oz	229	0.0	13.0
choice, 0-inch fat, braised	3 oz	225	0.0	12.5
choice, 1/4-inch fat, braised	3 oz	224	0.0	12.2
choice, 1/2-inch fat, braised	3 oz	234	0.0	13.4
prime, 1/2-inch fat, braised	3 oz	270	0.0	17.5
prime, 1/2-inch fat, raw	1 lb	921	0.0	60.8
prime, 1/2-inch fat, raw	1 oz	58	0.0	3.8
select, 0-inch fat, braised	3 oz	202	0.0	9.9
select, 1/4-inch fat, braised	3 oz	201	0.0	9.9
select, 1/2-inch fat, braised	3 oz	218	0.0	11.6

Food Name	Serv. Size	Total Cal.	Carbs GMS	Fat GMS
Untrimmed				
all grades, 0-inch fat, braised	3 oz	284	0.0	20.5
all grades, 1/4-inch fat, braised	3 oz	293	0.0	21.8
all grades, 1/4-inch fat, raw	1 lb	1152	0.0	91.2
all grades, 1/4-inch fat, raw	1 oz	72	0.0	5.7
all grades, 1/2-inch fat, braised	3 oz	326	0.0	25.8
all grades, 1/2-inch fat, raw	1 lb	1288	0.0	107.0
all grades, 1/2-inch fat, raw	1 oz	81	0.0	6.7
choice, 0-inch fat, braised	3 oz	296	0.0	22.0
choice, 1/4-inch fat, braised	3 oz	309	0.0	23.6
choice, 1/4-inch fat, raw	1 lb	1234	0.0	100.8
choice, 1/4-inch fat, raw	1 oz	77	0.0	6.3
choice, 1/2-inch fat, braised	3 oz	330	0.0	26.4
choice, 1/2-inch fat, raw	1 lb	1320	0.0	110.7
choice, 1/2-inch fat, raw	1 oz	83	0.0	6.9
prime, 1/2-inch fat, braised	3 oz	354	0.0	29.0
prime, 1/2-inch fat, raw	1 lb	1488	0.0	129.6
prime, 1/2-inch fat, raw	1 oz	93	0.0	8.1
select, 0-inch fat, braised	3 oz	266	0.0	18.4
select, 1/4-inch fat, braised	3 oz	277	0.0	19.9
select, 1/4-inch fat, raw	1 lb	1066	0.0	81.3
select, 1/4-inch fat, raw	1 oz	67	0.0	5.1
select, 1/2-inch fat, braised	3 oz	311	0.0	24.1
select, 1/2-inch fat, raw	1 lb	1179	0.0	94.4
select, 1/2-inch fat, raw	1 oz	74	0.0	5.9
FLANK				
Trimmed				
choice, 0-inch fat, braised	3 oz	201	0.0	11.0
choice, 0-inch fat, broiled	3 oz	176	0.0	8.6
Untrimmed				
choice, 0-inch fat, braised	3 oz	224	0.0	14.0
choice, 0-inch fat, broiled	3 oz	192	0.0	10.6
choice, 0-inch fat, raw	1 oz	51	0.0	3.0
choice, 0-inch fat, raw	4 oz	203	0.0	12.0
HEART				
raw	4 oz	132	2.9	4.3
simmered	3 oz	149	0.4	4.8
KIDNEY				
raw	4 oz	121	2.5	3.5
simmered	3 oz	122	0.8	2.9
LEAN CUTS				
bottom round steak, 'Lite' (Heritage Lifestyle) uncooked	3 oz	108	0.0	4.0
(Brae Beef) raw	4 oz	120	0.0	2.0

Food Name	Serv. Size	Total Cal.	Carbs GMS	Fat GMS
brisket 'Lite' (Heritage Lifestyle) uncooked	3 oz	98	0.0	3.0
burger (Lean and Free) raw	4 oz	174	0.0	9.3
chuck, arm pot roast, 'Lite' (Heritage Lifestyle) uncooked	3 oz	101	0.0	3.0
chuck blade roast, 'Lite' (Heritage Lifestyle) uncooked	3 oz	128	0.0	7.0
cube steak (Lean and Free) raw	4 oz	109	0.0	1.0
eye round steak, 'Lite' (Heritage Lifestyle) uncooked	3 oz	111	0.0	4.0
ground, lean, 'Lite' (Heritage Lifestyle) uncooked	3 oz	118	0.0	5.0
lean cuts, raw (Lean and Free)	4 oz	161	0.0	7.5
rib eye (Lean and Free) raw	4 oz	121	0.0	2.6
rib roast, large end, 'Lite' (Heritage Lifestyle) uncooked	3 oz	142	0.0	8.0
rib steak, small end, 'Lite' (Heritage Lifestyle) uncooked	3 oz	118	0.0	5.0
rolled (Lean and Free) raw	4 oz	125	0.0	2.8
round steak (Lean and Free) raw	4 oz	111	0.0	1.1
round tip roast, 'Lite' (Heritage Lifestyle) uncooked	3 oz	91	0.0	1.5
sirloin steak (Lean and Free) raw	4 oz	111	0.0	1.8
sirloin steak, 'Lite' (Heritage Lifestyle) uncooked	3 oz	103	0.0	3.0
sirloin tip (Lean and Free) raw	4 oz	110	0.0	1.2
strip loin steak (Lean and Free) raw	4 oz	113	0.0	1.8
T-bone (Lean and Free) raw	4 oz	125	0.0	2.7
tenderloin fillet steak (Lean and Free) raw	4 oz	116	0.0	2.4
tenderloin steak, 'Lite' (Heritage Lifestyle) uncooked	3 oz	109	0.0	4.0
top loin steak, 'Lite' (Heritage Lifestyle) uncooked	3 oz	114	0.0	4.0
top round (Lean and Free) raw	4 oz	134	0.0	4.5
top round steak, 'Lite' (Heritage Lifestyle) uncooked	3 oz	100	0.0	3.0
LIVER				
braised	3 oz	137	2.9	4.2
pan-fried	3 oz	184	6.7	6.8
pan-fried in vegetable oil	4 oz	246	8.9	9.1
raw	4 oz	162	6.6	4.3
LUNG				
braised	3 oz	102	0.0	3.2
raw	4 oz	104	0.0	2.8
PANCREAS				
braised	3 oz	230	0.0	14.6
raw	4 oz	266	0.0	21.0
PORTERHOUSE				
Trimmed				
choice, 1/4-inch fat, broiled	3 oz	185	0.0	9.2
choice, 1/2-inch fat, broiled	3 oz	185	0.0	9.2
Untrimmed				
choice, 1/4-inch fat, broiled	3 oz	259	0.0	18.8
choice, 1/4-inch fat, raw	1 lb	1229	0.0	98.4
choice, 1/4-inch fat, raw	1 oz	77	0.0	6.2

Food Name	Serv. Size	Total Cal.	Carbs GMS	Fat GMS
choice, 1/2-inch fat, broiled	3 oz	254	0.0	18.0
choice, 1/2-inch fat, raw	1 lb	1288	0.0	105.6
choice, 1/2-inch fat, raw	1 oz	81	0.0	6.6
RIB, LARGE END				
Trimmed				
all grades, ribs 6-9, 0-inch fat, roasted	3 oz	202	0.0	11.4
all grades, ribs 6-9, 1/4-inch fat, broiled	3 oz	190	0.0	11.0
all grades, ribs 6-9, 1/4-inch fat, roasted	3 oz	201	0.0	11.2
all grades, ribs 6-9, 1/2-inch fat, broiled	3 oz	198	0.0	12.1
all grades, ribs 6-9, 1/2-inch fat, roasted	3 oz	207	0.0	11.9
choice, ribs 6-9, 0-inch fat, roasted	3 oz	215	0.0	12.7
choice, ribs 6-9, 1/4-inch fat, broiled	3 oz	204	0.0	12.4
choice, ribs 6-9, 1/4-inch fat, roasted	3 oz	213	0.0	12.5
choice, ribs 6-9, 1/2-inch fat, broiled	3 oz	203	0.0	12.6
choice, ribs 6-9, 1/2-inch fat, roasted	3 oz	211	0.0	12.3
prime, ribs 6-9, 1/4-inch fat, broiled	3 oz	250	0.0	17.7
prime, ribs 6-9, 1/4-inch fat, roasted	3 oz	241	0.0	15.6
prime, ribs 6-9, 1/2-inch fat, broiled	3 oz	250	0.0	17.7
prime, ribs 6-9, 1/2-inch fat, roasted	3 oz	241	0.0	15.6
select, ribs 6-9, 0-inch fat, roasted	3 oz	187	0.0	9.7
select, ribs 6-9, 1/4-inch fat, broiled	3 oz	175	0.0	9.3
select, ribs 6-9, 1/4-inch fat, roasted	3 oz	187	0.0	9.7
select, ribs 6-9, 1/2-inch fat, broiled	3 oz	183	0.0	10.4
select, ribs 6-9, 1/2-inch fat, roasted	3 oz	197	0.0	10.8
Untrimmed				
all grades, ribs 6-9, 0-inch fat, roasted	3 oz	300	0.0	24.0
all grades, ribs 6-9, 1/4-inch fat, broiled	3 oz	295	0.0	24.2
all grades, ribs 6-9, 1/4-inch fat, raw	1 lb	1465	0.0	127.9
all grades, ribs 6-9, 1/4-inch fat, raw	1 oz	92	0.0	8.0
all grades, ribs 6-9, 1/4-inch fat, roasted	3 oz	310	0.0	25.3
all grades, ribs 6-9, 1/2-inch fat, broiled	3 oz	321	0.0	27.5
all grades, ribs 6-9, 1/2-inch fat, raw	1 lb	1588	0.0	142.3
all grades, ribs 6-9, 1/2-inch fat, raw	1 oz	99	0.0	8.9
all grades, ribs 6-9, 1/2-inch fat, roasted	3 oz	313	0.0	25.5
choice, ribs 6-9, 0-inch fat, roasted	10.2 oz	1080	0.0	88.4
choice, ribs 6-9, 0-inch fat, roasted	3 oz	316	0.0	25.9
choice, ribs 6-9, 1/4-inch fat, broiled	3 oz	312	0.0	26.2
choice, ribs 6-9, 1/4-inch fat, raw	1 lb	1565	0.0	139.8
choice, ribs 6-9, 1/4-inch fat, raw	1 oz	98	0.0	8.7
choice, ribs 6-9, 1/4-inch fat, roasted	3 oz	326	0.0	27.2
choice, ribs 6-9, 1/2-inch fat, broiled	3 oz	326	0.0	28.1
choice, ribs 6-9, 1/2-inch fat, raw	1 lb	1615	0.0	145.6
choice, ribs 6-9, 1/2-inch fat, raw	1 oz	101	0.0	9.1

Food Name	Serv. Size	Total Cal.	Carbs GMS	Fat GMS
choice, ribs 6-9, 1/2-inch fat, roasted	3 oz	316	0.0	25.9
prime, ribs 6-9, 1/4-inch fat, broiled	3 oz	351	0.0	30.8
prime, ribs 6-9, 1/4-inch fat, raw	1 lb	1710	0.0	156.5
prime, ribs 6-9, 1/4-inch fat, raw	1 oz	107	0.0	9.8
prime, ribs 6-9, 1/4-inch fat, roasted	3 oz	342	0.0	28.9
prime, ribs 6-9, 1/2-inch fat, broiled	3 oz	361	0.0	32.1
prime, ribs 6-9, 1/2-inch fat, raw	1 lb	1737	0.0	159.6
prime, ribs 6-9, 1/2-inch fat, raw	1 oz	109	0.0	10.0
prime, ribs 6-9, 1/2-inch fat, roasted	3 oz	346	0.0	29.4
select, ribs 6-9, 0-inch fat, roasted	3 oz	281	0.0	21.7
select, ribs 6-9, 1/4-inch fat, broiled	3 oz	275	0.0	21.9
select, ribs 6-9, 1/4-inch fat, raw	1 lb	1379	0.0	117.7
select, ribs 6-9, 1/4-inch fat, raw	1 oz	86	0.0	7.4
select, ribs 6-9, 1/4-inch fat, roasted	3 oz	289	0.0	22.7
select, ribs 6-9, 1/2-inch fat, broiled	3 oz	301	0.0	25.1
select, ribs 6-9, 1/2-inch fat, raw	1 lb	1488	0.0	130.7
select, ribs 6-9, 1/2-inch fat, raw	1 oz	93	0.0	8.2
select, ribs 6-9, 1/2-inch fat, roasted	3 oz	303	0.0	24.5
RIB, SHORTRIB				
Trimmed, choice, braised	3 oz	251	0.0	15.4
Untrimmed				
choice, braised	3 oz	400	0.0	35.7
choice, raw	1 lb	1760	0.0	164.3
choice, raw	1 oz	110	0.0	10.3
RIB, SMALL END				
Trimmed				
all grades, ribs 10-12, 0-inch fat, broiled	3 oz	181	0.0	8.8
all grades, ribs 10-12, 1/4-inch fat, roasted	3 oz	185	0.0	9.8
all grades, ribs 10-12, 1/2-inch fat, broiled	3 oz	188	0.0	9.5
all grades, ribs 10-12, 1/2-inch fat, roasted	3 oz	201	0.0	11.5
all grades, ribs 10-12, 1/4-inch fat, broiled	3 oz	188	0.0	9.5
choice, ribs 10-12, 0-inch fat, broiled	3 oz	191	0.0	9.9
choice, ribs 10-12, 1/4-inch fat, broiled	3 oz	198	0.0	10.7
choice, ribs 10-12, 1/4-inch fat, roasted	3 oz	197	0.0	11.1
choice, ribs 10-12, 1/2-inch fat, broiled	3 oz	191	0.0	9.9
choice, ribs 10-12, 1/2-inch fat, roasted	3 oz	207	0.0	12.1
prime, ribs 10-12, 1/4-inch fat, broiled	3 oz	221	0.0	13.2
prime, ribs 10-12, 1/4-inch fat, roasted	3 oz	258	0.0	17.9
prime, ribs 10-12, 1/2-inch fat, broiled	3 oz	221	0.0	13.2
prime, ribs 10-12, 1/2-inch fat, roasted	3 oz	258	0.0	17.9
select, ribs 10-12, 0-inch fat, broiled	3 oz	168	0.0	7.4
select, ribs 10-12, 1/4-inch fat, broiled	3 oz	176	0.0	8.2
select, ribs 10-12, 1/4-inch fat, roasted	3 oz	173	0.0	8.3

Food Name	Serv. Size	Total Cal.	Carbs GMS	Fat GMS
select, ribs 10-12, 1/2-inch fat, broiled	3 oz	178	0.0	8.4
select, ribs 10-12, 1/2-inch fat, roasted	3 oz	184	0.0	9.6
Untrimmed				
all grades, ribs 10-12, 0-inch fat, broiled	3 oz	252	0.0	17.9
all grades, ribs 10-12, 1/4-inch fat, broiled	3 oz	286	0.0	22.1
all grades, ribs 10-12, 1/4-inch fat, raw	1 lb	1352	0.0	113.9
all grades, ribs 10-12, 1/4-inch fat, raw	1 oz	84	0.0	7.1
all grades, ribs 10-12, 1/4-inch fat, roasted	3 oz	295	0.0	23.8
all grades, ribs 10-12, 1/2-inch fat, broiled	3 oz	277	0.0	21.1
all grades, ribs 10-12, 1/2-inch fat, raw	1 lb	1388	0.0	117.8
all grades, ribs 10-12, 1/2-inch fat, raw	1 oz	87	0.0	7.4
all grades, ribs 10-12, 1/2-inch fat, roasted	3 oz	305	0.0	24.9
choice, ribs 10-12, 0-inch fat, broiled	3 oz	265	0.0	19.4
choice, ribs 10-12, 1/4-inch fat, broiled	3 oz	297	0.0	23.5
choice, ribs 10-12, 1/4-inch fat, raw	1 lb	1429	0.0	122.8
choice, ribs 10-12, 1/4-inch fat, raw	1 oz	89	0.0	7.7
choice, ribs 10-12, 1/4-inch fat, roasted	3 oz	312	0.0	25.7
choice, ribs 10-12, 1/2-inch fat, broiled	3 oz	282	0.0	21.6
choice, ribs 10-12, 1/2-inch fat, raw	1 lb	1415	0.0	121.2
choice, ribs 10-12, 1/2-inch fat, raw	1 oz	88	0.0	7.6
choice, ribs 10-12, 1/2-inch fat, roasted	3 oz	312	0.0	25.7
prime, ribs 10-12, 1/4-inch fat, broiled	3 oz	307	0.0	24.4
prime, ribs 10-12, 1/4-inch fat, raw	1 lb	1551	0.0	136.4
prime, ribs 10-12, 1/4-inch fat, raw	1 oz	97	0.0	8.5
prime, ribs 10-12, 1/4-inch fat, roasted	3 oz	354	0.0	30.5
prime, ribs 10-12, 1/2-inch fat, broiled	3 oz	309	0.0	24.7
prime, ribs 10-12, 1/2-inch fat, raw	1 lb	1583	0.0	140.2
prime, ribs 10-12, 1/2-inch fat, raw	1 oz	99	0.0	8.8
prime, ribs 10-12, 1/2-inch fat, roasted	3 oz	357	0.0	30.8
select, ribs 10-12, 0-inch fat, broiled	3 oz	242	0.0	16.8
select, ribs 10-12, 1/4-inch fat, broiled	3 oz	273	0.0	20.6
select, ribs 10-12, 1/4-inch fat, raw	1 lb	1297	0.0	107.4
select, ribs 10-12, 1/4-inch fat, raw	1 oz	81	0.0	6.7
select, ribs 10-12, 1/4-inch fat, roasted	3 oz	281	0.0	22.2
select, ribs 10-12, 1/2-inch fat, broiled	3 oz	263	0.0	19.4
select, ribs 10-12, 1/2-inch fat, raw	1 lb	1288	0.0	106.4
select, ribs 10-12, 1/2-inch fat, raw	1 oz	81	0.0	6.7
select, ribs 10-12, 1/2-inch fat, roasted	3 oz	283	0.0	22.3
RIB, WHOLE				
Trimmed				
all grades, ribs 6-12, 1/4-inch fat, broiled	3 oz	190	0.0	10.4
all grades, ribs 6-12, 1/4-inch fat, roasted	3 oz	195	0.0	10.6
all grades, ribs 6-12, 1/2-inch fat, broiled	3 oz	194	0.0	11.0

Food Name	Serv. Size	Total Cal.	Carbs GMS	Fat GMS
all grades, ribs 6-12, 1/2-inch fat, roasted	3 oz	204	0.0	11.7
choice, ribs 6-12, 1/4-inch fat, broiled	3 oz	201	0.0	11.7
choice, ribs 6-12, 1/4-inch fat, roasted	3 oz	207	0.0	11.9
choice, ribs 6-12, 1/2-inch fat, broiled	3 oz	198	0.0	11.5
choice, ribs 6-12, 1/2-inch fat, roasted	3 oz	209	0.0	12.2
prime, ribs 6-12, 1/4-inch fat, broiled	3 oz	238	0.0	15.9
prime, ribs 6-12, 1/4-inch fat, roasted	3 oz	248	0.0	16.5
prime, ribs 6-12, 1/2-inch fat, broiled	3 oz	238	0.0	15.9
prime, ribs 6-12, 1/2-inch fat, roasted	3 oz	248	0.0	16.5
select, ribs 6-12, 1/4-inch fat, broiled	3 oz	175	0.0	8.9
select, ribs 6-12, 1/4-inch fat, roasted	3 oz	181	0.0	9.1
select, ribs 6-12, 1/2-inch fat, broiled	3 oz	181	0.0	9.6
select, ribs 6-12, 1/2-inch fat, roasted	3 oz	191	0.0	10.3
Untrimmed				
all grades, ribs 6-12, 1/4-inch fat, broiled	3 oz	291	0.0	23.3
all grades, ribs 6-12, 1/4-inch fat, raw	1 lb	1420	0.0	122.4
all grades, ribs 6-12, 1/4-inch fat, raw	1 oz	89	0.0	7.7
all grades, ribs 6-12, 1/4-inch fat, roasted	3 oz	304	0.0	24.7
all grades, ribs 6-12, 1/2-inch fat, broiled	3 oz	308	0.0	25.5
all grades, ribs 6-12, 1/2-inch fat, raw	1 lb	1501	0.0	132.2
all grades, ribs 6-12, 1/2-inch fat, raw	1 oz	94	0.0	8.3
all grades, ribs 6-12, 1/2-inch fat, roasted	3 oz	324	0.0	27.0
choice, ribs 6-12, 1/4-inch fat, broiled	3 oz	306	0.0	25.1
choice, ribs 6-12, 1/4-inch fat, raw	1 lb	1510	0.0	133.2
choice, ribs 6-12, 1/4-inch fat, raw	1 oz	94	0.0	8.3
choice, ribs 6-12, 1/4-inch fat, roasted	3 oz	320	0.0	26.5
choice, ribs 6-12, 1/2-inch fat, broiled	3 oz	313	0.0	26.1
choice, ribs 6-12, 1/2-inch fat, raw	1 lb	1533	0.0	135.5
choice, ribs 6-12, 1/2-inch fat, raw	1 oz	96	0.0	8.5
choice, ribs 6-12, 1/2-inch fat, roasted	3 oz	328	0.0	27.6
prime, ribs 6-12, 1/4-inch fat, broiled	3 oz	333	0.0	28.2
prime, ribs 6-12, 1/4-inch fat, raw	1 lb	1651	0.0	149.0
prime, ribs 6-12, 1/4-inch fat, raw	1 oz	103	0.0	9.3
prime, ribs 6-12, 1/4-inch fat, roasted	3 oz	348	0.0	29.6
prime, ribs 6-12, 1/2-inch fat, broiled	3 oz	347	0.0	29.9
prime, ribs 6-12, 1/2-inch fat, raw	1 lb	1678	0.0	152.4
prime, ribs 6-12, 1/2-inch fat, raw	1 oz	105	0.0	9.5
prime, ribs 6-12, 1/2-inch fat, roasted	3 oz	361	0.0	31.4
select, ribs 6-12, 1/4-inch fat, broiled	3 oz	275	0.0	21.4
select, ribs 6-12, 1/4-inch fat, raw	1 lb	1347	0.0	113.7
select, ribs 6-12, 1/4-inch fat, raw	1 oz	84	0.0	7.1
select, ribs 6-12, 1/4-inch fat, roasted	3 oz	286	0.0	22.5
select, ribs 6-12, 1/2-inch fat, broiled	3 oz	289	0.0	23.3

Food Name	Serv. Size	Total Cal.	Carbs GMS	Fat GMS
select, ribs 6-12, 1/2-inch fat, raw	1 lb	1411	0.0	121.2
select, ribs 6-12, 1/2-inch fat, raw	1 oz	88	0.0	7.6
select, ribs 6-12, 1/2-inch fat, roasted	3 oz	306	0.0	24.9
RIB EYE, SMALL END				
Trimmed				
choice, ribs 10-12, 0-inch fat, broiled	3 oz	191	0.0	9.9
choice, ribs 10-12, 1/4-inch fat, broiled	4 oz	255	0.0	13.3
Untrimmed				
choice, ribs 10-12, 0-inch fat, broiled	3 oz	261	0.0	18.9
choice, ribs 10-12, 0-inch fat, raw	1 lb	1243	0.0	100.1
choice, ribs 10-12, 0-inch fat, raw	1 oz	78	0.0	6.3
ROUND, BOTTOM				
Trimmed				
all grades, 0-inch fat, braised	3 oz	173	0.0	6.5
all grades, 0-inch fat, roasted	3 oz	156	0.0	5.7
all grades, 1/4-inch fat, braised	3 oz	178	0.0	7.0
all grades, 1/4-inch fat, roasted	3 oz	161	0.0	6.3
all grades, 1/2-inch fat, braised	3 oz	189	0.0	8.2
choice, 0-inch fat, braised	3 oz	181	0.0	7.4
choice, 0-inch fat, roasted	3 oz	164	0.0	6.6
choice, 1/4-inch fat, braised	3 oz	187	0.0	8.0
choice, 1/4-inch fat, roasted	3 oz	168	0.0	7.1
choice, 1/2-inch fat, braised	3 oz	191	0.0	8.5
prime, 1/2-inch fat, braised	3 oz	212	0.0	10.8
prime, 1/2-inch fat, raw	1 lb	721	0.0	33.1
prime, 1/2-inch fat, raw	1 oz	45	0.0	2.1
select, 0-inch fat, braised	3 oz	163	0.0	5.3
select, 0-inch fat, roasted	3 oz	145	0.0	4.6
select, 1/4-inch fat, braised	3 oz	167	0.0	5.8
select, 1/4-inch fat, roasted	10.5 oz	534	0.0	18.5
select, 1/4-inch fat, roasted	3 oz	152	0.0	5.3
select, 1/2-inch fat, braised	3 oz	182	0.0	7.4
Untrimmed				
all grades, 0-inch fat, braised	3 oz	181	0.0	7.5
all grades, 0-inch fat, roasted	3 oz	160	0.0	6.3
all grades, 1/4-inch fat, braised	3 oz	234	0.0	14.4
all grades, 1/4-inch fat, raw	1 lb	943	0.0	60.9
all grades, 1/4-inch fat, raw	1 oz	59	0.0	3.8
all grades, 1/4-inch fat, roasted	3 oz	211	0.0	12.7
all grades, 1/2-inch fat, braised	3 oz	222	0.0	12.6
all grades, 1/2-inch fat, raw	1 lb	1021	0.0	70.5
all grades, 1/2-inch fat, raw	1 oz	64	0.0	4.4
choice, 0-inch fat, braised	3 oz	193	0.0	9.0

Food Name	Serv. Size	Total Cal.	Carbs GMS	Fat GMS
choice, 0-inch fat, roasted	3 oz	173	0.0	7.7
choice, 1/4-inch fat, braised	3 oz	241	0.0	15.2
choice, 1/4-inch fat, raw	1 lb	989	0.0	66.7
choice, 1/4-inch fat, raw	1 oz	62	0.0	4.2
choice, 1/4-inch fat, roasted	3 oz	221	0.0	13.9
choice, 1/2-inch fat, braised	3 oz	224	0.0	12.9
choice, 1/2-inch fat, raw	1 lb	1030	0.0	71.5
choice, 1/2-inch fat, raw	1 oz	64	0.0	4.5
prime, 1/2-inch fat, braised	3 oz	252	0.0	16.2
prime, 1/2-inch fat, raw	1 lb	1021	0.0	69.8
prime, 1/2-inch fat, raw	1 oz	64	0.0	4.4
select, 0-inch fat, braised	3 oz	171	0.0	6.4
select, 0-inch fat, roasted	3 oz	150	0.0	5.1
select, 1/4-inch fat, braised	3 oz	220	0.0	12.8
select, 1/4-inch fat, raw	1 lb	885	0.0	54.3
select, 1/4-inch fat, raw	1 oz	55	0.0	3.4
select, 1/4-inch fat, roasted	3 oz	199	0.0	11.3
select, 1/2-inch fat, braised	3 oz	215	0.0	11.8
select, 1/2-inch fat, raw	1 lb	984	0.0	66.0
select, 1/2-inch fat, raw	1 oz	62	0.0	4.1

ROUND, EYE OF

Trimmed

Food Name	Serv. Size	Total Cal.	Carbs GMS	Fat GMS
all grades, 0-inch fat, roasted	3 oz	141	0.0	4.0
all grades, 1/4-inch fat, roasted	3 oz	143	0.0	4.2
all grades, 1/2-inch fat, roasted	3 oz	156	0.0	5.5
choice, 0-inch fat, roasted	3 oz	149	0.0	4.8
choice, 1/4-inch fat, roasted	3 oz	149	0.0	4.8
choice, 1/2-inch fat, roasted	3 oz	156	0.0	5.7
prime, 1/2-inch fat, roasted	3 oz	213	0.0	12.7
prime, 1/2-inch fat, raw	1 lb	676	0.0	28.4
prime, 1/2-inch fat, raw	1 oz	42	0.0	1.8
prime, 1/2-inch fat, roasted	3 oz	168	0.0	7.0
select, 0-inch fat, roasted	3 oz	132	0.0	3.0
select, 0-inch fat, roasted	10.4 oz	460	0.0	10.4
select, 1/4-inch fat, roasted	3 oz	136	0.0	3.4
select, 1/2-inch fat, roasted	3 oz	151	0.0	5.1

Untrimmed

Food Name	Serv. Size	Total Cal.	Carbs GMS	Fat GMS
all grades, 0-inch fat, roasted	3 oz	145	0.0	4.6
all grades, 1/4-inch fat, raw	1 lb	966	0.0	64.8
all grades, 1/4-inch fat, raw	1 oz	60	0.0	4.1
all grades, 1/4-inch fat, roasted	3 oz	195	0.0	10.8
all grades, 1/2-inch fat, raw	1 lb	903	0.0	57.1
all grades, 1/2-inch fat, raw	1 oz	56	0.0	3.6

Food Name	Serv. Size	Total Cal.	Carbs GMS	Fat GMS
all grades, 1/2-inch fat, roasted	3 oz	207	0.0	12.1
choice, 0-inch fat, braised	3 oz	176	0.0	4.9
choice, 0-inch fat, roasted	3 oz	153	0.0	5.4
choice, 1/4-inch fat, raw	1 lb	989	0.0	67.1
choice, 1/4-inch fat, raw	1 oz	62	0.0	4.2
choice, 1/4-inch fat, roasted	3 oz	205	0.0	12.0
choice, 1/2-inch fat, raw	1 lb	916	0.0	58.8
choice, 1/2-inch fat, raw	1 oz	57	0.0	3.7
choice, 1/2-inch fat, roasted	3 oz	207	0.0	12.2
prime, 1/2-inch fat, raw	1 lb	1002	0.0	68.3
prime, 1/2-inch fat, raw	1 oz	63	0.0	4.3
select, 0-inch fat, roasted	3 oz	137	0.0	3.5
select, 1/4-inch fat, raw	1 lb	916	0.0	59.1
select, 1/4-inch fat, raw	1 oz	57	0.0	3.7
select, 1/4-inch fat, roasted	1 oz	184	0.0	9.6
select, 1/4-inch fat, roasted	4 oz	246	0.0	12.8
select, 1/2-inch fat, raw	1 lb	853	0.0	51.4
select, 1/2-inch fat, raw	1 oz	53	0.0	3.2
select, 1/2-inch fat, roasted	3 oz	201	0.0	11.5
ROUND, FULL CUT				
Trimmed				
choice, 1/4-inch fat, broiled	3 oz	162	0.0	6.2
select, 1/4-inch fat, broiled	3 oz	146	0.0	4.4
select, 1/2-inch fat, broiled	3 oz	156	0.0	5.9
Untrimmed				
choice, 1/4-inch fat, broiled	3 oz	204	0.0	11.6
choice, 1/4-inch fat, raw	1 lb	921	0.0	58.1
choice, 1/4-inch fat, raw	1 oz	58	0.0	3.6
choice, 1/2-inch fat, broiled	3 oz	233	0.0	15.5
choice, 1/2-inch fat, raw	1 lb	1093	0.0	79.6
choice, 1/2-inch fat, raw	1 oz	68	0.0	5.0
select, 1/4-inch fat, broiled	3 oz	190	0.0	10.0
select, 1/4-inch fat, raw	1 lb	866	0.0	52.6
select, 1/4-inch fat, raw	1 oz	54	0.0	3.3
select, 1/2-inch fat, broiled	3 oz	223	0.0	14.3
select, 1/2-inch fat, raw	1 lb	1048	0.0	74.1
select, 1/2-inch fat, raw	1 oz	65	0.0	4.6
ROUND, TIP				
Trimmed				
all grades, 0-inch fat, roasted	3 oz	150	0.0	5.0
all grades, 1/4-inch fat, roasted	3 oz	157	0.0	5.9
all grades, 1/2-inch fat, roasted	3 oz	161	0.0	6.4
choice, 0-inch fat, roasted	3 oz	153	0.0	5.4

Food Name	Serv. Size	Total Cal.	Carbs GMS	Fat GMS
choice, 1/4-inch fat, roasted	3 oz	160	0.0	6.2
choice, 1/2-inch fat, roasted	3 oz	164	0.0	6.6
prime, 1/4-inch fat, roasted	3 oz	181	0.0	8.6
prime, 1/2-inch fat, roasted	3 oz	181	0.0	8.6
select, 0-inch fat, roasted	3 oz	144	0.0	4.5
select, 1/4-inch fat, roasted	3 oz	153	0.0	5.4
select, 1/2-inch fat, roasted	3 oz	156	0.0	5.7
Untrimmed				
all grades, 0-inch fat, roasted	3 oz	162	0.0	6.7
all grades, 1/4-inch fat, raw	1 lb	912	0.0	59.8
all grades, 1/4-inch fat, raw	1 oz	57	0.0	3.7
all grades, 1/4-inch fat, roasted	3 oz	199	0.0	11.3
all grades, 1/2-inch fat, raw	1 lb	934	0.0	62.4
all grades, 1/2-inch fat, raw	1 oz	58	0.0	3.9
all grades, 1/2-inch fat, roasted	3 oz	213	0.0	13.0
choice, 0-inch fat, roasted	3 oz	170	0.0	7.6
choice, 1/4-inch fat, raw	1 lb	962	0.0	65.2
choice, 1/4-inch fat, raw	1 oz	60	0.0	4.1
choice, 1/4-inch fat, roasted	3 oz	210	0.0	12.6
choice, 1/2-inch fat, raw	1 lb	948	0.0	64.0
choice, 1/2-inch fat, raw	1 oz	59	0.0	4.0
choice, 1/2-inch fat, roasted	3 oz	216	0.0	13.3
prime, 1/4-inch fat, raw	1 lb	971	0.0	66.1
prime, 1/4-inch fat, raw	1 oz	61	0.0	4.1
prime, 1/4-inch fat, roasted	3 oz	233	0.0	15.2
prime, 1/2-inch fat, raw	1 lb	1012	0.0	72.9
prime, 1/2-inch fat, raw	1 oz	63	0.0	4.6
prime, 1/2-inch fat, roasted	3 oz	241	0.0	16.3
select, 0-inch fat, roasted	3 oz	158	0.0	6.2
select, 1/4-inch fat, raw	1 lb	848	0.0	51.2
select, 1/4-inch fat, raw	1 oz	53	0.0	3.2
select, 1/4-inch fat, roasted	3 oz	191	0.0	10.3
select, 1/2-inch fat, raw	1 lb	875	0.0	55.7
select, 1/2-inch fat, raw	1 oz	55	0.0	3.5
select, 1/2-inch fat, roasted	3 oz	205	0.0	12.0
ROUND, TOP				
Trimmed				
all grades, 0-inch fat, braised	3 oz	169	0.0	4.3
all grades, 1/4-inch fat, braised	3 oz	174	0.0	4.8
all grades, 1/4-inch fat, broiled	3 oz	153	0.0	4.2
all grades, 1/2-inch fat, broiled	3 oz	162	0.0	5.3
choice, 1/4-inch fat, braised	3 oz	181	0.0	5.5
choice, 1/4-inch fat, broiled	3 oz	161	0.0	5.0

Food Name	Serv. Size	Total Cal.	Carbs GMS	Fat GMS
choice, 1/4-inch fat, pan-fried	3 oz	193	0.0	7.3
choice, 1/4-inch fat, pan-fried in vegetable oil	4 oz	257	0.0	9.7
choice, 1/2-inch fat, broiled	3 oz	165	0.0	5.5
choice, 1/2-inch fat, pan-fried	3 oz	193	0.0	7.3
prime, 1/4-inch fat, broiled	3 oz	183	0.0	7.5
prime, 1/2-inch fat, broiled	3 oz	183	0.0	7.5
select, 0-inch fat, braised	3 oz	161	0.0	3.4
select, 1/4-inch fat, braised	3 oz	167	0.0	3.9
select, 1/4-inch fat, broiled	3 oz	144	0.0	3.2
select, 1/2-inch fat, broiled	3 oz	156	0.0	4.6
Untrimmed				
all grades, 0-inch fat, braised	3 oz	178	0.0	5.4
all grades, 1/4-inch fat, braised	3 oz	211	0.0	9.7
all grades, 1/4-inch fat, broiled	3 oz	184	0.0	8.2
all grades, 1/4-inch fat, raw	1 lb	798	0.0	42.5
all grades, 1/4-inch fat, raw	1 oz	50	0.0	2.7
all grades, 1/2-inch fat, broiled	3 oz	179	0.0	7.5
all grades, 1/2-inch fat, raw	1 lb	780	0.0	39.7
all grades, 1/2-inch fat, raw	1 oz	49	0.0	2.5
choice, 0-inch fat, braised	3 oz	184	0.0	6.0
choice, 1/4-inch fat, broiled	3 oz	190	0.0	9.0
choice, 1/4-inch fat, pan-fried	3 oz	235	0.0	13.1
choice, 1/4-inch fat, pan-fried in vegetable oil	4 oz	314	0.0	17.4
choice, 1/4-inch fat, raw	1 lb	821	0.0	45.0
choice, 1/4-inch fat, raw	1 oz	51	0.0	2.8
choice, 1/2-inch fat, braised	3 oz	221	0.0	10.9
choice, 1/2-inch fat, broiled	3 oz	181	0.0	7.7
choice, 1/2-inch fat, pan-fried	3 oz	247	0.0	14.5
choice, 1/2-inch fat, raw	1 lb	789	0.0	40.7
choice, 1/2-inch fat, raw	1 oz	49	0.0	2.5
prime, 1/4-inch fat, broiled	3 oz	195	0.0	9.1
prime, 1/4-inch fat, raw	1 lb	816	0.0	42.9
prime, 1/4-inch fat, raw	1 oz	51	0.0	2.7
prime, 1/2-inch fat, broiled	3 oz	201	0.0	9.9
prime, 1/2-inch fat, raw	1 lb	853	0.0	47.9
prime, 1/2-inch fat, raw	1 oz	53	0.0	3.0
select, 0-inch fat, braised	3 oz	170	0.0	4.5
select, 1/4-inch fat, braised	3 oz	199	0.0	8.4
select, 1/4-inch fat, broiled	3 oz	175	0.0	7.2
select, 1/4-inch fat, raw	1 lb	744	0.0	36.2
select, 1/4-inch fat, raw	1 oz	46	0.0	2.3
select, 1/2-inch fat, broiled	3 oz	176	0.0	7.1
select, 1/2-inch fat, raw	1 lb	748	0.0	36.3

Food Name	Serv. Size	Total Cal.	Carbs GMS	Fat GMS
select, 1/2-inch fat, raw	1 oz	47	0.0	2.3

SIRLOIN, TOP

Trimmed

Food Name	Serv. Size	Total Cal.	Carbs GMS	Fat GMS
all grades, 0-inch fat, broiled	3 oz	162	0.0	5.8
all grades, 1/4-inch fat, broiled	3 oz	166	0.0	6.1
all grades, 1/2-inch fat, broiled	3 oz	177	0.0	7.4
choice, 0-inch fat, broiled	4 oz	227	0.0	8.8
choice, 0-inch fat, broiled	3 oz	170	0.0	6.6
choice, 1/4-inch fat, broiled	4 oz	229	0.0	9.1
choice, 1/4-inch fat, broiled	3 oz	172	0.0	6.8
choice, 1/4-inch fat, pan-fried	3 oz	202	0.0	9.3
choice, 1/4-inch fat, pan-fried in vegetable oil	4 oz	270	0.0	12.4
choice, 1/2-inch fat, broiled	3 oz	179	0.0	7.7
choice, 1/2-inch fat, pan-fried	3 oz	202	0.0	9.3
prime, 1/2-inch fat, broiled	3 oz	201	0.0	10.1
prime, 1/2-inch fat, raw	1 lb	703	0.0	32.1
prime, 1/2-inch fat, raw	1 oz	44	0.0	2.0
select, 0-inch fat, broiled	3 oz	153	0.0	4.8
select, 1/4-inch fat, broiled	3 oz	158	0.0	5.3
select, 1/2-inch fat, broiled	3 oz	170	0.0	6.6

Untrimmed

Food Name	Serv. Size	Total Cal.	Carbs GMS	Fat GMS
all grades, 0-inch fat, broiled	3 oz	183	0.0	8.5
all grades, 1/4-inch fat, broiled	3 oz	219	0.0	13.1
all grades, 1/4-inch fat, raw	1 lb	984	0.0	68.2
all grades, 1/4-inch fat, raw	1 oz	62	0.0	4.3
all grades, 1/2-inch fat, broiled	3 oz	238	0.0	15.3
all grades, 1/2-inch fat, raw	1 lb	1179	0.0	91.5
all grades, 1/2-inch fat, raw	1 oz	74	0.0	5.7
choice, 0-inch fat, broiled	3 oz	195	0.0	9.8
choice, 1/4-inch fat, broiled	3 oz	229	0.0	14.2
choice, 1/4-inch fat, pan-fried	3 oz	277	0.0	19.4
choice, 1/4-inch fat, pan-fried in vegetable oil	4 oz	370	0.0	25.9
choice, 1/4-inch fat, raw	1 lb	1030	0.0	73.5
choice, 1/4-inch fat, raw	1 oz	64	0.0	4.6
choice, 1/2-inch fat, broiled	3 oz	241	0.0	15.7
choice, 1/2-inch fat, pan-fried	3 oz	288	0.0	20.9
choice, 1/2-inch fat, raw	1 lb	1198	0.0	93.8
choice, 1/2-inch fat, raw	1 oz	75	0.0	5.9
prime, 1/2-inch fat, broiled	3 oz	271	0.0	19.4
prime, 1/2-inch fat, raw	1 lb	1320	0.0	108.0
prime, 1/2-inch fat, raw	1 oz	83	0.0	6.8
select, 0-inch fat, broiled	3 oz	166	0.0	6.4
select, 1/4-inch fat, broiled	3 oz	208	0.0	11.8

Food Name	Serv. Size	Total Cal.	Carbs GMS	Fat GMS
select, 1/4-inch fat, raw	1 lb	939	0.0	62.5
select, 1/4-inch fat, raw	1 oz	59	0.0	3.9
select, 1/2-inch fat, broiled	3 oz	232	0.0	14.8
select, 1/2-inch fat, raw	1 lb	1116	0.0	84.0
select, 1/2-inch fat, raw	1 oz	70	0.0	5.3
SHANK CROSSCUTS				
Trimmed				
choice, 1/4-inch fat, simmered	4 oz	228	0.0	7.2
choice, 1/4-inch fat, simmered	3 oz	171	0.0	5.4
choice, 1/2-inch fat, simmered	3 oz	171	0.0	5.4
Untrimmed				
choice, 1/4-inch fat, raw	1 oz	50	0.0	2.8
choice, 1/4-inch fat, raw	3 oz	150	0.0	8.4
choice, 1/4-inch fat, simmered	3 oz	224	0.0	12.5
choice, 1/2-inch fat, raw	1 lb	721	0.0	35.1
choice, 1/2-inch fat, raw	1 oz	45	0.0	2.2
choice, 1/2-inch fat, simmered	3 oz	207	0.0	10.3
SPLEEN				
braised	3 oz	123	0.0	3.6
calf, raw	100 gm	104	0.0	3.0
raw	4 oz	119	0.0	3.4
T-BONE				
Trimmed				
choice, 1/4-inch fat, broiled	3 oz	182	0.0	8.8
choice, 1/2-inch fat, broiled	3 oz	182	0.0	8.8
Untrimmed				
choice, 1/4-inch fat, broiled	3 oz	253	0.0	18.0
choice, 1/4-inch fat, raw	1 lb	1234	0.0	99.2
choice, 1/4-inch fat, raw	1 oz	77	0.0	6.2
choice, 1/2-inch fat, broiled	3 oz	275	0.0	20.9
choice, 1/2-inch fat, raw	1 lb	1393	0.0	118.5
choice, 1/2-inch fat, raw	1 oz	87	0.0	7.4
TENDERLOIN				
Trimmed				
all grades, 0-inch fat, broiled	3 oz	175	0.0	8.1
all grades, 1/4-inch fat, broiled	3 oz	179	0.0	8.5
all grades, 1/4-inch fat, roasted	3 oz	189	0.0	9.8
all grades, 1/2-inch fat, broiled	3 oz	173	0.0	7.9
all grades, 1/2-inch fat, roasted	3 oz	186	0.0	9.6
choice, 0-inch fat, broiled	3 oz	180	0.0	8.6
choice, 1/4-inch fat, broiled	3 oz	189	0.0	9.5
choice, 1/4-inch fat, roasted	4 oz	262	0.0	14.2
choice, 1/4-inch fat, roasted	3 oz	196	0.0	10.6

Food Name	Serv. Size	Total Cal.		
choice, 1/2-inch fat, broiled	3 oz	176	0.0	8.
choice, 1/2-inch fat, roasted	3 oz	190	0.0	9.9
prime, 1/4-inch fat, broiled	3 oz	197	0.0	10.5
prime, 1/4-inch fat, roasted	3 oz	217	0.0	13.0
prime, 1/2-inch fat, broiled	3 oz	197	0.0	10.5
prime, 1/2-inch fat, roasted	3 oz	217	0.0	13.0
select, 0-inch fat, broiled	3 oz	170	0.0	7.5
select, 1/4-inch fat, broiled	3 oz	169	0.0	7.4
select, 1/4-inch fat, roasted	3 oz	179	0.0	8.8
select, 1/2-inch fat, broiled	3 oz	167	0.0	7.1
select, 1/2-inch fat, roasted	3 oz	177	0.0	8.6
Untrimmed				
all grades, 0-inch fat, broiled	3 oz	200	0.0	11.2
all grades, 1/4-inch fat, broiled	3 oz	247	0.0	17.2
all grades, 1/4-inch fat, raw	1 lb	1284	0.0	104.4
all grades, 1/4-inch fat, raw	1 oz	80	0.0	6.5
all grades, 1/4-inch fat, roasted	3 oz	282	0.0	21.8
all grades, 1/2-inch fat, broiled	3 oz	226	0.0	14.6
all grades, 1/2-inch fat, raw	1 lb	1093	0.0	81.6
all grades, 1/2-inch fat, roasted	3 oz	258	0.0	18.7
choice, 0-inch fat, broiled	3 oz	207	0.0	12.2
choice, 1/4-inch fat, broiled	4 oz	356	0.0	25.6
choice, 1/4-inch fat, broiled	3 oz	258	0.0	18.6
choice, 1/4-inch fat, raw	1 lb	1306	0.0	106.8
choice, 1/4-inch fat, raw	1 oz	82	0.0	6.7
choice, 1/4-inch fat, roasted	3 oz	288	0.0	22.4
choice, 1/2-inch fat, broiled	3 oz	230	0.0	15.1
choice, 1/2-inch fat, raw	1 lb	1116	0.0	83.9
choice, 1/2-inch fat, roasted	3 oz	262	0.0	19.2
prime, 1/4-inch fat, broiled	3 oz	269	0.0	19.9
prime, 1/4-inch fat, raw	1 lb	1288	0.0	104.6
prime, 1/4-inch fat, raw	1 oz	81	0.0	6.5
prime, 1/4-inch fat, roasted	3 oz	300	0.0	23.7
prime, 1/2-inch fat, broiled	3 oz	270	0.0	19.9
prime, 1/2-inch fat, raw	1 lb	1306	0.0	106.8
prime, 1/2-inch fat, roasted	3 oz	304	0.0	24.4
select, 0-inch fat, broiled	3 oz	195	0.0	10.6
select, 1/4-inch fat, broiled	3 oz	230	0.0	15.2
select, 1/4-inch fat, raw	1 lb	1261	0.0	101.6
select, 1/4-inch fat, raw	1 oz	79	0.0	6.3
select, 1/4-inch fat, roasted	3 oz	275	-0.0	21.0
select, 1/2-inch fat, broiled	3 oz	216	0.0	13.4
select, 1/2-inch fat, raw	1 lb	1043	0.0	75.7

Food Name	Serv. Size	Total Cal.	Carbs GMS	Fat GMS
select, 1/2-inch fat, roasted	3 oz	245	0.0	17.3
THYMUS				
braised	3 oz	271	0.0	21.2
raw	4 oz	267	0.0	23.0
TONGUE				
potted or deviled	100 gm	290	0.7	23.0
raw	4 oz	253	4.2	18.2
simmered	3 oz	241	0.3	17.6
smoked	100 gm	328	0.9	28.8
whole, canned or pickled	100 gm	267	0.3	20.3
TOP LOIN				
Trimmed				
all grades, 0-inch fat, broiled	3 oz	168	0.0	7.1
all grades, 1/4-inch fat, broiled	3 oz	176	0.0	8.0
all grades, 1/2-inch fat, broiled	3 oz	173	0.0	7.6
choice, 0-inch fat, broiled	4 oz	237	0.0	10.9
choice, 0-inch fat, broiled	3 oz	178	0.0	8.2
choice, 1/4-inch fat, broiled	4 oz	243	0.0	11.5
choice, 1/4-inch fat, broiled	3 oz	182	0.0	8.6
choice, 1/2-inch fat, broiled	3 oz	176	0.0	8.0
prime, 1/4-inch fat, broiled	3 oz	208	0.0	11.6
prime, 1/2-inch fat, broiled	3 oz	208	0.0	11.6
select, 0-inch fat, broiled	3 oz	156	0.0	5.9
select, 1/4-inch fat, broiled	3 oz	164	0.0	6.6
select, 1/2-inch fat, broiled	3 oz	161	0.0	6.4
Untrimmed				
all grades, 0-inch fat, broiled	3 oz	180	0.0	8.7
all grades, 1/4-inch fat, broiled	3 oz	244	0.0	16.8
all grades, 1/4-inch fat, raw	1 lb	1102	0.0	81.3
all grades, 1/2-inch fat, broiled	3 oz	238	0.0	16.0
all grades, 1/2-inch fat, raw	1 lb	1284	0.0	103.6
choice, 0-inch fat, broiled	3 oz	194	0.0	10.2
choice, 1/4-inch fat, broiled	3 oz	253	0.0	17.8
choice, 1/4-inch fat, raw	1 lb	1179	0.0	90.4
choice, 1/2-inch fat, broiled	3 oz	243	0.0	16.6
choice, 1/2-inch fat, raw	1 lb	1311	0.0	106.7
prime, 1/4-inch fat, broiled	3 oz	275	0.0	20.3
prime, 1/4-inch fat, raw	1 lb	1383	0.0	114.2
prime, 1/2-inch fat, broiled	3 oz	288	0.0	22.0
prime, 1/2-inch fat, raw	1 lb	1461	0.0	123.7
select, 0-inch fat, broiled	3 oz	169	0.0	7.5
select, 1/4-inch fat, broiled	3 oz	226	0.0	14.6
select, 1/4-inch fat, raw	1 lb	1043	0.0	74.6

Food Name	Serv. Size	Total Cal.	Gm.	
select, 1/2-inch fat, broiled	3 oz	223	0.0	14.2
select, 1/2-inch fat, raw	1 lb	1198	0.0	93.0
TRIPE				
canned (Armour)	6 oz	180	1.0	4.0
pickled	100 gm	62	0.0	1.3
raw	4 oz	111	0.0	4.5
BEEF, ALTERNATIVE				
(Heartline) 'Beef Fillet Style'	2 oz	176	9.0	7.0
(Heartline) 'Beef Fillet Style' lite	.5 oz	22	1.0	0.0
(Heartline) 'Ground Beef Style'	2 oz	176	9.0	7.0
(Heartline) 'Ground Beef Style' lite	.5 oz	22	1.0	0.0
(Heartline) 'Teriyaki Beef Style'	2 oz	176	9.0	7.0
Canned				
(Worthington) 'Prime Stakes'	3.25-oz piece	160	7.0	10.0
(Worthington) 'Savory Slices' 2-oz slices	2 slices	100	4.0	6.0
(Worthington) 'Vegetable Steaks' approx 1.28-oz pieces	3.2 oz	110	5.0	2.0
Frozen				
(Worthington) roll, approx 1.25-oz slices	2 slices	130	7.0	6.0
(Worthington) roll, smoked, frozen, approx 2/3-oz slices	3 slices	120	7.0	6.0
(Worthington) 'Stakelets'	2.5 oz	150	7.0	8.0
BEEF, CANNED, chopped (Armour)	3 oz	280	3.0	24.0
BEEF, CORNED				
(Healthy Deli)	1 oz	35	0.7	1.0
(Hillshire Farm)	1 oz	31	<1.0	0.4
(Oscar Mayer)	.6 oz	17	0.1	0.3
brisket, cured, cooked	3 oz	213	0.4	16.1
brisket, cured, raw	1 lb	898	0.6	67.6
brisket, cured, raw	1 oz	56	0.0	4.2
canned (Dinty Moore)	2 oz	130	0.0	8.0
canned, cured	1 oz	71	0.0	4.2
canned, '7-oz can' (Libby's)	2.3 oz	160	2.0	9.0
canned, '12-oz can' (Libby's)	2.4 oz	160	2.0	9.0
'St. Paddy's' (Healthy Deli)	1 oz	24	1.1	0.4
'Slender Sliced' (Eckrich)	1 oz	40	1.0	1.0
BEEF, CORNED, ALTERNATIVE				
roll, frozen (Worthington)	2.5 oz	150	9.0	7.0
roll, frozen (Worthington) approx .5-oz slices	4 slices	120	8.0	6.0
BEEF, CORNED, HASH				
canned (Armour)	7.5 oz	390	18.0	27.0
canned, '15-oz can' (Libby's)	7 1/2 oz	400	20.0	27.0
canned, '15-oz can' (Mary Kitchen)	7 1/2 oz	360	19.0	24.0
canned (Mary Kitchen)	1 oz	47	2.0	3.0
canned (Nalley's)	8 oz	420	27.0	27.0

Food Name	Serv. Size	Total Cal.	Carbs GMS	Fat GMS
canned, 'No Frills' (Pathmark)	7 1/2 oz	410	27.0	26.0
canned, '25-oz can' (Mary Kitchen)	8 1/3 oz	400	19.0	27.0
canned, '24-oz can' (Libby's)	8 oz	420	21.0	28.0
canned, w/potato	1 cup	398	23.5	24.9
microwave cup (Dinty Moore)	7.5 oz	350	19.0	22.0
25% less salt, 'Premium' (Armour)	7.5 oz	350	21.0	21.0
BEEF, CORNED, SPREAD, canned (Hormel)	.5 oz	35	0.0	3.0
BEEF, DRIED				
chipped, cooked, creamed	1 cup	377	17.4	25.2
cured	1 oz	47	0.4	1.1
sliced (Armour)	1.1 oz	60	2.0	2.0
BEEF, GROUND				
Extra lean				
baked, medium-cooked	3 oz	213	0.0	13.7
baked, well-done	3 oz	233	0.0	13.6
broiled, medium-cooked	3 oz	218	0.0	13.9
broiled, well-done	3 oz	225	0.0	13.4
pan-fried, medium-cooked	3 oz	217	0.0	14.0
pan-fried, well-done	3 oz	224	0.0	13.6
raw	1 oz	66	0.0	4.8
raw	4 oz	264	0.0	19.3
Lean				
baked, medium-cooked	3 oz	228	0.0	15.6
baked, well-done	3 oz	248	0.0	15.6
broiled, medium-cooked	3 oz	231	0.0	15.7
broiled, well-done	3 oz	238	0.0	15.0
pan-fried, medium-cooked	3 oz	234	0.0	16.2
pan-fried, well-done	3 oz	235	0.0	15.0
raw	1 oz	75	0.0	5.9
raw	4 oz	298	0.0	23.4
Regular				
baked, medium-cooked	3 oz	244	0.0	17.8
baked, well-done	3 oz	269	0.0	18.3
broiled, frozen patty, medium-cooked	3 oz	240	0.0	16.7
broiled, medium-cooked	3 oz	246	0.0	17.6
broiled, well-done	3 oz	248	0.0	16.5
pan-fried, medium-cooked	3 oz	260	0.0	19.2
pan-fried, well-done	3 oz	243	0.0	16.1
raw	1 oz	88	0.0	7.5
raw	4 oz	350	0.0	30.0
raw, frozen patty	3 oz	240	0.0	19.7
BEEF DINNER, FROZEN. See also BEEF ENTRÉE, FROZEN.				
and gravy (Swanson)	11.25 oz	310	38.0	6.0

Food Name	Serv. Size	Total Cal.	Carbs GMS	Fat GMS
chopped *(Banquet)*	11 oz	420	14.0	32.0
chopped steak, 'Hungry Man' *(Swanson)*	16.75 oz	640	41.0	37.0
'Extra Helping' *(Banquet)*	16 oz	870	50.0	61.0
in barbecue sauce *(Swanson)*	11 oz	460	51.0	17.0
Mexicana *(Budget Gourmet)*	12.8 oz	560	56.0	23.0
patty, charbroiled *(Freezer Queen)*	10 oz	300	20.0	17.0
Salisbury steak *(Banquet)*	11 oz	500	26.0	34.0
Salisbury steak *(Freezer Queen)*	10 oz	380	28.0	22.0
Salisbury steak *(Healthy Choice)*	11.5 oz	300	41.0	7.0
Salisbury steak *(Le Menu)*	10.5 oz	370	28.0	20.0
Salisbury steak *(Morton)*	10 oz	300	23.0	17.0
Salisbury steak *(Swanson)*	10.75 oz	400	43.0	17.0
Salisbury steak, charbroiled flavor 'Healthy Balance' *(Banquet)*	10.5 oz	270	34.0	8.0
Salisbury steak 'Classics' *(Armour)*	11.25 oz	350	26.0	17.0
Salisbury steak 'Classics Lite' *(Armour)*	11.5 oz	300	29.0	2.0
Salisbury steak 'Extra Helping' *(Banquet)*	18 oz	910	49.0	60.0
Salisbury steak 'Hungry Man' *(Swanson)*	16.5 oz	680	37.0	41.0
Salisbury steak 'Lightstyle' *(Le Menu)*	10 oz	280	31.0	9.0
Salisbury steak, parmigiana 'Classics' *(Armour)*	11.5 oz	410	32.0	21.0
Salisbury steak, sirloin *(Budget Gourmet)*	11.5 oz	410	28.0	22.0
Salisbury steak, w/mushroom gravy 'Extra Helping' *(Banquet)*	18 oz	890	48.0	58.0
sirloin, chopped *(Le Menu)*	12.25 oz	430	28.0	24.0
sirloin, chopped *(Swanson)*	10.75 oz	340	28.0	16.0
sirloin, roast, 'Classics' *(Armour)*	10.45 oz	190	21.0	4.0
sirloin, w/barbecue sauce *(Healthy Choice)*	11 oz	280	44.0	4.0
sirloin tips *(Healthy Choice)*	11.25 oz	270	29.0	7.0
sliced *(Morton)*	10 oz	220	20.0	5.0
sliced, 'Hungry Man' *(Swanson)*	15.25 oz	450	49.0	12.0
sliced, w/gravy *(Freezer Queen)*	10 oz	210	18.0	7.0
steak Diane, 'Classics Lite' *(Armour)*	10 oz	290	25.0	9.0
tips *(Le Menu)*	11.5 oz	400	29.0	18.0
tips 'Classics' *(Armour)*	10.25 oz	230	20.0	7.0
tips, in Burgundy sauce *(Budget Gourmet)*	11 oz	310	28.0	11.0
BEEF ENTRÉE, ALTERNATIVE				
'Country Stew' *(Worthington)*	9.5 oz	220	23.0	10.0
pie, frozen *(Worthington)*	8 oz	360	44.0	16.0
BEEF ENTRÉE, CANNED				
chow mein *(LaChoy)*	3/4 cup	40	5.0	2.0
chow mein, 'Bi-Pack' *(LaChoy)*	8.748 oz	83	11.1	0.9
chow mein, 'Bi-Pack' *(LaChoy)*	3/4 cup	70	8.0	1.0
Oriental, w/noodles, 'Bi-Pack' *(LaChoy)*	9 oz	148	24.3	1.2

Food Name	Serv. Size	Total Cal.	Carbs GMS	Fat GMS
pepper, 'Bi-Pack' (LaChoy)	3/4 cup	80	10.0	2.0
pepper Oriental, 'Bi-Pack' (LaChoy)	8.783 oz	101	12.7	2.0
pepper Oriental, 'Bi-Pack' (LaChoy)	3/4 cup	80	10.0	2.0
stew (Armour)	8 oz	210	16.0	11.0
stew (Dinty Moore)	8 oz	220	16.0	13.0
stew (Estee)	7.5 oz	210	15.0	11.0
stew (Featherweight)	7.5 oz	160	17.0	3.0
stew (Wolf Brand)	1 cup	179	18.3	7.5
stew, 'Big Chunk' (Nalley's)	7.5 oz	200	24.0	7.0
stew, '15-oz can' (Dinty Moore)	7.5 oz	200	15.0	12.0
stew, '15-oz pkg' (Libby's)	7.5 oz	160	18.0	5.0
stew, 'Homestyle' (Nalley's)	8 oz	180	22.0	5.0
stew, '40-oz can' (Dinty Moore)	8 oz	210	16.0	11.0
stew, 'No Frills' (Pathmark)	8 oz	190	25.0	4.0
stew, '24-oz can' (Dinty Moore)	8 oz	220	15.0	12.0
stew, '24-oz pkg' (Libby's)	8 oz	170	19.0	6.0
pepper Oriental (LaChoy)	3/4 cup	100	12.0	4.0
BEEF ENTRÉE, FREEZE-DRIED				
beef and rice w/onions, prepared (Mountain House)	1 cup	330	42.0	12.0
stew, prepared (Mountain House)	1 cup	260	26.0	9.0
BEEF ENTRÉE, FROZEN. See also BEEF DINNER, FROZEN.				
and broccoli, w/rice, 'Fresh & Lite' (LaChoy)	11 oz	260	42.0	5.0
Cantonese, w/rice, 'Stir Fry' (Weight Watchers)	9 oz	200	27.0	4.0
casserole, 'Microwave Classic' (Pillsbury)	1 pkg	430	34.0	25.0
champignon, 'Gourmet Selection' (Tyson)	10.5 oz	370	31.0	15.0
creamed, chipped (Myers)	3.5 oz	136	7.0	8.0
creamed, chipped (Stouffer's)	5.5 oz	230	9.0	17.0
creamed, chipped, 'Cookin' Bag' (Banquet)	4 oz	100	9.0	4.0
creamed, chipped, 'Cook-In-Pouch' (Freezer Queen)	5 oz	80	11.0	2.0
Dijon, w/pasta and vegetables (Right Course)	9.5 oz	290	31.0	9.0
fiesta, w/corn pasta (Right Course)	8 7/8 oz	270	33.0	7.0
homestyle, w/noodles, gravy, and vegetable (Stouffer's)	8 3/8 oz	230	26.0	7.0
Jade garden, 'Stir Fry' (Weight Watchers)	9 oz	150	17.0	3.0
London broil (Ultimate 200)	7.5 oz	110	4.0	3.0
London broil, in mushroom sauce (Weight Watchers)	7.37 oz	140	9.0	3.0
Oriental, w/vegetables and rice (Lean Cuisine)	8 5/8 oz	290	31.0	9.0
patty, charbroiled, w/mushroom and onion gravy (Banquet)	8 oz	300	14.0	21.0
patty, charbroiled, w/ mushroom and onion gravy (Freezer Queen)	7 oz	200	10.0	12.0
patty, charbroiled, w/mushroom gravy (Banquet)	8 oz	290	13.0	21.0
patty, charbroiled, w/mushroom gravy (Banquet)	5 oz	210	8.0	15.0
patty, charbroiled, w/ mushroom gravy (Freezer Queen)	7 oz	180	9.0	11.0
patty, charbroiled, w/ mushroom gravy (Freezer Queen)	5 oz	90	7.0	3.0

Food Name	Serv. Size	Total Cal.	Carbs GMS	Fat GMS
pepper, Oriental *(Chun King)*	13 oz	310	53.0	3.0
pie *(Banquet)*	7 oz	510	39.0	33.0
pie *(Myers)*	3.5 oz	123	10.0	6.0
pie *(Stouffer's)*	10 oz	460	37.0	27.0
pie, 'Supreme Microwave' *(Banquet)*	7 oz	440	30.0	29.0
'Platters' *(Banquet)*	10 oz	460	20.0	34.0
pot pie *(Swanson)*	7 oz	370	36.0	19.0
pot pie, 'Hungry Man' *(Swanson)*	16 oz	610	58.0	31.0
ragoût, w/rice pilaf *(Right Course)*	10 oz	300	38.0	8.0
rib, boneless, seasoned, w/barbecue sauce *(Healthy Choice)*	11 oz	330	40.0	6.0
Romanoff supreme, w/pasta and vegetables *(Weight Watchers)*	9 oz	230	29.0	7.0
Salisbury steak *(Dining Lite)*	9 oz	200	14.0	8.0
Salisbury steak, charbroiled, w/vegetable medley 'Single Serve' *(Freezer Queen)*	9 oz	330	14.0	22.0
Salisbury steak, homestyle, w/gravy, macaroni and cheese *(Stouffer's)*	9 5/8 oz	350	23.0	17.0
Salisbury steak, 'Homestyle Recipe' *(Swanson)*	10 oz	320	22.0	16.0
Salisbury steak, supreme 'Gourmet Selection' *(Tyson)*	10 oz	430	34.0	26.0
Salisbury steak, w/gravy 'Cook-In-Pouch' *(Freezer Queen)*	5 oz	160	7.0	11.0
Salisbury steak, w/gravy 'Cookin' Bags' *(Banquet)*	5 oz	190	8.0	14.0
Salisbury steak, w/gravy 'Family Entrées' *(Banquet)*	8 oz	300	12.0	22.0
Salisbury steak, w/gravy 'Family Suppers' *(Freezer Queen)*	7 oz	200	9.0	13.0
Salisbury steak, w/gravy and scalloped potatoes *(Lean Cuisine)*	9.5 oz	240	22.0	7.0
Salisbury steak, w/mushroom gravy 'Classics' *(Healthy Choice)*	11 oz	280	35.0	6.0
sirloin roast *(Budget Gourmet)*	9.5 oz	330	36.0	14.0
sirloin tips *(Ultimate 200)*	7.5 oz	200	20.0	6.0
sirloin tips, w/Burgundy sauce, Homestyle Recipe *(Swanson)*	7 oz	160	16.0	5.0
sirloin tips, w/country-style vegetables *(Budget Gourmet)*	10 oz	310	21.0	18.0
sliced beef, w/barbecue sauce, 'Cookin' Bag' *(Banquet)*	4 oz	100	11.0	2.0
sliced beef, w/gravy, 'Cookin' Bag' *(Banquet)*	4 oz	100	5.0	5.0
sliced beef, w/gravy, 'Cook-In-Pouch' *(Freezer Queen)*	4 oz	60	4.0	1.0
sliced beef, w/gravy, 'Deluxe Family Suppers' *(Freezer Queen)*	7 oz	130	10.0	3.0
sliced beef, w/gravy, 'Family Entrées' *(Banquet)*	8 oz	160	8.0	5.0
steak, breaded *(Hormel)*	4 oz	370	13.0	30.0
steak and mushroom hand-held pie, 'Aussie Pie' *(Mrs. Paterson's)*	5.5 oz	410	43.0	20.0
Szechuan *(Chun King)*	13 oz	340	57.0	3.0

Food Name	Serv. Size	Total Cal.	Carbs GMS	Fat GMS
teriyaki *(Chun King)*	13 oz	380	68.0	2.0
teriyaki *(Dining Lite)*	9 oz	270	36.0	5.0
teriyaki, w/rice and vegetables, 'Fresh & Lite' *(LaChoy)*	10 oz	240	39.9	5.0
stew, 'Family Entrées' *(Banquet)*	7 oz	140	18.0	5.0
stew, 'Family Suppers' *(Freezer Queen)*	7 oz	150	15.0	6.0
BEEF ENTRÉE, MICROWAVE				
beef and mushrooms, 'Health Selections' micro cup *(Hormel)*	7 oz	210	25.0	3.0
ribs, boneless, microwave bowl *(Top Shelf)*	1 serving	440	29.0	24.0
roast, tender, microwave bowl *(Top Shelf)*	1 serving	240	18.0	7.0
roast beef, w/gravy and potatoes, 'American Classics' *(Dinty Moore)*	10 oz	260	26.0	6.0
Salisbury steak, w/potatoes, microwave bowl *(Top Shelf)*	1 serving	254	22.0	6.0
stew *(Armour)*	7.5 oz	150	15.0	5.0
stew, chunky, microwave cup *(Weight Watchers)*	7.5 oz	120	14.0	2.0
stew, 'Diner' microwave cup *(Libby's)*	7.75 oz	240	22.0	12.0
stew, hearty, 'Microeasy,' 1/4 pkg prepared w/1.5 lbs beef *(Lipton)*	1 serving	370	14.0	20.0
stew, hearty, microwave cup *(Lunch Bucket)*	7.5 oz	180	13.0	11.0
stew, micro cup *(Hormel)*	7.5 oz	230	11.0	15.0
stew, microwave bowl *(Dinty Moore)*	10 oz	260	19.0	14.0
stew, microwave cup *(Dinty Moore)*	7.5 oz	180	15.0	9.0
sukiyaki, microwave bowl *(Top Shelf)*	1 serving	330	36.0	10.0
w/macaroni, 'Diner' microwave cup *(Libby's)*	7.75 oz	230	34.0	6.0
BEEF ENTRÉE, PACKAGED				
Salisbury steak *(Top Shelf)*	10 oz	320	22.0	15.0
Salisbury steak, w/mushroom gravy *(Ultra Slim Fast)*	10.5 oz	290	44.0	5.0
BEEF JERKY				
'Arrowhead' *(Pemmican)*	.7-oz piece	70	2.0	3.0
'Big Jerk' *(Slim Jim)*	.25-oz piece	25	1.0	1.0
'Giant Jerk' *(Slim Jim)*	.63-oz piece	60	2.0	2.0
jalapeño *(Pemmican)*	1.3-oz piece	110	5.0	3.0
jalapeño *(Pemmican)*	1.1 oz	90	4.0	2.0
jalapeño flavored steak *(Pemmican)*	.25 oz	25	1.0	1.0
'Lumberjack' *(Hormel)*	1 oz	101	0.0	9.0
natural *(Pemmican)*	1.3-oz piece	110	5.0	3.0
natural *(Pemmican)*	1.1 oz	90	4.0	2.0
natural *(Pemmican)*	1 oz	80	4.0	2.0
natural flavored steak *(Pemmican)*	.25 oz	25	1.0	1.0
peppered *(Pemmican)*	1.3-oz piece	110	5.0	3.0
peppered *(Pemmican)*	1.1 oz	90	4.0	2.0
peppered steak *(Pemmican)*	.25 oz	25	1.0	1.0
regular *(Frito-Lay's)*	.21 oz	25	1.0	1.0

Food Name	Serv. Size	Total Cal.	Carbs GMS	Fat GMS
regular *(Hickory Farms)*	1 oz	100	4.0	3.0
regular *(Slim Jim)*	.14-oz piece	20	1.0	1.0
regular 'Super Jerk' approx .31 oz *(Slim Jim)*	1 piece	30	1.0	1.0
'Steakers' *(Pemmican)*	1.1-oz pouch	80	4.0	1.0
'Steakers' *(Pemmican)*	1 strip	40	2.0	1.0
Tabasco *(Pemmican)*	1.3-oz piece	110	5.0	3.0
Tabasco *(Pemmican)*	1.1 oz	90	4.0	2.0
Tabasco flavored steak *(Pemmican)*	.25 oz	25	1.0	1.0
Tabasco 'Super Jerk' *(Slim Jim)*	.31-oz piece	30	1.0	1.0
'Tender' *(Frito-Lay's)*	.7 oz	120	2.0	10.0
'Tender Brave' *(Pemmican)*	1 oz	80	2.0	2.0
'Tender Chief' *(Pemmican)*	1 oz	80	2.0	2.0
'Tender Tomahawk' *(Pemmican)*	.25-oz piece	20	1.0	1.0
'Tender Trail' *(Pemmican)*	1 oz	80	2.0	2.0
'Tender Tribe' *(Pemmican)*	1 oz	80	2.0	2.0
teriyaki, natural style *(Pemmican)*	1 oz	80	4.0	2.0
teriyaki, natural style *(Pemmican)*	.25-oz piece	20	1.0	1.0
teriyaki, natural style, slab *(Pemmican)*	1.3 oz	100	5.0	2.0
BEEF JERKY, ALTERNATIVE				
'Jerquee' vegetable protein product *(Stonewall's)*	.5 oz	50	2.0	2.0
'Spicy Italian Style' *(Cajun Jerky)*	.5 oz	50	2.0	2.0
BEEF POT PIE. See BEEF ENTRÉE, FROZEN.				
BEEF SEASONING MIX				
(French's) dry ground, w/onions	1/4 pkg	25	6.0	0.0
(Lawry's) marinade	1 pkg	49	10.7	0.2
(Schilling) Stroganoff	1/4 pkg	32	6.0	0.3
BEEF STEW. See BEEF ENTRÉE, CANNED; BEEF ENTRÉE, FREEZE-DRIED; BEEF ENTRÉE, FROZEN; BEEF ENTRÉE, MICROWAVE.				
BEEF STEW MIX, hearty, 'Microeasy' *(Lipton)* dry	1/4 pkg	70	14.0	<1.0
BEEF STEW SEASONING MIX				
(French's) dry mix	1/6 pkg	25	5.0	0.0
(Lawry's) 'Seasoning Blends'	1 pkg	131	25.7	0.7
(Schilling)	1/2 pkg	33	6.0	0.3
(Schilling) 'Bag'n Season'	1 pkg	87	11.0	1.0
BEEF SUET, raw	1 oz	242	0.0	26.7
BEEF TALLOW				
	1 cup	1849	0.0	205.0
	1 oz	256	0.0	28.4
	1 tbsp	115	0.0	12.8
BEEFALO				
composite of cuts, diced, roasted	1 cup	263	0.0	8.8
composite of cuts, roasted	4 oz	213	0.0	7.2
raw	1 lb	649	0.0	21.8

Food Name	Serv. Size	Total Cal.	Carbs GMS	Fat GMS
raw	1 oz	40	0.0	1.3
roasted	3 oz	160	0.0	5.4

BEER. See ALCOHOLIC BEVERAGES.

BEER, NONALCOHOLIC. See ALCOHOL-FREE BEVERAGES.

BEER SALAMI. See LUNCHEON MEAT.

BEERWURST

Food Name	Serv. Size	Total Cal.	Carbs GMS	Fat GMS
beef	1 oz	92	0.5	8.3
beef, 4-inch diam	1/8-inch slice	76	0.4	6.9
beef, 2.75-inch diam	1/16-inch slice	20	0.1	1.8
pork	1 oz	67	0.6	5.3
pork, 4-inch diam	1/8-inch slice	55	0.5	4.3
pork, 2.75-inch diam	1/16-inch slice	14	0.1	1.1
pork, cured, 4-inch diam	1/8-inch slice	55	0.5	4.3
pork, cured, 2.75-inch diam	1/16-inch slice	14	0.1	1.1

BEET

Food Name	Serv. Size	Total Cal.	Carbs GMS	Fat GMS
boiled, drained	4 oz	35	7.6	0.1
boiled, drained, sliced	1/2 cup	37	8.5	0.2
raw, sliced	1/2 cup	29	6.5	0.1
raw, trimmed	1 oz	12	2.8	<.1
raw, untrimmed	1 lb	133	30.4	0.4

BEET, CANNED

Food Name	Serv. Size	Total Cal.	Carbs GMS	Fat GMS
cut *(Stokely)*	1/2 cup	40	8.0	0.0
diced *(S&W)*	1/2 cup	40	9.0	0.0
diced *(Stokely)*	1/2 cup	35	7.0	0.0
Harvard *(Stokely)*	1/2 cup	70	18.0	0.0
Harvard, sliced, w/liquid	1/2 cup	90	22.4	0.1
julienne *(S&W)*	1/2 cup	40	9.0	0.0
'No Salt or Sugar Added' *(Stokely)*	1/2 cup	40	8.0	0.0
pickled *(Freshlike)*	1/2 cup	40	9.0	0.0
pickled *(Stokely)*	1/2 cup	100	25.0	0.0
pickled *(Veg•All)*	1/2 cup	100	25.0	0.0
pickled, crinkle sliced, w/liquid *(Del Monte)*	1/2 cup	80	19.0	0.0
pickled 'Jars' *(Stokely)*	1/2 cup	90	22.0	0.0
pickled, sliced, w/liquid	1/2 cup	74	18.6	0.1
pickled, sliced, w/red wine vinegar 'Party' *(S&W)*	1/2 cup	70	16.0	0.0
pickled, sliced, w/red wine vinegar 'Regular' *(S&W)*	1/2 cup	70	16.0	0.0
pickled, whole, extra small *(S&W)*	1/2 cup	70	16.0	0.0
regular pack, w/liquid	1/2 cup	36	8.3	0.1
sliced *(A&P)*	1/2 cup	40	9.0	<1.0
sliced *(Featherweight)*	1/2 cup	45	10.0	0.0
sliced *(Finast)*	1/2 cup	40	9.0	0.0
sliced *(Pathmark)*	1/2 cup	45	10.0	0.0
sliced *(S&W Nutradiet)*	1/2 cup	35	9.0	0.0

Food Name	Serv. Size	Total Cal.	Carbs GMS	Fat GMS
sliced *(Stokely)*	1/2 cup	40	8.0	0.0
sliced, drained	1/2 cup	26	6.1	0.1
sliced, 'No Salt Added' *(A&P)*	1/2 cup	35	8.0	<1.0
sliced, 'No Salt Added' *(Finast)*	1/2 cup	40	9.0	0.0
sliced, 'No Salt Added' *(Pathmark)*	1/2 cup	35	7.0	0.0
sliced, water packed, w/o salt *(Freshlike)*	1/2 cup	40	9.0	0.0
sliced, water packed, w/o sugar or salt *(Freshlike)*	1/2 cup	40	9.0	0.0
sliced, w/liquid, 'No Salt Added' *(Del Monte)*	1/2 cup	35	8.0	0.0
small, sliced *(Freshlike)*	1/2 cup	40	9.0	0.0
small, sliced, 'Premium' *(S&W)*	1/2 cup	40	9.0	0.0
small, whole *(Freshlike)*	1/2 cup	40	9.0	0.0
small, whole *(S&W)*	1/2 cup	40	9.0	0.0
special dietary pack, w/liquid	1/2 cup	36	8.3	0.1
tiny, whole, w/liquid *(Del Monte)*	1/2 cup	35	8.0	0.0
whole *(A&P)*	1/2 cup	40	9.0	<1.0
whole *(IGA)*	1/2 cup	40	9.0	0.0
whole *(Stokely)*	1/2 cup	40	8.0	0.0
whole, sliced, w/liquid *(Del Monte)*	1/2 cup	35	8.0	0.0
BEET GREENS				
boiled, drained	4 oz	31	6.2	0.2
boiled, drained, 1-inch pieces	1/2 cup	19	3.9	0.1
raw, approx 2 oz	1 leaf	6	1.3	<.1
raw, 1-inch pieces	1/2 cup	4	0.8	0.0
raw, untrimmed	1 lb	49	10.1	0.2
raw, untrimmed	1 oz	5	1.1	<.1
BEET ROOT JUICE, bottled *(Biotta)*	6 oz	75	15.9	0.1
BELLYFISH. See MONKFISH.				
BERLINER				
beef and pork	1 oz	65	0.7	4.9
beef and pork, 2.5-inch diam	1/4-inch slice	53	0.6	4.0
BERRY DRINK				
'Berries & Berries' *(Tropicana)*	6 oz	90	23.0	<1.0
'Berries & Berries' juice *(Tropicana)*	10 oz	156	39.0	0.0
'Berry B. Wild' *(Squeezit)*	6.75 oz	120	29.0	0.0
berry blend juice, 'Fruit Box' *(Tang)*	8.45 oz	140	36.0	0.0
berry citrus drink, frozen, prepared *(Five Alive)*	6 oz	90	22.0	0.0
berry juice, bottled *(Juicy Juice)*	6 oz	90	22.0	0.0
berry juice, boxed *(Juicy Juice)*	8.45 oz	130	30.0	0.0
berry juice, canned *(Juicy Juice)*	6 oz	90	22.0	0.0
berry nectar, organic *(Santa Cruz Natural)*	8 oz	90	22.0	<1.0
berry punch, aseptic box or chilled *(Minute Maid)*	6 oz	90	23.0	0.0
berry punch, frozen concentrate *(Minute Maid)*	6 oz	90	23.0	0.0
'Bopin' Berry' *(Hi-C)*	6 oz	90	23.0	0.0

Food Name	Serv. Size	Total Cal.	Carbs GMS	Fat GMS
'Great Bluedini' *(Kool-Aid)* 'Kool Bursts'	6.75 oz	110	28.0	0.0
'Great Bluedini' *(Kool-Aid)* 'Koolers'	8.45 oz	110	29.0	0.0
Mountain Berry Punch *(Kool-Aid)* 'Koolers'	8.45 oz	140	37.0	0.0
'Very Berry' *(Hawaiian Punch)*	6 oz	90	22.0	0.0
BERRY DRINK MIX				
berry blend, sugar-free w/NutraSweet, prepared *(Crystal Light)*	8 oz	4	0.0	0.0
'Berry Blue' sugar-free w/NutraSweet, prepared *(Kool-Aid)*	8 oz	4	0.0	0.0
'Berry Blue' sugar-sweetened, prepared *(Kool-Aid)*	8 oz	80	21.0	0.0
'Berry Blue' unsweetened, prepared w/sugar *(Kool-Aid)*	8 oz	100	25.0	0.0
'Berry Blue' unsweetened, prepared w/o sugar *(Kool-Aid)*	8 oz	2	0.0	0.0
'Great Bluedini' sugar-free w/NutraSweet, prepared *(Kool-Aid)*	8 oz	4	0.0	0.0
'Great Bluedini' sugar-sweetened, prepared *(Kool-Aid)*	8 oz	70	18.0	0.0
'Great Bluedini' unsweetened, prepared w/sugar *(Kool-Aid)*	8 oz	100	25.0	0.0
'Great Bluedini' unsweetened, prepared w/o sugar *(Kool-Aid)*	8 oz	2	0.0	0.0
Mountain Berry Punch, sugar-free w/NutraSweet, prepared *(Kool-Aid)*	8 oz	4	0.0	0.0
Mountain Berry Punch, sugar-sweetened, prepared *(Kool-Aid)*	8 oz	80	20.0	0.0
Mountain Berry Punch, unsweetened, prepared w/sugar *(Kool-Aid)*	8 oz	100	25.0	0.0
Mountain Berry Punch, unsweetened, prepared w/o sugar *(Kool-Aid)*	8 oz	2	0.0	0.0
'Surfin' Berry' sugar-free w/NutraSweet, prepared *(Kool-Aid)*	8 oz	4	0.0	0.0
'Surfin' Berry' unsweetened, prepared w/sugar *(Kool-Aid)*	8 oz	100	25.0	0.0
'Surfin' Berry' unsweetened, prepared w/o sugar *(Kool-Aid)*	8 oz	2	0.0	0.0

BEVERAGES. See ALCOHOL-FREE BEVERAGES; ALCOHOLIC BEVERAGES; COFFEE; DIET DRINK; MILK; SOFT DRINKS AND MIXERS; SPORTS DRINK; TEA; WATER; and individual listings.

BIBB LETTUCE. See LETTUCE.

BISCUIT

Food Name	Serv. Size	Total Cal.	Carbs GMS	Fat GMS
buttermilk, commercially baked	1 oz	103	13.8	4.7
mixed grain, dough, baked	1 oz	86	15.6	1.8
plain, commercially baked	1 oz	103	13.8	4.7
(Awrey's) country	3-inch biscuit	160	23.0	5.0
(Awrey's) round	1 oz	80	12.0	3.0
(Awrey's) sliced	2 oz	160	23.0	5.0
(Awrey's) square	1 oz	80	12.0	3.0

Food Name	Serv. Size	Total Cal.	Carbs GMS	Fat GMS
(Awrey's) unsliced	2 oz	160	23.0	5.0
(Mrs. Winner's)	1 biscuit	245	45.0	5.0
(Weight Watchers) buttermilk	1.8 oz	100	23.0	1.0
(Wonder)	1 biscuit	80	14.0	1.0
BISCUIT, FROZEN (Bridgford)	2 oz	180	28.0	6.0
BISCUIT, REFRIGERATED				
(Ballard) buttermilk, extra lights, 'Ovenready'	1 biscuit	50	10.0	0.0
(Ballard) buttermilk, 'Ovenready'	1 biscuit	50	10.0	1.0
(Ballard) extra lights, 'Ovenready'	1 biscuit	50	10.0	0.0
(Ballard) 'Ovenready'	1 biscuit	50	10.0	1.0
(Big Country) 'Butter Tastin''	1 biscuit	100	14.0	4.0
(Big Country) buttermilk	1 biscuit	100	14.0	4.0
(Big Country) Southern style	1 biscuit	100	14.0	4.0
(1869 Brand) baking powder	1 biscuit	100	12.0	5.0
(1869 Brand) 'Butter Tastin'	1 biscuit	100	12.0	5.0
(1869 Brand) buttermilk	1 biscuit	100	12.0	5.0
(Good 'N Buttery) fluffy	1 biscuit	90	11.0	5.0
(Grands Inch) 'Butter Tastin'	1 biscuit	190	22.0	9.0
(Grands Inch) cinnamon raisin	1 biscuit	190	27.0	7.0
(Grands Inch) flaky	1 biscuit	190	23.0	8.0
(Hungry Jack) buttermilk, 'Extra Rich'	1 biscuit	50	9.0	1.0
(Hungry Jack) buttermilk, flaky	1 biscuit	90	12.0	4.0
(Hungry Jack) buttermilk, fluffy	1 biscuit	90	12.0	4.0
(Hungry Jack) flaky, 'Butter Tastin''	1 biscuit	90	11.0	4.0
(Hungry Jack) flaky	1 biscuit	80	12.0	4.0
(Hungry Jack) honey, flaky, 'Honey Tastin''	1 biscuit	90	13.0	4.0
(Hungry Jack) Southern style, flaky	1 biscuit	80	12.0	4.0
(Pillsbury) 'Big Premium Heat 'n Eat'	2 biscuits	280	32.0	15.0
(Pillsbury) butter	1 biscuit	50	10.0	1.0
(Pillsbury) buttermilk, 'Heat 'n Eat'	2 biscuits	170	27.0	5.0
(Pillsbury) buttermilk	1 biscuit	50	10.0	1.0
(Pillsbury) buttermilk, 'Tender Layer'	1 biscuit	50	9.0	1.0
(Pillsbury) 'Country'	1 biscuit	50	10.0	1.0
(Roman Meal) oat bran, honey nut	1 biscuit	131	19.7	4.7
(Roman Meal) white	2 biscuits	180	32.2	3.8
(Roman Meal) white, 'Premium'	1 biscuit	127	18.8	4.7
BISCUIT, TOASTER				
(Oroweat) 'Australian'	1 biscuit	180	30.0	5.0
(Oroweat) cinnamon raisin	1 biscuit	200	34.0	5.0
(Oroweat) cornbread	1 biscuit	200	39.0	3.0
BISCUIT MIX				
(Arrowhead Mills)	2 oz	100	19.0	1.0
(Bisquick)	1/2 cup	240	37.0	8.0

Food Name	Serv. Size	Total Cal.	Carbs GMS	Fat GMS
(Gold Medal) 'Pouch Mix,' prepared w/skim milk	1/8 recipe	90	14.0	3.0
(Health Valley) buttermilk, 'Biscuit & Pancake'	1 oz	100	20.0	1.0
(Krusteaz) cinnamon raisin, w/glaze, prepared from mix	3-inch biscuit	200	39.0	4.0
(Krusteaz) prepared from mix	2-inch biscuit	90	14.0	3.0
(Martha White) prepared from mix, 'BixMix,' made w/2% milk, rolled	2-inch biscuit	90	15.0	2.0
(Robin Hood) 'Pouch Mix,' prepared w/skim milk	1/8 recipe	90	14.0	3.0

BISON. See BUFFALO, AMERICAN.

BLACK BEAN

boiled	4 oz	150	26.9	0.6
boiled	1/2 cup	114	20.4	0.5
raw	1/2 cup	331	60.5	1.4
raw	1 oz	97	17.7	0.4
raw *(Arrowhead Mills)*	2 oz	190	35.0	1.0

BLACK BEAN, CANNED

(Eden Foods) organic, very low sodium, no salt added	1/2 cup	70	17.0	<1.0
(Green Giant)	1/2 cup	90	21.0	0.0
(Joan of Arc)	1/2 cup	90	21.0	0.0
(Progresso)	1/2 cup	90	19.0	1.0

BLACK BEAN DINNER, CANNED

Western, w/garden vegetables, 'Fast Menu' *(Health Valley)*	7.5 oz	120	14.0	1.0

BLACK BEAN MIX, INSTANT

prepared w/o added ingredients *(Fantastic Foods)*	1/2 cup	157	28.0	2.0
prepared w/2 tbsp salted butter *(Fantastic Foods)*	1/2 cup	207	28.0	8.0

BLACK CHERRY DRINK MIX

unsweetened, prepared w/sugar *(Kool-Aid)*	8 oz	100	25.0	0.0
unsweetened, prepared w/o sugar *(Kool-Aid)*	8 oz	2	0.0	0.0

BLACK CHERRY JUICE

(Knudsen & Sons)	8 oz	150	38.0	0.0
(Smucker's) 'Naturally 100%'	8 oz	130	31.0	0.0

BLACK PUDDING. See BLOOD SAUSAGE.

BLACK TURTLE BEAN

boiled	1/2 cup	120	22.4	0.3
canned	1/2 cup	109	19.9	0.4
raw	1/2 cup	312	58.2	0.8

BLACK WALNUT FLAVOR DRINK

canned, liquid nutrition *(Ensure)*	8 oz	250	34.3	8.8

BLACKBERRY

raw	1/2 cup	37	9.2	0.3
trimmed	1 oz	15	3.6	0.1
untrimmed	1 lb	225	56.0	1.7

Food Name	Serv. Size	Total Cal.	Carbs GMS	Fat GMS
BLACKBERRY, CANNED				
in heavy syrup	4 oz	104	26.2	0.2
in heavy syrup, w/liquid	1/2 cup	118	29.6	0.2
in water (Allens)	1/2 cup	25	4.0	<1.0
BLACKBERRY, FROZEN				
unsweetened	18-oz pkg	326	79.9	2.2
unsweetened	1 cup	97	23.7	0.7
unsweetened	1/2 cup	49	11.8	0.3
BLACKBERRY SYRUP (Knott's Berry Farm)	1 oz	120	30.0	0.0
BLACK-EYED PEAS/cowpeas/yellow-eyed peas				
boiled, drained	1/2 cup	79	16.7	0.3
boiled, drained	4 oz	110	23.1	0.4
leafy tips, boiled, drained	4 oz	25	3.2	0.1
leafy tips, raw, chopped	1/2 cup	5	0.9	<.1
leafy tips, raw, trimmed	1 oz	8	1.4	0.1
leafy tips, raw, untrimmed	1 lb	68	11.4	0.6
raw, in pods	1 lb	208	43.7	0.8
raw, trimmed	1 oz	26	5.4	0.1
raw, trimmed	1/2 cup	65	13.6	0.3
young pods w/seeds, raw, approx 11 7/8 inches x 5/16 inch	1 pod	5	1.1	<.1
young pods, w/seeds, raw, trimmed	1 oz	12	2.7	0.1
young pods, w/seeds, raw, trimmed	1/2 cup	21	4.5	0.1
young pods, w/seeds, raw, untrimmed	1 lb	182	39.2	1.2
BLACK-EYED PEAS, CANNED				
(A&P) mature	7.5 oz	120	20.0	1.0
(Allens)	1/2 cup	100	18.0	<1.0
(Allens) mature	1/2 cup	105	18.0	1.0
(Allens) w/snaps	1/2 cup	100	20.0	<1.0
(Bush's Best) packed from fresh shelled	1/2 cup	70	16.0	0.0
(Bush's Best) packed from soaked dry	1/2 cup	70	16.0	0.0
(Bush's Best) seasoned w/bacon	1/2 cup	90	16.0	1.0
(Green Giant) mature	1/2 cup	90	18.0	1.0
(Joan of Arc) mature	1/2 cup	90	18.0	1.0
(Luck's) mature, w/pork	1/2 cup	200	25.0	6.0
BLACK-EYED PEAS, DRIED				
mature, boiled	1/2 cup	100	17.9	0.5
mature, boiled	4 oz	132	23.6	0.6
mature, boiled (A&P)	1 cup	230	41.0	1.0
mature, raw	1 oz	95	17.0	0.4
mature, raw	1/2 cup	283	50.4	1.1
BLACK-EYED PEAS, FROZEN				
	10-oz pkg	396	71.4	2.0

Food Name	Serv. Size	Total Cal.	Carbs GMS	Fat GMS
boiled, drained	1/2 cup	112	20.2	0.6
boiled, drained	4 oz	150	26.9	0.7
(Freshlike)	3.3 oz	130	23.0	1.0
(Frosty Acres)	3.3 oz	130	23.0	1.0
(Seabrook)	3.3 oz	130	23.0	1.0
(Southern)	3.5 oz	136	24.2	0.7
(Veg•All)	3.3 oz	130	23.0	1.0
BLINTZ				
(Golden) blueberry	1 blintz	90	18.0	1.0
(Golden) cheese, low fat	1 blintz	80	13.0	2.0
(Golden) cherry	1 blintz	95	18.0	1.0
(King Kold) frozen	2.5 oz	113	18.9	1.6
(King Kold) frozen 'No Salt Added'	1.5 oz	96	18.6	0.5
BLOOD PUDDING. See BLOOD SAUSAGE.				
BLOOD SAUSAGE/black pudding/blood pudding				
	1 oz	107	0.4	9.8
approx 5 inches x 4 5/8 inches	1/16-inch slice	94	0.3	8.6
BLOODY MARY. See ALCOHOLIC BEVERAGES.				
BLOODY MARY MIX. See ALCOHOL-FREE BEVERAGES.				
BLUEBERRY				
trimmed	1 pint	225	56.8	1.5
trimmed	1 cup	81	20.5	0.6
trimmed	1/2 cup	41	10.2	0.3
trimmed	1 oz	16	4.0	0.1
untrimmed	1 lb	250	62.8	1.7
untrimmed	1 pint	226	56.8	1.5
BLUEBERRY, CANNED				
in heavy syrup	4 oz	100	25.0	0.4
in heavy syrup (A&P)	1/2 cup	110	28.0	<1.0
in heavy syrup (S&W)	1/2 cup	111	30.0	0.0
in heavy syrup, w/liquid	1/2 cup	113	28.2	0.4
in water (Lucky Leaf)	4 oz	40	9.0	0.0
in water (Musselman's)	4 oz	40	9.0	0.0
BLUEBERRY, FROZEN				
sweetened	10-oz pkg	230	62.3	0.4
sweetened	1/2 cup	94	25.2	0.2
unsweetened	20-oz pkg	289	69.0	3.6
unsweetened	1 cup	79	18.9	1.0
unsweetened	1/2 cup	39	9.4	0.5
BLUEBERRY NECTAR (Knudsen & Sons)	8 oz	135	34.0	0.0
BLUEBERRY SYRUP				
(Estee) 'Breakfast'	1 tbsp	12	3.0	0.0
(Featherweight)	1 tbsp	16	4.0	0.0

Food Name	Serv. Size	Total Cal.	Carbs GMS	Fat GMS
(Knott's Berry Farm)	1 oz	120	30.0	0.0
(Knott's Berry Farm) 'Light'	1 oz	50	12.0	0.0
(Knudsen & Sons)	1 oz	75	19.0	<1.0
BLUEFISH				
dry-heat cooked	3 oz	135	0.0	4.6
raw	1 lb	562	0.0	19.2
raw	3 oz	105	0.0	3.6
raw	1 oz	35	0.0	1.2
BLUEGILL				
raw	1 lb	404	0.0	3.2
raw	1.7-oz fillet	43	0.0	0.3
raw	1 oz	25	0.0	0.2
BOAR, WILD				
raw	1 lb	553	0.0	15.1
raw	1 oz	34	0.0	0.9
roasted	3 oz	136	0.0	3.7
roasted, diced	1 cup	224	0.0	6.1
BOBWHITE. See QUAIL.				
BOCKWURST				
	1 oz	87	0.1	7.8
7 links per lb	1 link	200	0.3	17.9
BOK CHOY				
boiled, drained	4 oz	14	2.0	0.2
boiled, drained, shredded	1/2 cup	10	1.5	0.1
raw, shredded	1 cup	9	1.5	0.1
raw, shredded	1/2 cup	5	0.8	0.1
raw, shredded *(Dole)*	1/2 cup	5	1.0	0.1
raw, trimmed	1 oz	4	0.6	0.1
raw, untrimmed	1 lb	52	8.7	0.8
BOLOGNA. See LUNCHEON MEAT.				
BONITO. See also TUNA, SKIPJACK.				
Caribbean, raw	1 lb	626	0.0	19.1
Caribbean, raw	1 oz	39	0.0	1.2
Japanese, raw	1 lb	585	1.8	9.1
Japanese, raw	1 oz	37	0.1	0.6
BORAGE				
boiled, drained	4 oz	28	4.0	0.9
boiled, drained	3.5 oz	25	3.5	0.8
raw, 1-inch pieces	1/2 cup	9	1.4	0.3
raw, trimmed	1 oz	6	0.9	0.2
raw, untrimmed	1 lb	76	11.1	2.5
BORECOLE. See KALE.				
BORLOTTI BEAN. See CRANBERRY BEAN.				

Food Name	Serv. Size	Total Cal.	Carbs GMS	Fat GMS
BOSTON CREAM PIE. See CAKE.				
BOTTLE GOURD. See GOURD, BOTTLE.				
BOUILLON. See SOUP.				
BOURBON. See ALCOHOLIC BEVERAGES.				
BOYSENBERRY, CANNED, in heavy syrup	1/2 cup	113	28.6	0.2
BOYSENBERRY, FROZEN				
unsweetened, unthawed	10-oz pkg	142	34.6	0.7
unsweetened, unthawed	1 cup	66	16.1	0.3
BOYSENBERRY DRINK				
boysenberry juice, 'Naturally 100%' (Smucker's)	8 oz	120	30.0	0.0
boysenberry nectar (Knudsen & Sons)	8 oz	110	33.0	0.0
BOYSENBERRY SYRUP				
(Knott's Berry Farm)	1 oz	120	30.0	0.0
(Knott's Berry Farm) 'Light'	1 oz	50	12.0	0.0
BRAMBLE. See RASPBERRY.				
BRANDY. See ALCOHOLIC BEVERAGES.				
BRATWURST				
(Eckrich)	1 link	310	1.0	30.0
(Hickory Farms) 'Brotwurst'	1 oz	90	1.0	8.0
(Hickory Farms) cheddar, 'Cheddy Brots'	1 oz	98	1.0	9.0
(Hillshire Farm) fresh	2 oz	190	1.0	17.0
(Hillshire Farm) 'Fully Cooked'	2 oz	170	1.0	16.0
(Hickory Farms) hot, 'Hot Brots'	1 oz	96	1.0	9.0
(Hillshire Farm) smoked	2 oz	190	1.0	17.0
(Hillshire Farm) spicy	2 oz	180	1.0	17.0
(Kahn's)	1 link	190	2.0	17.0
BRAUNSCHWEIGER				
(Hormel)	1 oz	80	0.0	7.0
(JM)	1 oz	80	2.0	6.0
(Oscar Mayer) 'German Brand'	1 oz	96	0.5	8.7
(Oscar Mayer) liver sausage	1 oz	100	<1.0	9.0
(Oscar Mayer) 'Slices'	1 oz	96	0.6	8.7
(Oscar Mayer) 'Tube'	1 oz	97	0.7	8.7
BRAZIL NUT / butternut / cream nut / paranut				
in shell, unblanched	1 lb	1428	27.9	144.2
shelled, unblanched, approx 6–8 kernels	1 oz	186	3.6	18.8
shelled, unblanched, approx 32 kernels	1 cup	919	17.9	92.7
BREAD. See also BAGEL; BISCUIT; BUN; CROISSANT; ENGLISH MUFFIN; ROLL; MUFFIN/PASTRY, TOASTER.				
APPLE-WALNUT (Arnold)	1 slice	64	12.6	1.3
BARBECUE, 'BBQ Loaf' (Colombo Brand)	2 oz	139	23.5	1.6
BRAN				
and oat, 'Light' (Oatmeal Goodness)	1 slice	40	6.0	<1.0

Food Name	Serv. Size	Total Cal.	Carbs GMS	Fat GMS
'Bran'nola' (Brownberry)	1 slice	85	17.5	1.4
'Bran'nola Original' (Arnold)	1 slice	85	17.5	1.4
'Gold'N Bran' (Earth Grains)	1 oz	70	12.0	1.0
honey bran, '1.5-lb loaf' (Pepperidge Farm)	1 slice	90	18.0	1.0
original, natural 'Bran'nola' (Oroweat)	1 slice	100	19.0	1.0
raisin (Brownberry)	1 slice	61	12.4	1.3
BROWN				
Boston, w/white corn meal, 3.25 inch diam	1/2-inch slice	95	20.5	0.6
Boston, w/yellow corn meal, 3.25 inch diam	1/2-inch slice	95	20.5	0.6
canned (B&M)	1.6 oz	94	22.0	0.0
canned (Friends)	1.6 oz	94	22.0	0.0
canned, Boston	1 oz	55	12.3	0.4
canned, 'New England' (S&W)	2 slices	76	17.0	0.0
canned, raisin (B&M)	1.6 oz	92	21.0	0.0
canned, raisin (Friends)	1.6 oz	92	21.0	0.0
plain (B&M)	1/2-inch slice	92	21.0	0.0
plain (Friends)	1/2-inch slice	92	21.0	0.0
raisin (B&M)	1/2-inch slice	94	22.0	0.0
raisin (Friends)	1/2-inch slice	94	22.0	0.0
BUTTERMILK				
(Grant's Farm)	1-oz slice	70	12.0	1.0
(Oroweat)	1 slice	100	20.0	1.0
CRESCENT (Pillsbury)	1 serving	100	11.0	6.0
CRISP, hard crispbread or toast	4 oz	473	80.2	9.8
EGG	1 oz	81	13.5	1.7
FRENCH				
enriched	1 oz	78	14.7	0.9
enriched, 5 inches x 2.5 inches	1 slice	101	19.4	1.0
extra sour (Colombo Brand)	2 oz	150	26.9	1.3
extra sour, sliced (Colombo Brand)	2 oz	153	27.2	1.6
'Hearth' (Pepperidge Farm)	1 oz	75	14.0	1.0
'Parisian' (DiCarlo)	1 slice	70	13.0	1.0
sweet, 'French Stick' (Colombo Brand)	2 oz	154	27.1	1.9
twin (Farm Hearth)	1 oz	80	15.0	1.0
unenriched, 5 inches x 2.5 inches	1 slice	101	19.4	1.0
GARLIC (Colombo Brand)	2 oz	185	17.3	10.1
GRAIN				
'Bran'nola' (Arnold)	1 slice	85	17.4	1.6
'Bran'nola Nutty Grains' (Brownberry)	1 slice	85	17.4	1.6
honey grain (Grant's Farm)	1-oz slice	70	13.0	1.0
honey grain, 'Family Recipe' (Colonial)	1-oz slice	70	14.0	1.0
honey grain, 'Family Recipe' (Kilpatrick's)	1-oz slice	70	14.0	1.0
honey grain, 'Family Recipe' (Rainbo)	1-oz slice	70	14.0	1.0

Food Name	Serv. Size	Total Cal.	Carbs GMS	Fat GMS
5-grain, organic *(BreadMill Bakery)*	1 slice	122	23.0	1.0
mixed grain, 'Round Top' *(Roman Meal)*	1 slice	67	13.2	0.8
mixed grain, 'Thin Sliced Sandwich' *(Roman Meal)*	1 slice	55	10.7	0.7
mixed grain, toasted	1 oz	77	14.3	1.2
mixed grain, whole grain	1 oz	71	13.1	1.1
multi-grain *(Hearty Grains)*	1 slice	80	15.0	2.0
multi-grain *(Weight Watchers)*	1 slice	40	9.0	<1.0
9-grain, 'Light' *(Oroweat)*	1 slice	40	10.0	0.0
7-grain *(Aunt Hattie's)*	1 slice	100	17.0	2.0
7-grain *(Grant's Farm)*	1-oz slice	60	13.0	1.0
7-grain, 'Hearty Slice' *(Pepperidge Farm)*	2 slices	180	36.0	2.0
7-grain, 'Light' *(Grant's Farm)*	.75-oz slice	40	9.0	<1.0
'Sun Grain' *(Roman Meal)*	1 slice	68	12.3	1.4
12-grain *(Earth Grains)*	1 oz	70	13.0	1.0
12-grain *(Oroweat)*	1 slice	110	20.0	2.0
GRANOLA, oat and honey *(Pepperidge Farm)*	1 slice	60	12.0	2.0
HAWAIIAN *(King's Hawaiian Bread)*	2 oz	180	30.0	4.0
HEALTH NUT				
(Brownberry)	1 slice	71	12.4	2.6
(Oroweat)	1 slice	110	20.0	2.0
HIGH-CALCIUM				
dark	1 oz	69	13.9	0.7
light	1 oz	64	12.5	0.6
HOLLYWOOD				
'Dark' *(Hollywood)*	1 slice	70	13.0	1.0
'Light' *(Hollywood)*	1 slice	70	13.0	1.0
HONEY NUT, and oat bran *(Aunt Hattie's)*	1 slice	100	16.0	na
HONEY OAT NUT *(Earth Grains)*	1 oz	80	14.0	2.0
HONEY WHEAT BRAN *(Grant's Farm)*	1-oz slice	70	14.0	1.0
HONEY WHEATBERRY				
(Earth Grains)	1 oz	70	12.0	1.0
(Oroweat)	1 slice	90	17.0	1.0
INDIAN FRY, Navajo, 5 inch diam	1 slice	296	48.0	8.6
ITALIAN				
'Family' *(Wonder)*	1 slice	70	13.0	1.0
'Francisco International' *(Arnold)*	1-oz slice	72	14.1	1.1
'Hearth' *(Pepperidge Farm)*	1 oz	80	14.0	1.0
'Hi-Fibre' *(Monk's)*	1 slice	70	13.0	1.0
light, 'Bakery' *(Arnold)*	1 slice	45	9.9	0.5
'Light' *(Brownberry)*	1 slice	44	9.9	0.5
thick sliced, 'Francisco International' *(Arnold)*	1 slice	66	13.7	0.8
OAT				
'Bran'nola Country' *(Arnold)*	1 slice	90	17.8	2.0

Food Name	Serv. Size	Total Cal.	Carbs GMS	Fat GMS
'Bran'nola Country' (Brownberry)	1 slice	90	17.8	2.0
country oat, 'Light' (Oroweat)	1 slice	40	10.0	0.0
crunchy (Pepperidge Farm)	2 slices	190	34.0	4.0
split-top, 'Family Recipe' (Colonial)	1-oz slice	70	13.0	1.0
split-top, 'Family Recipe' (Kilpatrick's)	1-oz slice	70	13.0	1.0
split-top, 'Family Recipe' (Rainbo)	1-oz slice	70	13.0	1.0
OAT BRAN				
country oat, natural, 'Bran'nola' (Oroweat)	2 slices	230	39.0	4.0
honey (Roman Meal)	1 slice	71	12.7	1.2
honey (Earth Grains)	1 oz	80	13.0	1.0
honey, w/whole wheat, organic (BreadMill Bakery)	1 slice	121	23.0	1.0
honey nut (Roman Meal)	1 slice	72	12.1	1.6
organic, 'Light' (BreadMill Bakery)	1 slice	113	22.0	1.0
plain (Awrey's)	1 slice	50	10.0	0.0
plain (Grant's Farm)	1-oz slice	70	14.0	1.0
plain (Weight Watchers)	1 slice	40	10.0	<1.0
'Split-Top' (Roman Meal)	1 slice	68	13.2	0.9
OATMEAL				
cinnamon (Oatmeal Goodness)	1 slice	90	15.0	2.0
country twists (Hearty Grains)	1 slice	80	15.0	2.0
light, 'Bakery' (Arnold)	1 slice	44	9.6	0.6
light, 'Light Style' (Pepperidge Farm)	1 slice	45	9.0	0.0
'1.5-lb loaf' (Pepperidge Farm)	1 slice	90	17.0	1.0
plain (Pepperidge Farm)	1 slice	70	12.0	1.0
raisin, 'Hearty Grain' (Pillsbury)	1 slice	90	16.0	2.0
toasted almond (Grant's Farm)	1-oz slice	80	14.0	1.0
'Very Thin' (Pepperidge Farm)	1 slice	40	8.0	1.0
w/bran (Oatmeal Goodness)	1 slice	90	15.0	2.0
w/sunflower seed (Oatmeal Goodness)	1 slice	90	15.0	2.0
OATNUT (Oroweat)	1 slice	100	18.0	2.0
PITA				
oat bran (Sahara)	1/2 pita	66	15.3	0.3
onion, no fats, no oils, pre-sliced, 1.2 oz (Kangaroo)	1 pocket	75	15.0	0.0
white (Sahara)	1/2 pita	79	15.6	0.5
white, enriched	1 oz	78	15.8	0.3
white, enriched	1 pita	165	33.4	0.7
white, mini (Sahara)	1 pita	79	15.6	0.5
white, unenriched	1 oz	78	15.8	0.3
white, unenriched	1 pita	165	33.4	0.7
whole-wheat	1 oz	75	15.6	0.7
whole-wheat	1 pita	170	35.2	1.7
whole-wheat, approx 2 oz (Sahara)	1 pita	150	28.0	2.0
PROTEIN, includes gluten	1 oz	69	12.4	0.6

Food Name	Serv. Size	Total Cal.	Carbs GMS	Fat GMS
PUMPERNICKEL				
....	1 oz	71	13.5	0.9
'Family' (Pepperidge Farm)	1 slice	80	15.0	1.0
plain (Arnold)	1 slice	70	14.7	0.9
small, 'Party' (Pepperidge Farm)	4 slices	60	12.0	1.0
RAISIN				
cinnamon (Arnold)	1 slice	67	12.9	1.4
cinnamon (Brownberry)	1 slice	66	12.8	1.3
cinnamon (Monk's)	1 slice	70	10.0	2.0
cinnamon (Pepperidge Farm)	1 slice	90	16.0	2.0
cinnamon swirl (Pepperidge Farm)	1 slice	90	16.0	2.0
orange (Brownberry)	1 slice	67	13.0	1.2
unenriched	1 oz	84	16.1	1.4
walnut (Brownberry)	1 slice	68	11.4	2.7
walnut, royal (Northridge)	1 slice	90	16.0	2.0
whole wheat, organic (BreadMill Bakery)	1 slice	120	24.0	1.0
RICE BRAN				
golden (Monk's)	1 slice	70	14.0	1.0
honey nut (Roman Meal)	1 slice	71	12.8	1.6
plain (Roman Meal)	1 slice	70	12.4	1.5
RYE				
caraway, 'Natural' (Brownberry)	1 slice	73	15.4	0.8
Dijon (Pepperidge Farm)	1 slice	50	9.0	1.0
Dijon, 'Hearty' (Pepperidge Farm)	1 slice	70	15.0	1.0
dill (Arnold)	1 slice	71	14.4	1.0
'Hearty' (Beefsteak)	1 slice	70	13.0	1.0
hearty rye, 'Light' (Oroweat)	1 slice	40	10.0	0.0
honey cracked (Grant's Farm)	1-oz slice	70	13.0	1.0
Jewish, seeded (Levy's)	1 slice	76	15.9	0.9
Jewish, seedless (Levy's)	1 slice	75	16.0	0.8
'Mild' (Beefsteak)	1 slice	70	13.0	1.0
'Old Allegheny' (Braun's)	1 slice	70	13.0	1.0
onion (Beefsteak)	1 slice	70	12.0	1.0
plain (Weight Watchers)	1 slice	40	10.0	<1.0
seeded, 'Family' (Pepperidge Farm)	1 slice	80	16.0	1.0
seedless, 'Family' (Pepperidge Farm)	1 slice	80	16.0	1.0
seedless, 'Natural Thin Sliced' (Brownberry)	1 slice	45	9.8	0.6
small, 'Party' (Pepperidge Farm)	4 slices	60	12.0	1.0
'Soft' (Beefsteak)	1 slice	70	13.0	1.0
very thin, light (Earth Grains)	1 oz	70	14.0	1.0
wheatberry (Beefsteak)	1 slice	70	13.0	1.0
SOURDOUGH				
French (Boudin), approx 2-oz slices	2 slices	130	27.0	1.0

Food Name	Serv. Size	Total Cal.	Carbs GMS	Fat GMS
'Light' (Earth Grains)	.75 oz	40	9.0	1.0
'Light' (Rainbo)	.75-oz slice	40	9.0	<1.0
plain (DiCarlo)	1 slice	70	12.0	1.0
SUNFLOWER				
and bran (Monk's)	1 slice	70	12.0	1.0
'Texas Toast' (Golden Corral)	1 serving	170	26.0	6.0
whole wheat, organic (BreadMill Bakery)	1 slice	129	21.0	2.0
VIENNA				
light, 'Light Style' (Pepperidge Farm)	1 slice	45	10.0	0.0
thick sliced, 'Hearth' (Pepperidge Farm)	1 slice	70	13.0	1.0
WHEAT				
	1 oz	74	13.4	1.2
apple honey (Brownberry)	1 slice	69	11.4	1.9
'Brick Oven' (Arnold)	1 slice	57	10.6	1.5
'Butter Top' (Home Pride)	1 slice	70	13.0	1.0
buttertop (Aunt Hattie's)	1 slice	70	13.0	1.0
cracked	1 oz	74	14.0	1.1
cracked (Earth Grains)	1 oz	70	12.0	1.0
cracked (Pepperidge Farm)	1 slice	70	13.0	1.0
cracked (Wonder)	1 slice	70	13.0	1.0
cracked wheat and honey twists (Hearty Grains)	1 serving	80	14.0	2.0
dark, 'Bran'nola' (Arnold)	1 slice	83	17.6	1.0
'Family Recipe' (Colonial)	1-oz slice	70	14.0	1.0
'Family Recipe' (Kilpatrick's)	1-oz slice	70	14.0	1.0
'Family Recipe' (Rainbo)	1-oz slice	70	14.0	1.0
'Family,' 2-lb loaf (Pepperidge Farm)	1 slice	70	13.0	1.0
fat-free, 'Light' (Wonder)	1 slice	40	7.0	<1.0
'Hearth' (Brownberry)	1 oz	70	13.6	1.4
'Hearty' (Beefsteak)	1 slice	70	11.0	1.0
hearty, 'Bran'nola' (Arnold)	1 slice	88	17.1	1.9
hearty, 'Bran'nola' (Brownberry)	1 slice	88	17.1	1.9
honey buttered, split-top, 'Family Recipe' (Colonial)	1-oz slice	70	14.0	1.0
honey buttered, split-top, 'Family Recipe' (Kilpatrick's)	1-oz slice	70	14.0	1.0
honey buttered, split-top, 'Family Recipe' (Rainbo)	1-oz slice	70	14.0	1.0
honey wheatberry (Arnold)	1 slice	77	16.5	1.2
'Light' (Grant's Farm)	.75-oz slice	40	9.0	<1.0
'Light' (Rainbo)	.75-oz slice	40	9.0	<1.0
light, golden, 'Bakery' (Arnold)	1 slice	44	9.5	0.5
'Light Style' (Pepperidge Farm)	1 slice	45	9.0	0.0
'Light 35' (Earth Grains)	1 oz	35	8.0	<1.0
loaf (Pipin' Hot)	1-inch slice	70	12.0	2.0
multi-grain (Beefsteak)	1 slice	70	11.0	1.0
'Natural' (Brownberry)	1 slice	80	17.0	1.3

Food Name	Serv. Size	Total Cal.	Carbs GMS	Fat GMS
oatmeal (Oatmeal Goodness)	1 slice	90	15.0	2.0
oatmeal, 'Light' (Oatmeal Goodness)	1 slice	40	6.0	<1.0
1.5-lb loaf (Pepperidge Farm)	1 slice	90	18.0	2.0
plain (Country Grain)	1 slice	70	12.0	1.0
plain (Fresh & Natural)	1 slice	70	13.0	1.0
plain (Weight Watchers)	1 slice	40	9.0	<1.0
sesame, 'Hearty' (Pepperidge Farm)	2 slices	190	36.0	3.0
'7-Grain' (Home Pride)	1 slice	70	12.0	1.0
'Soft' (Beefsteak)	1 slice	70	12.0	1.0
soft (Brownberry)	1 slice	74	13.1	1.8
soft, made w/buttermilk (Aunt Hattie's)	1 slice	70	12.0	1.0
sprouted (Pepperidge Farm)	1 slice	70	11.0	2.0
stone-ground (Grant's Farm)	1-oz slice	60	12.0	1.0
stone-ground, 'Family Recipe' (Colonial)	1-oz slice	70	14.0	1.0
stone-ground, 'Family Recipe' (Kilpatrick's)	1-oz slice	70	14.0	1.0
stone-ground, 'Family Recipe' (Rainbo)	1-oz slice	70	14.0	1.0
'Stoneground' (Home Pride)	1 slice	70	12.0	1.0
very thin (Earth Grains)	1 oz	70	13.0	1.0
WHEAT GERM	1 oz	74	13.7	0.8
WHEATBERRY (Grant's Farm)	1-oz slice	70	13.0	1.0
WHITE				
	1 oz	76	14.0	1.0
'Brick Oven' (Arnold)	1 slice	61	11.3	1.2
'Butter Top' (Home Pride)	1 slice	70	13.0	1.0
buttermilk (Wonder)	1 slice	70	13.0	1.0
buttertop, 'Homestyle' (Aunt Hattie's)	1 slice	70	13.0	1.0
'Country White' (Arnold)	1 slice	98	18.6	1.8
enriched, 'Country Style' (Holsum)	1 slice	70	14.0	1.0
extra fiber, 'Brick Oven' (Arnold)	1 slice	55	12.1	0.8
'Hearty Country' (Pepperidge Farm)	2 slices	190	38.0	2.0
'High Fiber' (Wonder)	1 slice	40	6.0	0.0
honey buttered, split-top, 'Family Recipe' (Colonial)	1-oz slice	80	14.0	1.0
honey buttered, split-top, 'Family Recipe' (Kilpatrick's)	1-oz slice	80	14.0	1.0
honey buttered, split-top, 'Family Recipe' (Rainbo)	1-oz slice	80	14.0	1.0
'Large Family,' 2-lb loaf (Pepperidge Farm)	1 slice	70	13.0	1.0
'Light' (Grant's Farm)	.75-oz slice	40	9.0	<1.0
'Light' (Rainbo)	.75-oz slice	40	9.0	<1.0
'Light' (Wonder)	1 slice	40	7.0	0.0
'Light Premium' (Arnold)	1 slice	42	9.6	0.5
'Light Premium' (Brownberry)	1 slice	42	9.6	0.5
'Light 35' (Earth Grains)	1 oz	35	8.0	<1.0
'Natural' (Brownberry)	1 slice	59	11.1	1.1
old fashioned (Northridge)	1 slice	70	13.0	1.0

Food Name	Serv. Size	Total Cal.	Carbs GMS	Fat GMS
plain *(Monk's)*	1 slice	60	10.0	1.0
plain *(Weight Watchers)*	1 slice	40	10.0	<1.0
plain *(Wonder)*	1 slice	70	13.0	1.0
'Robust' *(Beefsteak)*	1 slice	70	13.0	1.0
sandwich *(Pepperidge Farm)*	2 slices	130	24.0	2.0
special recipe, 'Iron Kids' *(Rainbo)*	1 slice	60	13.0	1.0
thin *(Holsum)*	1 slice	70	14.0	1.0
'Thin Sliced' *(Wonder)*	1 slice	50	10.0	1.0
'Thin Sliced,' 1-lb size *(Pepperidge Farm)*	1 slice	80	14.0	2.0
toasting *(Pepperidge Farm)*	1 slice	90	17.0	1.0
very thin *(Earth Grains)*	1 oz	80	14.0	1.0
'Very Thin' *(Pepperidge Farm)*	1 slice	40	8.0	0.0
white loaf *(Pipin' Hot)*	1-inch slice	70	12.0	2.0
w/buttermilk, 'Homestyle' *(Aunt Hattie's)*	1 slice	80	13.0	1.0
WHOLE BRAN, 'Natural' *(Brownberry)*	1 slice	58	11.7	1.4
WHOLE WHEAT				
	1 oz	70	13.1	1.2
'Family' *(Wonder)*	1 slice	70	13.0	1.0
'High Fiber' *(Wonder)*	1 slice	40	6.0	0.0
'Light' *(Wonder)*	1 slice	40	7.0	0.0
100% *(Northridge)*	1 slice	60	11.0	1.0
'100% Stone Ground' *(Monk's)*	1 slice	70	13.0	1.0
100%-whole-wheat *(Earth Grains)*	1 oz	70	11.0	1.0
'100%' *(Wonder)*	1 slice	70	12.0	1.0
plain *(Aunt Hattie's)*	1 slice	90	14.0	2.0
plain *(Daily)*	2-oz slice	140	26.0	0.0
'Soft 100%' *(Wonder)*	1 slice	70	10.0	1.0
'Stoneground 100%' *(Arnold)*	1 slice	48	9.9	0.7
stoneground, 100% *(Oroweat)*	1 slice	60	11.0	1.0
'Thin Sliced,' 1-lb loaf *(Pepperidge Farm)*	1 slice	60	12.0	1.0
'Very Thin' *(Pepperidge Farm)*	1 slice	35	7.0	0.0
BREAD, BROWN AND SERVE				
'Austrian' *(Du Jour)*	1 oz	70	13.0	1.0
'French' *(Du Jour)*	1 oz	70	13.0	1.0
'Italian' *(Pepperidge Farm)*	1 oz	80	14.0	1.0
BREAD, QUICK, MIX				
APPLE CINNAMON				
(Pillsbury) mix only, dry	1/12 pkg	140	30.0	1.0
(Pillsbury) prepared as directed	1/12 loaf	170	27.0	6.0
(Pillsbury) prepared w/1/4 cup oil, 1/4 cup egg substitute	1/12 loaf	190	31.0	6.0
(Pillsbury) prepared w/water, 1/4 cup oil, 1 egg	1/12 loaf	180	31.0	6.0
(Pillsbury) prepared w/water, 1/4 cup oil, 1/4 cup egg substitute	1/12 loaf	190	31.0	6.0

Food Name	Serv. Size	Total Cal.	Carbs GMS	Fat GMS
BANANA				
(Pillsbury) mix only, dry	1/12 pkg	120	27.0	1.0
(Pillsbury) prepared w/water, 3 tbsp oil, 1/2 cup egg substitute	1/12 loaf	170	27.0	6.0
(Pillsbury) prepared w/water, 3 tbsp oil, and 2 eggs	1/12 loaf	170	27.0	5.0
BANANA NUT (Krusteaz) prepared as directed	3/4-inch slice	190	33.0	6.0
BLUEBERRY NUT				
(Pillsbury) mix only, dry	1/12 pkg	130	29.0	1.0
(Pillsbury) prepared as directed	1/12 loaf	150	26.0	4.0
(Pillsbury) prepared w/1/4 cup oil,1/4 cup egg substitute	1/12 loaf	180	30.0	6.0
(Pillsbury) prepared w/water, 1/4 cup oil, 1 egg	1/12 loaf	180	30.0	6.0
(Pillsbury) prepared w/water, 1/4 cup oil, 1/4 cup egg substitute	1/12 loaf	180	30.0	6.0
CHERRY NUT (Pillsbury) prepared as directed	1/12 loaf	180	29.0	5.0
CORNBREAD				
(Aunt Jemima) 'Easy,' prepared as directed	1 piece	196	32.7	6.3
(Ballard) mix only, dry	1/16 pkg	120	24.0	2.0
(Ballard) prepared as directed	1/8 pan	140	25.0	3.0
(Ballard) prepared w/1 cup milk, 1 egg	1/16 pan	150	25.0	3.0
(Dromedary) mix only, dry	3 tbsp	100	19.0	2.0
(Dromedary) prepared as directed	2-inch square	130	20.0	3.0
(Gold Medal) white, 'Pouch Mix, prepared w/egg and whole milk	1/6 pan	150	22.0	5.0
(Gold Medal) yellow, 'Pouch Mix,' prepared w/egg and whole milk	1/6 pan	150	23.0	5.0
(Krusteaz) honey, prepared as directed	1/16 pan	120	21.0	3.0
(Krusteaz) Southern, prepared as directed	2-inch square	140	27.0	3.0
(Martha White) buttermilk, prepared w/water	1/6 pan	110	21.0	2.0
(Martha White) 'Cotton Pickin' prepared as directed	1/4 pan	170	31.0	3.0
(Martha White) 'Cotton Pickin' prepared w/water	1/6 pan	110	21.0	2.0
(Martha White) Mexican, prepared w/2% milk	1/6 pan	140	24.0	4.0
(Martha White) yellow, 'Light Crust,' prepared as directed	2 oz	140	21.0	4.0
(Robin Hood) white, 'Pouch Mix,' prepared w/egg and whole milk	1/6 pan	150	22.0	5.0
CRANBERRY				
(Pillsbury) mix only, dry	1/12 pkg	140	30.0	1.0
(Pillsbury) prepared as directed	1/12 loaf	160	30.0	4.0
(Pillsbury) prepared w/water, 2 tbsp oil, 1 egg	1/12 loaf	160	30.0	4.0
(Pillsbury) prepared w/water, 2 tbsp oil, 1/4 cup egg substitute	1/12 loaf	170	30.0	4.0
DATE				
(Pillsbury) prepared w/water, 1 tbsp oil, 1 egg	1/12 pkg	160	32.0	3.0

Food Name	Serv. Size	Total Cal.	Carbs GMS	Fat GMS
(Pillsbury) prepared w/water, 1 tbsp oil, 1/4 cup egg substitute	1/12 loaf	160	32.0	3.0
DATE NUT				
(Dromedary) mix only, dry	1/12 pkg	166	26.0	7.0
(Dromedary) prepared as directed	1/12 loaf	183	26.0	8.0
GINGERBREAD				
(Betty Crocker) 'Classic' mix only, dry	1/9 pkg	200	35.0	6.0
(Betty Crocker) 'Classic,' prepared w/cholesterol-free egg product	1/9 pan	210	35.0	6.0
(Betty Crocker) 'Classic,' prepared w/egg	1/9 pan	220	35.0	7.0
(Dromedary) mix only, dry	3 tbsp	100	19.0	2.0
(Pillsbury) mix only, dry	1/9 pkg	180	32.0	5.0
(Pillsbury) prepared as directed	3-inch square	190	36.0	4.0
NUT				
(Pillsbury) mix only, dry	1/12 pkg	150	27.0	3.0
(Pillsbury) prepared w/water, 2 tbsp oil, 1 egg	1/12 loaf	170	27.0	6.0
(Pillsbury) prepared w/water, 2 tbsp oil, 1/4 cup egg substitute	1/12 loaf	170	28.0	6.0
OATMEAL RAISIN				
(Pillsbury) mix only, dry	1/12 pkg	140	30.0	2.0
(Pillsbury) prepared w/water, 1/4 cup oil, 1 egg	1/12 loaf	190	30.0	7.0
(Pillsbury) prepared w/water, 1/4 cup oil, 1/4 cup egg substitute	1/12 loaf	190	30.0	7.0
BREAD CRUMBS				
Italian-style *(Devonsheer)*	1 oz	104	21.1	1.3
Italian-style *(Progresso)*	2 tbsp	60	11.0	<1.0
Italian-style, whole-wheat *(Jaclyn's)*	.5 oz	28	13.0	1.0
plain	1 cup	427	78.3	5.8
plain	1 oz	112	20.6	1.5
plain *(Devonsheer)*	1 oz	108	21.6	1.4
plain *(Progresso)*	2 tbsp	60	11.0	<1.0
seasoned	1 cup	440	84.5	3.1
seasoned	1 oz	104	20.0	0.7
seasoned *(Contadina)*	1 cup	426	81.5	3.6
seasoned *(Contadina)*	1 tbsp	35	7.0	<1.0
BREAD DOUGH				
cornbread twists, refrigerated *(Pillsbury)*	1 twist	70	8.0	4.0
French, crusty, refrigerated *(Pillsbury)*	1-inch slice	60	11.0	<1.0
honey walnut, frozen *(Bridgford)*	1 oz	76	13.8	0.9
refrigerated *(Roman Meal)*	1 oz	85	12.6	2.8
wheat, refrigerated *(Pipin' Hot)*	1-inch slice	70	12.0	2.0
white, frozen *(Bridgford)*	1 oz	76	13.8	1.2
white, frozen *(Rich's)*	2 slices	120	23.0	1.0

Food Name	Serv. Size	Total Cal.	Carbs GMS	Fat GMS
white, refrigerated *(Pipin' Hot)* .... 1-inch slice		70	12.0	2.0
BREADFRUIT				
raw .... 1 cup		227	59.7	0.5
raw .... 1/4 small		99	26.0	0.2
trimmed .... 1/2 cup		114	29.8	0.3
trimmed .... 1 oz		29	7.7	0.1
untrimmed .... 1 lb		365	96.0	0.8
BREADFRUIT SEEDS				
boiled .... 1 oz		48	9.1	0.7
Pacific, in soft shell, boiled .... 1 lb		274	52.3	3.8
Pacific, shelled, boiled .... 1 oz		48	9.1	0.7
raw .... 1 oz		54	8.3	1.6
roasted .... 1 oz		59	11.4	0.8
shelled, raw .... 1 oz		54	8.3	1.6
South American, in shell, raw .... 1 lb		590	90.2	17.2
South American, shelled, roasted .... 1 oz		59	11.4	0.8
BREADNUT TREE SEEDS/Jamaican breadnut				
dried .... 1 oz		104	22.5	0.5
raw .... 1 oz		62	13.1	0.3
BREADSTICK				
garlic, Italian-style *(Barbara's Bakery)* ...... 1 oz		120	18.0	3.0
onion *(Stella D'oro)* .... 1 stick		40	6.1	1.3
pizza *(Fattorie & Pandea)* .... 3 stick s		59	10.0	1.0
pizza *(Stella D'oro)* .... 1 stick		43	6.9	1.2
plain *(Stella D'oro)* .... 1 stick		41	6.5	1.2
plain, dietetic *(Stella D'oro)* .... 1 stick		46	7.3	1.4
regular *(Barbara's Bakery)* .... 1 oz		120	18.0	3.0
sesame *(Fattorie & Pandea)* .... 3 sticks		65	10.0	2.0
sesame *(Stella D'oro)* .... 1 stick		51	6.3	2.2
sesame, dietetic *(Stella D'oro)* .... 1 stick		49	6.1	2.1
sesame, Italian-style *(Barbara's Bakery)* .... 1 oz		120	18.0	3.0
soft, refrigerated *(Pillsbury)* .... 1 stick		100	17.0	2.0
soft, refrigerated *(Roman Meal)* .... 1 stick		117	17.4	3.9
wheat *(Stella D'oro)* .... 1 stick		42	6.1	1.4
whole wheat *(Fattorie & Pandea)* .... 3 sticks		57	10.0	1.0
BREAKFAST BAR. See SNACK BAR				
BREAKFAST DRINK MIX, INSTANT				
CHOCOLATE FLAVOR				
(Carnation) 'Instant Breakfast' dry mix .... 1 pouch		130	24.0	2.0
(Carnation) 'Instant Breakfast' dry mix, no sugar added ... 1 pouch		70	12.0	1.0
(Pillsbury) 'Instant Breakfast' from variety pack, dry mix ... 1/10 pkg		130	25.0	0.0
(Pillsbury) 'Instant Breakfast' from variety pack, prepared w/ 8 oz 2% milk .... 1 cup		250	37.0	5.0

Food Name	Serv. Size	Total Cal.	Carbs GMS	Fat GMS
(Pillsbury) 'Instant Breakfast' from variety pack, prepared w/ 8 oz whole milk	1 cup	290	38.0	9.0
CHOCOLATE MALT FLAVOR				
(Carnation) 'Instant Breakfast' dry mix	1 pouch	130	24.0	2.0
(Carnation) 'Instant Breakfast' dry mix, no sugar added	1 pouch	70	8.0	2.0
(Pillsbury) 'Instant Breakfast' dry mix	1 pouch	130	26.0	0.0
COFFEE FLAVOR				
(Carnation) 'Instant Breakfast' dry mix	1 pouch	130	25.0	0.2
VANILLA FLAVOR				
(Carnation) 'Instant Breakfast' dry mix	1 pouch	130	25.0	0.2
(Carnation) 'Instant Breakfast' dry mix, no sugar added	1 pouch	70	10.0	0.0
(Pillsbury) 'Instant Breakfast' dry mix	1 pouch	140	29.0	0.0
(Pillsbury) 'Instant Breakfast' prepared w/whole milk	1 cup	300	41.0	9.0
(Pillsbury) 'Instant Breakfast' from variety pack, dry mix	1/10 pkg	130	28.0	0.0
(Pillsbury) 'Instant Breakfast' from variety pack, prepared w/ 8 oz 2% milk	1 cup	260	40.0	5.0
BREAKFAST JUICE. See also individual listings.				
(Health Valley)	1/2 cup	26	5.0	0.0
(Knudsen & Sons) 'Natural'	8 oz	90	21.0	0.0
(Smucker's) orange banana, 'Naturally 100%'	8 oz	120	30.0	0.0
BREAKFAST STRIPS. See also BACON; BACON, ALTERNATIVE.				
beef, cured, cooked	6 oz	763	2.4	58.5
beef, cured, cooked	3 slices	153	0.5	11.7
beef, cured, raw	3 slices	276	0.5	26.4
beef, cured, unheated	3 slices	276	0.5	26.4
BREATH MINT. See CANDY, HARD.				
BROAD BEAN				
boiled, drained	4 oz	64	11.5	0.6
immature, boiled, drained	100 gm	56	10.1	0.5
immature, raw	1 cup	78	12.7	0.7
mature, boiled	1/2 cup	94	16.7	0.3
mature, raw	1/2 cup	256	43.7	1.1
raw, trimmed	1 oz	20	3.3	0.2
raw, untrimmed	1 lb	317	51.5	2.6
BROAD BEAN, DRIED				
mature, boiled	1/2 cup	93	16.7	0.3
mature, boiled	4 oz	125	22.3	0.5
mature, raw	1/2 cup	256	43.7	1.2
mature, raw	1 oz	97	16.5	0.4
BROCCOLI				
boiled, drained	4 oz	32	5.7	0.4
boiled, drained, chopped	1/2 cup	22	4.0	0.3
florets, raw, chopped	1/2 cup	12	2.3	0.2

Food Name	Serv. Size	Total Cal.	Carbs GMS	Fat GMS
fresh *(Dole)*	1 med spear	40	4.0	1.0
leaves, raw, chopped	1/2 cup	12	2.3	0.2
raw, chopped	1/2 cup	12	2.3	0.2
raw, trimmed	1 oz	8	1.5	0.1
raw, untrimmed	1 lb	77	14.5	1.0
BROCCOLI, FROZEN. See also BROCCOLI DISHES, FROZEN; BROCCOLI ENTRÉE, FROZ				
chopped *(A&P)*	3.3 oz	25	5.0	<1.0
chopped *(Birds Eye)*	3.3 oz	25	5.0	0.0
chopped *(Finast)*	3.3 oz	25	5.0	0.0
chopped *(Frosty Acres)*	3.3 oz	25	5.0	0.0
chopped *(Seabrook)*	3.3 oz	25	5.0	0.0
chopped *(Southern)*	3.5 oz	28	4.4	0.3
chopped, boiled, drained	4 oz	32	6.1	0.1
chopped, boiled, drained	1/2 cup	26	4.9	0.1
chopped, unprepared	10-oz pkg	74	13.6	0.8
cuts *(A&P)*	3.3 oz	25	5.0	<1.0
cuts *(Birds Eye)*	3.2 oz	25	5.0	0.0
cuts *(Frosty Acres)*	3.3 oz	25	5.0	0.0
cuts *(Seabrook)*	3.3 oz	25	5.0	0.0
cuts, 'Harvest Fresh' *(Green Giant)*	1/2 cup	16	3.0	0.0
cuts, 'Plain Polybag' *(Green Giant)*	1/2 cup	18	5.0	0.0
cuts, 'Portion Pack' *(Birds Eye)*	3 oz	20	4.0	0.0
cuts, 'Singles' *(Stokely)*	3 oz	25	5.0	1.0
florets *(Frosty Acres)*	3.3 oz	30	5.0	0.0
florets, 'Deluxe' *(Birds Eye)*	3.3 oz	25	5.0	0.0
spears *(A&P)*	3.3 oz	25	5.0	<1.0
spears *(Birds Eye)*	3.3 oz	25	5.0	0.0
spears *(Frosty Acres)*	3.3 oz	25	5.0	0.0
spears *(Seabrook)*	3.3 oz	25	5.0	0.0
spears *(Southern)*	3.5 oz	30	4.8	0.2
spears, baby *(Seabrook)*	3.3 oz	30	5.0	0.0
spears, baby, 'Deluxe' *(Birds Eye)*	3.3 oz	30	5.0	0.0
spears, boiled, drained	4 oz	32	6.1	0.1
spears, boiled, drained	10-oz pkg	70	13.4	0.3
spears, boiled, drained	1/2 cup	26	4.9	0.1
spears, 'Harvest Fresh' *(Green Giant)*	1/2 cup	20	4.0	0.0
spears, mini, 2 1/2 inch x 1/4 inch, approx .6 oz *(Green Giant)*	1/5 pkg	18	5.0	0.0
spears, unprepared	10-oz pkg	82	15.2	1.0
spears, whole, 'Farm Fresh' *(Birds Eye)*	4 oz	30	6.0	0.0
spears and florets, 'Deluxe' *(Birds Eye)*	3.3 oz	25	5.0	0.0
BROCCOLI DISHES, FROZEN				
cuts, in butter sauce, 'One Serving' *(Green Giant)*	4.5 oz	45	7.0	2.0

Food Name	Serv. Size	Total Cal.	Carbs GMS	Fat GMS
cuts, in cheese sauce, *(Finast)*	3.3 oz	45	6.0	0.0
cuts, in cheese sauce, 'One Serving' *(Green Giant)*	5 oz	80	13.0	2.0
cuts, in cheese sauce, 'Singles' *(Stokely)*	4 oz	80	7.0	4.0
fanfare, 'Valley Combinations' *(Green Giant)*	1/2 cup	80	14.0	2.0
in cheese flavored sauce *(Green Giant)*	1/2 cup	60	9.0	2.0
in cheese sauce, 'Family Side Dishes' *(Freezer Queen)*	4.5 oz	48	8.0	1.0
spears, 'Butter Sauce' *(Green Giant)*	1/2 cup	40	6.0	2.0
spears, 'Butter Sauce Combinations' *(Birds Eye)*	3.3 oz	45	5.0	2.0
w/baby carrots and water chestnuts, 'Farm Fresh' *(Birds Eye)*	4 oz	45	10.0	0.0
w/cauliflower *(A&P)*	3.2 oz	25	4.0	<1.0
w/cauliflower, 'Valley Combinations' medley *(Green Giant)*	1/2 cup	30	10.0	1.0
w/cauliflower, 'Singles' *(Stokely)*	3 oz	20	4.0	1.0
w/cauliflower, 'Swiss Mix' *(Frosty Acres)*	3 oz	25	5.0	0.0
w/red peppers, 'Select' *(Green Giant)*	1/2 cup	25	4.0	0.0
w/whole baby carrots and chestnuts, 'Singles' *(Stokely)*	3 oz	30	6.0	1.0

BROCCOLI ENTRÉE, FROZEN

and baked potato wedges w/cheese sauce, 9.5-oz pkg *(Healthy Choice)*	1 serving	240	41.0	5.0
au gratin w/rice, 'For One' *(Birds Eye)*	5.75 oz	180	27.0	6.0
in pastry, w/cheese *(Pepperidge Farm)*	1 pastry	230	18.0	16.0
pot pie w/cheddar cheese, organic *(Amy's Kitchen)*	8 oz	390	46.0	18.0

BROTH. See SOUP.

BROWN BREAD. See BREAD.

BRUSSELS SPROUTS

boiled, drained	4 oz	44	9.8	0.6
boiled, drained	1/2 cup	30	6.8	0.4
boiled, drained	1 sprout	8	1.8	0.1
fresh *(Dole)*	1/2 cup	19	4.0	0.1
'Plain Polybag' *(Green Giant)*	1/2 cup	25	6.0	0.0
raw	1/2 cup	19	3.9	0.1
raw	1 sprout	8	1.7	0.1
raw, trimmed	1 oz	12	2.5	0.1
raw, untrimmed	1 lb	174	36.6	1.2

BRUSSELS SPROUTS, FROZEN

boiled, drained	4 oz	48	9.4	0.4
boiled, drained	1/2 cup	33	6.5	0.3
(A&P)	3.3 oz	35	7.0	<1.0
(Birds Eye)	3.3 oz	35	7.0	0.0
(Birds Eye) baby, 'Cheese Sauce Combinations'	4.5 oz	130	12.0	7.0
(Frosty Acres)	3.3 oz	35	7.0	0.0
(Green Giant) in butter sauce	1/2 cup	40	8.0	1.0

Food Name	Serv. Size	Total Cal.	Carbs GMS	Fat GMS
(Seabrook)	3.3 oz	35	7.0	0.0
(Seabrook) baby	3.3 oz	40	7.0	0.0
(Southern)	3.5 oz	37	7.5	0.0
(Stokely) in butter sauce, 'Singles'	4 oz	50	10.0	1.0
(Stokely) 'Singles'	3 oz	35	7.0	0.0
BUBBLE GUM. See CANDY.				
BUCKWHEAT				
whole-grain	1/2 cup	292	60.8	2.9
whole-grain	1 oz	97	20.3	<1.0
BUCKWHEAT FLOUR				
whole-grain	1 cup	402	84.7	3.7
whole-grain	1 oz	95	20.0	0.9
whole-grain *(Arrowhead Mills)*	2 oz	190	41.0	1.0
whole-groat	1/2 cup	201	42.4	1.9
BUCKWHEAT GROATS/kasha				
brown *(Arrowhead Mills)*	2 oz	190	41.0	1.0
roasted, cooked	1/2 cup	91	19.7	0.6
roasted, cooked	4 oz	104	22.6	0.7
roasted, dry	1/2 cup	284	61.5	2.2
roasted, dry	1 oz	98	21.2	0.8
white *(Arrowhead Mills)*	2 oz	190	41.0	1.0
BUFFALO, AMERICAN/bison				
raw	1 lb	494	0.0	8.4
raw	1 oz	31	0.0	0.5
roasted	4 oz	162	0.0	2.7
roasted, diced	1 cup	200	0.0	3.4
roasted, yield from 1 lb raw	12 oz	487	0.0	8.2
BULGUR. See also TABBOULEH MIX.				
cooked	4 oz	94	21.1	0.3
cooked	1/2 cup	76	16.9	0.2
dry	1/2 cup	239	53.1	0.9
dry	1 oz	97	21.5	0.4
BULLOCK'S HEART. See CUSTARD APPLE.				
BUN. See also BISCUIT; CROISSANT; ENGLISH MUFFIN; ROLL.				
brown and serve, partially baked	2.5-inch roll	85	14.2	2.0
brown and serve, partially baked, unbrowned	2.5-inch roll	78	13.2	1.8
enriched, browned	2.5-inch roll	85	14.2	2.0
enriched, unbrowned	2.5-inch roll	84	14.2	1.9
hard, enriched, ready to cook	3.75-inch roll	156	29.7	1.6
hard, enriched, ready to cook	2.5-inch roll	78	14.9	0.8
hard, unenriched, ready to cook	3.75-inch roll	156	29.7	1.6
hard, unenriched, ready to cook	2.5-inch roll	78	14.9	0.8
Kaiser, 'Big' *(Holsum)*	1 bun	200	38.0	3.0

Food Name	Serv. Size	Total Cal.	Carbs GMS	Fat GMS
sesame seed, 'Big BBQ Buns' (Holsum)	1 bun	200	38.0	3.0
'Sof-Buns' (Holsum)	1 bun	120	23.0	2.0
BUN, FRANKFURTER				
Dijon (Pepperidge Farm)	1 bun	160	23.0	5.0
'Light' (Wonder)	1 bun	80	13.0	1.0
'New England Style' (Arnold)	1 bun	108	20.9	2.0
mixed grain	1 bun	113	19.2	2.6
oat bran (Awrey's)	1 bun	110	20.0	2.0
'Original' (Roman Meal)	1 bun	104	19.5	1.9
plain	1 bun	123	21.6	2.2
plain (Arnold)	1 bun	100	19.6	1.8
plain (Country Grain)	1 bun	100	18.0	1.0
plain (Pepperidge Farm)	1 bun	140	24.0	3.0
plain (Wonder)	1 bun	80	14.0	1.0
potato (Aunt Hattie's)	1 bun	150	23.0	4.0
reduced calorie	1 bun	84	18.1	0.9
reduced calorie	1 oz	56	11.9	0.6
whole-grain (Roman Meal)	1 bun	120	19.0	3.0
BUN, HAMBURGER				
'Light' (Wonder)	1 bun	80	13.0	1.0
mixed grain	1 bun	113	19.2	2.6
mixed grain	1 oz	75	12.6	1.7
'Original' (Roman Meal)	1 bun	113	21.1	1.9
plain	1 bun	123	21.6	2.2
plain	1 oz	81	14.3	1.5
plain (Arnold)	1 bun	115	22.0	2.2
plain (Pepperidge Farm)	1 bun	130	22.0	2.0
plain (Wonder)	1 bun	120	21.0	2.0
potato (Aunt Hattie's)	1 bun	150	23.0	4.0
reduced calorie	1 bun	84	18.1	0.9
reduced calorie	1 oz	56	11.9	0.6
whole-grain (Roman Meal)	1 bun	130	20.0	3.0
BUN, SWEET				
apple honey, multi pak, 1.5 oz (Break Cake)	1 bun	170	20.0	10.0
cheese-topped (Entenmann's)	1 bun	240	29.0	12.0
cinnamon (Entenmann's)	1 bun	230	31.0	10.0
cinnamon, frozen 'Ever Fresh' 2.5 oz (Rich's)	1 bun	293	38.0	14.6
cinnamon, frozen '2/pkg' (Pepperidge Farm)	1 bun	280	34.0	14.0
cinnamon, homestyle (Awrey's)	1 bun	240	40.0	7.0
cinnamon, iced, refrigerated (Hungry Jack)	2 buns	290	37.0	14.0
cinnamon swirl 'Grande' (Awrey's)	1 bun	340	46.0	16.0
honey (Aunt Fanny's)	3 oz	360	42.0	30.0
honey (Break Cake) 3 oz	1 bun	420	38.0	28.0

Food Name	Serv. Size	Total Cal.	Carbs GMS	Fat GMS
honey, apple bear *(Aunt Fanny's)*	4 oz	460	50.0	26.0
honey, birdie, jelly-filled *(Aunt Fanny's)*	4 oz	450	53.0	24.0
honey, bogie, creme-filled *(Aunt Fanny's)*	4 oz	460	49.0	27.0
honey, frozen, mini, 'Ever Fresh', 1.36 oz *(Rich's)*	1 bun	133	17.5	6.6
honey, lemon bear *(Aunt Fanny's)*	4 oz	440	52.0	23.0
honey, multi pak *(Break Cake)*	1 bun	380	34.0	24.0
honey, snow bear *(Aunt Fanny's)*	4 oz	480	60.0	24.0
honey-glazed *(Tastykake)*	3.25 oz	362	42.3	20.4
honey-glazed *(Hostess)*	1 bun	360	38.0	21.0
honey-iced *(Tastykake)*	3.25 oz	348	50.0	14.9
honey-iced *(Hostess)*	1 bun	430	55.0	22.0
pecan-caramel swirl *(Hostess)*	1 bun	240	23.0	15.0
BURBOT				
dry-heat cooked	3 oz	98	0.0	0.9
raw	1 lb	407	0.0	3.7
raw	1 oz	26	0.0	0.2
raw	3 oz	77	0.0	0.7
BURDOCK ROOT/gobo				
boiled, drained	4 oz	100	24.0	0.2
boiled, drained	1 root	146	35.1	0.2
boiled, drained	1 cup	110	26.4	0.2
raw	1 root	112	27.1	0.2
raw, 1-inch pieces	1 cup	85	20.5	0.2
raw, trimmed	1 oz	20	4.9	<.1
raw, untrimmed	1 lb	245	59.0	0.5
BURGER, VEGETARIAN				
canned 'Vegetarian Burger' *(Worthington)*	1/2 cup	150	9.0	4.0
canned 'Vegetarian Burger No Salt Added' *(Worthington)*	1/2 cup	160	9.0	6.0
frozen 'FriPats' *(Worthington)*	2.25-oz piece	180	5.0	12.0
frozen 'Grillers' *(Morningstar Farms)*	2.25-oz patty	180	5.0	12.0
frozen 'Harvest Burger' original flavor *(Green Giant)*	1 burger	140	8.0	4.0
frozen 'Harvest Burger' southwest style *(Green Giant)*	1 burger	140	9.0	4.0
frozen, organic *(Amy's Kitchen)*	2.5 oz	173	22.0	4.0
BURGER MIX, VEGETARIAN				
(Fantastic Foods) w/tofu, prep, excluding cooking fat	3.4-oz burger	133	14.0	5.0
(Love Natural Foods) 'Loveburger' prepared	4-oz burger	245	20.0	11.0
(Nature's Burger) barbecue, prepared, excluding cooking fat	3-oz burger	117	24.0	0.8
(Nature's Burger) 'Original' prepared, excluding cooking fat	3-oz burger	152	21.0	4.0
(Nature's Burger) pizza, prep, excluding cooking fat	3-oz burger	121	24.0	1.0
(Worthington) 'Granburger' prepared, excluding cooking fat	1 burger	110	7.0	1.0

Food Name	Serv. Size	Total Cal.	Carbs GMS	Fat GMS
BURRITO, FROZEN				
(Amy's Kitchen) bean and rice	6 oz	251	44.0	5.0
(Don Miguel) cheese, no beans	1 burrito	410	52.0	14.0
(Don Miguel) cheese and green chili	1 burrito	390	53.0	11.0
(Las Campanas) bean and cheese, no lard	1 burrito	272	42.0	7.0
(Las Campanas) beef and bean, no lard	1 burrito	304	39.0	12.0
(Maria's) jalapeño bean and cheese	1 burrito	360	54.0	11.0
(Marquez) beef, green chili, and cheese, 'Primera'	1 burrito	330	43.0	11.0
(Old El Paso) bean and cheese	1 burrito	330	45.0	11.0
(Swanson) hot and spicy 'Great Starts'	1 burrito	220	30.0	7.0
(Swanson) original, w/cheese and chili peppers 'Great Starts'	1 burrito	200	25.0	8.0
(Swanson) w/egg, bacon, cheese 'Great Starts'	1 burrito	250	27.0	11.0
(Swanson) w/egg, ham, cheese 'Great Starts'	1 burrito	210	29.0	6.0
(Swanson) w/egg, pizza sauce, cheese, pepperoni 'Great Starts'	1 burrito	240	28.0	9.0
BURRITO DINNER MIX				
(Amy's Kitchen) beans, rice, and cheese, organic	6 oz	279	43.0	8.0
(Hormel) beef	1 burrito	205	31.0	8.0
(Old El Paso) prepared, w/filling	1 burrito	299	36.0	13.0
(Patio)	12 oz	517	74.0	16.0
(Tio Sancho) 'Dinner Kit'	1 burrito	125	24.0	1.9
BURRITO DINNER, FROZEN				
beef and bean (Patio)	5 oz	370	43.0	16.0
beef and bean 'Britos' (Patio)	3.63 oz	250	33.0	10.0
beef and bean 'Festive Dinners' (Old El Paso)	11 oz	470	72.0	9.0
beef and bean, green chili (Patio)	5 oz	330	43.0	12.0
beef and bean, hot (Old El Paso)	1 burrito	310	41.0	11.0
beef and bean, medium (Old El Paso)	1 burrito	330	41.0	13.0
beef and bean, mild (Old El Paso)	1 burrito	320	42.0	11.0
beef and bean, nacho 'Britos' (Patio)	3.63 oz	270	30.0	13.0
beef and bean 'Quick Meals' 1 serving (Healthy Choice)	5.2 oz	270	42.0	7.0
beef and bean, red chili (Patio)	5 oz	340	44.0	13.0
beef steak fajita, 'Supreme' 5-oz pkg (Ruiz)	1 burrito	290	42.0	9.0
cheese (Hormel)	1 burrito	210	32.0	5.0
cheese, nacho, 'Britos' (Patio)	3.63 oz	250	32.0	10.0
chicken, spicy, 'Britos' (Patio)	3.63 oz	250	33.0	10.0
chicken and rice (Hormel)	1 burrito	200	32.0	4.0
chicken con queso 'Quick Meals' (Healthy Choice)	5.4 oz	280	40.0	8.0
chicken fajita, 'Supreme,' 5-oz pkg (Ruiz)	1 burrito	260	50.0	1.0
chili, hot (Hormel)	1 burrito	240	33.0	8.0
green chili 'Britos' (Patio)	3.63 oz	250	33.0	10.0
red chili 'Britos' (Patio)	3.63 oz	240	31.0	10.0

Food Name	Serv. Size	Total Cal.	Carbs GMS	Fat GMS
red hot *(Patio)*	5 oz	360	43.0	15.0
BURRITO FILLING FIX, beans *(Del Monte)*	1/2 cup	110	20.0	1.0
BURRITO SEASONING MIX				
(Lawry's) 'Seasoning Blends' dry mix	1 pkg	132	23.3	1.7
(Old El Paso)	1/8 pkg	17	3.0	0.0
(Tio Sancho) 'Dinner Kit'	3.25 oz	265	49.3	2.1
BUSH NUT. See MACADAMIA NUT.				
BUTTER, CLARIFIED. See GHEE.				
BUTTER, REGULAR				
lightly salted *(Breakstone's)*	1 tbsp	100	0.0	11.0
lightly salted *(Darigold)*	1 tsp	25	0.0	3.0
lightly salted *(Hotel Bar)*	1 tsp	35	0.0	4.0
lightly salted *(Kellers)*	1 tsp	35	0.0	4.0
lightly salted *(Land O'Lakes)*	1 tbsp	35	0.0	4.0
salted	4-oz stick	813	0.0	92.0
salted	1 tbsp	100	0.0	11.4
salted	1 tsp	34	0.0	3.8
salted *(Challenge)*	1 tbsp	100	0.0	11.0
salted *(Darigold)*	1 tsp	35	0.0	4.0
salted *(Hotel Bar)*	1 tsp	35	0.0	4.0
salted *(Kellers)*	1 tsp	35	0.0	4.0
salted *(Land O'Lakes)*	1 tbsp	35	0.0	4.0
salted *(Seal of Arizona)*	1 tbsp	100	0.0	11.0
salted, packed 90 pats per 1 lb	1 pat	36	0.0	4.1
unsalted	4-oz stick	813	0.1	92.0
unsalted	1 tbsp	100	0.0	11.4
unsalted	1 pat	36	0.0	4.1
unsalted	1 tsp	34	0.0	3.8
unsalted *(Breakstone's)*	1 tbsp	100	0.0	11.0
unsalted *(Challenge)*	1 tbsp	100	0.0	11.0
unsalted *(Land O'Lakes)*	1 tbsp	35	0.0	4.0
BUTTER, WHIPPED				
lightly salted *(Breakstone's)*	1 tbsp	70	0.0	7.0
lightly salted *(Land O'Lakes)*	1 tsp	25	0.0	3.0
salted	1 tbsp	67	tr	7.6
salted	1 tsp	23	tr	2.6
salted *(Land O'Lakes)*	1 tsp	25	0.0	3.0
salted, packed 120 pats per 1 lb	1 pat	27	tr	3.1
unsalted	1 tbsp	67	tr	7.6
unsalted	1 tsp	23	tr	2.6
unsalted *(Breakstone's)*	1 tbsp	70	0.0	7.0
unsalted *(Darigold)*	1 tsp	25	0.0	3.0
unsalted *(Land O'Lakes)*	1 tbsp	25	0.0	3.0

Food Name	Serv. Size	Total Cal.	Carbs GMS	Fat GMS
unsalted *(Land O'Lakes)*	1 tsp	25	0.0	3.0
BUTTER FLAVORED OIL *(Wesson)*	1 tbsp	122	0.0	13.6
BUTTER FLAVORED TOPPING *(Molly McButter)*	1/2 tsp	4.0	1.0	0.0
BUTTER OIL				
	1 oz	248	0.0	28.2
anhydrous	1 cup	1796	0.0	204.0
anhydrous	1 tbsp	112	0.0	12.7
BUTTERBEAN. See LIMA BEAN.				
BUTTERBUR/Fuki				
boiled, drained	4 oz	9	2.4	<.1
raw	1 cup	13	3.4	0.0
raw, approx .2 oz	1 stalk	1	0.2	tr
raw, trimmed	1/2 cup	7	1.7	<.1
raw, trimmed	1 oz	4	1.0	<.1
raw, untrimmed	1 lb	57	14.4	0.2
BUTTERBUR, CANNED				
	4 oz	12	0.4	0.1
chopped	1 cup	4	0.5	0.2
stalks	3 stalks	1	0.2	0.1
BUTTERFISH				
dry-heat cooked	3 oz	159	0.0	8.7
raw	1 lb	663	0.0	36.4
raw	3 oz	124	0.0	6.8
raw	1 oz	41	0.0	2.3
BUTTERHEAD LETTUCE. See LETTUCE.				
BUTTERMILK				
blend, cultured, dry *(Saco Foods)*	3.5 tbsp	79	10.7	0.7
cultured	1 cup	99	11.7	2.2
cultured	1 oz	11	1.4	0.2
cultured *(A&P)*	1 cup	90	12.0	1.0
cultured *(Crowley)*	1 cup	110	12.0	4.0
cultured, 1.5% 'Golden Churn' *(Borden)*	1 cup	120	11.0	4.0
cultured, 1.5% 'Unsalted' *(Friendship)*	1 cup	120	12.0	4.0
cultured, 2% *(Knudsen)*	1 cup	120	12.0	5.0
cultured, 'Unsalted' *(Crowley)*	1 cup	110	12.0	4.0
sweet cream, dry	1 cup	464	58.8	6.9
sweet cream, dry	1 oz	110	13.9	1.6
sweet cream, dry	1 tbsp	25	3.2	0.4
BUTTERNUT. See BRAZIL NUT.				
BUTTERNUT SQUASH. See SQUASH, BUTTERNUT				
BUTTERSCOTCH TOPPING				
	2 tbsp	103	27.0	0.0
(Kraft)	1 tbsp	60	13.0	1.0

Food Name	Serv. Size	Total Cal.	Carbs GMS	Fat GMS
(Mrs. Richardson's) caramel	2 tbsp	130	28.0	2.0
(Mrs. Richardson's) caramel fudge, microwavable	2 tbsp	130	28.0	2.0
(Smucker's)	2 tbsp	140	33.0	1.0
(Smucker's) caramel flavor 'Special Recipe'	2 tbsp	160	33.0	3.0

C

Food Name	Serv. Size	Total Cal.	Carbs GMS	Fat GMS
CABBAGE				
boiled, drained	1 head	278	56.3	5.4
boiled, drained	4 oz	24	5.4	0.3
boiled, drained, shredded	1/2 cup	16	3.3	0.3
raw, approx 2.5 lbs	1 head	227	49.3	2.5
raw, medium size *(Dole)*	1/12 head	18	3.0	0.0
raw, shredded	1/2 cup	9	1.9	0.1
raw, trimmed	1 oz	7	1.5	0.1
raw, untrimmed	1 lb	86	19.5	0.7
CABBAGE, DANISH				
fresh	1 head	218	48.8	1.6
fresh, shredded	1/2 cup	8	1.9	0.1
CABBAGE, NAPA/Chinese cabbage				
boiled, drained	1 leaf	2	0.3	0.0
boiled, drained, shredded	1/2 cup	10	1.5	0.1
bok-choy, boiled, drained	4 oz	14	2.0	0.2
bok-choy, boiled, drained, shredded	1/2 cup	10	1.5	0.1
bok-choy, raw, shredded	1/2 cup	5	0.8	0.1
bok-choy, raw, trimmed	1 oz	4	0.6	0.1
bok-choy, raw, untrimmed	1 lb	52	8.7	0.8
pe-tsai, boiled, drained	4 oz	16	2.7	0.2
pe-tsai, boiled, drained, shredded	1/2 cup	8	1.4	0.1
pe-tsai, raw, trimmed	1 oz	5	0.9	0.1
pe-tsai, raw, untrimmed	1 lb	68	13.6	0.8
raw, shredded	1/2 cup	5	0.8	0.1
CABBAGE, RED				
boiled, drained	4 oz	24	5.3	0.2
boiled, drained, shredded	1/2 cup	16	3.5	0.2
raw, shredded	1/2 cup	9	2.1	0.1
raw, trimmed	1 oz	8	1.7	0.1
CABBAGE, SAVOY				
boiled, drained	4 oz	27	6.1	0.1
boiled, drained, shredded	1/2 cup	18	4.0	0.1
raw, shredded	1/2 cup	9	2.1	0.0

Food Name	Serv. Size	Total Cal.	Carbs GMS	Fat GMS
raw, trimmed	1 oz	8	1.7	<.1
raw, untrimmed	1 lb	100	22.1	0.4
CABBAGE, SKUNK/swamp cabbage/water convolvulus				
boiled, drained	4 oz	23	4.2	0.3
boiled, drained, chopped	1/2 cup	10	1.8	0.1
raw	1 shoot	2	0.4	0.0
raw, chopped	1/2 cup	10	1.8	0.1
raw, trimmed, chopped	1/2 cup	6	0.9	0.1
raw, untrimmed	1 lb	67	11.0	0.7
CABBAGE ENTRÉE, FROZEN				
w/meat, and tomato sauce (Lean Cuisine)	9.5 oz	210	26.0	6.0
CABBAGE TURNIP. See KOHLRABI.				
CAESAR SALAD, 'Easy Caesar Kit' (Saco)	.75 oz	98	7.0	7.0
CAIMIT/star apple				
ripe, trimmed	1 oz	19	4.1	0.5
CAJUN SEASONING (Tone's)	1 tsp	9	2.1	0.2
CAJUN STYLE MARINADE, barbecue sauce (Golden Dipt)	1 oz	90	5.0	8.0
CAKE. See also BREAD, QUICK.				
'Best Wishes' 6 inch (Awrey's)	1/4 cake	150	18.0	9.0
'Four-in-One Occasion' (Awrey's)	1.3 oz	150	18.0	8.0
Banana				
loaf (Entenmann's)	1.3 oz	90	20.0	0.0
single-layer, iced, frozen (Sara Lee)	1/8 cake	170	28.0	6.0
Black forest				
torte (Awrey's)	1/14 cake	350	38.0	21.0
two-layer, frozen (Sara Lee)	1/8 cake	190	28.0	8.0
Blueberry crunch (Entenmann's)	1 oz	70	16.0	0.0
Boston cream, 'Supreme' frozen (Pepperidge Farm)	2.875 oz	290	39.0	14.0
Carrot				
cream cheese icing 'Old Fashioned' frozen (Pepperidge Farm)	1.5 oz	150	19.0	9.0
frozen (Weight Watchers)	3 oz	170	27.0	5.0
single-layer, iced, frozen (Sara Lee)	1/8 cake	250	30.0	13.0
supreme, iced (Awrey's)	1 piece	210	23.0	12.0
three-layer, cream cheese icing (Awrey's)	1/12 cake	390	44.0	23.0
Cheesecake				
brownie 'Sweet Celebrations' frozen (Weight Watchers)	3.5 oz	200	34.0	5.0
cream cheese, cherry, frozen (Sara Lee)	1/6 cake	243	35.0	8.0
cream cheese, frozen (Sara Lee)	1/6 cake	230	27.0	11.0
cream cheese, strawberry, frozen (Sara Lee)	1/6 cake	222	34.0	8.0
French 'Classics' frozen (Sara Lee)	1/8 cake	250	23.0	16.0
frozen (Weight Watchers)	3.9 oz	210	29.0	7.0
nondairy 'Better Than Cheesecake' frozen (Tofutti)	1/10 cake	160	16.0	10.0

Food Name	Serv. Size	Total Cal.	Carbs GMS	Fat GMS
strawberry, French 'Classics' frozen (Sara Lee)	1/8 cake	240	28.0	13.0
strawberry 'Sweet Celebrations' frozen (Weight Watchers)	3.9 oz	180	28.0	4.0
triple chocolate 'Sweet Celebrations' frozen (Weight Watchers)	1 cake	190	30.0	4.0
Cherry, and cream, frozen (Weight Watchers)	3 oz	190	32.0	6.0
Chocolate				
(Awrey's)	.8 oz	70	11.0	3.0
devil's food, fudge icing (Entenmann's)	1.2 oz	130	19.0	5.0
devil's food, layer, frozen (Pepperidge Farm)	1 5/8 oz	180	24.0	9.0
devil's food, white icing (Awrey's)	1 piece	150	17.0	8.0
double, iced (Awrey's)	1 piece	130	21.0	6.0
double, three-layer (Awrey's)	1/12 cake	310	48.0	14.0
double, three-layer, frozen (Sara Lee)	1/8 cake	220	26.0	11.0
double, torte (Awrey's)	1/14 cake	340	51.0	15.0
double, two-layer (Awrey's)	1/12 cake	250	38.0	11.0
double, fudge, frozen (Weight Watchers)	2.75 oz	200	34.0	5.0
'Free & Light' frozen (Sara Lee)	1/8 cake	110	26.0	0.0
frozen (Weight Watchers)	2.5 oz	180	31.0	5.0
fudge, layer, frozen (Pepperidge Farm)	1 5/8 oz	180	23.0	10.0
fudge stripe, layer, frozen (Pepperidge Farm)	1 5/8 oz	170	20.0	9.0
German, frozen (Weight Watchers)	2.5 oz	200	31.0	7.0
German, iced (Awrey's)	2-inch sq.	160	19.0	9.0
German, single-layer, frozen (Pepperidge Farm)	1 5/8 oz	180	22.0	10.0
German, three-layer (Awrey's)	1/12 cake	350	46.0	18.0
'Happy Birthday' (Awrey's)	1.4 oz	150	18.0	8.0
milk, and yellow, two-layer (Awrey's)	1/12 cake	290	33.0	17.0
mousse 'Classics' frozen (Sara Lee)	1/8 cake	260	23.0	17.0
'Supreme' frozen (Pepperidge Farm)	2 7/8 oz	300	37.0	16.0
two-layer, white icing (Awrey's)	1/12 cake	270	34.0	15.0
Cinnamon swirl, refrigerated (Pillsbury)	1/8 cake	180	22.0	9.0
Coconut				
butter cream (Awrey's)	1 piece	160	19.0	9.0
layer, frozen (Pepperidge Farm)	1 5/8 oz	180	24.0	8.0
and yellow, three-layer (Awrey's)	1/12 cake	350	40.0	21.0
Coffeecake				
all butter, cheese, frozen (Sara Lee)	1/8 cake	210	25.0	11.0
all butter, pecan, frozen (Sara Lee)	1/8 cake	160	19.0	8.0
all butter, streusel, frozen (Sara Lee)	1/8 cake	160	20.0	7.0
caramel nut (Awrey's)	1/12 cake	140	15.0	8.0
cheese (Entenmann's)	1.6 oz	150	20.0	7.0
cinnamon swirl, iced (Pillsbury)	1 piece	230	29.0	11.0
crumb (Entenmann's)	1.3 oz	160	21.0	7.0

Food Name	Serv. Size	Total Cal.	Carbs GMS	Fat GMS
crumb, cheese-filled *(Entenmann's)*	1.4 oz	130	18.0	6.0
'Long John' *(Awrey's)*	1/12 cake	160	19.0	8.0
pecan crumb, iced *(Pillsbury)*	1 piece	230	29.0	12.0
French crumb, all butter *(Entenmann's)*	1.6 oz	180	26.0	8.0
Golden				
layer, frozen *(Pepperidge Farm)*	1 5/8 oz	180	24.0	9.0
thick fudge icing *(Entenmann's)*	1.2 oz	130	20.0	6.0
Lemon				
coconut 'Supreme' frozen *(Pepperidge Farm)*	3 oz	280	38.0	13.0
cream 'Supreme' frozen *(Pepperidge Farm)*	1 5/8 oz	170	21.0	9.0
three-layer *(Awrey's)*	1/12 cake	320	38.0	19.0
yellow, two-layer *(Awrey's)*	1/12 cake	290	33.0	17.0
Louisiana crunch *(Entenmann's)*	1.7 oz	180	27.0	8.0
Neapolitan torte *(Awrey's)*	1/14 cake	380	43.0	22.0
Orange				
frosty, iced *(Awrey's)*	1 piece	150	19.0	8.0
three-layer *(Awrey's)*	1/12 cake	320	40.0	17.0
Peanut butter torte *(Awrey's)*	1/14 cake	380	44.0	22.0
Pecan streusel, refrigerated *(Pillsbury)*	1/8 cake	180	21.0	9.0
Pineapple				
cream 'Supreme' frozen *(Pepperidge Farm)*	2 oz	190	28.0	7.0
crunch *(Entenmann's)*	1 oz	70	16.0	0.0
Pistachio torte *(Awrey's)*	1/12 cake	370	41.0	22.0
Pound				
(Drake's)	1/10 cake	110	16.0	5.0
all butter 'Family Size Original' frozen *(Sara Lee)*	1/15 cake	130	14.0	7.0
all butter, loaf *(Entenmann's)*	1 oz	110	15.0	5.0
all butter 'Original' frozen *(Sara Lee)*	1/10 cake	130	14.0	7.0
'Free & Light' frozen *(Sara Lee)*	1/10 cake	70	17.0	0.0
golden *(Awrey's)*	1/14 loaf	130	19.0	5.0
'Old Fashioned Cholesterol Free' frozen *(Pepperidge Farm)*	1 oz	110	13.0	6.0
sour cream, loaf *(Entenmann's)*	1 oz	120	14.0	7.0
Raisin spice, iced *(Awrey's)*	1 piece	160	21.0	8.0
Raspberry nut *(Awrey's)*	1/16 cake	310	39.0	16.0
Shortcake				
strawberry 'Dessert Lights' frozen, 3 oz *(Pepperidge Farm)*	1 piece	170	30.0	5.0
strawberry, frozen *(Sara Lee)*	1/8 cake	190	26.0	8.0
Sponge *(Awrey's)*	2-inch sq.	80	11.0	3.0
Strawberry				
cream 'Supreme' frozen *(Pepperidge Farm)*	2 oz	190	30.0	7.0
stripe, layer, frozen *(Pepperidge Farm)*	1.5 oz	160	21.0	8.0

Food Name	Serv. Size	Total Cal.	Carbs GMS	Fat GMS
supreme, torte *(Awrey's)*	1/14 cake	270	38.0	12.0
Vanilla, layer, frozen *(Pepperidge Farm)*	1 5/8 oz	190	25.0	8.0
Walnut torte *(Awrey's)*	1/14 cake	320	38.0	19.0
Yellow				
(Awrey's)	.9 oz	80	12.0	3.0
white icing *(Awrey's)*	2-inch sq.	150	18.0	9.0
CUPCAKE				
Creme, 'Kreme Kup' *(Tastykake)*	1 cupcake	86	14.6	2.8
White *(Break Cake)*	1 cupcake	130	24.0	3.0
SNACK CAKE				
bar *(Sunbelt)*	1.31 oz	130	28.0	2.0
'Be My Valentine' *(Little Debbie)*	2.5 oz	330	44.0	17.0
'Best Wishes, Miniature' *(Awrey's)*	3 oz	320	33.0	22.0
'Caravella' *(Little Debbie)*	1.2 oz	200	26.0	9.0
'Christmas Tree' *(Little Debbie)*	1.6 oz	220	28.0	11.0
coconut covered 'Sno Balls' *(Hostess)*	1 piece	150	26.0	4.0
dessert cup *(Hostess)*	1 piece	90	18.0	2.0
dessert cup *(Little Debbie)*	.79 oz	80	4.0	1.0
'Doodle Dandies' *(Little Debbie)*	2.5 oz	320	44.0	16.0
'Easter Bunny' *(Little Debbie)*	2.5 oz	320	45.0	15.0
fancy *(Little Debbie)*	2.6 oz	340	46.0	16.0
filled twins, 3 oz *(Break Cake)*	2 pieces	310	53.0	10.0
filled twins, multi pak, 1.5 oz *(Break Cake)*	1 piece	150	26.0	5.0
'Funny Bones' *(Drake's)*	1.25 oz	150	18.0	8.0
'Lil' Angels' *(Hostess)*	1 piece	90	14.0	2.0
'Poppets' *(Erewhon)*	1 oz	110	24.0	1.0
'Star Crunch' *(Little Debbie)*	1.08 oz	150	22.0	6.0
Swiss roll *(Little Debbie)*	2.25 oz	280	40.0	12.0
'Tasty Twist' *(Tastykake)*	1 piece	18	2.7	0.6
'Tiger Tail' *(Hostess)*	1 piece	240	38.0	8.0
'Zoinks' *(Drake's)*	1.25 oz	130	20.0	5.0
Apple streusel *(Awrey's)*	1 piece	160	18.0	9.0
Banana, iced *(Awrey's)*	1 piece	140	17.0	8.0
Brownie				
À la mode 'Sweet Celebrations' frozen *(Weight Watchers)*	1 serving	180	35.0	4.0
chocolate 'Sweet Celebrations' frozen *(Weight Watchers)*	1/3 pkg	100	16.0	3.0
chocolate chip 'Toll House Ready to Bake' frozen *(Nestlé)*	1.4 oz	150	19.0	7.0
chocolate nut, mini *(Break Cake)*	.5 oz	70	9.0	4.0
Dutch chocolate 'Cake' *(Awrey's)*	1/16 cake	340	40.0	20.0
fudge *(Break Cake)*	2.8 oz	370	47.0	18.0
fudge *(Little Debbie)*	3 oz	350	57.0	12.0
fudge *(Little Debbie)*	2 oz	240	39.0	8.0
fudge nut *(Frito-Lay's)*	3 oz	360	56.0	14.0

Food Name	Serv. Size	Total Cal.	Carbs GMS	Fat GMS
fudge nut, iced 'Sheet Cake' (Awrey's)	2.5 oz	300	36.0	17.0
fudge nut 'Sheet Cake' (Awrey's)	1.25 oz	150	16.0	9.0
fudge walnut (Tastykake)	3 oz	335	53.4	14.2
hot fudge 'Newport' frozen (Pepperidge Farm)	1 ramekin	400	50.0	20.0
low-fat, fudge, chocolate icing 'Lights' (Hostess)	1 brownie	140	29.0	2.6
mint frosting 'Sweet Celebrations' frozen				
(Weight Watchers)	1.23 oz	100	18.0	2.0
peanut butter fudge 'Sweet Celebrations' frozen				
(Weight Watchers)	1.23 oz	100	18.0	3.0
Swiss mocha fudge 'Sweet Celebrations' frozen				
(Weight Watchers)	1.23 oz	90	18.0	2.0
Caramel				
fudge, À la mode, frozen (Weight Watchers)	1 serving	180	35.0	3.0
peanut filled, chocolate coated (Little Debbie)	1 piece	230	28.0	12.0
Carrot				
(Break Cake)	2 pieces	370	64.0	12.0
'Classic' frozen, 2.5 oz (Pepperidge Farm)	1 piece	260	32.0	16.0
'Deluxe' frozen, 1.8 oz (Sara Lee)	1 piece	180	26.0	7.0
'Lights' frozen, 2.5 oz (Sara Lee)	1 piece	170	30.0	4.0
multi pak, 1.2 oz (Break Cake)	1 piece	120	20.0	4.0
Cheesecake				
brownie 'Sweet Celebrations' frozen (Weight Watchers)	3.5 oz	200	34.0	5.0
classic, frozen, 2 oz (Sara Lee)	1 piece	200	16.0	14.0
French 'Lights' frozen, 3.2 oz (Sara Lee)	1 piece	150	24.0	4.0
French, strawberry 'Lights' frozen, 3.5 oz (Sara Lee)	1 piece	150	29.0	2.0
strawberry 'Manhattan' frozen (Pepperidge Farm)	1 piece	300	49.0	9.0
strawberry 'Sweet Celebrations' frozen				
(Weight Watchers)	3.9 oz	180	28.0	4.0
Cinnamon, twirl (Aunt Fanny's)	1 oz	110	16.0	4.0
Coffeecake				
(Little Debbie)	2.1 oz	250	39.0	9.0
apple cinnamon, individually wrapped, frozen				
(Sara Lee)	1 piece	290	40.0	13.0
butter streusel, individually wrapped, frozen				
(Sara Lee)	1 piece	230	27.0	12.0
cinnamon crumb (Drake's)	1.33 oz	150	22.0	6.0
cinnamon streusel 'Microwave' frozen				
(Weight Watchers)	1 piece	190	28.0	7.0
cream filled 'Koffee Kake' (Tastykake)	1 oz	110	17.5	4.0
crumb (Hostess)	1 piece	120	19.0	5.0
crumb 'Light' (Hostess)	1 piece	80	19.0	1.0
'Jr.' (Drake's)	1.1 oz	140	18.0	6.0
'Koffee Kake Juniors' (Tastykake)	2.5 oz	261	43.8	8.5

Food Name	Serv. Size	Total Cal.	Carbs GMS	Fat GMS
pecan, individually wrapped, frozen *(Sara Lee)*	1 piece	280	30.0	16.0
'Small' *(Drake's)*	2 oz	220	33.0	9.0
Oatmeal, creme pie, individually wrapped *(Little Debbie)*	1.35 oz	170	29.0	8.0
Shortcake				
strawberry, À la mode, frozen *(Weight Watchers)*	1 piece	170	33.0	2.0
strawberry 'Dessert Lights' frozen *(Pepperidge Farm)*	1 piece	170	30.0	5.0
CAKE, MICROWAVE				
apple streusel, prepared *(MicroRave)*	1/12 cake	240	33.0	11.0
banana, w/vanilla frosting 'Snack' prepared *(Pillsbury)*	1/9 cake	170	26.0	7.0
carrot, w/cream cheese frosting 'Snack' prepared *(Pillsbury)*	1/9 cake	170	25.0	7.0
cinnamon pecan, prepared *(MicroRave)*	1/6 cake	290	39.0	13.0
cinnamon streusel, prepared *(Streusel Swirl)*	1/8 cake	240	33.0	11.0
chocolate, prepared *(Pillsbury)*	1/8 cake	210	23.0	13.0
chocolate, w/chocolate frosting, prepared *(Pillsbury)*	1/8 cake	300	35.0	17.0
chocolate, w/vanilla frosting, prepared *(Pillsbury)*	1/8 cake	300	36.0	17.0
chocolate supreme, double, prepared *(Pillsbury)*	1/8 cake	330	39.0	19.0
devil's food, w/chocolate frosting, dry mix *(MicroRave)*	1/6 pkg	210	35.0	7.0
German chocolate, w/coconut pecan frosting, dry mix *(MicroRave)*	1/6 pkg	230	37.0	8.0
lemon, prepared *(Pillsbury)*	1/8 cake	220	23.0	13.0
lemon, w/lemon frosting, prepared *(MicroRave)*	1/6 cake	300	37.0	16.0
lemon, w/lemon frosting, prepared *(Pillsbury)*	1/8 cake	300	37.0	17.0
lemon supreme, double, prepared *(Pillsbury)*	1/8 cake	300	40.0	15.0
yellow, w/chocolate frosting, prepared *(Pillsbury)*	1/8 cake	300	36.0	17.0
yellow, w/chocolate frosting 'Singles' dry mix *(MicroRave)*	1/6 pkg	210	36.0	7.0
SNACK CAKE				
Brownie				
caramel 'Supreme' prepared *(Betty Crocker)*	1 brownie	110	21.0	2.0
caramel 'Supreme' prepared *(General Mills)*	1 brownie	110	21.0	2.0
caramel fudge chunk, prepared *(Pillsbury)*	1 brownie	170	25.0	7.0
carrot, dry mix *(Pillsbury)*	1/9 pkg	110	17.0	5.0
chocolate chip 'Supreme' prepared *(Betty Crocker)*	1 brownie	110	20.0	3.0
chocolate chip 'Supreme' prepared *(General Mills)*	1 brownie	110	20.0	3.0
double chocolate, prepared *(Great Additions)*	1 brownie	140	19.0	6.0
double fudge 'Brownies Plus' prepared *(Duncan Hines)*	1 brownie	150	22.0	6.0
double fudge, prepared *(Pillsbury)*	1 brownie	160	24.0	6.0
frosted, prepared *(MicroRave)*	1 brownie	180	27.0	7.0
frosted 'Supreme' prepared *(Betty Crocker)*	1 brownie	140	26.0	3.0
frosted 'Supreme' prepared *(General Mills)*	1 brownie	140	26.0	3.0

Food Name	Serv. Size	Total Cal.	Carbs GMS	Fat GMS
fudge, mix only *(Duncan Hines)*	1 brownie	100	18.0	18.0
fudge, 21.5-oz pkg, dry mix *(Pillsbury)*	1/24 pkg	100	20.0	2.0
fudge, 15-oz pkg, dry mix *(Pillsbury)*	1/16 pkg	110	21.0	2.0
fudge 'Family Size' prepared *(General Mills)*	1 brownie	110	22.0	2.0
fudge 'Light' prepared *(General Mills)*	1 brownie	100	21.0	1.0
fudge, prepared *(Pillsbury)*	1 brownie	190	25.0	9.0
fudge, prepared *(Duncan Hines)*	1 brownie	130	18.0	5.0
fudge, prepared *(Krusteaz)*	1 brownie	190	28.0	8.0
fudge, prepared *(Lovin' Lites)*	1/24 pkg	100	19.0	2.0
fudge 'Pouch Mix' dry mix *(Gold Medal)*	1/16 pkg	100	16.0	4.0
fudge 'Pouch Mix' dry mix *(Robin Hood)*	1/16 pkg	100	16.0	4.0
fudge 'Regular Size' prepared *(General Mills)*	1 brownie	110	23.0	2.0
fudge 'Ultra Moist' dry mix *(Finast)*	1/16 pkg	130	20.0	5.0
fudge, w/fudge frosting, prepared *(Pilsbury)*	1/9 pkg	240	32.0	11.0
fudge deluxe 'Family Size' prepared *(Pillsbury)*	1 brownie	150	20.0	7.0
fudge deluxe, prepared *(Pillsbury)*	1 brownie	150	21.0	6.0
fudge deluxe, w/walnuts, prepared *(Pillsbury)*	1 brownie	150	19.0	8.0
'Funfetti Frosted' prepared *(Great Additions)*	1 brownie	160	23.0	7.0
German chocolate 'Supreme' prepared *(Betty Crocker)*	1 brownie	130	24.0	3.0
German chocolate 'Supreme' prepared *(General Mills)*	1 brownie	130	24.0	3.0
'Gourmet Turtle' prepared *(Duncan Hines)*	1 brownie	200	27.0	9.0
milk chocolate 'Brownies Plus' prepared *(Duncan Hines)*	1 brownie	160	20.0	8.0
original 'Supreme' prepared *(Betty Crocker)*	1 brownie	120	22.0	3.0
original 'Supreme' prepared *(General Mills)*	1 brownie	120	22.0	3.0
party 'Supreme' prepared *(Betty Crocker)*	1 brownie	140	26.0	3.0
party 'Supreme' prepared *(General Mills)*	1 brownie	140	26.0	3.0
peanut butter 'Brownies Plus' prepared *(Duncan Hines)*	1 brownie	150	16.0	8.0
peanut butter candies 'Supreme' prepared *(Betty Crocker)*	1 brownie	140	21.0	5.0
prepared *(Estee)*	1 brownie	50	11.0	2.0
rocky road, fudge *(Pillsbury)*	1 brownie	170	24.0	8.0
'Singles' prepared *(MicroRave)*	1 brownie	250	39.0	9.0
triple fudge, chunky *(Pillsbury)*	1 brownie	170	25.0	7.0
walnut 'Brownies Plus' prepared *(Duncan Hines)*	1 brownie	150	19.0	7.0
walnut, prepared *(Great Additions)*	1 brownie	140	16.0	8.0
walnut, prepared *(MicroRave)*	1 brownie	160	21.0	7.0
walnut 'Supreme' prepared *(Betty Crocker)*	1 brownie	110	18.0	4.0
walnut 'Supreme' prepared *(General Mills)*	1 brownie	110	18.0	4.0
walnut 'Ultra Moist' prepared *(Finast)*	1 brownie	130	19.0	6.0
w/hot fudge topping 'Singles' prepared *(MicroRave)*	1 brownie	340	54.0	12.0

CAKE MIX

Angel food

| chocolate, dry mix *(General Mills)* | 1/12 pkg | 150 | 34.0 | 0.0 |

Food Name	Serv. Size	Total Cal.	Carbs GMS	Fat GMS
confetti, dry mix *(General Mills)*	1/12 pkg	150	34.0	0.0
dry mix *(Duncan Hines)*	1/12 pkg	140	30.0	0.0
dry mix *(Lovin' Loaf)*	1/8 pkg	90	20.0	0.0
lemon custard, dry mix *(General Mills)*	1/12 pkg	150	34.0	0.0
lemon pudding, dry mix *(General Mills)*	1/12 pkg	150	34.0	0.0
strawberry, dry mix *(General Mills)*	1/12 pkg	150	35.0	0.0
'Traditional' dry mix *(Betty Crocker)*	1/12 pkg	130	30.0	0.0
white, one-step, dry mix *(General Mills)*	1/12 pkg	150	34.0	0.0
Apple cinnamon, prepared *(SuperMoist)*	1/12 cake	250	36.0	10.0
Banana				
dry mix *(Duncan Hines)*	1/12 pkg	190	36.0	4.0
dry mix *(Pillsbury Plus)*	1/12 pkg	180	34.0	4.0
Black forest				
cherry 'Bundt Ring Cake' dry mix *(Pillsbury)*	1/16 pkg	200	40.0	4.0
mousse 'Tiarra' prepared *(Duncan Hines)*	1/12 cake	260	33.0	13.0
Blueberry streusel, dry mix *(Streusel Swirl)*	1/16 pkg	210	39.0	5.0
Boston cream, chocolate Eclair 'Bundt Ring Cake' dry mix *(Pillsbury)*	1/16 pkg	210	42.0	4.0
Butter brickle, prepared *(SuperMoist)*	1/12 cake	250	38.0	10.0
Butter pecan, dry mix *(SuperMoist)*	1/12 pkg	180	35.0	4.0
Butter recipe				
chocolate, dry mix *(Pillsbury Plus)*	1/12 pkg	170	32.0	4.0
chocolate, dry mix *(SuperMoist)*	1/12 pkg	190	35.0	5.0
dry mix *(Pillsbury Plus)*	1/12 pkg	170	35.0	3.0
fudge, dry mix *(Duncan Hines)*	1/12 pkg	190	34.0	4.0
golden, dry mix *(Duncan Hines)*	1/12 pkg	190	36.0	4.0
yellow, dry mix *(SuperMoist)*	1/12 pkg	170	37.0	2.0
Carrot				
dry mix *(SuperMoist)*	1/12 pkg	180	36.0	3.0
'n' spice, dry mix *(Pillsbury Plus)*	1/12 pkg	180	33.0	5.0
prepared *(Dromedary)*	1/12 cake	232	23.0	15.0
prepared *(Estee)*	1/10 cake	100	18.0	2.0
Cheesecake				
lemon 'No Bake' dry mix *(Jell-O)*	1 pkg	170	31.0	3.0
lite 'No-Bake' prepared *(Royal)*	1/8 cake	210	23.0	10.0
New York style 'No Bake' dry mix *(Jell-O)*	1 pkg	180	33.0	3.0
'No Bake' dry mix *(Jell-O)*	1 pkg	160	30.0	4.0
real 'No-Bake' prepared *(Royal)*	1/8 cake	280	31.0	9.0
Cherry, and cream 'Tiarra' prepared *(Duncan Hines)*	1/12 cake	250	34.0	11.0
Cherry chip, dry mix *(SuperMoist)*	1/12 pkg	180	37.0	3.0
Chocolate				
caramel 'Bundt Ring Cake' dry mix *(Pillsbury)*	1/16 pkg	220	43.0	5.0
chocolate chip, dry mix *(SuperMoist)*	1/12 pkg	190	34.0	5.0

Food Name	Serv. Size	Total Cal.	Carbs GMS	Fat GMS
dark, dry mix *(Pillsbury Plus)*	1/12 pkg	170	32.0	5.0
devil's food, dry mix *(Duncan Hines)*	1/12 pkg	190	33.0	5.0
devil's food, dry mix *(Lovin' Lites)*	1/12 pkg	160	32.0	2.0
devil's food, dry mix *(Pillsbury Plus)*	1/12 pkg	170	32.0	4.0
devil's food, dry mix *(SuperMoist)*	1/12 pkg	190	35.0	5.0
devil's food 'Light' dry mix *(SuperMoist)*	1/12 pkg	180	36.0	3.0
devil's food, prepared *(Krusteaz)*	1/12 cake	190	37.0	2.0
devil's food 'Ultra Moist' prepared *(Finast)*	1/12 cake	250	33.0	11.0
Dutch fudge, dark, dry mix *(Duncan Hines)*	1/12 pkg	190	33.0	5.0
fudge, dry mix *(SuperMoist)*	1/12 pkg	180	35.0	4.0
fudge 'Tunnel of Fudge' dry mix *(Pillsbury)*	1/16 pkg	210	42.0	4.0
fudge marble, dry mix *(Duncan Hines)*	1/12 pkg	190	36.0	4.0
fudge marble, dry mix *(SuperMoist)*	1/12 pkg	180	36.0	4.0
fudge swirl, dry mix *(Pillsbury Plus)*	1/12 pkg	180	36.0	5.0
German, dry mix *(Pillsbury Plus)*	1/12 pkg	170	33.0	4.0
German, dry mix *(SuperMoist)*	1/12 pkg	180	35.0	4.0
macaroon 'Bundt Ring Cake' dry mix *(Pillsbury)*	1/16 pkg	210	37.0	7.0
milk, dry mix *(SuperMoist)*	1/12 pkg	190	34.0	5.0
mousse, amaretto 'Tiarra' prepared *(Duncan Hines)*	1/12 cake	270	29.0	16.0
mousse 'Bundt Ring Cake' dry mix *(Pillsbury)*	1/16 pkg	180	37.0	4.0
mousse 'Tiarra' prepared *(Duncan Hines)*	1/12 cake	270	29.0	16.0
prepared *(Estee)*	1/10 cake	100	18.0	2.0
pudding 'Classic Dessert' dry mix *(Betty Crocker)*	1/6 pkg	220	44.0	4.0
Swiss, dry mix *(Duncan Hines)*	1/12 pkg	190	33.0	5.0
Chocolate chip				
dry mix *(Pillsbury Plus)*	1/12 pkg	180	34.0	5.0
dry mix *(SuperMoist)*	1/12 pkg	180	35.0	4.0
Cinnamon streusel, dry mix *(Streusel Swirl)*	1/16 pkg	200	38.0	5.0
Coffeecake				
apple cinnamon, prepared *(Pillsbury)*	1/8 cake	240	40.0	7.0
'Flako' prepared *(Quaker)*	1 piece	156	27.1	4.4
prepared *(Aunt Jemima)*	1 piece	156	27.1	4.4
Lemon				
'Bundt Tunnel of Lemon' dry mix *(Pillsbury)*	1/16 pkg	210	44.0	4.0
chiffon 'Classic Dessert' dry mix *(Betty Crocker)*	1/12 pkg	190	36.0	4.0
dry mix *(Pillsbury Plus)*	1/12 pkg	170	34.0	3.0
dry mix *(SuperMoist)*	1/12 pkg	180	36.0	4.0
prepared *(Estee)*	1/10 cake	100	18.0	2.0
pudding 'Classic Dessert' dry mix *(Betty Crocker)*	1/6 pkg	220	45.0	4.0
supreme, dry mix *(Duncan Hines)*	1/12 pkg	190	36.0	4.0
supreme, dry mix *(Streusel Swirl)*	1/16 pkg	200	37.0	6.0
Orange, supreme, dry mix *(Duncan Hines)*	1/12 pkg	190	36.0	4.0

Food Name	Serv. Size	Total Cal.	Carbs GMS	Fat GMS
Pineapple				
creme 'Bundt Ring Cake' dry mix *(Pillsbury)*	1/16 pkg	200	42.0	3.0
supreme, dry mix *(Duncan Hines)*	1/12 pkg	190	36.0	4.0
upside down 'Classic Dessert' dry mix *(Betty Crocker)*	1/9 pkg	240	43.0	7.0
Plain, 'Funfetti' dry mix *(Pillsbury Plus)*	1/12 pkg	180	35.0	4.0
Pound				
dry mix *(Dromedary)*	5 tbsp	130	20.0	5.0
golden 'Classic Dessert' dry mix *(Betty Crocker)*	1/12 pkg	190	28.0	8.0
prepared *(Estee)*	1/8 cake	120	23.0	2.5
prepared *(Martha White)*	1/10 cake	120	19.0	4.0
Rainbow chip, party cake, dry mix *(SuperMoist)*	1/12 pkg	180	35.0	4.0
Sour cream				
chocolate, dry mix *(SuperMoist)*	1/12 pkg	180	35.0	4.0
white, dry mix *(SuperMoist)*	1/12 pkg	180	36.0	3.0
Spice				
dry mix *(Duncan Hines)*	1/12 pkg	190	36.0	4.0
dry mix *(SuperMoist)*	1/12 pkg	180	36.0	4.0
prepared *(Estee)*	1/8 cake	120	23.0	3.0
Strawberry				
dry mix *(Pillsbury Plus)*	1/12 pkg	180	35.0	4.0
supreme, dry mix *(Duncan Hines)*	1/12 pkg	190	36.0	4.0
Swirl, party cake, prepared *(SuperMoist)*	1/12 cake	260	36.0	11.0
Vanilla				
French, dry mix *(Duncan Hines)*	1/12 pkg	190	36.0	4.0
golden, dry mix *(SuperMoist)*	1/12 pkg	180	36.0	4.0
golden, prepared *(MicroRave)*	1/6 cake	320	40.0	17.0
sunshine, dry mix *(Pillsbury Plus)*	1/12 pkg	180	34.0	5.0
White				
dry mix *(Duncan Hines)*	1/12 pkg	190	36.0	4.0
dry mix *(Lovin' Lites)*	1/12 pkg	170	35.0	2.0
dry mix *(Lovin' Loaf)*	1/12 pkg	170	35.0	2.0
dry mix *(Pillsbury Plus)*	1/12 pkg	180	34.0	4.0
dry mix *(SuperMoist)*	1/12 pkg	180	34.0	4.0
'Light' dry mix *(SuperMoist)*	1/12 pkg	180	37.0	3.0
'n fudge swirl, dry mix *(Pillsbury Plus)*	1/12 pkg	190	36.0	4.0
prepared *(Estee)*	1/10 cake	100	18.0	2.0
prepared *(Krusteaz)*	1/12 cake	190	37.0	3.0
Yellow				
dry mix *(Duncan Hines)*	1/12 pkg	190	36.0	4.0
dry mix *(Pillsbury Plus)*	1/12 pkg	180	34.0	5.0
dry mix *(SuperMoist)*	1/12 pkg	180	36.0	4.0
'Light' dry mix *(SuperMoist)*	1/12 pkg	180	37.0	3.0
prepared *(Krusteaz)*	1/12 cake	200	36.0	5.0

Food Name	Serv. Size	Total Cal.	Carbs GMS	Fat GMS
prepared *(Lovin' Loaf)*	1/12 cake	180	35.0	3.0
'Ultra Moist' prepared *(Finast)*	1/12 cake	240	34.0	10.0
CALAMANSI PUNCH, 'Rain Forest' *(Knudsen & Sons)*	8 oz	115	27.0	0.0
CALAMARI. See SQUID, MIXED SPECIES.				
CALICO BASS. See SUNFISH.				
CALIFORNIA SHEEPSHEAD. See SHEEPSHEAD.				
CANADIAN BACON. See BACON, CANADIAN-STYLE.				
CANDLEFISH/eulachon				
dry-heat cooked	4 oz	141	0.0	3.5
raw	1 lb	440	0.0	11.0
raw	1 oz	27	0.0	0.7
CANDY				
'Bridge Mix' *(Brach's)*	1 oz	140	17.0	7.0
'Estee-ets' *(Estee)*	5 pieces	35	4.0	2.0
'Home Fashioned Favorites' *(Russell Stover)*	1.4 oz	170	27.0	7.0
'Smoothie' 1.6 oz *(Boyer)*	2 pieces	250	24.0	15.0
'Smoothie' .5 oz *(Boyer)*	1 piece	75	12.5	7.5
'Smoothie' .275 oz *(Boyer)*	1 piece	38	6.3	3.8
ALMOND				
'Almond Delights' *(Russell Stover)*	1.4 oz	210	22.0	12.0
chocolate covered *(Estee)*	2 squares	60	4.5	4.5
chocolate covered *(Featherweight)*	1 section	90	6.0	7.0
'Golden Almond Solitaires' chocolate covered *(Hershey's)*	1.5 oz	240	19.0	16.0
'Golden Almond Solitaires' chocolate covered *(Hershey's)*	3 oz	455	40.0	31.5
'Jordan Almonds' candy coated *(Brach's)*	1 oz	120	23.0	2.0
'Kisses w/Almonds' chocolate w/almonds, 1 oz *(Hershey's)*	6 pieces	160	14.0	10.0
'M&M's' candy coated almonds *(M&M/Mars)*	1 oz	150	17.0	8.0
'Solitaires' chocolate covered, 1.6 oz *(Hershey's)*	1/2 bar	260	20.0	17.0
AMARETTO CHOCOLATE, 'Buffalo Ball' confection *(Great Cakes)*	1 ball	105	27.0	3.5
BAR				
'Aero' milk chocolate, dark chocolate *(Nestlé)*	1 bar	210	20.0	12.0
'Aero' milk chocolate, dark chocolate, bite size *(Nestlé)*	2 bars	85	10.0	5.0
'Almond Crunch' date sweetened, carob *(Carafection)*	1 oz	139	17.0	7.0
'Almond Joy' 1.76 oz *(Hershey's)*	1 bar	232	29.2	13.9
'Almond Joy' miniatures *(Hershey's)*	2 pieces	120	14.0	7.0
'Almond Joy' snack size *(Hershey's)*	1 bar	93	11.7	5.5
'Alpine White' white chocolate w/almonds *(Nestlé)*	1 bar	197	17.6	12.9
'Alpine White' white chocolate w/almonds, 2.2 oz *(Nestlé)*	1 bar	350	31.3	22.9
'A-Ok' fruit juice sweetened *(Natures Warehouse)*	1 oz	130	16.5	6.2
'Baby Ruth' chocolate w/peanuts *(Nestlé)*	1 bar	277	37.2	13.3
'Baby Ruth' chocolate w/peanuts, fun size *(Nestlé)*	1 bar	110	15.0	5.0

Food Name	Serv. Size	Total Cal.	Carbs GMS	Fat GMS
'Bar None' 1.5 oz *(Bar None)*	1 bar	224	22.5	14.6
'Bounty' dark chocolate *(M&M/Mars)*	1 oz	140	17.0	8.0
'Bounty' milk chocolate *(M&M/Mars)*	1 oz	140	17.0	7.0
'Brazil Nut Crunch' *(Yogafection)*	1 oz	180	17.0	10.0
'Butterfinger' 2.16 oz *(Nestlé)*	1 bar	267	40.5	11.3
'Butterfinger' snack size *(Nestlé)*	1 bar	92	13.9	3.9
'Caramello' 5 oz *(Cadbury)*	1 bar	694	93.7	35.9
'Caramello' 1.6 oz *(Cadbury)*	1 bar	220	29.7	11.4
carob *(Caroby)*	4 sections	150	13.0	9.0
carob candy, plain, date sweetened *(Carafection)*	1 oz	139	17.0	7.0
carob coated *(Tiger's Milk)*	1 bar	160	22.0	6.0
carob coated 'Light' *(Tiger's Milk)*	1 bar	110	24.0	3.0
'Cashew Coconut Crunch' carob candy *(Carafection)*	1 oz	139	17.0	7.0
'Cashew Nut Crunch' *(Yogafection)*	1 oz	180	17.0	10.0
'Chew!' nougat, chocolate coated, all flavors *(Charleston)*	1 oz	120	22.0	3.0
chocolate tofu truffle w/pralines *(Barat)*	1 oz	170	12.0	11.0
chocolate tofu w/almonds *(Barat)*	1 oz	170	13.0	11.0
chocolate tofu w/almonds and raisins *(Barat)*	1 oz	160	14.0	11.0
chocolate w/almonds, w/o sugar, extra thick *(Fifty 50)*	1 section	90	6.0	6.0
chocolate w/coconut *(Estee)*	2 squares	60	5.0	4.0
chocolate w/crisps and honey *(Cadbury)*	1 oz	150	18.0	7.0
chocolate w/fruit and nuts *(Cadbury)*	1 oz	150	17.0	8.0
chocolate w/fruit and nuts *(Estee)*	2 squares	60	4.5	4.5
chocolate w/fruit and nuts, w/o sugar, extra thick *(Fifty 50)*	1 section	80	6.0	5.0
chocolate w/roasted almonds *(Cadbury)*	1 oz	150	15.0	9.0
'Chunky' 1.4 oz *(Nestlé)*	1 bar	198	22.8	11.7
'Chunky' 1.25 oz *(Nestlé)*	1 bar	173	20.0	10.2
'Chunky' w/raisins, peanuts and cashews *(Nestlé)*	1.4 oz	170	21.0	12.0
'Cookies 'N' Mint' mint chocolate, cookie pieces *(Hershey's)*	1 bar	220	26.0	12.0
'Crispy Crunch' carob candy, date sweetened *(Carafection)*	1 oz	139	17.0	7.0
crunch *(Estee)*	2 squares	45	4.0	3.0
crunch, chocolate, w/o sugar, extra thick *(Fifty 50)*	1 section	70	6.0	5.0
'Crunch' milk chocolate w/crisp rice, 1.4 oz *(Nestlé)*	1 bar	210	26.0	10.0
'Crunch' milk chocolate w/crisp rice, fun size *(Nestlé)*	2 bars	100	13.0	5.0
'Crunch' milk chocolate w/crisp rice, snack size *(Nestlé)*	1 bar	49	6.4	2.6
'Dairy Milk' milk chocolate *(Cadbury)*	1 oz	150	17.0	8.0
dark chocolate, deluxe *(Estee)*	2 squares	50	6.0	3.0
'Dove' dark chocolate, miniatures *(M&M/Mars)*	4 pieces	130	14.0	8.0
'Dove' milk chocolate, miniatures *(M&M/Mars)*	4 pieces	130	14.0	8.0
'5th Avenue' 4.2 oz *(Hershey's)*	1 pkg	555	80.9	25.2
'5th Avenue' 2.1 oz *(Hershey's)*	1 bar	280	40.8	12.7
French chocolate *(Russell Stover)*	1 bar	200	20.0	13.0

Food Name	Serv. Size	Total Cal.	Carbs GMS	Fat GMS
French chocolate mint *(Russell Stover)*	1 bar	230	20.0	15.5
'Golden Almond' chocolate w/almonds, 3 oz *(Hershey's)*	1 bar	466	41.3	32.1
'Golden III' 3.2 oz	1 bar	471	50.8	30.0
'Halvah' *(Fantastic Foods)*	1.5 oz	232	17.0	10.0
'Hershey's Milk Chocolate Bar' *(Hershey's)*	1.55 oz	240	25.0	14.0
'Hershey's Milk Chocolate Bar w/Almonds' *(Hershey's)*	1.45 oz	230	20.0	14.0
'Kit Kat' chocolate covered wafer, 3.375 oz *(Hershey's)*	1 bar	490	59.4	27.4
'Kit Kat' chocolate covered wafer, 1.625 oz *(Hershey's)*	1 bar	235	28.5	13.1
'Kit Kat' chocolate covered wafer, snack size *(Hershey's)*	1.12 oz	170	20.0	9.0
'Krackel' chocolate w/rice crisps, 2.6 oz *(Hershey's)*	1 bar	371	45.8	20.6
'Krackel' chocolate w/rice crisps, 1.65 oz *(Hershey's)*	1 bar	236	29.1	13.1
'Mars Almond, 1.76 oz *(M&M/Mars)*	1 bar	233	31.4	11.5
milk chocolate *(Estee)*	2 squares	60	5.0	4.0
milk chocolate, mini *(Fifty 50)*	4 pieces	90	6.0	6.0
milk chocolate w/o sugar, extra thick *(Fifty 50)*	1 section	80	6.0	6.0
'Milky Way' dark chocolate *(M&M/Mars)*	1.76 oz	220	36.0	8.0
'Milky Way' milk chocolate, 2.1 oz *(M&M/Mars)*	1 bar	251	43.5	9.1
'Milky Way' milk chocolate, minis *(M&M/Mars)*	1 piece	40	6.0	1.0
'Milky Way' milk chocolate, snack size *(M&M/Mars)*	1 bar	75	13.1	2.7
mint *(Estee)*	2 squares	50	6.0	3.0
'Mint' date sweetened, carob candy *(Carafection)*	1 oz	139	17.0	7.0
'Mint Honey Graham' carob coated *(Carafection)*	1 oz	139	17.0	7.0
'Mounds' chocolate covered coconut, 1.9 oz *(Hershey's)*	1 pkg	195	31.3	11.7
'Mounds' chocolate covered coconut, minis *(Hershey's)*	2 pieces	110	13.0	6.0
'Mounds' chocolate covered coconut, snack size *(Hershey's)*	1 bar	72	11.6	4.3
'Mr. GoodBar' milk chocolate w/peanuts, 2.8 oz *(Hershey's)*	1 bar	406	40.5	25.5
'Mr. GoodBar' milk chocolate w/peanuts, 1.75 oz *(Hershey's)*	1 bar	257	25.6	16.1
'Munch' *(M&M/Mars)*	1.42 oz	220	19.0	14.0
'My O My' fruit juice sweetened *(Natures Warehouse)*	1 oz	103	20.5	1.4
'No How' peanut butter, fruit juice sweetened *(Natures Warehouse)*	1 oz	140	11.0	10.0
'Non Stop' fruit juice sweetened *(Natures Warehouse)*	1 oz	122	18.2	5.0
'Nut Wit' carob, caramel, and peanuts *(Natures Warehouse)*	1 oz	135	16.5	6.3
'Oh Henry!' chocolate covered caramel w/peanuts, 2 oz *(Nestlé)*	1 bar	246	36.9	9.6
'100 Grand' 1.5 oz *(Nestlé)*	1 bar	195	30.9	8.5
'Original' *(Cocofection)*	1 oz	155	15.0	10.0
'Original Honey Graham' carob coated *(Carafection)*	1 oz	139	17.0	7.0
'Pay Day' *(Pay Day)*	1.85 oz	250	28.0	12.0
peanut butter *(Russell Stover)*	1 bar	290	22.0	19.0
peanut butter, carob coated *(Tiger's Milk)*	1 bar	160	20.0	7.0
peanut butter, carob coated 'Light' *(Tiger's Milk)*	1 bar	110	24.0	3.0
peanut butter and honey, carob coated *(Tiger's Milk)*	1 bar	160	23.0	5.0

Food Name	Serv. Size	Total Cal.	Carbs GMS	Fat GMS
'Peanut Crunch' carob candy, date sweetened (Carafection)	1 oz	139	17.0	7.0
'Protein Blast' high-energy, chocolate (Weider)	1 bar	270	40.0	6.0
'Skor' toffee, 1.4 oz (Hershey's)	1 bar	211	22.0	13.8
'Sky Bar' (Necco)	1.5 oz	196	31.5	7.1
'Snickers' 2.16 oz (M&M/Mars)	1 bar	278	36.8	13.6
'Snickers,' minis (M&M/Mars)	1 piece	45	5.0	2.0
'Snickers' snack size (M&M/Mars)	1 bar	68	9.0	3.3
'Soft'n Crunchy Bar' 1 3/16 oz (Heath)	2 pieces	190	19.0	12.0
'Special Dark' sweet chocolate bar, 2.8 oz (Hershey's)	1 bar	376	48.7	23.9
'Special Dark' sweet chocolate bar, 1.45 oz (Hershey's)	1 bar	195	25.3	12.4
'Symphony' milk chocolate, 2.4 oz (Hershey's)	1 bar	355	38.6	22.0
'Symphony' milk chocolate, 1.4 oz (Hershey's)	1 bar	209	22.7	13.0
'Symphony' milk chocolate w/almonds and toffee chips (Hershey's)	1.4 oz	220	20.0	14.0
'3 Musketeers' 2.13 oz (M&M/Mars)	1 bar	250	46.1	7.7
'3 Musketeers' snack size (M&M/Mars)	1 bar	75	13.8	2.3
'Twix' caramel, 2.0 oz (M&M/Mars)	1 pkg	272	37.5	13.4
'Twix' cookies-n-creme (M&M/Mars)	1 bar	120	13.0	7.0
'Twix' peanut butter, 1.77 oz (M&M/Mars)	1 pkg	253	28.5	14.5
'Whatchamacallit' 1.8 oz (Hershey's)	1 bar	257	30.0	13.2
BUBBLE GUM				
(Beechies) candy coated	1 piece	6	2.0	0.0
(Bubble Yum)				
bananaberry split	1 piece	25	7.0	0.0
checkermint	1 piece	25	7.0	0.0
cherry	1 piece	25	7.0	0.0
fruit	1 piece	25	7.0	0.0
grape	1 piece	25	7.0	0.0
Hawaiian punch	1 piece	25	7.0	0.0
luscious lime	1 piece	25	7.0	0.0
strawberry stripe	1 piece	25	7.0	0.0
sugarless, fruit	1 piece	20	5.0	0.0
sugarless, grape	1 piece	20	5.0	0.0
sugarless, peppermint	1 piece	20	5.0	0.0
sugarless, strawberry	1 piece	20	5.0	0.0
3-flavor, grape, cherry and fruit	1 piece	25	7.0	0.0
wet 'n wild watermelon	1 piece	25	7.0	0.0
(Bubblicious)				
	1 piece	25	6.2	tr
'Sugarless'	1 piece	5	1.3	tr
(Care Free) sugarless				
fruit	1 piece	10	2.0	0.0
wild cherry	1 piece	10	2.0	0.0

Food Name	Serv. Size	Total Cal.	Carbs GMS	Fat GMS
wintergreen	1 piece	10	2.0	0.0
(Chiclets)				
candy coated	1 piece	6	1.5	tr
'Tiny' candy coated	1 pkg	8	<.1	tr
(Clorets) candy coated	1 piece	6	1.5	tr
(Extra)				
classic	1 piece	6	(mq)	(mq)
original	1 piece	7	(mq)	(mq)
(Fruit Stripe)				
cherry	1 piece	8	2.0	0.0
fruit	1 piece	8	2.0	0.0
grape	1 piece	8	2.0	0.0
lemon	1 piece	8	2.0	0.0
(Hubba Bubba)				
regular, all flavors	1 piece	23	5.8	0.0
'Sugar-free' grape	1 piece	13	(mq)	0.0
sugar-free, original	1 piece	14	(mq)	0.0
BUTTERSCOTCH, squares *(Russell Stover)*	1.4 oz	180	29.0	6.5
CARAMEL				
(Allen Wertz)	1 piece	37	6.0	2.0
(Featherweight)	1 piece	30	5.0	1.0
(Kraft)	1 piece	30	6.0	1.0
butter cream, squares *(Russell Stover)*	1.4 oz	170	26.0	7.5
chocolate *(Estee)*	1 piece	20	3.0	1.0
chocolate coated *(Pom Poms)*	1 oz	100	15.0	3.0
marshmallow, milk chocolate, squares *(Russell Stover)*	1.4 oz	190	25.0	10.0
milk chocolate coated, approx 1.93 oz *(Rolo)*	8 pieces	270	37.0	12.0
'Milk Maid' *(Brach's)*	1 oz	110	22.0	2.0
'Milk Maid' chocolate *(Brach's)*	1 oz	110	20.0	3.0
'Nip' *(Pearson)*	1 oz	120	23.0	3.0
nougat swirl *(Allen Wertz)*	1 piece	32	6.0	1.0
pop *(Sugar Daddy)*	1 3/8 oz	150	33.0	1.0
'Regular' 1 5/8 oz *(Sugar Babies)*	1 pkg	180	40.0	2.0
'Rolos' milk chocolate covered *(Hershey's)*	1.93 oz	270	37.0	12.0
'Tidbits' 1 5/8 oz *(Sugar Babies)*	1 pkg	180	40.0	2.0
vanilla *(Estee)*	1 piece	20	3.0	1.0
CHERRY				
'Cherry Cordials' *(Russell Stover)*	1.4 oz	170	25.0	7.5
chocolate cream *(Brach's)*	1 oz	110	21.0	2.0
dark chocolate coated *(Brach's)*	1 oz	110	22.0	2.0
'Nibs' *(Y&S)*	1 oz	106	26.2	0.7
squares *(Russell Stover)*	1.4 oz	160	28.0	5.5
'Villa' milk chocolate covered *(Brach's)*	1 oz	110	22.0	2.0

Food Name	Serv. Size	Total Cal.	Carbs GMS	Fat GMS
CHEWING GUM				
(Beech-Nut)				
cinnamon	1 piece	10	2.0	0.0
fruit	1 piece	10	2.0	0.0
peppermint	1 piece	10	2.0	0.0
spearmint	1 piece	10	2.0	0.0
(Brach's) 'Gumdinger' balls, all flavors	1 oz	110	24.0	2.0
(Care Free) sugarless				
cinnamon	1 piece	8	2.0	0.0
peppermint	1 piece	8	2.0	0.0
spearmint	1 piece	8	2.0	0.0
(Chewels) all flavors	1 piece	8	2.0	tr
(Clorets) stick, all flavors	1 piece	9	2.3	tr
(Dentyne)				
all flavors	1 piece	6	1.5	tr
'Sugarless' all flavors	1 piece	5	1.1	tr
(Estee) gumdrops	4 pieces	25	6.0	0.0
(Extra)				
cinnamon	1 stick	8	(mq)	(mq)
peppermint	1 stick	8	(mq)	(mq)
spearmint	1 stick	8	(mq)	(mq)
winter fresh	1 stick	8	(mq)	(mq)
(Freedent)				
cinnamon	1 stick	10	2.0	(mq)
peppermint	1 stick	10	2.0	(mq)
spearmint	1 stick	10	2.0	(mq)
(Freshen-Up) all flavors	1 piece	13	3.1	tr
(Fruit Stripe)				
cherry	1 piece	10	2.0	0.0
lemon	1 piece	10	2.0	0.0
lime	1 piece	10	2.0	0.0
orange	1 piece	10	2.0	0.0
(Sticklets) all flavors	1 piece	7	1.9	tr
(Wrigley's)				
'Big Red'	1 piece	10	2.3	0.0
'Doublemint'	1 piece	10	2.3	0.0
'Juicy Fruit'	1 piece	10	2.3	0.0
'Spearmint'	1 piece	10	2.3	0.0
CHOCOLATE				
assorted, wrapped, 1-lb bag *(Brach's)*	1 oz	110	23.0	2.0
'Bits' tofu pastilles *(Barat)*	.75 oz	120	11.0	8.0
chewy roll *(Tootsie Roll)*	1 oz	112	22.8	2.5
'Choc'Oh's' *(Saco Foods)*	1.5 oz	111	13.8	6.6

Food Name	Serv. Size	Total Cal.	Carbs GMS	Fat GMS
chunks (Saco Foods)	3.5 oz	466	66.8	26.4
coated, creme center (Spangler)	1 piece	80	15.0	2.0
coated, creme center caramel, w/nuts (Spangler)	1 piece	100	11.0	6.0
coated, creme center cherry, w/nuts (Spangler)	1 piece	110	12.0	5.0
coated, creme center fudge, w/nuts (Spangler)	1 piece	140	17.0	6.0
coated, creme center fudge, w/pecans (Spangler)	1 piece	140	18.0	7.0
coated, creme center maple, w/nuts (Spangler)	1 piece	110	12.0	5.0
coated, creme center vanilla, w/nuts (Spangler)	1 piece	110	13.0	5.0
cream (Callard & Bowser)	1 oz	120	22.3	3.7
creamy milk, w/almonds and toffee chips (Hershey's)	.75 oz	280	26.0	17.0
crunch (Featherweight)	1 section	80	7.0	6.0
'Gift Box' dark and milk mix (Russell Stover)	1.4 oz	180	26.0	8.5
'Gourmet' assortment (Allen Wertz)	11.9 grams	55	9.0	2.0
'Jots' (Brach's)	1 oz	130	21.0	5.0
'Kisses' (Hershey's)	6 pieces	150	16.0	9.0
'M&M's' plain (M&M/Mars)	10 pieces	33	4.8	1.5
'M&M's' plain, 1.69 oz (M&M/Mars)	1 pkg	228	32.7	10.7
'Malted Milk Balls' milk coated (Brach's)	1 oz	130	21.0	5.0
malted milk balls, milk coated (Whoppers)	1 oz	136	20.0	6.0
milk (Featherweight)	1 section	80	7.0	6.0
milk, assortment (Russell Stover)	1.4 oz	190	27.0	8.5
'Passionettes' tofu (Barat)	1 piece	70	6.0	5.0
'Stars' (Brach's)	1 oz	150	17.0	8.0
'Stars' approx 13 pieces (Nabisco)	1 oz	160	19.0	8.0
trail mix, premium (Cocofection)	1 oz	130	13.0	9.0
COCONUT				
'Macaroo' chocolate coated (Sunbelt)	2 oz	288	33.0	16.0
Neapolitan (Brach's)	1 oz	120	24.0	2.0
COFFEE				
(Brach's)	1 oz	120	25.0	2.0
'Coffee Time' (Allen Wertz)	1 piece	20	4.0	1.0
'Coffee Time' assorted (Allen Wertz)	1 piece	28	5.0	1.0
'Coffee Time' decaffeinated (Allen Wertz)	1 piece	20	4.0	1.0
'Nip' (Pearson)	1 oz	120	23.0	3.0
FONDANT, candy corn	1 cup	728	179.2	4.0
FRUIT				
(Bonkers!) chews, all flavors	1 piece	20	5.0	0.0
(Brach's)				
orange sticks, chocolate coated	1 oz	110	23.0	2.0
'Orangettes'	1 oz	100	24.0	0.0
(Featherweight)				
berry patch	1 piece	12	3.0	0.0
drops, all flavors	.33 oz	30	8.0	0.0

Food Name	Serv. Size	Total Cal.	Carbs GMS	Fat GMS
orchard	1 piece	12	3.0	0.0
tropical blend	1 piece	12	3.0	0.0
(Glenny's) 'Drops'				
black cherry	1 drop	6	1.0	<1.0
Mandarin orange	1 drop	6	1.0	<1.0
mixed fruit	1 drop	6	1.0	<1.0
twist of lemon	1 drop	6	1.0	<1.0
(Jujyfruits)	11 pieces	100	25.0	<1.0
(Rascals) chews, all flavors	1 piece	4	1.0	tr
(Russell Stover) lemon squares	1.4 oz	160	27.0	5.5
'Skittles' *(M&M/Mars)*				
candy coated, bite size	1 oz	120	26.0	1.0
candy coated, bite size, 2.3 oz	1 pkg	255	62.4	2.0
'Starburst' *(M&M/Mars)*				
original fruit chews	2 oz	240	48.0	5.0
tropical fruit chews	2 oz	240	48.0	5.0
(Soda-Licious) all flavors	1 pouch	100	22.0	1.0
(SweeTARTS) chewy	1 oz	113	25.0	1.0
'Twizzlers' *(Y&S)*				
strawberry sticks, 5 oz	1 pkg	525	131.6	2.3
strawberry sticks, 2.5 oz	1 pkg	263	65.8	1.1
FUDGE				
chocolate, w/walnuts *(Woodys)*	1 oz	120	18.0	4.0
'Fudgies' *(Kraft)*	1 piece	35	6.0	1.0
maple walnut *(Woodys)*	1 oz	120	19.0	4.0
mint, w/walnuts *(Woodys)*	1 oz	120	18.0	4.0
w/walnuts *(Woodys)*	1 oz	120	18.0	4.0
HARD CANDY				
(Brach's)				
'Cut Rock'	1 oz	110	27.0	0.0
'Disks' butterscotch	1 oz	110	27.0	0.0
'Disks' cinnamon	1 oz	110	27.0	0.0
filled, assorted	1 oz	110	27.0	0.0
'Imperials' cinnamon	1 oz	110	27.0	0.0
lemon drops	1 oz	110	27.0	0.0
raspberry filled	1 oz	110	27.0	0.0
ribbon, crimp	1 oz	110	27.0	0.0
'Royals'	1 oz	100	20.0	2.0
sour balls	1 oz	110	27.0	0.0
'Spicettes'	1 oz	100	26.0	0.0
(Breath Savers)				
cores, mint-cinnamon	1 piece	2	<1.0	0.0
cores, peppermint	1 piece	2	<1.0	0.0

Food Name	Serv. Size	Total Cal.	Carbs GMS	Fat GMS
cores, spearmint	1 piece	2	<1.0	0.0
cores, wintergreen	1 piece	2	<1.0	0.0
mint-cinnamon	1 piece	8	2.0	0.0
peppermint	1 piece	8	2.0	0.0
spearmint	1 piece	8	2.0	0.0
wintergreen	1 piece	8	2.0	0.0
(Callard & Bowser) butterscotch	1 oz	115	25.2	1.9
(Ce De) 'Smarties'	1 roll	25	6.0	0.0
(Certs)				
sugar-free, mini	1 piece	1	0.4	tr
sugar-free, mints	1 piece	6	1.6	tr
(Clorets)				
clear mint	1 piece	8	2.1	tr
pressed mints	1 piece	6	1.6	tr
(Estee)	2 pieces	25	6.0	0.0
(Featherweight)				
butterscotch	1 piece	25	6.0	0.0
'Sweet Pretenders' tropical blend	1 piece	12	3.0	0.0
(Fruit Juicers)				
citrus fruits	1 piece	8	2.0	0.0
fruit punch	1 piece	8	2.0	0.0
grape	1 piece	8	2.0	0.0
mixed berries	1 piece	8	2.0	0.0
strawberry	1 piece	8	2.0	0.0
(Glenny's)				
fruit	1 piece	19	4.0	<1.0
peppermint	1 piece	19	4.0	<1.0
(Jolly Joes)	1 piece	9	2.1	tr
(Jolly Rancher)				
apple	1 piece	23	6.0	0.0
butterscotch	1 piece	25	6.0	<1.0
cherry	1 piece	23	6.0	0.0
fire cinnamon	1 piece	23	6.0	0.0
fruit punch	1 piece	23	6.0	0.0
grape	1 piece	23	6.0	0.0
lemon	1 piece	23	6.0	0.0
orange	1 piece	23	6.0	0.0
peach	1 piece	23	6.0	0.0
peppermint	1 piece	23	6.0	0.0
pink lemonade	1 piece	23	6.0	0.0
raspberry	1 piece	23	6.0	0.0
strawberry	1 piece	23	6.0	0.0
watermelon	1 piece	23	6.0	0.0

Food Name	Serv. Size	Total Cal.	Carbs GMS	Fat GMS
(Jurassic Park)				
'Raptor Bites' wild cherry	13 pieces	60	15.0	0.0
'Spitters' tropical flavors	13 pieces	60	15.0	0.0
(Life Savers)				
butter creme mint	1 piece	8	2.0	0.0
butter rum	1 piece	8	2.0	0.0
butterscotch	1 piece	8	2.0	0.0
'Cin-O-Mon'	1 piece	8	2.0	0.0
'Cryst-O-Mint'	1 piece	8	2.0	0.0
fancy fruits	1 piece	8	2.0	0.0
five flavor	1 piece	8	2.0	0.0
holes, butter rum	1 piece	2	<1.0	0.0
holes, five flavor	1 piece	2	<1.0	0.0
holes, pepomint	1 piece	2	<1.0	0.0
candy coated, bite size	10 pieces	43	10.6	0.3
holes, sunshine fruits	1 piece	2	<1.0	0.0
holes, tangerine	1 piece	2	<1.0	0.0
holes, 'Wint-O-Green'	1 piece	2	<1.0	0.0
'Pep-O-Mint'	1 piece	8	2.0	0.0
root beer	1 piece	8	2.0	0.0
'Spear-O-Mint'	1 piece	8	2.0	0.0
sunshine fruits	1 piece	8	2.0	0.0
tropical fruits	1 piece	8	2.0	0.0
wild cherry	1 piece	8	2.0	0.0
'Wint-O-Green'	1 piece	8	2.0	0.0
(Mike & Ike)	1 piece	9	2.1	tr
(Pearson) 'Nip' butter rum	1 oz	120	24.0	3.0
(Russell Stover) sugar-free, mix	3 pieces	70	18.0	0.0
(Spree) fruit	1 oz	110	26.0	0.0
(SweeTARTS) fruit	1 oz	110	26.0	0.0
HOLIDAY				
assorted, chocolate *(Brach's)*	1 oz	110	23.0	2.0
autumn leaves *(Brach's)*	1 oz	100	26.0	0.0
bell, chocolate, in foil *(Brach's)*	1 oz	150	17.0	8.0
holiday mints *(Brach's)*	1 oz	110	26.0	1.0
holiday mix *(Brach's)*	1 oz	110	27.0	0.0
Christmas				
candy cane *(Brach's)*	1 oz	110	27.0	0.0
candy cane *(Spangler)*	1 piece	60	14.0	<1.0
jellies *(Brach's)*	1 oz	100	24.0	0.0
jellies, snowbase *(Brach's)*	1 oz	100	24.0	0.0
'Jots' *(Brach's)*	1 oz	130	21.0	5.0
nougat *(Brach's)*	1 oz	110	24.0	2.0

Food Name	Serv. Size	Total Cal.	Carbs GMS	Fat GMS
ornaments *(Brach's)*	1 oz	150	17.0	8.0
'Pearls' mint *(Brach's)*	1 oz	110	25.0	1.0
'Perkys' *(Brach's)*	1 oz	90	23.0	0.0
Santa, chocolate, in foil *(Brach's)*	1 oz	140	18.0	7.0
Santa, marshmallow *(Brach's)*	1 oz	120	23.0	3.0
snowmen, marshmallow, large pieces *(Just Born)*	1 piece	111	26.8	0.1
snowmen, marshmallow, small pieces *(Just Born)*	1 piece	37	8.9	<.1
'Starlight' mint *(Brach's)*	1 oz	110	27.0	0.0
trees, marshmallow, large pieces *(Just Born)*	1 piece	111	26.8	0.1
trees, marshmallow, small pieces *(Just Born)*	1 piece	37	8.9	<.1
Easter				
'Chicks & Rabbits' assorted *(Brach's)*	1 oz	100	26.0	0.0
corn *(Brach's)*	1 oz	100	26.0	0.0
'Easter Fun' assorted *(Brach's)*	1 oz	100	26.0	0.0
eggs, chocolate, in foil *(Brach's)*	1 oz	150	17.0	8.0
eggs, chocolate malted milk *(Brach's)*	1 oz	130	21.0	5.0
eggs, creme *(Cadbury)*	1.37 oz	190	26.0	8.0
eggs, creme, chocolate coated buttercream *(Brach's)*	1 oz	120	22.0	3.0
eggs, creme, chocolate coated cherry *(Brach's)*	1 oz	110	23.0	2.0
eggs, creme, chocolate coated coconut *(Brach's)*	1 oz	110	22.0	3.0
eggs, creme, chocolate coated fruit and nut *(Brach's)*	1 oz	110	23.0	2.0
eggs, creme, chocolate coated maple *(Brach's)*	1 oz	110	23.0	2.0
eggs, creme, chocolate coated vanilla *(Brach's)*	1 oz	110	23.0	2.0
eggs, creme, mini *(Cadbury)*	1 oz	140	20.0	7.0
eggs, 'Fiesta' pastel *(Brach's)*	1 oz	120	23.0	3.0
eggs 'Hide'n Seek' *(Brach's)*	1 oz	110	27.0	0.0
eggs, jelly *(Brach's)*	1 oz	100	24.0	0.0
eggs, jelly, speckled *(Brach's)*	1 oz	110	27.0	0.0
eggs, jelly, spiced *(Brach's)*	1 oz	90	22.0	0.0
eggs, jelly 'Tiny' *(Brach's)*	1 oz	100	26.0	0.0
eggs, marshmallow *(Brach's)*	1 oz	100	25.0	0.0
eggs, 'Robin's Eggs' *(Brach's)*	1 oz	140	20.0	6.0
nougats *(Brach's)*	1 oz	100	24.0	1.0
peeps, marshmallow *(Just Born)*	1 piece	27	6.6	<.1
rabbits, 'Jube' *(Brach's)*	1 oz	100	24.0	0.0
rabbits, marshmallow *(Brach's)*	1 oz	120	22.0	3.0
'Starlight' mint *(Brach's)*	1 oz	110	27.0	0.0
Halloween				
cats, marshmallow *(Just Born)*	1 piece	28	6.7	<.1
cats 'Scary Cats' *(Brach's)*	1 oz	100	26.0	0.0
corn, Indian *(Brach's)*	1 oz	100	26.0	0.0
corn, three color *(Brach's)*	1 oz	100	26.0	0.0
jelly beans *(Brach's)*	1 oz	100	26.0	0.0

Food Name	Serv. Size	Total Cal.	Carbs GMS	Fat GMS
lollipops 'Picture Pops' (Brach's)	1 oz	110	27.0	0.0
'Mellowcremes' (Brach's)	1 oz	100	26.0	0.0
pumpkin heads, crazy (Brach's)	1 oz	100	24.0	1.0
pumpkins (Brach's)	1 oz	100	26.0	0.0
pumpkins, marshmallow, large pieces (Just Born)	1 piece	111	26.8	0.1
pumpkins, marshmallow, small pieces (Just Born)	1 piece	14	3.4	<.1
'Trick or Treat Party Pack' (Brach's)	1 oz	110	27.0	0.0
witches' teeth (Brach's)	1 oz	100	26.0	0.0
Valentine's Day				
'Heart Box, 1-lb' (Brach's)	1 oz	110	23.0	2.0
'Heart Box, 1/2-lb' (Brach's)	1 oz	110	23.0	2.0
'Heart Box, 1/3-lb' (Brach's)	1 oz	110	23.0	2.0
hearts 'Conversation' large (Brach's)	1 oz	110	27.0	0.0
hearts 'Conversation' small (Brach's)	1 oz	110	27.0	0.0
hearts, fruity (Brach's)	1 oz	100	24.0	0.0
hearts 'Imperial' cinnamon (Brach's)	1 oz	110	27.0	0.0
hearts, 'Jube' cherry (Brach's)	1 oz	100	26.0	0.0
hearts, red jelly (Brach's)	1 oz	100	24.0	0.0
hearts 'Sassy Hearts' (Brach's)	1 oz	100	25.0	0.0
'I Luv U' chocolate (Brach's)	1 oz	150	17.0	8.0
kisses, nougat (Brach's)	1 oz	110	24.0	2.0
lollipop, pastels (Life Savers)	1 lollipop	40	10.0	0.0
'Love' (Brach's)	1 oz	150	17.0	8.0
'Mellowcremes' (Brach's)	1 oz	100	26.0	0.0
JELLIED AND GUMMED				
cinnamon bears (Brach's)	1 oz	80	21.0	0.0
eggs (Rodda)	1 piece	7	1.7	tr
'Fruit Bunch' (Brach's)	1 oz	100	24.0	0.0
gummi bears (Brach's)	1 oz	100	22.0	0.0
gummi dinosaurs, tropical (Jurassic Park)	15 pieces	140	31.0	0.0
gummi savers (Life Savers)	1 piece	12	3.0	0.0
gummi worms (Brach's)	1 oz	100	22.0	0.0
gummy bears (Estee)	4 pieces	20	4.0	0.0
gummy bears 'Amazin Fruit' approx 12 pieces (Hershey's)	1 oz	90	21.0	<1.0
gummy bears, tropical 'Amazin Fruit' (Hershey's)	1 oz	90	21.0	<1.0
hot cinnamon (Hot Tamales)	1 piece	9	2.1	tr
jelly beans (Brach's)	1 oz	100	26.0	0.0
jelly nougat (Brach's)	1 oz	100	24.0	1.0
'Jels' sour cherry (Brach's)	1 oz	100	26.0	0.0
'Jube Jels' (Brach's)	1 oz	100	24.0	0.0
juicy (Callard & Bowser)	1 oz	90	22.9	0.0
mint, assorted (Brach's)	1 oz	100	26.0	0.0
'Petite' eggs (Just Born)	1 piece	4	1.1	tr

Food Name	Serv. Size	Total Cal.	Carbs GMS	Fat GMS
'Rainbow Bears' (Brach's)	1 oz	100	24.0	0.0
'Spearmint Leaves' (Brach's)	1 oz	100	24.0	0.0
spicettes (Brach's)	1 oz	100	26.0	0.0
'Teenee Beanee Gourmet' (Just Born)	1 piece	4	1.1	tr
LICORICE				
candy coated (Good & Fruity)	1 oz	106	25.7	0.1
candy coated (Good & Plenty)	1 oz	106	25.9	<.1
'Cherry Nibs' (Y&S)	1 oz	100	23.0	<1.0
'Nip' (Pearson)	1 oz	120	23.0	3.0
'Red Laces' (Brach's)	1 oz	100	22.0	0.0
'Twin Twists' (Brach's)	1 oz	100	22.0	0.0
'Twists' (Brach's)	1 oz	100	22.0	1.0
'Twizzlers Bites' cherry (Y&S)	1 oz	100	23.0	<1.0
'Twizzlers' strawberry (Y&S)	1 oz	100	23.0	1.0
LOLLIPOP				
all flavors (Estee)	1 lollipop	30	7.0	0.0
all flavors (Life Savers)	1 lollipop	45	11.0	0.0
all flavors bubble gum center (Spangler)	1 lollipop	57	14.0	<1.0
all flavors 'Dum Dums' (Spangler)	1 lollipop	25	6.0	<1.0
all flavors except chocolate (Tootsie Pop)	1 oz	111	26.4	0.6
all fruit flavors (Sorbee)	1 lollipop	22	5.0	0.0
all flavors 'Pops' (Brach's)	1 oz	110	27.0	0.0
all flavors 'Saf-T-Pops' (Spangler)	1 lollipop	45	11.0	<1.0
black raspberry (Fruit Juicers)	1 lollipop	40	10.0	0.0
chocolate (Tootsie Pop)	1 oz	110	26.2	0.6
fruit (Glenny's)	1 lollipop	21	5.0	<1.0
fruit punch (Fruit Juicers)	1 lollipop	40	10.0	0.0
pineapple (Fruit Juicers)	1 lollipop	40	10.0	0.0
strawberry (Fruit Juicers)	1 lollipop	40	10.0	0.0
swirled (Life Savers)	1 lollipop	45	11.0	0.0
vitamin 'C' (Glenny's)	1 lollipop	35	8.0	<1.0
MARSHMALLOW				
'Circus Peanuts' approx 1 oz (Spangler)	4 pieces	110	26.0	<1.0
'Mallow Cup' 1.6 oz (Boyer)	2 pieces	224	30.0	11.0
'Mallow Cup' .5 oz (Boyer)	1 piece	71	15.0	5.0
'Mallow Cup' .275 oz (Boyer)	1 piece	36	7.5	2.5
'Perkys Circus Peanuts' (Brach's)	1 oz	100	26.0	0.0
toasted coconut (Just Born)	1 piece	30	6.1	0.6
MINT				
'After Dinner' tofu, chocolate (Barat)	1 piece	40	4.0	2.0
'After Eight' dark chocolate (Rowntree)	1 mint	35	6.0	1.0
all flavors except cocoamint (Velamints)	1 mint	7	1.7	0.0
'Bits' tofu, chocolate (Barat)	.75 oz	120	11.0	8.0

Food Name	Serv. Size	Total Cal.	Carbs GMS	Fat GMS
butter *(Kraft)*	1 piece	8	2.0	0.0
cocoamint *(Velamints)*	1 mint	7	1.5	0.3
'Cool Blue' *(Featherweight)*	1 piece	25	6.0	0.0
'Coolers/Starlight' *(Brach's)*	1 oz	110	27.0	0.0
creme, chocolate covered, regular *(Brach's)*	1 oz	110	24.0	2.0
'Creme de Menthe' *(Brach's)*	1 oz	150	16.0	9.0
'Creme de Menthe' chocolate *(Andes)*	6 pieces	150	16.0	9.0
dark chocolate coated *(Spangler)*	1 piece	80	14.0	2.0
'Dessert Mints' assorted *(Brach's)*	1 oz	110	27.0	0.0
'Drops' *(Glenny's)*	1 drop	6	1.0	<1.0
filled straws *(Brach's)*	1 oz	110	26.0	1.0
'Jots/Pearls' *(Brach's)*	1 oz	120	25.0	2.0
'Junior Mints' chocolate covered, 1 oz	12 pieces	120	24.0	3.0
'Kentucky Mints' *(Brach's)*	1 oz	110	27.0	0.0
'Meltaway' .33 oz *(Mint)*	1 piece	50	5.0	3.0
'Nip' chocolate *(Pearson)*	1 oz	120	23.0	3.0
'Mint Oh's' *(Saco Foods)*	1.5 oz	111	13.8	6.6
parfait *(Brach's)*	1 oz	150	16.0	9.0
party *(Kraft)*	1 piece	8	2.0	0.0
peppermint kisses *(Brach's)*	1 oz	100	24.0	1.0
'Peppermint Pattie' large patties *(York)*	1 piece	149	33.6	3.9
'Peppermint Pattie' small patties *(York)*	1 piece	38	8.6	1.0
peppermint swirls *(Featherweight)*	1 piece	20	5.0	0.0
squares *(Russell Stover)*	1.4 oz	160	28.0	5.0
thin, chocolate covered, regular *(Brach's)*	1 oz	110	24.0	2.0
NONPAREILS				
dark chocolate *(Brach's)*	1 oz	140	20.0	6.0
'Sno-Caps' *(Nestlé)*	1 oz	140	21.0	6.0
PEANUT				
'Bits' chocolate tofu, dipped *(Barat)*	1 oz	120	8.0	8.0
candy coated *(Estee)*	10 pieces	70	8.0	4.0
caramel cluster *(Brach's)*	1 oz	150	15.0	8.0
chocolate coated *(Cocofection)*	1 oz	140	10.0	12.0
chocolate coated *(Estee)*	2 squares	60	4.5	4.5
chocolate coated, approx 14 pieces *(Nabisco)*	1 oz	160	14.0	9.0
chocolate coated 'Small' *(Brach's)*	1 oz	140	15.0	7.0
filled *(Brach's)*	1 oz	110	25.0	1.0
French, burnt *(Brach's)*	1 oz	130	18.0	5.0
'Goobers' chocolate covered *(Nestlé)*	10 pieces	51	4.9	3.3
'Goobers' chocolate covered, 1 3/8 oz *(Nestlé)*	1 pkg	200	16.0	13.0
'Jots' *(Brach's)*	1 oz	140	18.0	6.0
'M&M's' candy coated chocolate peanuts *(M&M/Mars)*	10 pieces	99	11.8	5.4

Food Name	Serv. Size	Total Cal.	Carbs GMS	Fat GMS
'M&M's' candy coated chocolate peanuts, fun size				
(M&M/Mars)	1 pkg	110	13.0	5.0
milk chocolate coated (Brach's)	1 oz	150	15.0	9.0
'Nut Goodies' (Brach's)	1 oz	130	21.0	4.0
parfait (Brach's)	1 oz	160	14.0	10.0
'Peanut Clusters' (Brach's)	1 oz	150	15.0	9.0
'Peanut Delights' (Russell Stover)	1.4 oz	210	22.0	12.0
PEANUT BRITTLE				
(Estee)	.5 oz	60	10.0	2.0
(Estee)	.25 oz	35	5.0	1.0
(Kraft)	1 oz	130	20.0	5.0
(Sophie Mae)	1.4 oz	170	30.0	5.0
PEANUT BUTTER				
'Bar None' (Hershey's)	1.5 oz	240	23.0	14.0
cup (Estee)	1 cup	40	3.0	3.0
cup, 1.6 oz (Boyer)	2 pieces	250	23.0	15.0
cup, .5 oz (Boyer)	1 piece	75	12.0	7.5
cup, .275 oz (Boyer)	1 piece	38	6.0	3.8
kisses (Brach's)	1 oz	110	22.0	2.0
'Kudos' chocolate covered (M&M/Mars)	1.3 oz	200	19.0	12.0
'M&M's' candy coated (M&M/Mars)	1.63 oz	240	28.0	12.0
'M&M's' candy coated (M&M/Mars)	1 oz	150	17.0	7.0
'PB Max' chocolate covered cookie (M&M/Mars)	1 piece	240	20.0	15.0
'Reese's Crunchy Peanut Butter Cups' (Hershey's)	1.8 oz	280	24.0	18.0
'Reese's Peanut Butter Cups' (Hershey's)	1.6 oz	250	23.0	15.0
'Reese's Peanut Butter Cups' (Hershey's)	1.8 oz	247	24.4	15.9
'Reese's Peanut Butter Cups' miniatures (Hershey's)	6 cups	204	20.1	13.1
'Reese's Peanut Butter Cups' snack size (Hershey's)	1 cup	100	9.0	6.0
'Reese's Pieces' candy coated (Hershey's)	1.63 oz	230	28.0	10.0
'Reese's Pieces' candy coated (Hershey's)	10 pieces	38	5.0	1.7
'Reese's Pieces' candy coated, 1.95 oz (Hershey's)	1 pkg	258	34.2	11.4
toffee (Flavor House)	1 oz	150	17.0	7.0
PECAN				
'Demet's Turtles' milk chocolate, pecans, caramel (Demet's)	1 piece	82	9.9	4.7
'Pecan Crowns' (Russell Stover)	1.4 oz	200	19.0	13.0
'Pecan Delights' (Russell Stover)	1.4 oz	220	19.0	14.5
POWDER CANDY				
(Lik-m-aid Fun Dip)	1 oz	110	26.0	0.0
(Pixy Stix)	1 oz	100	26.0	0.0
RAISIN				
'Bits' chocolate tofu covered (Barat)	1 oz	120	14.0	7.0
chocolate coated (Brach's)	1 oz	130	20.0	5.0
chocolate coated (Cocofection)	1 oz	120	20.0	5.0

Food Name	Serv. Size	Total Cal.	Carbs GMS	Fat GMS
chocolate coated *(Estee)*	8 pieces	30	5.0	1.0
chocolate coated, approx 29 pieces *(Nabisco)*	1 oz	130	21.0	5.0
'Raisinets' chocolate covered *(Nestlé)*	1 3/8 oz	180	28.0	6.0
'Raisinets' chocolate covered *(Nestlé)*	10 pieces	41	7.1	1.6
'Raisinets' chocolate covered *(Nestlé)*	1.58 oz	185	32.0	7.2
TAFFY				
all flavors 'Salt Water Taffy' *(Brach's)*	1 oz	100	24.0	1.0
apple flavor 'Laffy Taffy' 1 oz *(Beich's)*	2 pieces	110	26.0	1.0
banana flavor 'Laffy Taffy' 1 oz *(Beich's)*	2 pieces	120	26.0	1.0
cherry flavor 'Laffy Taffy' 1 oz *(Beich's)*	2 pieces	110	26.0	1.0
grape flavor 'Laffy Taffy' 1 oz *(Beich's)*	2 pieces	110	26.0	1.0
honey flavor *(Bit-O-Honey)*	1.7 oz	200	39.0	4.0
passion punch flavor 'Laffy Taffy' 1 oz *(Beich's)*	2 pieces	120	26.0	1.0
strawberry flavor 'Laffy Taffy' 1 oz *(Beich's)*	2 pieces	110	26.0	1.0
tangy flavor *(Tangy Taffy)*	1 oz	120	23.0	2.5
watermelon flavor 'Laffy Taffy' 1 oz *(Beich's)*	2 pieces	110	26.0	1.0
TOFFEE				
(Brach's)	1 oz	110	23.0	2.0
(Callard & Bowser)	1 oz	135	19.2	6.5
'Bits'O Brickle' *(Heath)*	3 oz	448	50.0	28.0
English *(Bits'O Heath)*	3.5 oz	520	62.0	31.0
English, 'Heath Bar' 1 3/16 oz *(Heath)*	2 pieces	180	20.0	11.0
CANDY APPLE. See APPLE KIT.				
CANE SYRUP				
table blends	1/2 cup	397	102.4	0.0
table blends	1 tbsp	50	12.8	0.0
CANNELLINI BEAN, canned, white *(Pathmark)*	1/2 cup	100	18.0	0.0
CANNELLONI, CANNED, mini *(Chef Boyardee)*	7.5 oz	230	33.0	7.0
CANNELLONI ENTRÉE, frozen				
beef, w/tomato sauce *(Lean Cuisine)*	9 5/8 oz	200	28.0	3.0
cheese *(Dining Lite)*	9 oz	310	38.0	9.0
cheese, w/tomato sauce *(Lean Cuisine)*	9 1/8 oz	270	27.0	8.0
Florentine *(Celentano)*	12 oz	350	48.0	8.0
CANOLA AND VEGETABLE OIL, 'Best Blend' *(Wesson)*	1 tbsp	120	0.0	14.0
CANOLA OIL				
	1/2 cup	964	0.0	109.0
	1 oz	251	0.0	28.4
	1 tbsp	124	0.0	14.0
(Country Pure)	1 tbsp	120	0.0	14.0
(Hain)	1 tbsp	120	0.0	14.0
(Kroger)	1 tbsp	122	0.0	13.6
(Nucoa) 'Heart Beat'	1 tbsp	120	0.0	14.0
(Spectrum Naturals)	1 tbsp	120	0.0	14.0

Food Name	Serv. Size	Total Cal.	Carbs GMS	Fat GMS
(Spectrum Naturals) organic	1 tbsp	120	0.0	14.0
(Wesson)	1 tbsp	120	0.0	14.0
(Wesson) 'Food Service'	1 tbsp	122	0.0	13.6
CANOLA OIL SPRAY. See COOKING SPRAY.				
CANTALOUPE /muskmelon				
approx 5-inch diam	1/2 fruit	93	22.3	0.8
cubed	1/2 cup	29	6.7	0.2
pulp	1 oz	10	2.4	0.1
untrimmed	1 lb	82	19.3	0.6
untrimmed *(Dole)*	1/4 fruit	50	11.0	0.0
CAPE GOOSEBERRY/ground cherry /poha				
in husk	1 lb	226	47.8	3.0
raw	1/2 cup	37	7.8	0.5
trimmed	1/2 cup	37	7.8	0.5
trimmed	1 oz	15	3.2	0.2
CAPOCOLLA. See LUNCHEON MEAT.				
CAPPUCCINO. See COFFEE, FLAVORED.				
CARAMBOLA. See STAR FRUIT.				
CARAMEL TOPPING				
(Kraft)	1 tbsp	60	13.0	0.0
(Mrs. Richardson's) fat-free	2 tbsp	130	31.0	0.0
(Smucker's) hot	2 tbsp	150	28.0	4.0
CARAWAY SEED				
whole	1 oz	94	14.1	4.1
whole	1 tbsp	22	3.3	1.0
whole	1 tsp	7	1.0	0.3
whole *(Durkee)*	1 tsp	9	0.0	<0.1
whole *(Laurel Leaf)*	1 tsp	9	0.0	<0.1
whole *(Spice Islands)*	1 tsp	8	0.8	0.4
CARDAMOM				
ground	1 oz	88	19.4	1.9
ground	1 tbsp	18	4.0	0.4
ground	1 tsp	6	1.4	0.1
ground *(Durkee)*	1 tsp	7	0.0	tr
ground *(Laurel Leaf)*	1 tsp	7	0.0	tr
CARDAMOM SEED *(Spice Islands)*	1 tsp	6	1.3	0.1
CARDONI. See CARDOON.				
CARDOON/cardoni				
boiled, drained	4 oz	25	6.0	0.1
raw, shredded	1 cup	36	8.7	0.2
raw, shredded	1/2 cup	18	4.3	0.1
raw, trimmed	1 oz	6	1.4	<.1
raw, untrimmed	1 lb	44	10.9	0.2

Food Name	Serv. Size	Total Cal.	Carbs GMS	Fat GMS
CARIBOU				
raw	1 lb	576	0.0	15.2
raw	1 oz	36	0.0	0.9
roasted	4 oz	189	0.0	5.0
roasted	3 oz	142	0.0	3.8
roasted, diced	1 cup	234	0.0	6.2
CARISSA/natal plum				
raw, approx .8 oz	1 med	12	2.7	0.3
raw, sliced	1 cup	93	20.4	2.0
raw, w/o skin and seeds, approx .8 oz	1 fruit	12	2.7	0.3
trimmed	1 oz	18	3.9	0.4
untrimmed	1 lb	240	53.2	5.1
CAROB FLAVOR DRINK				
mix, powder	1 oz	105	26.5	0.1
mix, powder	3 tsp	45	11.2	0.0
mix, prepared w/1 cup whole milk	1 cup	195	22.6	8.2
mix, prepared w/1 cup 2% milk	1 cup	166	22.9	4.7
mix, prepared w/1 cup 1% milk	1 cup	147	22.9	2.6
mix, prepared w/1 cup skim milk	1 cup	131	23.1	0.4
CAROB FLOUR				
	1 cup	394	91.5	0.7
	1 oz	51	25.2	0.2
	1 tbsp	31	7.1	0.1
CARP				
dry-heat cooked	3 oz	138	0.0	6.1
dry-heat cooked, approx 7.7 oz raw wt	1 fillet	275	0.0	12.2
raw	1 lb	574	0.0	25.4
raw	3 oz	108	0.0	4.8
raw	1 oz	36	0.0	1.6
raw, approx 7.7 oz	1 fillet	277	0.0	12.2
CARROT				
baby, raw	1 large	6	1.2	0.1
baby, raw	1 med	4	0.8	0.1
boiled, drained	4 oz	51	11.9	0.2
boiled, drained	1 med	21	4.8	0.1
boiled, drained, sliced	1/2 cup	35	8.2	0.1
raw	1 med	31	7.3	0.1
raw *(Dole)*	1 med	40	8.0	1.0
raw, shredded	1/2 cup	24	5.6	0.1
raw, trimmed	1 oz	12	2.9	0.1
raw, untrimmed	1 lb	174	41.0	0.8

Food Name	Serv. Size	Total Cal.	Carbs GMS	Fat GMS
CARROT, CANNED				
Crinkle-sliced				
(A&P)	1/2 cup	30	6.0	<1.0
(Freshlike)	1/2 cup	30	6.0	0.0
(Veg•All)	1/2 cup	30	6.0	0.0
Diced				
(Allens)	1/2 cup	30	5.0	<1.0
'Fancy' (S&W)	1/2 cup	30	7.0	0.0
julienne 'Fancy' (S&W)	1/2 cup	30	7.0	0.0
'No Salt Added' (A&P)	1/2 cup	25	6.0	<1.0
'No Salt or Sugar Added' (Stokely)	1/2 cup	35	7.0	0.0
w/liquid (Del Monte)	1/2 cup	30	7.0	0.0
Sliced				
(Featherweight)	1/2 cup	30	6.0	0.0
(Finast)	1/2 cup	35	8.0	0.0
(IGA)	1/2 cup	30	6.0	0.0
(Pathmark)	1/2 cup	35	7.0	0.0
(S&W Nutradiet)	1/2 cup	30	7.0	0.0
(Stokely)	1/2 cup	35	7.0	0.0
'Fancy' (S&W)	1/2 cup	30	7.0	0.0
large (Allens)	1/2 cup	30	7.0	<1.0
medium (Allens)	1/2 cup	30	7.0	<1.0
'No Salt Added' (Finast)	1/2 cup	35	8.0	0.0
'No Salt Added' (Pathmark)	1/2 cup	35	8.0	0.0
regular pack, drained	1/2 cup	17	4.0	0.1
regular pack, w/liquid	1/2 cup	28	6.2	0.2
regular pack, w/liquid, low-sodium	1/2 cup	28	6.2	0.2
small (Allens)	1/2 cup	30	7.0	<1.0
special dietary pack, drained	1/2 cup	17	4.0	0.1
special dietary pack, w/liquid	1/2 cup	28	6.2	0.2
water-packed, w/o salt (Freshlike)	1/2 cup	30	6.0	0.0
water-packed, w/o sugar or salt (Freshlike)	1/2 cup	30	6.0	0.0
w/liquid (Del Monte)	1/2 cup	30	7.0	0.0
Whole				
baby (Allens)	1/2 cup	30	6.0	<1.0
tiny 'Fancy' (S&W)	1/2 cup	30	7.0	0.0
w/liquid	1/2 cup	26	5.7	0.2
CARROT, FROZEN				
	10 oz	112	25.5	0.6
(A&P)	3.3 oz	40	9.0	<1.0
(Seabrook)	3.3 oz	40	9.0	0.0
baby, whole 'Deluxe' (Bird's Eye)	3.3 oz	40	9.0	0.0
baby, whole, 'Harvest Fresh' (Green Giant)	1/2 cup	18	5.0	0.0

Food Name	Serv. Size	Total Cal.	Carbs GMS	Fat GMS
baby, whole 'Select' (Green Giant)	1/2 cup	20	7.0	0.0
baby whole, 'Singles' (Stokely)	3 oz	35	8.0	0.0
boiled, drained	4 oz	41	9.4	0.1
Parisienne 'Deluxe' (Deluxe)	2.6 oz	30	7.0	0.0
sliced (Birds Eye)	3.2 oz	35	8.0	0.0
sliced (Frosty Acres)	3.3 oz	40	9.0	0.0
sliced, boiled, drained	1/2 cup	26	6.0	0.1
sliced, unprepared	1/2 cup	25	5.8	0.1
whole (Southern)	3.5 oz	42	8.7	0.2
w/sweet peas, pearl onions 'Deluxe' (Birds Eye)	3.3 oz	50	10.0	0.0
CARROT JUICE				
canned	6 oz	74	17.1	0.3
canned	1/2 cup	49	11.4	0.2
canned (Biotta)	6 oz	51	11.3	0.1
canned (Hain)	6 oz	80	17.0	0.0
canned (Hollywood)	6 oz	80	17.0	0.0
CASABA MELON				
cubed	1 cup	44	10.5	0.2
1/10 of 7.75-inch melon	2-in. slice	43	10.2	0.2
pulp	1 oz	7	1.8	<.1
untrimmed	1 lb	71	16.9	0.3
CASHEW/heart nut				
(Beer Nuts)	1 oz	170	8.0	13.0
Dry-roasted				
halves (Fisher)	1 oz	160	8.0	13.0
lightly salted (Planters)	1 oz	160	9.0	13.0
salted	1 oz	163	9.3	13.2
salted (Pathmark)	1 oz	170	9.0	13.0
salted (Planters)	1 oz	160	9.0	13.0
salted, 'No Frills' (Pathmark)	1 oz	170	8.0	13.0
salted, wholes and halves	1 cup	787	44.8	63.5
unsalted	1 oz	163	9.3	13.2
'Unsalted' (Planters)	1 oz	160	9.0	13.0
unsalted, approx 14 large or 26 small kernels	1 oz	163	9.3	13.2
unsalted, wholes and halves	1 cup	787	44.8	63.5
wholes (Fisher)	1 oz	160	8.0	13.0
Honey-roasted				
(Frito-Lays)	1 oz	170	9.0	14.0
(Planters)	1 oz	170	11.0	12.0
halves (Fisher)	1 oz	150	7.0	13.0
wholes (Fisher)	1 oz	150	7.0	13.0
w/peanuts (Planters)	1 oz	170	9.0	12.0

Food Name	Serv. Size	Total Cal.	Carbs GMS	Fat GMS
Oil-roasted				
halves *(Fisher)*	1 oz	170	8.0	14.0
lightly salted *(Planters)*	1 oz	160	8.0	14.0
pieces *(Fisher)*	1 oz	170	8.0	14.0
salted	1 oz	164	8.1	13.7
salted *(Flavor House)*	1 oz	180	3.0	16.0
salted *(Pathmark)*	1 oz	170	8.0	14.0
salted, approx 14 large or 18 medium kernels	1 oz	163	8.1	13.7
salted, 'Fancy' *(Planters)*	1 oz	170	8.0	14.0
salted, halves *(Planters)*	1 oz	170	8.0	14.0
salted, 'No Frills' *(Pathmark)*	1 oz	170	8.0	14.0
salted, wholes *(Guy's)*	1 oz	170	5.0	14.0
salted, wholes and halves	1 cup	749	37.1	62.7
unsalted	1 oz	164	8.1	13.7
unsalted, approx 14 large or 18 medium kernels	1 oz	163	8.1	13.7
unsalted, 'Fancy' *(Planters)*	1 oz	170	8.0	14.0
unsalted, halves	1 cup	749	37.1	62.7
'Unsalted' halves *(Planters)*	1 oz	170	8.0	14.0
wholes *(Fisher)*	1 oz	170	8.0	14.0
w/almonds *(Fisher)*	1 oz	170	6.0	15.0
CASHEW BUTTER				
gourmet *(Roaster Fresh)*	1 oz	165	9.0	14.0
peanut date *(Maranatha Natural)*	2 tbsp	190	8.0	14.0
peanut date 'Natural' *(Westbrae)*	2 tbsp	200	8.0	15.0
plain	1 oz	167	7.8	14.0
plain	1 tbsp	94	4.4	7.9
raw *(Hain)*	2 tbsp	190	8.0	15.0
raw 'Natural' *(Westbrae)*	2 tbsp	300	8.0	28.0
raw, unsalted *(Hain)*	2 tbsp	210	8.0	19.0
roasted *(Maranatha Natural)*	2 tbsp	190	10.0	14.0
roasted 'Natural' *(Westbrae)*	2 tbsp	190	8.0	17.0
toasted *(Hain)*	2 tbsp	210	7.0	17.0
CASSAVA / manioc / yuca				
trimmed	1 lb	544	122.1	1.8
trimmed	1 oz	34	7.6	0.1
raw	100 gm	120	26.9	0.4
CATFISH, CHANNEL				
Farmed				
dry-heat cooked	3 oz	129	0.0	6.8
frozen, fillets *(Delta Pride)*	4 oz	132	4.8	4.9
raw	3 oz	115	0.0	6.4
raw	1 oz	33	0.0	1.2

Food Name	Serv. Size	Total Cal.	Carbs GMS	Fat GMS
Wild				
dry-heat cooked	3 oz	89	0.0	2.4
raw	3 oz	81	0.0	2.4
CATFISH, OCEAN. See WOLF FISH.				
CATSUP/ketchup				
	1 oz	29	7.7	0.1
	1 tbsp	16	4.1	0.1
	.2-oz pkt	6	1.6	0.0
(Del Monte)	1/4 cup	60	16.0	0.0
(Estee)	1 tbsp	6	0.0	0.0
(Featherweight)	1 tbsp	6	1.0	0.0
(Healthy Choice)	.5 oz	9	2.0	0.1
(Heinz)	1 tbsp	16	3.8	0.0
(Hunt's)	1 tbsp	16	3.7	0.1
(Smucker's)	1 tsp	8	2.0	0.0
(Snider's)	1 tbsp	16	3.7	0.1
(Stokely)	1 tbsp	20	5.0	0.0
(Weight Watchers)	2 tsp	8	2.0	0.0
'All Natural' (Life)	1 tbsp	17	4.0	0.0
'Food Service' (Hunt's)	1 tbsp	15	3.6	0.1
fruit-sweetened (Westbrae)	1 tbsp	12	2.0	0.0
fruit-sweetened, no salt (Westbrae)	1 tbsp	12	2.0	0.0
hot (Heinz)	1 tbsp	16	3.7	0.0
'Lite' (Heinz)	1 tbsp	8	1.7	0.0
low-sodium	1 oz	29	7.7	0.1
low-sodium	1 tbsp	16	4.1	0.1
low-sodium	.2-oz pkt	6	1.6	0.0
'Natural' (Hain)	1 tbsp	16	4.0	0.0
'Natural No Salt Added' (Hain)	1 tbsp	16	4.0	0.0
'No Salt Added' (Del Monte)	1/4 cup	60	16.0	0.0
'No Salt Added' (Hunt's)	1 tbsp	20	5.0	0.0
organic (Millina's Finest)	1 oz	17	4.0	0.1
portion pack (Hunt's)	.3175 oz	10	2.2	0.1
w/onions (Heinz)	1 tbsp	19	0.1	(tr)
CAULIFLOWER				
boiled, drained	4 oz	27	5.2	0.2
boiled, drained, approx 1.9 oz	3 flowerets	12	2.2	0.2
boiled, drained, 1-inch pieces	1/2 cup	14	2.5	0.3
fresh, medium size (Dole)	1/6 head	18	3.0	0.0
green, fresh (Dole)	1/5 head	35	7.0	0.0
raw, approx 5 oz	3 flowerets	14	2.9	0.1
raw, 1-inch pieces	1/2 cup	13	2.6	0.1
raw, trimmed	1 oz	7	1.4	0.1

Food Name	Serv. Size	Total Cal.	Carbs GMS	Fat GMS
raw, untrimmed	1 lb	42	8.7	0.3
Frozen				
	10 oz	68	13.3	0.8
(A&P)	3.3 oz	25	5.0	<1.0
(Birds Eye)	3.3 oz	25	5.0	0.0
(Finast)	3.3 oz	25	5.0	0.0
(Frosty Acres)	3.3 oz	25	5.0	0.0
(Kohl's)	3 oz	20	4.0	<1.0
(Seabrook)	3.3 oz	25	5.0	0.0
(Southern)	3.5 oz	26	4.8	0.2
boiled, drained	4 oz	22	4.3	0.2
boiled, drained, 1-inch pieces	1/2 cup	17	3.4	0.2
cuts (Green Giant)	1/2 cup	12	3.0	0.0
florets 'Plain Polybag' (Green Giant)	1/2 cup	12	3.0	0.0
in cheddar cheese sauce 'Side Dish' (Budget Gourmet)	5 oz	110	10.0	5.0
in cheese flavored sauce (Green Giant)	1/2 cup	60	10.0	2.0
in cheese sauce (Finast)	3.3 oz	40	5.0	0.0
in cheese sauce 'One Serving' (Green Giant)	5.5 oz	80	14.0	2.0
in cheese sauce 'Singles' (Stokely)	4 oz	70	7.0	3.0
'Singles' (Stokely)	3 oz	20	4.0	0.0
unprepared, 1-inch pieces	1/2 cup	16	3.1	0.2
Pickled				
'Hot & Spicy' (Vlasic)	1 oz	4	1.0	0.0
sweet (Vlasic)	1 oz	35	9.0	0.0
CAVIAR				
black, granular	1 oz	71	1.1	5.0
black, granular	1 tbsp	40	0.6	2.9
red, granular	1 oz	71	1.1	5.0
red, granular	1 tbsp	40	0.6	2.9
CAYENNE PEPPER				
ground	1 oz	90	16.1	4.9
ground	1 tbsp	17	3.0	0.9
ground	1 tsp	6	1.0	0.3
ground (Spice Islands)	1 tsp	9	1.1	0.3
CECI. See GARBANZO BEAN.				
CELERIAC/celery root				
boiled, drained	4 oz	28	6.7	0.2
boiled, drained	100 gm	25	5.9	0.2
raw	1/2 cup	30	7.2	0.2
raw (Frieda's)	3.5 oz	40	8.5	0.3
raw, trimmed	1 oz	11	2.6	0.1
raw, untrimmed	1 lb	154	35.9	1.2

Food Name	Serv. Size	Total Cal.	Carbs GMS	Fat GMS
CELERY				
boiled, drained	4 oz	20	4.5	0.1
boiled, drained, diced	1/2 cup	14	3.0	0.1
fresh, medium size *(Dole)*	2 stalks	20	4.0	0.0
raw, diced	1/2 cup	10	2.2	0.1
raw, trimmed	1 oz	5	1.0	<.1
raw, untrimmed	1 lb	65	14.7	0.6
CELERY FLAKES *(Tone's)*	1 tsp	9	0.9	0.5
CELERY ROOT. See CELERIAC.				
CELERY ROOT JUICE, bottled *(Biotta)*	6 oz	67	13.1	0.2
CELERY SALT *(Tone's)*	1 tsp	6	0.6	0.4
CELERY SEED				
whole	1 oz	111	11.7	7.2
whole	1 tbsp	25	2.7	1.6
whole	1 tsp	8	0.8	0.5
whole *(Durkee)*	1 tsp	9	0.0	<0.1
whole *(Laurel Leaf)*	1 tsp	9	0.0	<0.1
whole *(Spice Islands)*	1 tsp	11	1.1	0.5
CELLOPHANE NOODLES. See NOODLE, CHINESE.				
CELTUCE				
raw, approx .4 oz	1 leaf	2	0.3	0.0
trimmed	1 oz	6	1.0	0.1
untrimmed	1 lb	76	12.4	1.0
CEREAL, HOT				
(NOTE: All of the following hot cereals are dry unless otherwise noted.)				
BARLEY *(Erewhon)* organic plus	1 oz	110	22.0	1.0
BRAN *(H-O Brand)* 'Super Bran'	1/3 cup	110	18.0	2.0
BULGUR WHEAT				
(Arrowhead Mills)	2 oz	200	43.0	1.0
(Krusteaz) 'Ala'	1/4 cup	150	33.0	0.0
CORN GRITS. See GRITS.				
FARINA				
(H-O Brand) cream	3 tbsp	120	26.0	0.0
(H-O Brand) instant	1 pkt	110	22.0	0.0
(Krusteaz)	1 oz	100	22.0	0.0
(Malt•O•Meal) 'Maple Brown Sugar' 30% formulation	1 oz	100	22.0	0.0
GRAIN, MIXED				
(Arrowhead Mills) four grain	1 oz	94	18.0	1.0
(Arrowhead Mills) seven grain	1 oz	100	17.0	1.0
(Breadshop) 'Triple Bran'	1 oz	100	15.0	2.0
(Maltex) wheat and barley	1 oz	105	21.0	1.0
(Malt•O•Meal) wheat and barley, chocolate flavor	1 tbsp	38	8.0	0.1
(Malt•O•Meal) wheat and barley, plain	1 tbsp	38	8.0	0.1

Food Name	Serv. Size	Total Cal.	Carbs GMS	Fat GMS
(Pritikin) hearty multi-grain, microwave instant	1 pkt	150	32.0	na
(Quaker) multi-grain	1/2 cup	130	24.0	1.5
(Roman Meal) multi-grain, apple, and cinnamon	2/3 cup	112	23.8	2.8
(Roman Meal) oat, wheat, dates, raisins, and almonds	1.3 oz	140	26.0	3.0
(Roman Meal) oat, wheat, honey, coconut, and almonds	1.3 oz	150	21.0	6.0
(Roman Meal) oat, wheat, rye, bran, and flax	1.2 oz	116	25.0	1.7
OAT BRAN				
(Arrowhead Mills)	1 oz	110	17.0	1.0
(Breadshop) 'Oat Bran Muesli'	1 oz	100	20.0	2.0
(Breadshop) 'Oat Bran' 100% pure	1 oz	100	17.0	2.0
(Erewhon) toasted wheat germ	1 oz	115	18.0	2.0
(Health Valley) 'Natural' apple and cinnamon	1 oz	100	19.0	1.0
(Health Valley) 'Natural' raisins and spice	1 oz	110	19.0	1.0
(Malt•O•Meal) 'Plus 40% Oat Bran'	1.3 oz	130	25.0	2.0
(Mother's)	1/3 cup	92	16.6	2.1
(Quaker)	1 oz	92	16.6	2.1
(3-Minute Brand) instant	1 oz	90	17.0	2.0
(3-Minute Brand) 'Regular'	1 oz	90	17.0	2.0
(Wholesome 'N Hearty)	1 oz	100	18.0	2.0
(Wholesome 'N Hearty) instant, apple cinnamon	1 3/8 oz	130	30.0	2.0
(Wholesome 'N Hearty) instant, honey	1.25 oz	110	26.0	2.0
OATMEAL AND OATS				
(Arrowhead Mills) instant	1 oz	100	18.0	2.0
(Arrowhead Mills) instant, apple, date, and almond	1 oz	130	23.0	3.0
(Arrowhead Mills) instant, apple spice	1 oz	130	23.0	2.0
(Arrowhead Mills) instant, cinnamon, raisin, and almond	1 oz	140	23.0	3.0
(Erewhon) instant, apple and cinnamon	1.25 oz	145	25.0	3.0
(Erewhon) instant, apple and raisin	1.3 oz	150	27.0	3.0
(Erewhon) instant, maple spice	1.2 oz	140	24.0	3.0
(Erewhon) instant, oat bran	1.25 oz	125	23.0	3.0
(Erewhon) instant, raisins, dates, and walnuts	1.2 oz	130	24.0	3.0
(General Mills) instant, apple and cinnamon	1.5 oz	150	32.0	2.0
(General Mills) instant, cinnamon raisin	1.8 oz	170	38.0	2.0
(General Mills) 'Oatmeal Swirlers' instant, apple and cinnamon	1.7 oz	160	34.0	2.0
(General Mills) 'Oatmeal Swirlers' instant, cherry	1.7 oz	150	33.0	2.0
(General Mills) 'Oatmeal Swirlers' instant, cinnamon and spice	1.6 oz	160	35.0	2.0
(General Mills) 'Oatmeal Swirlers' instant, maple and brown sugar	1.6 oz	160	35.0	2.0
(General Mills) 'Oatmeal Swirlers' instant, milk chocolate	1.7 oz	170	37.0	2.0
(General Mills) 'Oatmeal Swirlers' instant, strawberry	1.6 oz	150	32.0	2.0
(H-O Brand) 'Gourmet'	1/3 cup	100	18.0	2.0

Food Name	Serv. Size	Total Cal.	Carbs GMS	Fat GMS
(H-O Brand) instant	1 pkt	110	18.0	2.0
(H-O Brand) instant, apple and cinnamon	1 pkt	130	26.0	2.0
(H-O Brand) instant, box	1/2 cup	130	22.0	2.0
(H-O Brand) instant, maple and brown sugar	1 pkt	160	32.0	2.0
(H-O Brand) instant, raisins and spice	1 pkt	150	32.0	2.0
(H-O Brand) instant, sweet 'n mellow	1 pkt	150	30.0	2.0
(H-O Brand) 'Quick'	1/2 cup	130	23.0	2.0
(H-O Brand) w/fiber, instant	1 pkt	110	18.0	2.0
(H-O Brand) w/fiber, instant, apple and bran	1 pkt	130	26.0	2.0
(H-O Brand) w/fiber, instant, box	1/3 cup	100	15.0	2.0
(H-O Brand) w/fiber, instant, raisin, and bran	1 pkt	150	32.0	2.0
(Maypo)	1 cup	362	67.7	5.0
(Maypo) '30 Second' quick	1 oz	100	19.0	1.0
(Maypo) 'Vermont Style' maple flavor	1 oz	105	20.0	1.0
(Mother's) instant	1 oz	110	18.0	2.0
(Quaker)	1/3 cup	99	18.6	2.0
(Quaker) 'Extra'	1 pkt	95	17.6	2.0
(Quaker) 'Extra' apples and spice	1 pkt	133	26.7	1.9
(Quaker) 'Extra' raisins and cinnamon	1 pkt	129	26.6	1.9
(Quaker) instant	1 pkt	94	18.0	2.0
(Quaker) instant, apple and cinnamon	1 pkt	118	26.0	1.5
(Quaker) instant, cinnamon and spice	1 pkt	164	34.9	2.1
(Quaker) instant, maple and brown sugar	1 pkt	152	31.6	2.1
(Quaker) instant, peaches and cream	1 pkt	129	26.3	2.2
(Quaker) instant, raisins and spice	1 pkt	149	31.5	2.0
(Quaker) instant, raisins, dates, and walnuts	1 pkt	141	25.1	3.8
(Quaker) instant, strawberries and cream	1 pkt	129	26.6	2.0
(Quaker) 'Kids' Choice' instant, cinnamon graham cookie	1 pkt	140	29.0	2.0
(Quaker) 'Kids' Choice' instant, maple and brown sugar	1 pkt	140	31.0	2.0
(Quaker) 'Kids' Choice' instant, radical raspberry	1 pkt	150	28.0	3.0
(Quaker) 'Kids' Choice' instant, strawberries and stuff	1 pkt	140	30.0	2.0
(Quaker) 'Old Fashioned'	1 oz	99	18.6	2.0
(Quaker) plus fiber	1/2 cup	130	21.0	2.5
(Quaker) plus fiber, oatmeal raisin bran	1 pkt	150	28.0	2.0
(Quaker) 'Quick'	1 oz	99	18.6	2.0
(Ralston)	1 cup	402	85.1	2.5
(Roman Meal)	1 cup	340	68.5	4.0
(3-Minute Brand) oat bran and raisins	1 oz	100	18.0	2.0
(3-Minute Brand) 'Old Fashioned'	1 oz	100	18.0	2.0
(3-Minute Brand) 'Quick'	1 oz	100	18.0	2.0
(3-Minute Brand) 'Quick' oat bran	1 oz	100	18.0	2.0
(3-Minute Brand) raisins	1 oz	100	18.0	2.0
(Total) instant	1.2 oz	110	22.0	2.0

Food Name	Serv. Size	Total Cal.	Carbs GMS	Fat GMS
(Total) instant, maple and brown sugar	1.6 oz	160	34.0	2.0
(Total) 'Quick'	1 oz	90	18.0	2.0
QUINOA *(Ancient Harvest)* steam-rolled flakes	1/3 cup	105	23.0	1.0
RICE				
(Cream of Rice)	1 tbsp	38	8.4	0.1
(Lundberg Family) 'Hot'n Creamy' cooked	1 oz	110	23.0	1.0
(Lundberg Family) 'Hot'n Creamy' almonds and dates, cooked	1 oz	110	24.0	1.0
RICE, BROWN				
(Arrowhead Mills) 'Rise & Shine'	1.5 oz	160	35.0	1.0
(Erewhon) cream of brown rice	1 oz	110	23.0	1.0
RYE				
(Breadshop) 'Rye Date Müesli'	1 oz	100	19.0	2.0
(Roman Meal) cream of rye	1.3 oz	110	27.0	<1.0
WHEAT				
(Arrowhead Mills) 'Bear Mush'	1 oz	100	21.0	0.0
(Arrowhead Mills) cracked wheat	2 oz	180	40.0	1.0
(Cream of Wheat)	1 tbsp	39	8.1	0.2
(Cream of Wheat) instant	1 oz	100	22.0	<1.0
(Cream of Wheat) instant	1 tbsp	42	8.7	0.2
(Cream of Wheat) 'Mix'n Eat' instant	1 oz	100	21.0	0.0
(Cream of Wheat) 'Mix'n Eat' instant, apple and cinnamon	1 oz	130	29.0	0.0
(Cream of Wheat) 'Mix'n Eat' instant, apple, banana, and maple	1 pkt	132	28.9	0.4
(Cream of Wheat) 'Mix'n Eat' instant, brown sugar and cinnamon	1 oz	130	29.0	0.0
(Cream of Wheat) 'Mix'n Eat' instant, maple and brown sugar	1 oz	130	29.0	0.0
(Cream of Wheat) 'Quick'	1 tbsp	38	7.9	0.1
(General Mills) 'Wheat Hearts'	1 oz	110	20.0	1.0
(Krusteaz) 'Zoom'	1/3 cup	120	24.0	0.0
(Maltex)	1 cup	532	116.7	3.2
(Mother's)	1/3 cup	92	20.9	0.6
(Quaker)	1/3 cup	92	20.9	0.6
(Wheatena)	1 oz	100	21.0	1.0
CEREAL, READY-TO-SERVE				
(NOTE: All of the following ready-to-serve cereals are in their dry form.)				
'Addam's Family' *(Ralston)*	1 oz	110	25.0	1.0
'All Bran' extra fiber *(Kellogg's)*	1 oz	50	22.0	0.0
'All Bran' wheat bran *(Kellogg's)*	1 oz	71	21.1	0.5
'Almond Flavor O's' fat-free *(Health Valley)*	1 oz	90	19.0	0.0
'Almond Raisin' low fat *(Golden Temple)*	1 oz	110	22.0	1.5
'Almond Raisin' nectarsweet premium *(Breadshop)*	1 oz	120	18.0	4.0
'Alpha Bits' oat and other grains *(Post)*	1 oz	111	24.6	0.7

Food Name	Serv. Size	Total Cal.	Carbs GMS	Fat GMS
'Alpha Bits' super swirl marshmallows *(Post)*	1 oz	150	31.0	1.0
'Apple Almond Müesli' *(Ralston)*	1.45 oz	150	31.0	2.0
'Apple & Cinnamon Toasted Oat' *(Malt•O•Meal)*	1 oz	110	22.0	2.0
'Apple Cinnamon Cheerios' *(General Mills)*	1 oz	110	22.0	2.0
'Apple Cinnamon Corn Flakes' *(Wonder)*	1 oz	110	25.0	0.0
'Apple Cinnamon' low fat *(Golden Temple)*	1 oz	110	22.0	1.5
'Apple Cinnamon O's' fat-free *(Health Valley)*	1 oz	90	19.0	0.0
'Apple Cinnamon Squares' *(Kellogg's)*	1 oz	90	23.0	0.0
'Apple Jacks' corn and other grains *(Kellogg's)*	1 oz	110	25.8	0.1
'Apple Raisin Crisp' *(Kellogg's)*	1 oz	130	32.0	0.0
'Aztec' *(Erewhon)*	1 oz	100	24.0	0.0
'Banana Nut Crunch' *(Post)*	1 oz	120	20.0	3.0
'Banana O's' *(Erewhon)*	1 oz	110	24.0	0.0
'Banana Walnut Müesli' *(Ralston)*	1.45 oz	150	30.0	3.0
'Basic 4' *(General Mills)*	3/4 cup	130	28.0	2.0
'Batman Returns' *(Ralston)*	1 oz	110	26.0	1.0
'Berry Berry Kix' *(General Mills)*	1 oz	110	25.0	1.0
'Blueberry 'N Cream' nectarsweet gourmet *(Breadshop)*	1 oz	115	18.7	3.0
'Blueberry Squares' *(Kellogg's)*	1 oz	90	23.0	0.0
'Body Buddies Natural Fruit' *(General Mills)*	1 oz	110	24.0	1.0
'Booberry' *(General Mills)*	1 oz	110	24.0	1.0
'Bran Buds' wheat bran *(Kellogg's)*	1 oz	73	21.6	0.7
'Bran Chex' wheat bran and corn *(Kellogg's)*	1 oz	91	22.6	0.8
'Bran Flakes' *(Arrowhead Mills)*	1 oz	100	21.0	1.0
'Bran Flakes' *(Kellogg's)*	1 oz	90	22.0	1.0
'Bran Flakes' *(Malt•O•Meal)*	1 oz	90	23.0	1.0
'Bran Flakes' *(Post)*	1 oz	90	23.0	0.0
'Breakfast O's' *(Barbara's Bakery)*	1 oz	120	21.0	2.0
Brown rice, crisp *(Erewhon)*	1 oz	110	24.0	1.0
Brown rice, crisp, low sodium *(Erewhon)*	1 oz	110	24.0	1.0
'Brown Rice Crisps' *(Barbara's Bakery)*	1 oz	120	26.0	1.0
'Buñuelitos' *(General Mills)*	1 oz	120	25.0	2.0
'C.W. Post Hearty Granola Cereal' *(Post)*	1 oz	130	21.0	4.0
'C.W. Post' oats and other grains *(Post)*	1 oz	126	20.3	4.4
'C.W. Post' oats and other grains, raisins *(Post)*	1 oz	123	20.4	4.1
'California Orange Crunch' honeysweet premium *(Breadshop)*	1 oz	130	18.0	5.0
'Captain Crunch' corn and other grains *(Quaker)*	1 oz	120	23.0	2.6
'Captain Crunch Crunchberries' corn and oat *(Quaker)*	1 oz	118	23.1	2.4
'Captain Crunch Peanut Butter' corn *(Quaker)*	1 oz	125	21.5	3.7
'Cashew Almond Granola' *(Golden Temple)*	1 oz	129	19.0	3.5
'Cheerios' oat and wheat *(General Mills)*	1 oz	111	19.6	1.8
'Cinnamon & Raisin' 100% natural *(Nature Valley)*	1 oz	120	20.0	4.0

Food Name	Serv. Size	Total Cal.	Carbs GMS	Fat GMS
'Cinnamon & Spice Crunch' psyllium and chia seed *(Golden Temple)*	1 oz	132	20.0	4.5
'Cinnamon Apple Raisin Granola' *(Golden Temple)*	1 oz	125	20.0	3.5
'Cinnamon Mini Buns' *(Kellogg's)*	1 oz	110	25.0	1.0
'Cinnamon Toast Crunch' *(General Mills)*	1 oz	120	22.0	3.0
'Cinnamon Toast Crunch' breakfast pack *(General Mills)*	1 oz	140	26.0	4.0
'Cinnapple Spice' honeysweet premium *(Breadshop)*	1 oz	125	18.5	4.5
'Clusters' *(General Mills)*	1 oz	110	22.0	2.0
'Cocoa Krispies' rice *(Kellogg's)*	1 oz	110	25.2	0.4
'Cocoa Pebbles' rice *(Post)*	1 oz	116	24.4	1.5
'Cocoa Puffs' *(General Mills)*	1 oz	110	25.0	1.0
'Coconut Almond Granola' *(Golden Temple)*	1 oz	145	18.0	7.0
'Common Sense Oat Bran' *(Kellogg's)*	1 oz	100	22.0	1.0
'Common Sense Oat Bran' raisins *(Kellogg's)*	3/4 cup	130	29.0	1.0
'Complete' bran flakes, beta carotene *(Kellogg's)*	1 oz	90	23.0	<1.0
'Cookie-Crisp' chocolate chip and vanilla *(Ralston)*	1 oz	114	24.9	1.0
'Corn Bran' corn bran and other grains *(Ralston)*	1 oz	98	23.9	1.0
'Corn Chex' *(Ralston)*	1 oz	111	24.9	0.1
'Corn Flakes' *(Arrowhead Mills)*	1 oz	100	25.0	0.0
'Corn Flakes' *(Barbara's Bakery)*	1 oz	110	24.0	0.0
'Corn Flakes' *(Kellogg's)*	1 oz	110	24.4	0.1
'Corn Flakes' *(Krusteaz)*	1 oz	110	24.0	1.0
'Corn Flakes' *(Malt•O•Meal)*	1 oz	110	25.0	0.0
'Corn Flakes' *(Ralston)*	1 oz	111	24.6	0.1
'Corn Flakes' sugar frosted *(Kellogg's)*	1 oz	108	25.7	0.1
'Corn Flakes' sugar frosted *(Ralston)*	1 oz	111	25.6	0.4
'Corn Pops' *(Kellogg's)*	1 oz	110	26.0	0.0
'Count Chocula' *(General Mills)*	1 oz	110	25.0	1.0
'Country Corn Flakes' *(General Mills)*	1 oz	110	25.0	1.0
'Cracklin' Bran' wheat bran and other grains *(Kellogg's)*	1 oz	108	19.5	4.2
'Cracklin' Oat Bran' *(Kellogg's)*	1 oz	110	21.0	3.0
'Cranberry Walnut Müesli' *(Ralston)*	1.45 oz	150	30.0	3.0
'Crisp N' Crackling Rice' *(Malt•O•Meal)*	1 oz	110	25.0	0.0
'Crisp Rice' *(Krusteaz)*	1 oz	110	25.0	0.0
'Crispix' *(Kellogg's)*	1 oz	110	25.0	0.0
'Crispy Wheats 'N Raisins' wheat *(General Mills)*	1 oz	99	23.2	0.5
'Crunch Graham Oat Rings' *(Wonder)*	1 oz	110	24.0	1.0
'Crunchies' brown rice *(Lundberg Family)*	1 cup	171	38.0	0.8
'Crunchy Oat Bran' nectarsweet gourmet *(Breadshop)*	1 oz	120	18.0	5.0
'Date Almond Müesli' *(Ralston)*	1.45 oz	140	32.0	2.0
'Dino Pebbles' *(Post)*	1 oz	110	25.0	1.0
'Double Chex' *(Ralston)*	1 oz	100	25.0	0.0
'Double Dip Crunch' *(Kellogg's)*	1 oz	120	23.0	2.0

Food Name	Serv. Size	Total Cal.	Carbs GMS	Fat GMS
'Fiber One' aspartame (General Mills)	1 oz	60	23.0	1.0
'Fiberwise' (Kellogg's)	1 oz	90	23.0	1.0
'Fingos' cinnamon (General Mills)	1 oz	110	22.0	3.0
'Fingos' honey toasted oat (General Mills)	1 oz	110	21.0	3.0
'40% Bran Flakes' wheat bran (Kellogg's)	1 oz	93	22.2	0.5
'40% Bran Flakes' wheat bran (Post)	1 oz	92	22.5	0.5
'40% Bran Flakes' wheat bran (Ralston)	1 oz	92	22.7	0.4
'Frankenberry' (General Mills)	1 oz	110	24.0	1.0
'Froot Loops' corn and other grains (Kellogg's)	1 oz	111	25.1	0.5
'Frosted Chex Juniors' (Ralston)	1 oz	110	25.0	0.0
'Frosted Flakes' (Kellogg's)	1 oz	110	26.0	0.0
'Frosted Funnies' (Barbara's Bakery)	1 cup	110	27.0	0.0
'Frosted Krispies' (Kellogg's)	1 oz	110	26.0	0.0
'Frosted Mini Wheats' (Kellogg's)	1 oz	100	24.0	0.0
'Frosted Mini Wheats' bite size (Kellogg's)	1 oz	100	24.0	0.0
'Frosted Mini Wheats' brown sugar and cinnamon (Kellogg's)	1 oz	102	23.4	0.3
'Frosted Rice Krinkles' rice	1 oz	109	25.9	0.1
'Frosted Rice Krispies' rice (Kellogg's)	1 oz	109	25.7	0.1
'Fruit & Fibre' oat, dates, raisins, and walnuts (Post)	1.25 oz	120	27.0	2.0
'Fruit & Fibre' oat, peaches, raisins, and almonds (Post)	1.25 oz	120	26.0	2.0
'Fruit & Fibre' oat, pineapple, banana, and coconut (Post)	1.25 oz	120	27.0	3.0
'Fruit & Fibre' oat, tropical fruit (Post)	1.25 oz	120	27.0	3.0
'Fruit & Frosted O's' mixed grain (Malt•O•Meal)	1 oz	110	25.0	1.0
'Fruit & Nut' 100%natural (Nature Valley)	1 oz	130	19.0	5.0
'Fruit 'N Nut Granola' (Golden Temple)	1 oz	129	19.0	4.5
'Fruit 'n Wheat' (Erewhon)	1 oz	100	21.0	1.0
'Fruit Wheats' apple (Nabisco)	1 oz	90	23.0	0.0
'Fruit Whirls' (Krusteaz)	1 oz	110	25.0	1.0
'Fruitful Bran' fruit (Kellogg's)	1 oz	120	31.0	0.0
'Fruity Marshmallow Krispies' (Kellogg's)	1 1/4 cups	140	32.0	0.0
'Fruity Pebbles' rice (Post)	1 oz	115	24.4	1.5
'Golden Crisp' (Post)	1 oz	110	26.0	0.0
'Golden Grahams' corn and wheat (General Mills)	1 oz	109	24.2	1.1
'Golden Granola' (Golden Temple)	1 oz	138	19.0	6.0
'Golden Maple Nut' honeysweet premium (Breadshop)	1 oz	130	17.0	5.0
'Gone Nuts!' nectarsweet premium (Breadshop)	1 oz	125	17.0	5.0
'Graham Chex' (Ralston)	1 oz	110	24.0	1.0
'Graham Crackos' wheat	1 oz	103	24.5	0.2
Granola, banana almond (Sunbelt)	1 oz	130	20.0	4.0
Granola, date and almond, fat-free (Health Valley)	1 oz	90	21.0	0.0
Granola, fruit and nut (Sunbelt)	1 oz	120	19.0	5.0
Granola, raisin cinnamon, fat-free (Health Valley)	1 oz	90	21.0	0.0
Granola, tropical fruit, fat-free (Health Valley)	1 oz	90	21.0	0.0

Food Name	Serv. Size	Total Cal.	Carbs GMS	Fat GMS
'Granola' toasted oat mix *(Nature Valley)*	1 oz	126	19.0	4.9
'Grape-Nuts' wheat and barley *(Post)*	1 oz	101	23.3	0.1
'Grape-Nuts Flakes' wheat and barley *(Post)*	1 oz	102	23.2	0.3
'Great Grains' double pecan *(Post)*	1 oz	120	20.0	3.0
'Great Grains' raisins, dates, and pecans *(Post)*	1.25 oz	140	27.0	3.0
'Hawaiian Granola' *(Golden Temple)*	1 oz	126	19.0	4.0
'Hazelnut Boysenberry' organic oats *(Golden Temple)*	1 oz	135	19.0	5.5
'Heritage O's' *(Natures Path)*	1 cup	165	34.0	<1.0
'High Fiber O's' fat-free *(Health Valley)*	1 oz	90	19.0	0.0
'High 5' *(Barbara's Bakery)*	3/4 cup	100	23.0	0.5
'High Protein Granola' *(Golden Temple)*	1 oz	124	19.0	3.5
'Honey Almond Delight' *(Ralston)*	1 oz	110	23.0	2.0
'Honey Almond Granola' *(Golden Temple)*	1 oz	130	20.0	3.5
'Honey & Nut Toasted Oat' *(Malt•O•Meal)*	1 oz	110	23.0	1.0
'Honey Apple Blueberry' honeysweet premium *(Breadshop)*	1 oz	125	18.0	5.0
'Honey Blueberry Apple Granola' *(Golden Temple)*	1 oz	128	20.0	3.5
'Honey Bunches of Oats' almonds *(Post)*	1 oz	120	22.0	3.0
'Honey Bunches of Oats' honey roasted *(Post)*	1 oz	110	24.0	2.0
'Honey Gone Nuts!' honeysweet premium *(Breadshop)*	1 oz	130	17.5	5.5
'Honey Nut' toasted oatmeal *(Quaker)*	1 oz	120	20.0	3.0
'Honey Nut Cheerios' oat and wheat *(General Mills)*	1 oz	107	22.8	0.7
'Honey Nut Cheerios' oat and wheat, breakfast pack *(General Mills)*	4/5 oz	100	21.0	1.0
'Honey Nut Crispy Rice' *(Wonder)*	1 oz	110	25.0	1.0
'Honey Nut O's' *(Krusteaz)*	1 oz	110	23.0	1.0
'HoneyComb' corn and oats *(Post)*	1 oz	111	25.3	0.5
'Just Right' fiber nuggets *(Kellogg's)*	1 oz	100	24.0	1.0
'Just Right' raisins, dates, and nuts *(Kellogg's)*	3/4 cup	140	30.0	1.0
'Kaboom' *(General Mills)*	1 oz	110	23.0	1.0
'Kamut Flakes' *(Erewhon)*	1 oz	90	18.0	0.0
'Kenmei Rice Bran' *(Kellogg's)*	1 oz	110	24.0	1.0
'King Vitaman' corn and other grains	1 oz	115	24.1	1.6
'Kix' corn and other grains *(General Mills)*	1 oz	110	23.5	0.7
'Life' oat and other grains *(Quaker Oat)*	1 oz	105	20.3	0.5
'Life' oat and other grains, cinnamon *(Quaker Oat)*	1 oz	105	20.3	0.5
'Lite Müesli' *(Golden Temple)*	1 oz	102	20.0	1.0
'Lite 'N Crunchy Granola' *(Golden Temple)*	1 oz	129	19.0	4.5
'Lucky Charms' oat and other grains *(General Mills)*	1 oz	111	23.2	1.1
'Lucky Charms' oat and other grains, breakfast pack *(General Mills)*	7/8 oz	110	24.0	1.0
'Maple Almond Granola' *(Golden Temple)*	1 oz	129	20.0	3.5
'Maple Corns' *(Arrowhead Mills)*	1 oz	100	23.0	1.0
'Maple Frosted Corn' mini puffs *(Glenny's)*	1 oz	109	20.0	<.5

Food Name	Serv. Size	Total Cal.	Carbs GMS	Fat GMS
'Marshmallow Alpha Bits' (Post)	1 oz	110	25.0	1.0
'Most' wheat bran and wheat	1 oz	96	21.6	0.3
'Müeslix Crispy Blend' (Kellogg's)	2/3 cup	150	32.0	2.0
'Müeslix Golden Crunch' (Kellogg's)	1/2 cup	120	25.0	2.0
'Multi Grain Cheerios' (General Mills)	1 oz	100	23.0	1.0
'Multi-Bran Chex' (Ralston)	1 oz	90	25.0	1.0
'Natural Blueberry Granola' (Golden Temple)	1 oz	132	19.0	5.0
'Natural Blueberry Granola' coconut-free (Golden Temple)	1 oz	131	19.0	4.5
'Natural Bran Flakes' (Post)	1 oz	90	23.0	0.0
'Natural Delite Granola' (Golden Temple)	1 oz	128	20.0	3.5
'Natural Foods Apple Cinnamon' low fat (Golden Temple)	1 oz	110	22.0	1.0
'Natural Foods Raisin Almond' low fat (Golden Temple)	1 oz	110	22.0	1.0
'Natural Foods Strawberry/Raspberry' low fat (Golden Temple)	1 oz	111	22.0	1.0
'Natural' oat and wheat germ (Heartland)	1 oz	123	19.4	4.4
'Natural' oat and wheat germ, coconut (Heartland)	1 oz	125	19.3	4.6
'Natural' oat and wheat germ, raisins (Heartland)	1 oz	121	19.6	4.0
'Natural Raisin Bran' (Post)	1.4 oz	120	31.0	1.0
'Nut & Honey Crunch' (Kellogg's)	1 oz	110	24.0	1.0
'Nut & Honey Crunch O's' (Kellogg's)	1 oz	110	22.0	2.0
'Nutri-Grain' barley (Kellogg's)	1 oz	106	23.5	0.2
'Nutri-Grain' corn (Kellogg's)	1 oz	108	24.0	0.7
'Nutri-Grain' rye (Kellogg's)	1 oz	102	24.0	0.2
'Nutri-Grain' wheat (Kellogg's)	1 oz	102	24.0	0.3
'Nutri-Grain Almond Raisin' (Kellogg's)	2/3 cup	140	31.0	2.0
'Nutri-Grain Raisin Bran' (Kellogg's)	1 cup	130	31.0	1.0
'Oat Bran Almond' (Golden Temple)	1 oz	120	20.0	3.5
'Oat Bran Apple' (Golden Temple)	1 oz	112	19.0	3.5
'Oat Bran Flakes' (Arrowhead Mills)	1 oz	100	19.0	2.0
'Oat Bran Granola' berries (Golden Temple)	1 oz	120	20.0	3.5
'Oat Bran Granola' raisins and almonds (Golden Temple)	1 oz	119	19.0	3.5
'Oat Bran Müesli' dates and almonds (Golden Temple)	1 oz	108	21.0	1.5
'Oat Bran Müesli' raisins and hazelnuts (Golden Temple)	1 oz	102	20.0	1.5
'Oat Bran Oregonberry' (Golden Temple)	1 oz	116	20.0	3.5
'Oat Flakes' (Arrowhead Mills)	2 oz	220	39.0	4.0
'Oat Flakes' (Post)	1 oz	110	21.0	1.0
'Oat Mini Puffs' (Glenny's)	1 oz	108	22.0	<.5
'Oat Mini Puffs' w/o salt, w/o sugar (Glenny's)	1 oz	108	22.0	<.5
'Oatbake Honey Bran' (Kellogg's)	1 oz	110	21.0	3.0
'Oatbake Raisin Nut' (Kellogg's)	1 oz	110	21.0	3.0
'Oatmeal Crisp' (General Mills)	1 oz	110	21.0	2.0
'Oatmeal Crisp With Apples' (General Mills)	1 oz	110	23.0	1.0
'Oatmeal Raisin Crisp' (General Mills)	1/2 cup	130	25.0	2.0
'100% Bran' wheat bran and barley (Nabisco)	1 oz	76	20.7	1.4

Food Name	Serv. Size	Total Cal.	Carbs GMS	Fat GMS
'100% Natural Almond' (Golden Temple)	1 oz	123	18.0	4.0
'100% Natural Apple/Cinnamon' (Golden Temple)	1 oz	120	18.0	4.0
'100% Natural' mixed grain (Quaker)	1 oz	127	18.0	5.5
'100% Natural' mixed grain, raisins, low fat (Quaker)	1 oz	110	21.0	2.0
'100% Natural Oat Bran' (Golden Temple)	1 oz	70	19.0	2.5
'100% Natural' oats and wheat (Quaker)	1 oz	133	17.8	6.1
'100% Natural' oats and wheat, apple and cinnamon (Quaker)	1 oz	130	19.1	5.3
'100% Natural' oats and wheat, raisins, low fat (Quaker)	1 oz	150	27.0	2.0
'100% Natural' oats and wheat, raisins and dates (Quaker)	1 oz	128	18.7	5.3
'100% Natural Raisin/Almond' (Golden Temple)	1 oz	120	19.0	4.0
'100% Organic Blue Corn Flakes' (Health Valley)	1 oz	90	19.0	<1.0
'Orange Almond' nectarsweet premium (Breadshop)	1 oz	120	18.0	4.0
'Orange Almond Granola' (Golden Temple)	1 oz	133	19.0	4.0
'Oregon Blueberry Crunch' honeysweet gourmet (Breadshop)	1 oz	125	18.0	5.0
'Organic Amaranth Flakes' (Health Valley)	1 oz	90	20.0	1.0
'Original' toasted oatmeal (Quaker)	1 oz	100	22.0	1.0
'Peach Pecan Müesli' (Ralston)	1.45 oz	150	30.0	3.0
'Peaches 'N Cream' nectarsweet gourmet (Breadshop)	1 oz	115	18.5	3.0
'Post Toasties Corn Flakes' (Post)	1 oz	110	24.0	0.0
'Product 19' corn and other grains (Kellogg's)	1 oz	108	23.6	0.2
'Puffed Corn' (Arrowhead Mills)	.5 oz	50	11.0	0.0
'Puffed Kamut' (Arrowhead Mills)	.5 oz	40	10.0	0.0
'Puffed Rice' (Arrowhead Mills)	.5 oz	50	12.0	0.0
'Puffed Rice' (Malt•O•Meal)	.5 oz	50	12.0	0.0
'Puffed Wheat' (Arrowhead Mills)	.5 oz	50	11.0	0.0
'Puffed Wheat' (Malt•O•Meal)	.5 oz	50	10.0	0.0
'Quisp' corn and oat	1 oz	118	23.7	2.0
'Raisin Apricot-Date Granola' (Golden Temple)	1 oz	127	20.0	3.5
'Raisin Bran' (Barbara's Bakery)	1 oz	170	36.0	1.0
'Raisin Bran' (Erewhon)	1 oz	100	22.0	0.0
'Raisin Bran' (Krusteaz)	3/4 cup	120	30.0	1.0
'Raisin Bran' wheat (Kellogg's)	1.3 oz	115	27.9	0.7
'Raisin Bran' wheat (Post)	1 oz	87	21.5	0.5
'Raisin Bran' wheat (Ralston)	1 1/3 oz	120	31.4	0.2
'Raisin Bran Flakes' (Malt•O•Meal)	1.4 oz	130	30.0	2.0
'Raisin Grape-Nuts' (Post)	1 oz	100	23.0	0.0
'Raisin Squares' (Kellogg's)	1 oz	90	23.0	0.0
'Raspberry Almond Müesli' (Ralston)	1.45 oz	150	30.0	3.0
'Raspberry 'N Cream' nectarsweet gourmet (Breadshop)	1 oz	115	18.5	3.0
'Rice Chex' (Ralston)	1 oz	112	25.3	0.1
'Rice Krispies' (Kellogg's)	1 oz	112	24.8	0.2
'Rice Krispies Treats' (Kellogg's)	1 oz	110	24.0	1.0
'Rice Mini Puffs' (Glenny's)	1 oz	109	20.0	<.5

Food Name	Serv. Size	Total Cal.	Carbs GMS	Fat GMS
'Right Start' (Erewhon)	1 oz	90	24.0	0.0
'Right Start With Raisins' (Erewhon)	1 oz	90	22.0	0.0
'Ripple Crisp' (General Mills)	1 oz	110	24.0	<1.0
'Ripple Crisp' honey bran (General Mills)	1 oz	100	24.0	<1.0
'Shredded Wheat' (Barbara's Bakery)	1.4 oz	140	31.0	1.0
'Shredded Wheat' (Nabisco)	1 biscuit	80	19.0	1.0
'Shredded Wheat 'n Bran' (Nabisco)	1 oz	90	23.0	0.0
'Shredded Wheat With Oat Bran' (Nabisco)	1 oz	100	22.0	1.0
'6-Grain Crisp' fruit and flaxseed (Golden Temple)	1 oz	118	20.0	3.5
'Smacks' (Kellogg's)	1 oz	110	25.0	1.0
'Smacks' wheat (Kellogg's)	1 oz	106	24.8	0.5
'S'Mores Grahams' (General Mills)	1 oz	120	24.0	2.0
'Smurf-Magic Berries' (Post)	1 oz	120	26.0	1.0
'Special K' rice and wheat (Kellogg's)	1 oz	111	21.3	0.1
'Spelt Flakes' (Arrowhead Mills)	1 oz	100	21.0	1.0
'Spoon Size Shredded Wheat' (Nabisco)	1 oz	90	23.0	1.0
'Sprinkle Spangles' corn puffs, sprinkles (General Mills)	1 oz	110	25.0	1.0
'Sprouts 7' bananas and Hawaiian fruit (Health Valley)	1 oz	90	16.0	0.0
'Sprouts 7' raisins, fat-free (Health Valley)	1 oz	90	16.0	0.0
'Startoons' cocoa (Barbara's Bakery)	1 cup	110	26.0	0.5
'Startoons' honey (Barbara's Bakery)	1 cup	110	26.0	0.0
'Strawberry 'N Cream' nectarsweet gourmet (Breadshop)	1 oz	110	16.0	4.0
'Strawberry Squares' (Kellogg's)	1 oz	90	23.0	0.0
'Sugar Corn Pops' (Kellogg's)	1 oz	108	25.7	0.1
'Sugar Frosted Flakes' (Krusteaz)	1 oz	110	26.0	0.0
'Sugar Frosted Flakes' (Malt•O•Meal)	1 oz	110	26.0	0.0
'Sugar Puffs' (Malt•O•Meal)	1 oz	110	25.0	0.0
'Sunflakes Multi-Grain' (Ralston)	1 oz	100	24.0	1.0
'Super Nutty Granola' (Golden Temple)	1 oz	135	19.0	5.0
'Super O's' (Erewhon)	1 oz	110	24.0	0.0
'Super Sugar Crisp' wheat (Post)	1 oz	106	25.6	0.3
'Supernatural' honeysweet gourmet (Breadshop)	1 oz	100	17.5	5.0
'Supernatural New England' honeysweet gourmet (Breadshop)	1 oz	130	18.0	5.0
'Sweet Home Farm Almond' (Golden Temple)	1 oz	123	18.0	4.0
'Sweet Home Farm Crunchy Müesli' low fat (Golden Temple)	1 oz	105	21.0	2.0
'Sweet Home Farm Granola' low fat (Golden Temple)	1 oz	110	22.0	2.0
'Sweet Home Farm Raisin' (Golden Temple)	1 oz	120	19.0	4.0
'Sweetened Puffed Wheat' (Malt•O•Meal)	1 oz	110	25.0	0.0
'Swiss Style Müesli' (Golden Temple)	1 oz	105	19.0	1.5
'Tasteeos' oat and other grains	1 oz	112	22.5	0.8
'Team' rice and other grains (Nabisco)	1 oz	111	24.4	0.5
'Team Flakes' (Nabisco)	1 oz	110	24.0	1.0
'Teenage Mutant Ninja Turtles' (Ralston)	1 oz	110	26.0	0.0

Food Name	Serv. Size	Total Cal.	Carbs GMS	Fat GMS
'35% Fruit Müesli' *(Golden Temple)*	1 oz	97	19.0	1.0
'Toasted Oat' 100% natural *(Nature Valley)*	1 oz	130	20.0	5.0
'Toasted Oats' *(Krusteaz)*	1 oz	110	22.0	1.0
'Toasted Oats' *(Malt•O•Meal)*	1 oz	110	20.0	2.0
'Toasties' corn *(Post)*	1 oz	110	24.4	0.1
'Tootie Fruities' *(Malt•O•Meal)*	1 oz	110	25.0	1.0
'Total Corn Flakes' *(General Mills)*	1 oz	110	24.0	1.0
'Total Raisin Bran' *(General Mills)*	1.5 oz	140	33.0	1.0
'Total' wheat *(General Mills)*	1 oz	100	22.4	0.6
'Triples' *(General Mills)*	1 oz	110	24.0	1.0
'Triples' breakfast pack *(General Mills)*	1 oz	110	23.0	1.0
'Trix' corn and other grains *(General Mills)*	1 oz	109	25.2	0.4
'Uncle Sam' *(US Mills)*	1 oz	110	20.0	1.0
'Urkel-O's' *(Ralston)*	1 oz	110	25.0	1.0
'Waffelos' wheat and other grains	1 oz	115	24.5	1.2
'Wheat Chex' *(Ralston)*	1 oz	104	23.3	0.7
'Wheat Flakes' *(Erewhon)*	1 oz	110	22.0	0.0
'Wheat 'n Raisin Chex' *(Ralston)*	1 1/3 oz	130	30.1	0.3
'Wheaties' *(General Mills)*	1 oz	99	22.6	0.5
'Wheaties Honey Gold' *(General Mills)*	1 oz	100	25.0	1.0
'Whole-Grain Shredded Wheat' *(Kellogg's)*	1 oz	90	23.0	0.0
'Whole-Grain Wheat Chex' *(Ralston)*	1 oz	100	23.0	1.0
CEREAL SNACK. See also GRANOLA AND CEREAL BAR; GRANOLA SNACK.				
'Cheerios-to-Go' *(General Mills)*	1 pouch	80	15.0	2.0
'Cheerios-to-Go' apple cinnamon *(General Mills)*	1 pouch	110	22.0	2.0
'Cheerios-to-Go' honey nut *(General Mills)*	1 pouch	110	23.0	1.0
'Fingos' cinnamon *(General Mills)*	1 oz	110	22.0	3.0
'Fingos' honey toasted oat *(General Mills)*	1 oz	110	21.0	3.0
CHARD. See SWISS CHARD.				
CHAYOTE				
boiled, drained	4 oz	27	5.8	0.5
boiled, drained, 1-inch pieces	1/2 cup	19	4.1	0.4
raw, approx 7.2 oz	1 med	49	11.0	0.6
raw, 1-inch pieces	1/2 cup	16	3.6	0.2
raw, trimmed	1 oz	7	1.5	0.1
raw, untrimmed	1 lb	108	24.3	1.4
CHEDDARWURST				
'Bun Size' *(Hillshire Farm)*	2 oz	200	1.0	18.0
'Links' *(Hillshire Farm)*	2 oz	190	1.0	17.0
CHEESE. See also CHEESE, ALTERNATIVE; CHEESE BALL; CHEESE FOOD; CHEESE LOG;				
CHEESE NUGGET; CHEESE NUT; CHEESE PRODUCT; CHEESE SPREAD; CHEESE STICK.				
AMERICAN				
(Borden) fat-free, low-cholesterol	1 oz	40	4.0	0.0

Food Name	Serv. Size	Total Cal.	Carbs GMS	Fat GMS
(Borden) 'Light'	1 oz	70	1.0	4.0
(Borden) 'Loaf'	1 oz	110	1.0	9.0
(Borden) 'Slices'	1 oz	110	1.0	9.0
(Borden) slices 'Premium'	1 oz	110	1.0	9.0
(Dorman's)	1 oz	110	1.0	9.0
(Dorman's) 'Loaf Low Sodium'	1 oz	110	1.0	9.0
(Healthy Favorites)	2/3 oz	45	2.0	2.0
(Hoffman's)	1 oz	110	1.0	9.0
(Kraft) 'Deluxe Loaf'	1 oz	110	1.0	9.0
(Kraft) 'Deluxe Slices'	1 oz	110	1.0	9.0
(Land O'Lakes)	1 oz	110	<1.0	9.0
(Land O'Lakes) sharp	1 oz	100	1.0	9.0
(Old English) sharp 'Loaf'	1 oz	110	1.0	9.0
(Old English) sharp 'Slices'	1 oz	110	1.0	9.0
(Sargento) hot pepper	1 oz	110	0.5	9.0
ASIAGO (Frigo) wheel	1 oz	110	1.0	9.0
BABYBEL				
(Laughing Cow)	1 oz	91	tr	7.0
(Laughing Cow) mini	3/4 oz	74	tr	6.0
BLUE				
crumbled, not packed	1 cup	477	3.2	38.8
(Dorman's) 'Castello 70%'	1 oz	134	0.1	12.3
(Dorman's) 'Danablu 60%'	1 oz	108	0.3	9.7
(Dorman's) 'Danablu 50%'	1 oz	100	0.3	8.2
(Dorman's) 'Saga 70%'	1 oz	134	0.1	12.3
(Frigo)	1 oz	100	1.0	8.0
(Hickory Farms) 'Domestic'	1 oz	101	0.7	8.3
(Kraft)	1 oz	100	1.0	9.0
(Sargento)	1 oz	100	1.0	8.0
BONBEL				
(Laughing Cow)	1 oz	100	tr	8.0
(Laughing Cow) mini, 3/4 oz	1 oz	74	tr	6.0
BONBINO (Laughing Cow)	1 oz	103	tr	9.0
BRICK				
(Dorman's)	1 oz	110	1.0	8.0
(Kraft)	1 oz	110	0.0	9.0
(Land O'Lakes)	1 oz	110	1.0	8.0
BRIE				
(Dorman's)	1 oz	81	0.3	6.6
(Sargento)	1 oz	100	0.1	8.0
BURGER (Sargento)	1 oz	110	0.5	9.0
BUTTERNIP (Hickory Farms)	1 oz	110	1.1	9.4
CAJUN (Sargento)	1 oz	110	0.3	9.0

Food Name	Serv. Size	Total Cal.	Carbs GMS	Fat GMS
CALJACK *(Churny)*	1 oz	100	1.0	8.0
CAMEMBERT				
domestic	1 oz	84	0.1	6.8
(Dorman's) '50%'	1 oz	89	0.3	7.3
(Dorman's) '45%'	1 oz	82	0.3	6.3
(Hickory Farms)	1 oz	90	0.1	7.0
(Sargento)	1 oz	90	0.1	7.0
CARAWAY	1 oz	105	0.9	8.2
CHEDDAR				
American domestic	1 oz	113	0.4	9.3
American domestic, shredded, not packed	1 cup	455	1.5	37.5
(Alpine Lace) 'Cheddar Flavored'	1 oz	100	1.0	8.0
(Alpine Lace) shredded 'Ched-R-Lo' milk cheese	1 oz	80	1.0	5.0
(Alta•Dena) mild	1 oz	110	1.0	9.0
(Alta•Dena) sharp	1 oz	110	1.0	9.0
(Axelrod) extra sharp	1 oz	110	1.0	9.0
(Boar's Head) sliced	1 oz	110	1.0	9.0
(Darigold)	1 oz	110	<1.0	9.0
(Dorman's)	1 oz	110	1.0	9.0
(Dorman's) 'Chedda-Delite'	1 oz	90	1.0	7.0
(Dorman's) reduced fat 'Low Sodium'	1 oz	80	1.0	5.0
(Dorman's) w/Monterey Jack 'Chedda-Jack'	1 oz	90	1.0	7.0
(Featherweight) 'Low Sodium'	1 oz	110	1.0	9.0
(Frigo)	1 oz	110	1.0	9.0
(Golden Balance) mild, shredded 'Natural Shreds'	1 oz	90	1.0	6.0
(Golden Balance) sharp, shredded 'Natural Shreds'	1 oz	90	1.0	6.0
(Healthy Choice) shredded, fat-free	1 oz	40	1.0	0.0
(Healthy Favorites) mild, fancy shredded	1 oz	70	0.0	4.0
(Hickory Farms)	1 oz	110	1.0	9.0
(Hickory Farms) raw milk 'Light Choice Low Sodium'	1 oz	114	0.0	8.0
(Hoffman's) super sharp processed	1 oz	110	2.0	8.0
(Kraft)	1 oz	110	1.0	9.0
(Kraft) mild, finely shredded 'Light Naturals'	1 oz	80	1.0	5.0
(Kraft) mild, reduced fat 'Light Naturals'	1 oz	80	0.0	5.0
(Kraft) mild, shredded 'Light Naturals'	1 oz	80	0.0	5.0
(Kraft) sharp, shredded 'Light Naturals'	1 oz	80	1.0	5.0
(Land O'Lakes)	1 oz	110	<1.0	9.0
(Land O'Lakes) 'Chedarella'	1 oz	100	<1.0	8.0
(Laughing Cow)	1 oz	110	tr	9.0
(Sargento)	1 oz	110	0.4	9.0
(Sargento) mild, fancy shredded 'Preferred Light'	1 oz	90	1.0	5.0
(Sargento) 'New York'	1 oz	110	0.4	9.0
(Weight Watchers) mild, 'Natural'	1 oz	80	1.0	5.0

Food Name	Serv. Size	Total Cal.	Carbs GMS	Fat GMS
(Weight Watchers) mild, 'Natural Low Sodium'	1 oz	80	1.0	5.0
(Weight Watchers) mild, shredded 'Natural'	1 oz	80	1.0	5.0
CHESHIRE	1 oz	108	1.3	8.6
CHUTTER *(Hickory Farms)* 'Cold Pack'	1 oz	87	2.6	5.8
COLBY				
(Alpine Lace) 'Colby-Lo'	1 oz	80	1.0	5.0
(Dorman's)	1 oz	110	1.0	9.0
(Hickory Farms) 'Light Choice Low Sodium'	1 oz	100	1.0	6.0
(Hickory Farms) 'Longhorn'	1 oz	112	0.7	8.6
(Hickory Farms) lowfat, calcium-enriched 'Light Choice'	1 oz	100	1.0	8.0
(Kraft)	1 oz	110	1.0	9.0
(Kraft) reduced fat 'Light Naturals'	1 oz	80	0.0	5.0
(Kraft) w/Monterey Jack, reduced fat 'Light Naturals'	1 oz	80	1.0	5.0
(Land O'Lakes)	1 oz	110	1.0	9.0
(Sargento)	1 oz	110	1.0	9.0
(Sargento) Jack	1 oz	110	0.5	9.0
(Weight Watchers) 'Natural'	1 oz	80	1.0	5.0
COTTAGE CHEESE				
Creamed				
large curd	4 oz	117	3.0	5.1
large curd, not packed	1 cup	217	5.6	9.5
lowfat 1%	1 oz	20	0.8	0.3
lowfat 2%	1 oz	25	1.0	0.5
small curd	4 oz	117	3.0	5.1
small curd, not packed	1 cup	217	5.6	9.5
(Bison) chive	1/2 cup	120	4.0	5.0
(Bison) 4% fat	1/2 cup	120	4.0	5.0
(Bison) garden salad	1/2 cup	110	4.0	4.0
(Bison) lowfat 1%	1/2 cup	90	4.0	2.0
(Bison) w/pineapple	1/2 cup	140	18.0	4.0
(Borden) 4% fat	1/2 cup	120	4.0	5.0
(Borden) 4% fat, unsalted	1/2 cup	120	4.0	5.0
(Breakstone's)	4 oz	110	3.0	5.0
(Breakstone's) lowfat 2%	4 oz	100	4.0	2.0
(Carnation) 4% fat, large curd	1/2 cup	115	4.0	5.0
(Carnation) 4% fat, small curd	1/2 cup	115	4.0	5.0
(Carnation) 4% fat, w/pineapple	1/2 cup	130	12.0	5.0
(Crowley) 4% fat	1/2 cup	120	4.0	5.0
(Crowley) 4% fat, w/peaches	1/2 cup	140	17.0	3.0
(Crowley) 4% fat, w/pineapple	1/2 cup	140	15.0	4.0
(Crowley) lowfat 1%	1/2 cup	90	4.0	1.0
(Crowley) lowfat 1%, calcium-fortified	1/2 cup	90	4.0	1.0
(Crowley) lowfat 1% 'No Salt Added'	1/2 cup	90	4.0	1.0

Food Name	Serv. Size	Total Cal.	Carbs GMS	Fat GMS
(Crowley) lowfat 1%, w/pineapple	1/2 cup	110	15.0	1.0
(Darigold) 4% fat	4 oz	120	4.0	4.2
(Darigold) lowfat 2% 'Trim'	4 oz	100	4.0	3.2
(Friendship) 'California Style 4%'	1/2 cup	120	4.0	5.0
(Friendship) 4% fat, w/pineapple	1/2 cup	140	15.0	4.0
(Friendship) lowfat 1%	1/2 cup	90	4.0	1.0
(Friendship) lowfat 1%, lactose-reduced	1/2 cup	90	4.0	1.0
(Friendship) lowfat 1% 'No Salt Added'	1/2 cup	90	4.0	1.0
(Friendship) lowfat 1%, w/pineapple	1/2 cup	110	15.0	1.0
(Friendship) lowfat 2%, pot style, large curd	1/2 cup	100	4.0	2.0
(Knudsen) 4% fat, large curd	4 oz	120	4.0	5.0
(Knudsen) 4% fat, small curd	4 oz	120	4.0	5.0
(Knudsen) 4% fat, w/pineapple	4 oz	140	14.0	5.0
(Lite-Line) lowfat 1.5%	1/2 cup	90	4.0	2.0
(Weight Watchers) lowfat 1%	1/2 cup	90	4.0	1.0
(Weight Watchers) lowfat 2%	1/2 cup	100	4.0	2.0
Lowfat				
1% not packed	1 cup	164	6.2	2.3
2%, not packed	1 cup	203	8.2	4.4
(Carnation) 1.5% 'Slender'	1/2 cup	90	4.0	2.0
(Knudsen) 2%	4 oz	100	4.0	2.0
(Knudsen) 2%, w/fruit cocktail	4 oz	130	16.0	2.0
(Knudsen) 2%, w/Mandarin orange	4 oz	110	11.0	2.0
(Knudsen) 2%, w/peach	6 oz	170	19.0	2.0
(Knudsen) 2%, w/pear	4 oz	110	12.0	2.0
(Knudsen) 2%, w/pineapple	6 oz	170	18.0	2.0
(Knudsen) 2%, w/spiced apple	6 oz	180	20.0	2.0
(Knudsen) 2%, w/strawberry	6 oz	170	19.0	2.0
(Light n' Lively) 1%	4 oz	80	4.0	2.0
(Light n' Lively) 1%, garden salad	4 oz	80	5.0	2.0
(Sealtest) 2%	4 oz	100	4.0	2.0
Nonfat				
(Knudsen)	4 oz	70	3.0	0.0
(Light n' Lively)	4 oz	90	7.0	0.0
Uncreamed				
dry, large curd	4 oz	96	2.1	0.5
dry, large curd, not packed	1 cup	123	2.7	0.6
dry, small curd	4 oz	96	2.1	0.5
dry, small curd, not packed	1 cup	123	2.7	0.6
dry curd, unsalted *(Borden)*	1/2 cup	80	3.0	1.0
dry curd, unsalted *(Darigold)*	4 oz	80	3.0	1.0
dry curd, unsalted, nonfat *(Breakstone's)*	4 oz	90	6.0	0.0

Food Name	Serv. Size	Total Cal.	Carbs GMS	Fat GMS
CREAM CHEESE				
natural	1 oz	98	0.7	9.8
(Alta•Dena) pasteurized	1 oz	100	2.0	10.0
(Crowley)	1 oz	110	1.0	9.0
(Darigold)	1 oz	99	0.8	9.9
(Dorman's) '70%'	1 oz	102	0.6	9.9
(Dorman's) '65%'	1 oz	90	0.6	8.4
(Healthy Choice) fat-free	1 oz	30	2.0	0.0
(Healthy Choice) herb and garlic, fat-free	1 oz	30	2.0	0.0
(Healthy Favorites)	1 oz	60	2.0	5.0
(Philadelphia Brand)	1 oz	100	1.0	10.0
(Philadelphia Brand) 'Free'	1 oz	25	1.0	0.0
(Philadelphia Brand) pasteurized process 'Light'	1 oz	60	2.0	5.0
(Philadelphia Brand) w/chives	1 oz	90	1.0	9.0
(Philadelphia Brand) w/olive and pimento, fat-free	1 oz	90	2.0	8.0
(Philadelphia Brand) w/pimento	1 oz	90	1.0	9.0
Soft				
(Friendship)	1 oz	103	0.8	10.0
(Philadelphia Brand)	1 oz	100	2.0	10.0
(Philadelphia Brand) w/chives and onion	1 oz	100	2.0	9.0
(Philadelphia Brand) w/herb and garlic	1 oz	100	2.0	9.0
(Philadelphia Brand) w/olives and pimento	1 oz	90	2.0	8.0
(Philadelphia Brand) w/pineapple	1 oz	90	4.0	8.0
(Philadelphia Brand) w/smoked salmon	1 oz	90	1.0	9.0
(Philadelphia Brand) w/strawberries	1 oz	90	4.0	8.0
Whipped				
(Philadelphia Brand)	1 oz	100	1.0	10.0
(Philadelphia Brand) w/chives	1 oz	90	1.0	8.0
(Philadelphia Brand) w/onions	1 oz	90	2.0	8.0
(Philadelphia Brand) w/smoked salmon	1 oz	90	2.0	8.0
(Temp-Tee)	1 oz	100	1.0	10.0
DANBO				
(Dorman's) 20%	1 oz	62	0.3	2.8
(Dorman's) 45%	1 oz	98	0.3	7.5
EDAM				
(Dorman's)	1 oz	100	1.0	8.0
(Dorman's) 45%	1 oz	91	0.3	7.0
(Hickory Farms) 'Domestic'	1 oz	100	0.9	8.4
(Kaukauna)	1 oz	100	<1.0	8.0
(Kraft)	1 oz	90	0.0	7.0
(Land O'Lakes)	1 oz	100	<1.0	8.0
(Laughing Cow)	1 oz	100	tr	8.0
(May-Bud)	1 oz	100	0.0	8.0

Food Name	Serv. Size	Total Cal.	Carbs GMS	Fat GMS
(Sargento)	1 oz	100	0.4	8.0
EFORT, sheep's milk	1 oz	314	1.7	26.0
FARMER				
(Friendship)	1/2 cup	160	4.0	12.0
(Friendship) 'No Salt Added'	1/2 cup	160	4.0	12.0
(Hickory Farms)	1 oz	90	1.0	7.0
(Hickory Farms) 'Light Choice'	1 oz	90	1.0	7.0
(Kaukauna)	1 oz	100	<1.0	8.0
(May-Bud)	1 oz	90	1.0	7.0
(Sargento)	1 oz	100	1.0	8.0
FETA				
sheep's milk	1 oz	75	1.2	6.0
(Churny) 'Natural'	1 oz	75	1.2	6.5
(Dorman's) 45%	1 oz	91	0.4	7.3
(Sargento)	1 oz	80	1.0	6.0
FONTINA (Sargento)	1 oz	110	0.4	9.0
FRENCH ONION (Alouette)	1 oz	95	2.0	9.0
GJETOST				
goat's milk, fresh	1 oz	82	0.9	6.8
(Sargento)	1 oz	130	12.0	8.0
GOAT				
hard type	1 oz	128	0.6	10.1
semisoft type	1 oz	103	0.7	8.5
soft type	1 oz	76	0.3	6.0
GOUDA				
(Dorman's)	1 oz	100	1.0	8.0
(Kaukauna)	1 oz	100	1.0	8.0
(Kaukauna) w/caraway seed	1 oz	100	<1.0	8.0
(Kaukauna) w/hickory smoke flavor	1 oz	100	<1.0	8.0
(Kraft)	1 oz	110	0.0	9.0
(Land O'Lakes)	1 oz	100	1.0	8.0
(Laughing Cow)	1 oz	110	tr	9.0
(Laughing Cow) mini	3/4 oz	80	tr	6.4
(May-Bud)	1 oz	100	1.0	8.0
(Sargento)	1 oz	100	1.0	8.0
GRATED. See also PARMESAN; ROMANO.				
(Polly-O)	1 oz	130	1.0	10.0
(Sargento) Italian style	1 oz	110	1.0	8.0
GRUYERE	1 oz	116	0.1	9.1
HAVARTI				
(Casino)	1 oz	120	0.0	11.0
(Dorman's) 45%	1 oz	91	0.3	7.0
(Dorman's) 60%	1 oz	118	0.3	10.6

Food Name	Serv. Size	Total Cal.	Carbs GMS	Fat GMS
(Hickory Farms) 'Danish Special'	1 oz	117	0.3	10.5
(Sargento)	1 oz	120	0.3	11.0
HORSERADISH *(Kaukauna)* hearty, cold pack 'Cup'	1 oz	100	3.0	7.0
HOT PEPPER *(Hickory Farms)*	1 oz	106	0.5	8.9
JARLSBERG				
(Hickory Farms)	1 oz	100	1.0	7.0
(Norseland)	1 oz	97	1.0	7.0
LIMBURGER				
(Mohawk Valley) 'Little Gem'	1 oz	90	0.0	8.0
(Sargento)	1 oz	90	0.1	8.0
MASCARPONE 'Imported' *(Galbani)*	1 oz	128	1.2	13.1
MONTEREY	1 oz	105	0.2	8.5
MONTEREY JACK				
(Alpine Lace) 'Monti-Jack-Lo'	1 oz	80	1.0	5.0
(Alpine Lace) 'Monti-Jack-Lo' sliced	1 oz	80	1.0	5.0
(Alta•Dena)	1 oz	100	1.0	8.0
(Alta•Dena) w/jalapeño pepper	1 oz	100	1.0	8.0
(Axelrod)	1 oz	100	1.0	8.0
(Axelrod) w/jalapeño pepper	1 oz	100	1.0	8.0
(Darigold)	1 oz	110	<1.0	8.0
(Dorman's)	1 oz	100	1.0	8.0
(Dorman's) reduced fat 'Low Sodium'	1 oz	80	1.0	5.0
(Hickory Farms) 'Light Choice Low Sodium'	1 oz	110	0.0	8.0
(Kaukauna)	1 oz	110	<1.0	9.0
(Kraft)	1 oz	110	0.0	9.0
(Kraft) reduced fat 'Light Naturals'	1 oz	80	0.0	5.0
(Kraft) reduced fat 'Light Naturals' w/peppers	1 oz	80	1.0	5.0
(Kraft) 'Singles'	1 oz	90	2.0	7.0
(Kraft) w/caraway	1 oz	100	1.0	8.0
(Kraft) w/jalapeño pepper	1 oz	110	1.0	9.0
(Land O'Lakes)	1 oz	110	<1.0	9.0
(Land O'Lakes) hot pepper	1 oz	110	<1.0	9.0
(Land O'Lakes) processed 'Jalapeño Jack'	1 oz	90	1.0	8.0
(May-Bud)	1 oz	110	0.0	9.0
(Sargento)	1 oz	110	0.2	9.0
(Weight Watchers) 'Natural'	1 oz	80	1.0	5.0
MOZZARELLA. See also CHEESE NUGGET.				
(Dorman's)	1 oz	90	1.0	6.0
(Healthy Choice) fat-free, chunk	1 oz	40	1.0	0.0
(Hickory Farms)	1 oz	72	0.8	4.5
(Hickory Farms) 'Light Choice Low Sodium'	1 oz	80	1.0	5.0
(Kraft)	1 oz	90	1.0	7.0
(Polly-O) 'Fior di Latte'	1 oz	80	1.0	6.0

Food Name	Serv. Size	Total Cal.	Carbs GMS	Fat GMS
(Polly-O) 'Lite'	1 oz	70	1.0	4.0
(Weight Watchers) 'Natural'	1 oz	70	1.0	4.0
Part skim milk				
(Alpine Lace) low moisture	1 oz	70	1.0	5.0
(Crowley)	1 oz	70	1.0	4.0
(Dorman's) low moisture 'Low Sodium'	1 oz	80	1.0	5.0
(Frigo) low moisture	1 oz	80	1.0	5.0
(Frigo) low moisture, reduced fat	1 oz	60	1.0	3.0
(Kraft) low moisture	1 oz	80	1.0	5.0
(Kraft) w/jalapeño pepper	1 oz	80	1.0	5.0
(Land O'Lakes) low moisture	1 oz	80	1.0	5.0
(Polly-O)	1 oz	80	1.0	5.0
(Sargento) low moisture	1 oz	80	1.0	5.0
Reduced fat				
(Dorman's) 'Low Sodium'	1 oz	80	1.0	4.0
(Kraft) 'Light Naturals'	1 oz	80	1.0	4.0
Shredded				
(Alpine Lace)	1 oz	70	1.0	5.0
(Alpine Lace) sliced	1 oz	70	1.0	5.0
(Healthy Choice) fat-free	1 oz	40	1.0	0.0
(Kraft) 'Light Naturals'	1 oz	80	1.0	4.0
(Sargento) fancy 'Preferred Light'	1 oz	60	<1.0	3.0
(Weight Watchers) 'Natural'	1 oz	80	1.0	4.0
Whole milk				
(Crowley)	1 oz	90	1.0	7.0
(Frigo) low moisture	1 oz	90	1.0	7.0
(Sargento)	1 oz	90	1.0	7.0
(Polly-O)	1 oz	90	1.0	6.0
MOZZARELLA CHEDDAR				
(Precious) shredded 'Pizza Cheese'	1 oz	95	1.0	7.0
MUENSTER				
(Alpine Lace)	1 oz	100	1.0	8.0
(Alpine Lace) sliced 'Low Sodium'	1 oz	100	1.0	9.0
(Dorman's)	1 oz	110	0.0	9.0
(Dorman's) 50%	1 oz	100	0.3	8.2
(Dorman's) 'Low Sodium'	1 oz	110	0.0	9.0
(Dorman's) reduced fat 'Low Sodium'	1 oz	80	0.0	5.0
(Hickory Farms)	1 oz	100	0.3	8.5
(Hickory Farms) 'Light Choice Low Sodium'	1 oz	110	0.0	9.0
(Kaukauna)	1 oz	110	<1.0	9.0
(Land O'Lakes)	1 oz	100	<1.0	9.0
(Sargento) red rind	1 oz	100	0.3	9.0

Food Name	Serv. Size	Total Cal.	Carbs GMS	Fat GMS
NEUFCHATEL				
(Hickory Farms) chocolate	1 oz	110	8.0	8.0
(Hickory Farms) orange	1 oz	100	4.0	8.0
(Hickory Farms) peach	1 oz	90	3.0	8.0
(Hickory Farms) pineapple	1 oz	90	2.0	8.0
(Hickory Farms) rum date nut	1 oz	100	4.0	8.0
(Hickory Farms) strawberry	1 oz	90	3.0	8.0
(Kaukauna) garden vegetable	1 oz	80	1.0	7.0
(Kaukauna) garlic and herbs	1 oz	80	1.0	7.0
(Philadelphia Brand) 'Light'	1 oz	80	1.0	7.0
NEW HOLLAND *(Hickory Farms)* w/herbs 'Light Choice'	1 oz	90	1.0	8.0
PARMESAN				
natural, piece	1 oz	110	0.9	7.2
natural, shredded	1 oz	116	1.0	7.7
natural, shredded	1 tbsp	21	0.2	1.4
(Churny) 'Natural'	1 oz	110	1.0	7.0
(Hickory Farms)	1 oz	110	1.0	7.0
(Kraft)	1 oz	100	1.0	7.0
(Sargento) fresh	1 oz	110	1.0	7.0
Grated				
natural	1 oz	128	1.0	8.4
natural	1 tbsp	23	0.2	1.5
(Frigo)	1 oz	130	1.0	9.0
(Frigo) fresh	1 oz	110	1.0	7.0
(Kraft)	1 oz	130	1.0	9.0
(Polly-O)	1 oz	130	1.0	9.0
(Progresso)	1 tbsp	23	<1.0	2.0
(Sargento)	1 oz	130	2.0	9.0
Hard	1 oz	111	0.9	7.3
Wheel *(Frigo)*	1 oz	110	1.0	7.0
W/Romano cheese, grated				
(Frigo)	1 oz	130	1.0	9.0
(Sargento)	1 oz	110	1.0	7.0
PARMESAN REGGIANO *(Galbani)* 'Imported'	1 oz	105	1.0	7.1
PIZZA				
(Frigo) shredded	1 oz	90	1.0	7.0
(Frigo) shredded, lowfat	1 oz	65	1.0	3.0
(Healthy Choice) fancy, shredded, fat-free	1 oz	40	1.0	0.0
PORT DU SALUT	1 oz	98	0.2	7.9
PORT WINE *(Hickory Farms)*	1 oz	97	2.4	6.9
POT *(Sargento)*	1 oz	25	1.0	0.2
PRIMAVERA *(Bel Paese)* 'Lite'	1 oz	68	2.0	4.0

Food Name	Serv. Size	Total Cal.	Carbs GMS	Fat GMS
PROVOLONE				
(Alpine Lace) 'Provo-Lo'	1 oz	70	1.0	5.0
(Dorman's)	1 oz	90	1.0	7.0
(Frigo)	1 oz	100	1.0	7.0
(Frigo) smoked	1 oz	100	1.0	7.0
(Hickory Farms) 'Light Choice Low Sodium'	1 oz	90	1.0	7.0
(Kraft)	1 oz	100	1.0	7.0
(Land O'Lakes)	1 oz	100	1.0	8.0
(Sargento)	1 oz	100	1.0	8.0
PUB (Hickory Farms)	1 oz	94	2.4	6.9
QUESO BLANCO (Sargento)	1 oz	100	0.3	9.0
QUESO DE PAPA (Sargento)	1 oz	110	0.4	9.0
QUESO DE TACO (Hickory Farms)	1 oz	106	0.5	8.9
RICOTTA				
Light/lowfat				
(Gardenia) '95% Fat-free'	1 oz	30	2.0	1.0
(Polly-O) 'Lite'	2 oz	80	3.0	4.0
(Precious) 'Lowfat'	1 oz	40	2.0	2.0
(Sargento) 'Lite'	1 oz	23	1.0	1.0
Part skim milk				
(Crowley)	2 oz	80	3.0	4.0
(Frigo)	1 oz	45	1.0	3.0
(Frigo) 'Truly Lite' fat-free	1 oz	20	2.0	0.0
(Polly-O)	2 oz	90	2.0	6.0
(Sargento)	1 oz	30	1.0	2.0
Whole milk				
(Breakstone's)	4 oz	200	6.0	15.0
(Crowley)	2 oz	100	3.0	7.0
(Frigo)	1 oz	50	1.0	4.0
(Polly-O)	2 oz	100	2.0	7.0
ROMANO				
Grated				
(Frigo)	1 oz	130	1.0	9.0
(Kraft)	1 oz	130	1.0	9.0
(Kraft) 'Natural'	1 oz	100	1.0	7.0
(Polly-O)	1 oz	130	1.0	10.0
(Progresso)	1 tbsp	23	<1.0	2.0
(Sargento)	1 oz	110	1.0	8.0
Loaf (Hickory Farms)	1 oz	110	1.0	8.0
Wedge (Frigo)	1 oz	110	1.0	8.0
ROQUEFORT				
	1 oz	103	0.6	8.6
sheep's milk	1 oz	105	0.6	8.7

Food Name	Serv. Size	Total Cal.	Carbs GMS	Fat GMS
SLIM JACK *(Dorman's)*	1 oz	90	1.0	7.0
SMOKED				
(Hickory Farms) 'Light Choice Smoky Lyte'	1 oz	80	1.0	6.0
(Hoffman's) sharp, processed	1 oz	110	1.0	9.0
(Sargento) 'Smokestick'	1 oz	100	1.0	7.0
STRING				
(Frigo)	1 oz	80	1.0	5.0
(Kraft) low moisture	1 oz	80	1.0	5.0
(Polly-O)	1 oz	90	2.0	6.0
(Sargento)	1 oz	80	1.0	5.0
(Sargento) smoked	1 oz	80	1.0	5.0
SWISS				
domestic	1 oz	105	1.0	7.7
domestic	1-inch cube	56	0.5	4.1
(Boar's Head) 'Domestic'	1 oz	110	1.0	8.0
(Boar's Head) 'No Salt Added'	1 oz	100	<1.0	8.0
(Casino)	1 oz	110	1.0	8.0
(Cracker Barrel) baby 'Natural'	1 oz	110	0.0	9.0
(Dorman's)	1 oz	100	0.0	8.0
(Dorman's) 'No Salt Added'	1 oz	100	0.0	8.0
(Hickory Farms) creamy 'Cold Pack'	1 oz	92	2.5	7.2
(Hickory Farms) 'Domestic'	1 oz	110	1.0	7.8
(Hickory Farms) 'Light Choice Lorraine'	1 oz	100	0.0	7.8
(Hickory Farms) 'Light Choice Low Sodium'	1 oz	100	0.0	8.0
(Kraft)	1 oz	110	1.0	8.0
(Kraft) aged	1 oz	110	1.0	8.0
(Kraft) 'Light Naturals'	1 oz	90	1.0	5.0
(Land O'Lakes)	1 oz	110	1.0	8.0
(Sargento) 'Finland'	1 oz	110	1.0	8.0
(Weight Watchers) 'Natural'	1 oz	90	1.0	5.0
Processed				
(Alpine Lace) sliced, milk cheese 'Swiss-Lo'	1 oz	90	1.0	6.0
(Alpine Lace) 'Swiss-Lo'	1 oz	100	1.0	7.0
(Borden)	1 oz	100	1.0	8.0
(Borden) fat-free, low-cholesterol	1 oz	40	4.0	0.0
(Dorman's) 'Reduced Fat'	1 oz	90	0.0	5.0
(Dorman's) smoked	1 oz	100	1.0	7.0
(Healthy Favorites) sliced, reduced fat	1 oz	80	1.0	4.0
(Hoffman's) smoky, w/cheddar	1 oz	110	1.0	8.0
(Kraft) 'Deluxe'	1 oz	90	1.0	7.0
(Kraft) 'Light'	1 oz	70	2.0	3.0
(Kraft) reduced fat 'Light Naturals'	1 oz	90	1.0	5.0
(Kraft) '75% Very Low Sodium'	1 oz	110	1.0	8.0

Food Name	Serv. Size	Total Cal.	Carbs GMS	Fat GMS
(Sargento)	1 oz	110	1.0	8.0
TACO				
(Frigo) shredded	1 oz	110	1.0	9.0
(Kraft) shredded	1 oz	110	1.0	9.0
(Sargento)	1 oz	110	0.5	9.0
TALEGGIO (Tal-Fino) 'Brand Imported'	1 oz	89	0.2	7.4
TILSIT				
whole milk	1 oz	95	0.5	7.3
(Sargento)	1 oz	100	1.0	7.0
TYBO				
(Dorman's) 45%	1 oz	98	0.3	7.5
(Sargento) red wax	1 oz	100	0.3	7.0
VERMONT (Churny)	1 oz	110	1.0	9.0
CHEESE, ALTERNATIVE				
(Cheeztwin)	1 oz	90	3.0	6.0
American cheddar style (Soya Kaas)	1 oz	79	1.6	5.4
American style (Delicia)	1 oz	80	1.0	6.0
American style (Golden Image)	1 oz	90	2.0	6.0
American style, hickory smoked (Delicia)	1 oz	80	0.0	6.0
American style, lactose-free, singles (Formägg)	3/4 oz	70	<1.0	5.0
American style, 'Low Sodium Slices' (Weight Watchers)	1 oz	50	2.0	2.0
American style, 'Slices' (Weight Watchers)	1 oz	50	2.0	2.0
American style, w/caraway (Delicia)	1 oz	80	1.0	6.0
American style, w/hot pepper (Delicia)	1 oz	80	1.0	6.0
American style, w/salami (Delicia)	1 oz	80	1.0	6.0
California cheddar style 'AlmondRella' (Sharon's Finest)	1 oz	50	1.0	1.4
California cheddar style 'Zero-Fat Rella' (Sharon's Finest)	1 oz	45	3.0	0.0
cheddar style (Frigo)	1 oz	90	1.0	7.0
cheddar style (Sargento)	1 oz	90	<1.0	6.0
cheddar style, fancy shredded (Formägg)	1 oz	70	1.0	5.0
cheddar style, shredded 'Ched-O-Mate' (Fisher)	1 oz	90	1.0	7.0
colby style (Golden Image)	1 oz	110	1.0	9.0
colby style 'LoChol' (Dorman's)	1 oz	90	1.0	6.0
colby style, Longhorn style (Delicia)	1 oz	80	1.0	6.0
cream cheese style (Soya Kaas)	1 oz	90	0.1	9.4
cream cheese style (Weight Watchers)	1 oz	35	1.0	2.0
cream cheese style, all flavors 'Better than Cream Cheese' (Tofutti)	1 oz	80	1.0	8.0
garlic-herb style 'AlmondRella' (Sharon's Finest)	1 oz	50	1.0	1.4
'Heart Beat' (Nucoa)	1 oz	50	2.0	2.0
jalapeño jack style 'Zero-Fat Rella' (Sharon's Finest)	1 oz	45	3.0	0.0
'Jalapeño Mexi Kaas' (Soya Kaas)	1 oz	77	0.3	5.3
'Low Cholesterol' (Lite-Line)	1 oz	90	2.0	7.0

Food Name	Serv. Size	Total Cal.	Carbs GMS	Fat GMS
mild cheddar style *(Golden Image)*	1 oz	110	0.0	9.0
mild cheddar style 'TofuRella' *(Sharon's Finest)*	1 oz	80	1.0	5.0
mild cheddar style 'TofuRella' slices *(Sharon's Finest)*	3/4 oz	60	1.0	4.0
mozzarella style *(Frigo)*	1 oz	90	1.0	7.0
mozzarella style *(Sargento)*	1 oz	80	<1.0	6.0
mozzarella style *(Soya Kaas)*	1 oz	78	1.8	5.6
mozzarella style 'AlmondRella' *(Sharon's Finest)*	1 oz	50	1.0	1.4
mozzarella style, shredded 'Pizza-Mate' *(Fisher)*	1 oz	90	1.0	7.0
mozzarella style 'TofuRella' *(Sharon's Finest)*	1 oz	80	1.0	5.0
mozzarella style 'TofuRella' slices *(Sharon's Finest)*	3/4 oz	60	1.0	4.0
mozzarella style 'Zero-Fat Rella' *(Sharon's Finest)*	1 oz	45	3.0	0.0
Muenster style 'LoChol' *(Dorman's)*	1 oz	100	1.0	7.0
'Sandwich-Mate' *(Fisher)*	1 oz	90	3.0	6.0
sharp cheddar style 'Slices' *(Weight Watchers)*	1 oz	50	2.0	2.0
Swiss style, lactose-free, singles *(Formägg)*	3/4 oz	70	<1.0	5.0
Swiss style 'LoChol' *(Dorman's)*	1 oz	100	1.0	7.0
Swiss style 'Slices' *(Weight Watchers)*	1 oz	50	2.0	2.0

CHEESE BALL

Food Name	Serv. Size	Total Cal.	Carbs GMS	Fat GMS
cheddar, w/almonds and bacon *(Kaukauna)*	1 oz	100	3.0	7.0
green onion flavor, w/almonds *(Kaukauna)*	1 oz	100	3.0	7.0
Port wine, w/almonds *(Kaukauna)*	1 oz	100	3.0	7.0
sharp cheddar, w/almonds *(Kaukauna)*	1 oz	100	3.0	7.0

CHEESE BLINTZ. See BLINTZ.

CHEESE FLAVORED SNACKS

(Barbara's Bakery)

Food Name	Serv. Size	Total Cal.	Carbs GMS	Fat GMS
'Pinta Puffs' tangy triple cheese	1 oz	70	10.0	2.0
puff lights	1 oz	40	3.0	3.0
(Bearitos) puffs, cheddar, baked, original	.5 oz	80	7.0	5.0
(Chee•tos)				
cheddar valley	1 oz	160	16.0	9.0
crunchy	1 oz	150	17.0	9.0
crunchy, light	1 oz	140	19.0	6.0
curls	1 oz	150	17.0	9.0
flamin' hot	1 oz	150	16.0	9.0
light	1 oz	140	19.0	6.0
paws	1 oz	160	15.0	10.0
puffed balls	1 oz	160	16.0	10.0
puffs	1 oz	160	16.0	9.0
(Flavor Tree) sticks, cheddar	1/4 cup	129	11.9	8.1
(Health Valley)				
'Cheddar Lite' puffs, w/organic corn, baked	.25 oz	40	4.0	2.0
puffs, fat-free	1 oz	100	21.0	0.0
puffs, w/chili, fat-free	1 oz	100	21.0	0.0

Food Name	Serv. Size	Total Cal.	Carbs GMS	Fat GMS
puffs, w/green onion, fat-free	1 oz	100	21.0	0.0
(Keebler) 'RC Ricers' zesty cheddar	1 oz	140	17.0	8.0
(Planter)				
'Cheez Balls'	1 oz	160	14.0	11.0
'Cheez Balls' nacho	1 oz	160	15.0	10.0
'Cheez Curls'	1 oz	160	14.0	11.0
'Cheez Curls' nacho	1 oz	160	15.0	10.0
(Weight Watchers) curls, crunchy	.5-oz pkg	70	10.0	2.0
(Wise)				
'Cheez Doodles' baked, puffed	1 oz	150	16.0	9.0
'Cheez Doodles' fried, crunchy	1 oz	160	16.0	10.0
'Cheez Waffies'	1 oz	140	14.0	8.0
corn spirals,nacho	1 oz	160	16.0	10.0
corn twists,nacho, crispy	1 oz	160	16.0	10.0

CHEESE FOOD

AMERICAN

Food Name	Serv. Size	Total Cal.	Carbs GMS	Fat GMS
(Darigold)	1 oz	80	2.0	6.0
cold pack	1 oz	94	2.4	6.9
colored (Hoffman's)	1 oz	100	3.0	7.0
grated (Kraft)	1 oz	130	8.0	7.0
'Light' (Kraft)	1 oz	70	2.0	4.0
sharp, 'Singles' (Borden)	1 oz	90	2.0	7.0
'Singles' (Borden)	1 oz	90	3.0	7.0
'Singles' (Kraft)	1 oz	90	2.0	7.0
'Slices' (Borden)	1 oz	100	2.0	7.0
white, 'Singles' (Kraft)	1 oz	90	2.0	7.0
w/Swiss cheese (Land O'Lakes)	1 oz	100	1.0	8.0

BACON

Food Name	Serv. Size	Total Cal.	Carbs GMS	Fat GMS
(Cracker Barrel)	1 oz	90	3.0	7.0
'Chees'N Bacon' (Hoffman's)	1 oz	90	3.0	6.0
'Cheez'N Bacon' (Kraft)	1 oz	90	2.0	7.0
CARAWAY, 'Swisson Rye' (Hoffman's)	1 oz	90	2.0	7.0

CHEDDAR

Food Name	Serv. Size	Total Cal.	Carbs GMS	Fat GMS
extra sharp (Cracker Barrel)	1 oz	90	3.0	7.0
extra sharp (Land O'Lakes)	1 oz	100	1.0	9.0
extra sharp, cold pack 'Cup' (Kaukauna)	1 oz	100	3.0	7.0
'La Chedda' (Land O'Lakes)	1 oz	90	2.0	7.0
nacho, cold pack, 'Cup' (Kaukauna)	1 oz	100	3.0	7.0
Port wine (Cracker Barrel)	1 oz	100	3.0	7.0
sharp (Cracker Barrel)	1 oz	100	4.0	7.0
sharp, cold pack (Wispride)	1 oz	100	2.0	7.0
sharp, cold pack 'Cup' (Kaukauna)	1 oz	100	3.0	7.0
sharp, cup 'Lite 50' (Kaukauna)	1 oz	70	5.0	3.0

Food Name	Serv. Size	Total Cal.	Carbs GMS	Fat GMS
sharp 'Lite' *(Kaukauna)*	1 oz	70	5.0	4.0
smoky 'Lite' *(Kaukauna)*	1 oz	70	5.0	4.0
w/bacon *(Land O'Lakes)*	1 oz	110	1.0	9.0
w/bacon and horseradish, cold pack, 'Cup' *(Kaukauna)*	1 oz	100	3.0	7.0
GARLIC *(Kraft)*	1 oz	90	2.0	7.0
ITALIAN HERB *(Land O'Lakes)*	1 oz	90	2.0	7.0
JALAPEÑO				
(Hoffman's)	1 oz	90	2.0	7.0
(Kraft)	1 oz	90	2.0	7.0
(Land O'Lakes)	1 oz	90	2.0	7.0
hot, 'Mexican' *(Velveeta)*	1 oz	100	3.0	7.0
mild, 'Mexican' *(Velveeta)*	1 oz	100	3.0	7.0
'Singles' *(Kraft)*	1 oz	90	2.0	7.0
MEXICAN				
hot, shredded *(Velveeta)*	1 oz	100	3.0	7.0
mild, shredded *(Velveeta)*	1 oz	100	3.0	7.0
ONION				
(Land O'Lakes)	1 oz	90	2.0	7.0
'Chees'N Onion' *(Hoffman's)*	1 oz	100	3.0	7.0
PEPPPERONI *(Land O'Lakes)*	1 oz	90	1.0	7.0
PIMIENTO				
'Deluxe' *(Kraft)*	1 oz	100	1.0	8.0
'Singles' *(Kraft)*	1 oz	90	2.0	7.0
PORT WINE				
cold pack *(Wispride)*	1 oz	100	3.0	7.0
cold pack, 'Cup' *(Kaukauna)*	1 oz	100	3.0	7.0
cup, 'Lite 50' *(Kaukauna)*	1 oz	70	5.0	3.0
PROCESSED				
(Land O'Lakes)	1 oz	90	2.0	6.0
singles, fat-free *(Healthy Choice)*	1 oz	40	3.0	0.0
singles, 'Free' *(Kraft)*	1 oz	45	4.0	0.0
slices *(Land O'Lakes)*	3/4 oz	70	2.0	5.0
slices *(Land O'Lakes)*	2/3 oz	60	2.0	4.0
SALAMI				
(Land O'Lakes)	1 oz	90	2.0	7.0
'Chees'N Salami' *(Hoffman's)*	1 oz	90	3.0	6.0
SHARP, 'Singles' *(Kraft)*	1 oz	100	1.0	8.0
SHREDDED *(Velveeta)*	1 oz	100	3.0	7.0
SMOKY, cold pack, 'Cup' *(Kaukauna)*	1 oz	100	3.0	7.0
SWISS				
(Velveeta)	1 oz	100	3.0	7.0
almond, cup, 'Lite 50' *(Kaukauna)*	1 oz	70	5.0	3.0
country, cold pack, 'Cup' *(Kaukauna)*	1 oz	100	3.0	7.0

Food Name	Serv. Size	Total Cal.	Carbs GMS	Fat GMS
country, 'Lite' (Kaukauna)	1 oz	70	5.0	4.0
singles (Kraft)	1 oz	90	2.0	7.0
singles, 'Free' (Kraft)	1 oz	45	4.0	0.0
slices, 'Singles' (Borden)	1 oz	100	2.0	7.0
CHEESE LOG				
hickory smoke/white sharp cheddar, double (Kaukauna)	1 oz	100	3.0	7.0
Port wine (Sargento)	1 oz	100	3.0	7.0
Port wine, w/almonds (Kaukauna)	1 oz	100	3.0	7.0
sharp cheddar (Sargento)	1 oz	100	3.0	7.0
sharp cheddar, w/almonds (Cracker Barrel)	1 oz	90	4.0	6.0
sharp cheddar, w/almonds (Kaukauna)	1 oz	100	3.0	7.0
smoky, w/almonds (Cracker Barrel)	1 oz	90	4.0	6.0
Swiss almond (Sargento)	1 oz	90	2.0	7.0
Swiss almond, w/almonds (Kaukauna)	1 oz	100	3.0	7.0
white sharp cheddar/green onion, double (Kaukauna)	1 oz	100	3.0	7.0
CHEESE NUGGET				
mozzarella, breaded, frozen 'Hot Bites' (Banquet)	2.63 oz	240	16.0	13.0
CHEESE NUT				
Port wine (Cracker Barrel)	1 oz	90	4.0	6.0
sharp, w/bell and jalapeño peppers (Kaukauna)	1 oz	100	3.0	7.0
sharp cheddar (Cracker Barrel)	1 oz	100	4.0	7.0
CHEESE PASTRY, pocket (Tastykake)	3 oz	325	40.8	16.7
CHEESE PRODUCT				
(Alpine Lace)	1 oz	90	2.0	7.0
'Free N' Lean' singles (Alpine Lace)	1 oz	40	1.0	0.0
'Free Singles' (Kraft)	1 oz	45	4.0	0.0
'Light' (Velveeta)	1 oz	70	3.0	4.0
sandwich slices (Lunch Wagon)	1 oz	90	2.0	7.0
'Singles' fat-free (Borden)	1 oz	40	4.0	0.0
'Slices' (Velveeta)	1 oz	90	3.0	6.0
slices, fat-free (Lite-Line)	1 slice	25	3.0	0.0
AMERICAN FLAVOR				
(Harvest Moon)	1 oz	70	2.0	4.0
(Lite-Line)	1 oz	50	1.0	2.0
'Light' (Borden)	1 oz	70	1.0	5.0
'Light Singles' (Kraft)	1 oz	70	2.0	4.0
'Reduced Sodium' (Lite-Line)	1 oz	70	2.0	4.0
'Singles' (Light n' Lively)	1 oz	70	2.0	4.0
'Sodium Lite' (Lite-Line)	1 oz	70	2.0	4.0
white 'Light Singles' (Kraft)	1 oz	70	2.0	4.0
white 'Singles' (Light n' Lively)	1 oz	70	2.0	4.0
CHEDDAR FLAVOR				
medium-sharp (Spreadery)	1 oz	70	3.0	4.0

Food Name	Serv. Size	Total Cal.	Carbs GMS	Fat GMS
mild *(Lite-Line)*	1 oz	50	1.0	2.0
sharp *(Lite-Line)*	1 oz	50	1.0	2.0
sharp *(Spreadery)*	1 oz	70	3.0	4.0
sharp, 'Free' *(Kraft)*	1 oz	45	4.0	0.0
sharp, 'Light' *(Kraft)*	1 oz	70	2.0	4.0
sharp, 'Singles' *(Kraft)*	1 oz	100	1.0	8.0
sharp, 'Singles' *(Light n' Lively)*	1 oz	70	2.0	4.0
sharp, slices *(Lite-Line)*	1 slice	35	1.0	2.0
Vermont white *(Spreadery)*	1 oz	70	3.0	4.0
CREAM CHEESE FLAVOR 'Light' *(Philadelphia Brand)*	1 oz	60	2.0	5.0
MEXICAN FLAVOR mild, w/jalapeños *(Spreadery)*	1 oz	70	3.0	4.0
MOZZARELLA FLAVOR *(Lite-Line)*	1 oz	50	1.0	2.0
MUENSTER FLAVOR *(Lite-Line)*	1 oz	50	1.0	2.0
NACHO FLAVOR *(Spreadery)*	1 oz	70	3.0	4.0
NEUFCHATEL				
classic ranch *(Spreadery)*	1 oz	70	1.0	7.0
French onion *(Spreadery)*	1 oz	70	2.0	6.0
garden vegetable *(Spreadery)*	1 oz	70	2.0	6.0
garlic and herb *(Spreadery)*	1 oz	70	1.0	6.0
w/strawberries *(Spreadery)*	1 oz	70	1.0	5.0
PORT WINE FLAVOR *(Spreadery)*	1 oz	70	3.0	4.0
SWISS FLAVOR				
(Lite-Line)	1 oz	50	1.0	2.0
'Free Singles' *(Kraft)*	1 oz	45	4.0	0.0
'Light' *(Kraft)*	1 oz	70	2.0	3.0
'Singles' *(Light n' Lively)*	1 oz	70	2.0	3.0
CHEESE SPREAD				
AMERICAN				
(Kraft)	1 oz	80	2.0	6.0
'Easy Cheese American' *(Nabisco)*	1 oz	80	2.0	6.0
sharp 'Cracker Snacks' *(Sargento)*	1 oz	110	0.5	9.0
w/pimiento 'Cracker Snacks' *(Sargento)*	1 oz	110	0.5	9.0
BACON				
(Kraft)	1 oz	80	1.0	7.0
(Squeez-A-Snak)	1 oz	80	1.0	7.0
BLUE *(Roka)*	1 oz	70	2.0	6.0
BRICK 'Cracker Snacks' *(Sargento)*	1 oz	100	1.0	9.0
CHEDDAR				
'Easy Cheese Cheddar' *(Nabisco)*	1 oz	80	2.0	6.0
'Easy Cheese Cheddar 'n Bacon' *(Nabisco)*	1 oz	80	2.0	6.0
'Easy Cheese Sharp Cheddar' *(Nabisco)*	1 oz	80	2.0	6.0
sharp, 'Cup' *(Weight Watchers)*	1 oz	70	7.0	3.0
FRENCH ONION *(Alouette)*	1 oz	95	2.0	9.0

Food Name	Serv. Size	Total Cal.	Carbs GMS	Fat GMS
GARLIC				
(Squeez-A-Snak)	1 oz	80	1.0	7.0
and herbs, soft 'Lite' (Rondel)	1 oz	70	2.0	6.0
and spices (Alouette)	1 oz	95	2.0	9.0
HERB				
and garlic, soft 'Light' (Alouette)	1 oz	60	2.0	4.5
soft, 'Fines Herbes' (Rondel)	1 oz	90	2.0	8.0
HICKORY (Squeez-A-Snak)	1 oz	80	1.0	7.0
HORSERADISH, and chive (Alouette)	1 oz	85	1.0	8.0
JALAPEÑO				
(Cheez Whiz)	1 oz	80	2.0	6.0
(Kraft)	1 oz	70	3.0	5.0
(Squeez-A-Snak)	1 oz	80	1.0	6.0
loaf (Kraft)	1 oz	80	2.0	6.0
LIMBURGER (Mohawk Valley)	1 oz	70	0.0	6.0
MEXICAN				
'Easy Cheese Nacho' (Nabisco)	1 oz	80	2.0	6.0
hot (Velveeta)	1 oz	80	3.0	6.0
mild (Cheez Whiz)	1 oz	80	2.0	6.0
mild (Velveeta)	1 oz	80	3.0	6.0
OLIVE, and pimiento (Kraft)	1 oz	60	2.0	5.0
PIMIENTO				
(Kraft)	1 oz	70	3.0	5.0
(Velveeta)	1 oz	80	3.0	6.0
PINEAPPLE (Kraft)	1 oz	70	4.0	5.0
PORT WINE, 'Cup' (Weight Watchers)	1 oz	70	7.0	3.0
SALMON (Alouette)	1 oz	70	2.0	6.0
SHARP				
(Old English)	1 oz	80	1.0	7.0
(Squeez-A-Snak)	1 oz	80	1.0	7.0
SPINACH, creamy (Alouette)	1 oz	90	2.0	8.0
SWISS, 'Cracker Snacks' (Sargento)	1 oz	100	1.0	7.0
VEGETABLE				
garden, soft (Rondele)	1 oz	90	3.0	8.0
spring, soft 'Light' (Alouette)	1 oz	60	1.0	4.5
CHEESE STICK				
cheddar, breaded, frozen (Farm Rich)	3 oz	300	19.0	21.0
cheddar, snack (Flavor Tree)	1/4 cup	129	11.9	8.1
hot pepper, breaded, frozen (Farm Rich)	3 oz	260	20.0	17.0
mozzarella, breaded, frozen (Farm Rich)	3 oz	240	19.0	13.0
provolone, breaded, frozen (Farm Rich)	3 oz	270	22.0	16.0
CHEESE STRAW				
made w/lard, 5 x 3/8 x 3/8 inches	10 straws	272	20.7	17.9

Food Name	Serv. Size	Total Cal.	Carbs GMS	Fat GMS
made w/vegetable shortening, 5 x 3/8 x 3/8 inches	10 straws	272	20.7	17.9
CHEESE TOPPING, cheddar, w/bacon *(Tone's)*	1 tsp	10	0.7	1.0
CHEESECAKE. See CAKE.				
CHEESECAKE FILLING				
'No-Bake' lite *(Royal)*	1/8 pie	130	22.0	3.0
'No-Bake' real *(Royal)*	1/8 pie	160	29.0	3.0
CHERIMOYA. See CUSTARD APPLE.				
CHERRY				
SOUR, RED				
trimmed, w/pits	1 cup	52	12.6	0.3
trimmed, w/pits	1 oz	14	3.5	0.1
trimmed, w/o pits	1 cup	78	18.9	0.5
untrimmed	1 lb	203	49.7	1.2
SWEET				
trimmed, w/pits	1 cup	104	24.0	1.4
trimmed, w/pits	1 oz	20	4.7	0.3
trimmed, w/pits, approx 2.6 oz	10 med	49	11.3	0.7
untrimmed	1 lb	293	67.6	3.9
untrimmed *(Dole)*	1 cup	90	19.0	1.0
CHERRY, CANNED				
SOUR, RED				
(A&P)	1/2 cup	50	12.0	<1.0
in extra heavy syrup	1/2 cup	148	38.0	0.1
in heavy syrup	1/2 cup	116	29.8	0.1
in light syrup	1/2 cup	94	24.3	0.1
in water	1/2 cup	44	10.9	0.1
Pitted				
in extra heavy syrup	1/2 cup	129	33.1	0.1
in heavy syrup	1/2 cup	103	26.4	0.1
in light syrup	1/2 cup	85	21.9	0.1
in water	1/2 cup	41	10.0	0.1
in water *(Stokely)*	1/2 cup	45	10.0	0.0
tart *(Lucky Leaf)*	4 oz	50	11.0	0.0
tart *(Musselman's)*	4 oz	50	11.0	0.0
(White House)	3.5 oz	43	11.0	0.0
SWEET				
dark *(Del Monte)*	1/2 cup	90	23.0	0.0
in extra heavy syrup	1/2 cup	116	29.7	0.2
in heavy syrup	1/2 cup	94	24.1	0.2
in juice	1/2 cup	61	15.7	<.1
in light syrup	1/2 cup	76	19.6	0.2
in light syrup *(Del Monte)*	1/2 cup	100	26.0	0.0
in water	1/2 cup	52	13.3	0.1

Food Name	Serv. Size	Total Cal.	Carbs GMS	Fat GMS
Pitted				
dark *(Del Monte)*	1/2 cup	90	24.0	0.0
in extra heavy syrup	1/2 cup	133	34.1	0.2
in heavy syrup	1/2 cup	107	27.4	0.2
in juice	1/2 cup	68	17.3	0.0
in light syrup	1/2 cup	84	21.8	0.2
in water	1/2 cup	57	14.6	0.2
CHERRY, FROZEN				
SOUR, RED				
unsweetened	4 oz	52	12.5	0.5
unsweetened	1/2 cup	36	8.5	0.3
SWEET				
sweetened	10-oz pkg	253	63.5	0.4
sweetened	1 cup	231	57.9	0.3
sweetened	4 oz	101	25.4	0.1
sweetened *(Lucky Leaf)*	4 oz	130	31.0	0.0
CHERRY, MARASCHINO, in jar, w/liquid	1 oz	33	8.3	0.1
CHERRY, PUERTO RICAN				
approx .2 oz	1 med	2	0.4	<.1
trimmed	1/2 cup	16	3.8	0.1
trimmed	1 oz	9	2.2	0.1
untrimmed	1 lb	114	27.9	1.1
CHERRY CIDER *(Knudsen & Sons)*	8 oz	100	24.0	0.0
CHERRY DRINK				
(Hi-C) aseptic box	6 oz	100	24.0	0.0
(Hi-C) chilled	6 oz	100	24.0	0.0
(Kool-Aid) 'Koolers'	8.45 oz	140	38.0	0.0
(Squeezit) 'Chuckin Cherry'	6.75 oz	110	27.0	0.0
CHERRY DRINK MIX				
(Finast) prepared	8 oz	80	21.0	0.0
(Kool-Aid) sugar-sweetened, prepared	8 oz	80	20.0	0.0
(Kool-Aid) unsweetened, prepared w/sugar	8 oz	100	25.0	0.0
(Kool-Aid) unsweetened, prepared w/o sugar	8 oz	2	0.0	0.0
(Kool-Aid) w/NutraSweet, prepared	8 oz	4	0.0	0.0
(Pathmark) 'No Frills' prepared	8 oz	90	22.0	0.0
(Wyler's) 'Fruit Slush' prepared	4 oz	157	39.3	0.0
CHERRY JUICE				
(Dole) 'Pure and Light Mountain Cherry'	6 oz	87	22.0	0.1
(Juicy Juice) bottled	6 oz	90	23.0	0.0
(Juicy Juice) boxed	8.45 oz	130	32.0	0.0
(Knudsen & Sons) tart	8 oz	125	30.0	0.0
(Santa Cruz Natural) 'Cruz' organic	8 oz	125	29.0	<1.0
(Welch's) 'Orchard'	6 oz	180	45.0	0.0

Food Name	Serv. Size	Total Cal.	Carbs GMS	Fat GMS
CHERRY JUICE DRINK				
(Hi-C)	8.45 oz	141	34.8	0.1
(Hi-C)	6 oz	100	24.7	0.1
(Tang) 'Fruit Box'	8.45 oz	130	34.0	0.0
CHERRY LEMONADE				
(Knudsen & Sons)	8 oz	105	31.0	0.0
(Santa Cruz Natural) dark, sweet, organic	8 oz	60	20.0	<1.0
CHERRY PASTRY				
(Hormel) frozen 'Cherry Dulcita'	4 oz	300	48.0	9.0
(Tastykake) pocket	3 oz	325	40.8	16.7
CHERRY PIE FILLING. See PIE FILLING.				
CHERRY STRUDEL, individual (Aunt Fanny's)	3 oz	320	39.0	16.0
CHERVIL				
dried	1 oz	67	13.9	1.1
dried	1 tbsp	4	0.9	0.1
dried	1 tsp	1	0.3	0.0
CHESTNUT, CHINESE				
boiled or steamed	1 oz	43	9.6	0.2
dried	1 oz	103	22.6	0.5
raw	1 oz	64	13.9	0.3
raw, in shell	1 lb	852	187.0	4.2
roasted	1 oz	68	14.9	0.3
CHESTNUT, EUROPEAN/Italian chestnut/sweet chestnut				
boiled or steamed, shelled	1 oz	37	7.9	0.4
dried, in shell	1 lb	1357	280.5	16.1
dried, shelled, peeled	1 oz	105	22.3	1.1
dried, shelled, unpeeled	1 oz	106	22.0	1.3
raw, in shell	1 lb	714	152.8	7.6
raw, shelled, peeled	1 oz	56	12.5	0.4
raw, shelled, unpeeled	1 cup	309	66.0	3.3
raw, shelled, unpeeled	1 oz	60	12.9	0.6
roasted, in shell	1 lb	700	151.3	6.3
roasted, in shell	1 cup	350	75.7	3.2
roasted, in shell	1 oz	70	15.0	0.6
roasted, shelled	1 oz	70	15.0	0.6
roasted, shelled, approx 17 nuts	1 cup	350	75.7	3.2
CHESTNUT, ITALIAN. See CHESTNUT, EUROPEAN.				
CHESTNUT, JAPANESE				
boiled or steamed	1 oz	16	3.6	0.1
dried, in shell	1 lb	1078	243.7	3.7
dried, shelled	1 oz	102	23.1	0.4
dried, shelled	1 cup	558	126.2	1.9
raw, in shell	1 lb	462	104.5	1.6

Food Name	Serv. Size	Total Cal.	Carbs GMS	Fat GMS
raw, shelled	1 oz	44	9.9	0.2
roasted	1 oz	57	12.8	0.2
CHESTNUT, SWEET. See CHESTNUT, EUROPEAN.				
CHESTNUT FLOUR	100 gm	362	76.2	3.7
CHEWING GUM. See CANDY.				
CHIA SEEDS, dried	1 oz	134	13.6	7.4
CHICK PEA. See GARBANZO BEAN.				
CHICK PEA FLOUR. See GARBANZO FLOUR.				
CHICKEN. For fresh chicken see CHICKEN, BROILER-FRYER; CHICKEN, CAPON; CHICKEN, ROASTER; CHICKEN, STEWING.				
CHICKEN, ALTERNATIVE				
(Heartline) 'Chicken Fillet Style'	2 oz	176	9.0	7.0
(Heartline) 'Chicken Fillet Style' lite	.5 oz	22	1.0	0.0
Canned				
(Worthington) diced, drained	1/4 cup	90	2.0	8.0
(Worthington) 'FriChik' 1.6-oz pieces	2 pieces	180	4.0	13.0
(Worthington) sliced, drained, 1.05-oz slices	2 slices	90	2.0	8.0
Frozen				
(Morningstar Farms) nuggets, homestyle 'Country Crisps'	3 oz	250	18.0	16.0
(Morningstar Farms) nuggets, zesty 'Country Crisps'	3 oz	280	17.0	19.0
(Morningstar Farms) patty 'Country Crisps'	2.5 oz	220	13.0	15.0
(Worthington) 'Crispy Chik'	3 oz	280	17.0	19.0
(Worthington) diced 'Meatless Chicken'	1/2 cup	190	5.0	13.0
(Worthington) patty 'Crispy Chik'	2.5 oz	220	13.0	15.0
(Worthington) roll 'Chic-ketts'	1/2 cup	160	6.0	7.0
(Worthington) roll 'Meatless Chicken'	2.5 oz	150	4.0	10.0
(Worthington) sliced 'Meatless Chicken' 1-oz slices	2 slices	130	3.0	9.0
(Worthington) sticks 'Chik Stiks' approx 1.7-oz pieces	1 stick	110	4.0	7.0
CHICKEN, BONELESS BREAST, PREPARED				
(Hillshire Farm) smoked 'Deli Select'	1 oz	31	<1.0	0.2
(Louis Rich) hickory-smoked	1 oz	30	0.6	0.8
(Louis Rich) hickory-smoked, 97% fat-free	1 oz	30	<1.0	<1.0
(Louis Rich) oven-roasted 'Deluxe'	1 oz	30	0.6	0.8
(Louis Rich) oven-roasted, 'Deluxe' 96% fat-free	1 oz	30	<1.0	1.0
(Oscar Mayer) oven-roasted	1 oz	29	0.6	0.7
(Oscar Mayer) smoked	1 oz	25	0.2	0.4
CHICKEN, BROILER-FRYER				
BACK MEAT AND SKIN				
fried, flour-coated	4 oz	375	7.4	23.5
raw	1 oz	90	0.0	8.1
roasted	4 oz	340	0.0	23.8
stewed	4 oz	293	0.0	20.6

Food Name	Serv. Size	Total Cal.	Carbs GMS	Fat GMS
BACK MEAT ONLY				
raw	1 lb	624	0.0	28.8
raw	1 oz	39	0.0	1.7
roasted	4 oz	271	0.0	14.9
stewed	4 oz	237	0.0	12.7
BREAST MEAT AND SKIN				
fried, batter-dipped	4 oz	295	10.2	15.0
fried, flour-coated	4 oz	252	1.9	10.1
raw	1 lb	784	0.0	41.6
raw	1 oz	49	0.0	2.6
roasted	4 oz	223	0.0	8.8
stewed	4 oz	209	0.0	8.4
BREAST MEAT ONLY				
raw	1 lb	496	0.0	6.4
raw	1 oz	31	0.0	0.4
roasted	4 oz	187	0.0	4.0
stewed	4 oz	171	0.0	3.4
DARK MEAT AND SKIN				
fried, batter-dipped	4 oz	338	10.6	21.1
fried, flour-coated	4 oz	323	4.6	19.2
raw	1 lb	1072	0.0	83.2
raw	1 oz	67	0.0	5.2
roasted	4 oz	287	0.0	17.9
stewed	4 oz	264	0.0	16.6
DARK MEAT ONLY				
fried, chopped, or diced	1 cup	335	3.6	16.3
raw	1 lb	560	0.0	19.2
raw	1 oz	35	0.0	1.2
roasted	1 cup	287	0.0	13.6
roasted	4 oz	232	0.0	11.0
roasted, chopped, or diced	1 cup	286	0.0	13.6
stewed	1 cup	269	0.0	12.6
stewed	4 oz	218	0.0	10.2
stewed, chopped, or diced	1 cup	269	0.0	12.6
DRUMSTICK MEAT AND SKIN				
fried, batter-dipped	4 oz	304	9.4	17.9
fried, flour-coated	4 oz	278	1.8	15.6
raw	1 lb	736	0.0	40.0
raw	1 oz	46	0.0	2.5
roasted	4 oz	245	0.0	12.6
stewed	4 oz	231	0.0	12.1
DRUMSTICK MEAT ONLY				
raw	1 lb	544	0.0	16.0

Food Name	Serv. Size	Total Cal.	Carbs GMS	Fat GMS
raw	1 oz	34	0.0	1.0
roasted	4 oz	195	0.0	6.4
stewed	4 oz	192	0.0	6.5
LEG MEAT AND SKIN				
fried, batter-dipped	4 oz	310	9.9	18.3
fried, flour-coated	4 oz	285	2.8	16.2
raw	1 lb	848	0.0	54.4
raw	1 oz	53	0.0	3.4
stewed	4 oz	249	0.0	14.7
LEG MEAT ONLY				
raw	1 lb	544	0.0	17.6
raw	1 oz	34	0.0	1.1
roasted	4 oz	217	0.0	9.6
stewed	4 oz	210	0.0	9.1
LIGHT MEAT AND SKIN				
fried, batter-dipped	4 oz	312	10.7	17.4
fried, flour-coated	4 oz	279	2.1	13.7
raw	1 lb	848	0.0	49.6
raw	1 oz	53	0.0	3.1
roasted	4 oz	252	0.0	12.3
stewed	4 oz	228	0.0	11.3
LIGHT MEAT ONLY				
fried	8 oz	269	0.6	7.8
raw	1 lb	512	0.0	8.0
raw	1 oz	32	0.0	0.5
roasted	1 cup	242	0.0	6.3
roasted	4 oz	196	0.0	5.1
roasted, chopped, or diced	1 cup	242	0.0	6.3
stewed, chopped, or diced	1 cup	223	0.0	5.6
stewed	4 oz	180	0.0	4.5
NECK MEAT AND SKIN				
fried, batter-dipped	4 oz	374	9.9	26.7
fried, flour-coated	4 oz	376	4.8	26.8
raw	1 lb	1344	0.0	118.4
raw	1 oz	84	0.0	7.4
simmered	4 oz	280	0.0	20.5
NECK MEAT ONLY				
raw	1 lb	704	0.0	40.0
raw	1 oz	44	0.0	2.5
simmered	4 oz	203	0.0	9.3
SKIN ONLY				
fried, batter-dipped	1 oz	112	6.6	8.2
roasted	1 oz	129	0.0	11.5

Food Name	Serv. Size	Total Cal.	Carbs GMS	Fat GMS
stewed	1 oz	103	0.0	9.4
THIGH MEAT AND SKIN				
fried, batter-dipped	4 oz	314	10.3	18.7
fried, flour-coated	4 oz	297	3.6	17.0
raw	1 lb	960	0.0	68.8
raw	1 oz	60	0.0	4.3
roasted	4 oz	280	0.0	17.6
stewed	4 oz	263	0.0	16.7
THIGH MEAT ONLY				
raw	1 lb	544	0.0	17.6
raw	1 oz	34	0.0	1.1
roasted	4 oz	237	0.0	12.3
stewed	4 oz	221	0.0	11.1
WING MEAT AND SKIN				
fried, batter-dipped	4 oz	367	12.4	24.7
fried, flour-coated	4 oz	364	2.7	25.1
raw	1 lb	1008	0.0	72.0
raw	1 oz	63	0.0	4.5
roasted	4 oz	329	0.0	22.1
stewed	4 oz	282	0.0	19.1
WING MEAT ONLY				
raw	1 lb	576	0.0	16.0
raw	1 oz	36	0.0	1.0
roasted	4 oz	230	0.0	9.2
stewed	4 oz	205	0.0	8.1
CHICKEN, CANNED				
Chunk				
(Featherweight)	3 oz	90	0.0	3.0
(Hormel) breast	6.75 oz	350	0.0	20.0
(Hormel) breast	2.5 oz	90	0.0	3.0
(Hormel) breast, no salt	2.5 oz	90	0.0	3.0
(Hormel) dark	6.75 oz	327	0.0	18.0
(Hormel) white and dark	6.75 oz	340	0.0	20.0
(Hormel) white and dark, unsalted	6.75 oz	330	0.0	18.0
(Swanson) 'Mixin' Chicken'	2.5 oz	130	1.0	8.0
(Swanson) white and dark	2.5 oz	100	0.0	4.0
Loaf (Hormel)	2 oz	130	0.0	10.0
White (Swanson)	2.5 oz	100	0.0	4.0
CHICKEN, CAPON				
GIBLETS				
raw	1 lb	592	6.4	24.0
raw	1 oz	37	0.4	1.5
simmered	1 cup	238	1.1	7.8

Food Name	Serv. Size	Total Cal.	Carbs GMS	Fat GMS
simmered	4 oz	186	0.9	6.1
MEAT AND SKIN				
raw	1 lb	1056	0.0	76.8
raw	1 oz	66	0.0	4.8
roasted	4 oz	260	0.0	13.2
CHICKEN, FROZEN. See also CHICKEN DINNER/ENTRÉE, FROZEN.				
BREAST				
Boneless				
(Pilgrim's Pride)	3 oz	195	10.8	10.2
(Tyson)	3 oz	190	15.0	9.0
(Tyson) barbecue	3 oz	110	6.0	3.0
(Tyson) chunks	3 oz	240	10.0	17.0
(Tyson) grilled	2.75 oz	100	4.0	3.0
(Tyson) hot and spicy	2.75 oz	110	7.0	3.0
(Tyson) skinless, Wholesale Club Item	3.5 oz	110	1.0	2.0
Halves, Wholesale Club Item (Tyson)	3.5 oz	230	0.0	13.0
Pieces				
(Banquet) fried	5.75 oz	220	13.0	11.0
(Tyson) mesquite, Wholesale Club Item	3.5 oz	170	1.0	7.0
Portions (Swanson) fried, 'Plump & Juicy'	4.5 oz	360	21.0	20.0
Strips (Weaver)	3.3 oz	200	14.0	10.0
Tenders				
(Banquet) Southern fried	2.25 oz	160	13.0	7.0
(Pilgrim's Pride)	3 oz	181	11.1	9.5
(Tyson) blanched, wholesale club item	3.5 oz	200	12.0	8.0
(Tyson) breaded, wholesale club item	3.5 oz	200	12.0	8.0
(Tyson) Southern fried	3 oz	220	15.0	11.0
(Tyson) unbreaded, wholesale club item	3.5 oz	120	0.0	1.0
Whole				
(Tyson) wholesale club item	3.5 oz	210	0.0	12.0
(Weaver)	4.5 oz	270	18.0	13.0
(Weaver) batter-dipped	4.4 oz	310	13.0	20.0
CHUNKS				
(Country Pride)	3 oz	240	15.0	15.0
(Country Pride) Southern fried	3 oz	280	14.0	20.0
(Tyson) diced	3 oz	150	0.0	5.0
(Tyson) mesquite flavor 'Hors D'Oeuvres'	3.5 oz	100	1.0	1.0
(Tyson) microwave, boneless	3.5 oz	220	11.0	15.0
LEG MEAT				
(Banquet) thighs and drumsticks, fried	6.25 oz	250	14.0	14.0
(Pilgrim's Pride) drumsters	3 oz	200	10.5	12.5
(Tyson) drums and thighs, wholesale club item	3.5 oz	270	0.0	17.0
(Tyson) 'Julienne Leg Meat' wholesale club item	3.5 oz	160	0.0	6.0

Food Name	Serv. Size	Total Cal.	Carbs GMS	Fat GMS
(Tyson) thighs, skinless, wholesale club item	3.5 oz	200	0.0	10.0
(Weaver) batter-dipped	3 oz	210	11.0	14.0
(Weaver) drums and thighs, 'Crispy Dutch Frye'	3.5 oz	290	14.0	19.0
NUGGETS				
(Country Pride)	3 oz	250	14.0	16.0
(Pilgrim's Pride)	3 oz	202	10.4	12.3
(Weaver)	2.6 oz	190	10.0	12.0
(Weight Watchers)	5.9 oz	220	23.0	7.0
PORTIONS				
(Pilgrim's Pride) fried	3 oz	255	11.9	17.7
(Swanson) 'Homestyle Recipe'	7 oz	390	33.0	21.0
(Swanson) 'Take-Out Pre-Fried'	3.25 oz	270	16.0	16.0
ROASTER *(Tyson)* wholesale club item	3.5 oz	230	0.0	13.0
WINGS				
(Pilgrim's Pride) Southern fried	3 oz	228	5.1	17.2
(Pilgrim's Pride) 'Wing Zappers'	3 oz	187	1.8	12.8
(Tyson) all varieties, 'Flyers'	3.5 oz	220	0.0	14.0
(Tyson) drummettes, wholesale club item	3.5 oz	260	2.0	17.0
(Tyson) barbecue 'Hors D'Oeuvres' wholesale club item	3.5 oz	210	3.0	12.0
(Tyson) raw, hot, wholesale club item	3.5 oz	280	1.0	19.0
(Tyson) roaster 'Hors D'Oeuvres' wholesale club item	3.5 oz	210	0.0	12.0
(Weaver) batter-dipped	4 oz	400	20.0	28.0
(Weaver) 'Crispy Dutch Frye'	4 oz	400	20.0	28.0
(Weaver) hot	2.7 oz	170	1.0	11.0
CHICKEN, ROASTER				
DARK MEAT ONLY				
raw	1 lb	512	0.0	16.0
raw	1 oz	32	0.0	1.0
roasted	4 oz	202	0.0	9.9
GIBLETS, simmered	1 cup	239	1.3	7.6
LIGHT MEAT ONLY				
raw	1 lb	496	0.0	8.0
raw	1 oz	31	0.0	0.5
roasted	1 cup	214	0.0	5.7
roasted	4 oz	174	0.0	4.6
MEAT AND SKIN				
raw	1 lb	976	0.0	72.0
raw	1 oz	61	0.0	4.5
roasted	4 oz	253	0.0	15.2
CHICKEN, STEWING				
DARK MEAT ONLY				
raw	1 lb	720	0.0	36.8
raw	1 oz	45	0.0	2.3

Food Name	Serv. Size	Total Cal.	Carbs GMS	Fat GMS
stewed	1 cup	361	0.0	21.4
stewed	4 oz	293	0.0	17.3
GIBLETS				
raw	1 lb	560	8.0	20.8
raw	1 oz	35	0.5	1.3
simmered	1 cup	281	0.2	13.5
LIGHT MEAT ONLY				
raw	1 lb	624	0.0	19.2
raw	1 oz	39	0.0	1.2
stewed	1 cup	298	0.0	11.2
stewed	4 oz	242	0.0	9.0
MEAT AND SKIN				
raw	1 lb	1168	0.0	92.8
raw	1 oz	73	0.0	5.8
stewed	4 oz	323	0.0	21.4
CHICKEN DINNER/ENTRÉE, CANNED				
(Featherweight) and dumplings	7.5 oz	160	18.0	5.0
(LaChoy)				
chow mein	3/4 cup	240	47.0	2.0
chow mein 'Bi-Pack'	8.642 oz	97	9.5	3.8
chow mein 'Bi-Pack'	3/4 cup	80	8.0	3.0
Oriental 'Bi-Pack'	3/4 cup	240	47.0	2.0
Oriental w/noodles 'Bi-Pack'	9 oz	160	23.0	3.8
sweet and sour	3/4 cup	240	47.0	2.0
sweet and sour 'Bi-Pack'	8.959 oz	161	28.6	2.5
sweet and sour 'Bi-Pack'	3/4 cup	120	18.0	2.0
teriyaki 'Bi-Pack'	8.642 oz	110	14.9	3.0
teriyaki 'Bi-Pack'	3/4 cup	85	8.0	2.0
(Luck's) and dumplings	7.25 oz	240	18.0	11.0
(Swanson)				
à la king	5 1/4 oz	190	9.0	12.0
and dumplings	7.5 oz	220	19.0	11.0
CHICKEN DINNER/ENTRÉE, FROZEN				
(Armour)				
à la king 'Classics Lite'	11.25 oz	290	38.0	7.0
and noodles 'Classics'	11 oz	230	23.0	7.0
breast, Marsala 'Classics Lite'	10.5 oz	250	27.0	7.0
Burgundy 'Classics Lite'	10 oz	210	25.0	2.0
fettuccini 'Classics'	11 oz	260	28.0	9.0
glazed 'Classics'	10.75 oz	300	24.0	16.0
mesquite 'Classics'	9.5 oz	370	42.0	16.0
Oriental 'Classics Lite'	10 oz	180	24.0	1.0
parmigiana 'Classics'	11.5 oz	370	27.0	19.0

Food Name	Serv. Size	Total Cal.	Carbs GMS	Fat GMS
sweet and sour 'Classics Lite'	11 oz	240	39.0	2.0
w/wine and mushroom sauce 'Classics'	10.75 oz	280	24.0	11.0
(Banquet)				
à la king 'Cookin' Bags'	4 oz	110	9.0	5.0
and dumplings	10 oz	430	34.0	24.0
and dumplings 'Family Entrées'	7 oz	280	28.0	14.0
drumsnackers 'Platters'	7 oz	430	49.0	19.0
fettuccini 'Healthy Balance'	11.25 oz	320	47.0	7.0
fried	10 oz	400	45.0	22.0
fried 'Extra Helping'	16 oz	570	70.0	28.0
fried, white meat 'Extra Helping'	16 oz	570	70.0	28.0
fried, white meat 'Platter'	9 oz	430	21.0	22.0
fried, white meat, hot'n spicy 'Platter'	9 oz	430	21.0	22.0
hot'n spicy 'Snack'n'	3.75 oz	140	8.0	9.0
nuggets, breast, Southern fried w/barbecue sauce	4.5 oz	370	20.0	23.0
nuggets, hot'n spicy, w/barbecue sauce	4.5 oz	360	23.0	21.0
nuggets, 'Platters'	6.4 oz	430	46.0	21.0
nuggets, Southern fried, w/barbecue sauce	4.5 oz	370	20.0	23.0
nuggets, w/barbecue sauce 'Extra Helping'	10 oz	640	56.0	36.0
nuggets, w/sweet and sour sauce 'Extra Helping'	10 oz	650	64.0	34.0
nuggets, w/sweet and sour sauce 'Microwave'	4.5 oz	360	22.0	21.0
parmesan, w/vermicelli 'Healthy Balance'	10.8 oz	290	30.0	10.0
patties, breast, Southern fried, w/biscuit	4 oz	320	37.0	14.0
patties 'Platters'	7.5 oz	380	34.0	21.0
pie	7 oz	550	39.0	36.0
pie 'Supreme Microwave'	7 oz	430	30.0	28.0
primavera and vegetable 'Cookin' Bags'	4 oz	100	14.0	2.0
primavera and vegetable 'Family Entrées'	7 oz	140	18.0	3.0
sweet and sour 'Cookin' Bags'	4 oz	130	22.0	2.0
(Budget Gourmet)				
and egg noodles, w/broccoli	10 oz	450	31.0	26.0
cacciatore	11 oz	300	27.0	13.0
Marsala	10 oz	250	37.0	5.0
Mexicana	12.8 oz	510	70.0	15.0
Oriental, and vegetables 'Light and Healthy'	9 oz	280	44.0	6.0
roast	11.2 oz	280	34.0	7.0
sweet and sour, w/rice	10 oz	350	53.0	7.0
teriyaki	12 oz	360	44.0	12.0
w/fettuccini	10 oz	400	29.0	21.0
(Celentano)				
parmigiana	9 oz	330	15.0	20.0
primavera	11.5 oz	270	18.0	10.0

Food Name	Serv. Size	Total Cal.	Carbs GMS	Fat GMS
(Chun King)				
chow mein	13 oz	370	53.0	6.0
imperial	13 oz	300	54.0	1.0
walnut, crunchy	13 oz	310	49.0	5.0
(Country Pride) primavera sticks	3 oz	240	16.0	15.0
(Dining Lite)				
à la king	9 oz	240	30.0	7.0
and noodles	9 oz	240	28.0	7.0
chow mein	9 oz	180	31.0	2.0
glazed	9 oz	220	30.0	4.0
(Freezer Queen)				
à la king 'Cook-In-Pouch'	4 oz	70	6.0	1.0
à la king, w/rice 'Single Serve'	9 oz	270	37.0	5.0
cacciatore 'Single Serve'	9 oz	270	33.0	6.0
croquettes, breaded, w/gravy 'Family Suppers'	7 oz	240	20.0	12.0
nuggets 'Deluxe Family Suppers'	3 oz	270	15.0	17.0
nuggets platter	6 oz	410	36.0	23.0
pattie 'Platter'	7.5 oz	360	33.0	17.0
primavera, sliced, w/gravy 'Cook-In-Pouch'	5 oz	80	6.0	3.0
sweet and sour, w/rice 'Single Serve'	9 oz	300	48.0	4.0
(Green Giant) and broccoli 'Entrées'	9.5 oz	340	28.0	15.0
(Healthy Choice)				
à l'orange	9 oz	260	38.0	2.0
and pasta divan	11.5 oz	300	41.0	4.0
and vegetables	11.5 oz	210	31.0	1.0
breast, glazed	8.5 oz	220	27.0	3.0
cacciatore 'Classics'	12.5 oz	310	47.0	3.0
chow mein	9 oz	240	29.0	5.0
chow mein, low fat, low cholesterol	9 oz	240	29.0	5.0
Dijon	11 oz	260	38.0	3.0
herb roasted	11 oz	380	56.0	7.0
honey mustard, low fat, low cholesterol	9.5 oz	250	37.0	3.0
Mandarin	10 oz	240	35.0	2.0
mesquite	10.5 oz	300	54.0	3.0
Oriental	11.25 oz	200	32.0	1.0
parmigiana	11.5 oz	290	41.0	6.0
roasted	12.3 oz	290	39.0	4.0
'Salsa Chicken Dinner'	11.25 oz	240	36.0	2.0
southwestern style, low fat, low cholesterol	12.5 oz	340	51.0	5.0
stir fry, w/vermicelli 'Extra Portion'	12 oz	300	42.0	5.0
sweet and sour	11.5 oz	280	52.0	2.0
teriyaki, low fat, low cholesterol	12.25 oz	290	39.0	4.0
w/barbecue sauce, low fat, low cholesterol	12.75 oz	410	65.0	6.0

Food Name	Serv. Size	Total Cal.	Carbs GMS	Fat GMS
(Hot Bites)				
drumsnackers	2.63 oz	220	13.0	15.0
nuggets	2.63 oz	210	11.0	14.0
nuggets, hot'n spicy	2.63 oz	250	10.0	19.0
nuggets, Southern fried	2.63 oz	220	13.0	14.0
nuggets, w/cheddar	2.63 oz	250	11.0	18.0
primavera sticks	2.63 oz	220	11.0	15.0
tenders, breast	2.25 oz	150	12.0	6.0
tenders, breast 'Microwave'	4 oz	260	24.0	10.0
(Kid Cuisine)				
fried	7.25 oz	420	41.0	22.0
fried 'Mega Meal'	10.8 oz	720	53.0	41.0
nuggets	6.25 oz	400	46.0	19.0
nuggets 'Mega Meal'	8.4 oz	470	51.0	20.0
(LaChoy)				
almond, w/rice and vegetables 'Fresh & Lite'	9.75 oz	270	40.1	8.0
imperial, w/rice 'Fresh & Lite'	11 oz	260	45.0	6.0
Oriental, spicy 'Fresh & Lite'	9.75 oz	270	52.0	4.0
sweet and sour, w/rice and vegetables 'Fresh & Lite'	10 oz	260	50.1	3.0
(LeMenu)				
à la king	10.25 oz	330	29.0	13.0
à la king, w/seasoned rice 'LightStyle'	8.25 oz	240	29.0	5.0
breast, glazed 'LightStyle'	10 oz	230	25.0	3.0
breast, herb roasted, w/rice and vegetables	7.75 oz	260	29.0	6.0
cordon bleu	11 oz	460	47.0	20.0
Dijon, w/pasta and vegetables 'LightStyle'	8.5 oz	240	21.0	7.0
empress, w/seasoned rice 'LightStyle'	8.25 oz	210	26.0	5.0
herb-roasted 'LightStyle'	10 oz	240	18.0	7.0
in wine sauce	10 oz	280	27.0	7.0
Kiev	8 oz	530	24.0	39.0
parmigiana	11.75 oz	410	31.0	20.0
sweet and sour	11.25 oz	400	41.0	18.0
sweet and sour 'LightStyle'	10 oz	250	29.0	7.0
(Mrs. Paterson's) 'Aussie Pie'	5.5 oz	440	43.0	24.0
(Myers)				
à la gratin	3.5 oz	129	9.0	7.0
à la king	3.5 oz	137	6.0	9.0
and noodles	3.5 oz	136	9.0	8.0
creamed	3.5 oz	151	5.0	10.0
croquettes	3.5 oz	168	10.0	7.0
pie	3.5 oz	129	10.0	7.0
(Pilgrim's Pride) Cajun style	3 oz	241	8.6	17.0

Food Name	Serv. Size	Total Cal.	Carbs GMS	Fat GMS
(Pillsbury)				
and cheese casserole 'Microwave Classic'	1 pkg	480	33.0	29.0
casserole 'Microwave Classic'	1 pkg	400	30.0	22.0
(Right Course)				
Italiano, w/fettuccini and vegetables	9 5/8 oz	280	29.0	8.0
sesame primavera	10 oz	320	34.0	9.0
tenderloins in barbecue sauce	8.75 oz	270	35.0	6.0
tenderloins in peanut sauce	9.25 oz	330	32.0	10.0
(Shanghai) stir fry	10.3 oz	190	19.0	3.0
(Smart Ones)				
a l'orange	8 oz	190	34.0	<1.0
chow mein	9 oz	170	27.0	1.0
fiesta, w/Spanish rice	8 oz	210	37.0	1.0
Francais, w/garlic vegetables	8.5 oz	150	18.0	1.0
grilled, glazed, and sauce	8 oz	130	17.0	1.0
honey mustard, and sauce	7.5 oz	140	20.0	1.0
Mirabella	9.2 oz	160	26.0	1.0
piccata, lemon herb	7.5 oz	160	25.0	1.0
(Stouffer's)				
à la king, w/rice	9.5 oz	270	38.0	5.0
a l'orange, w/almond rice, 'Lean Cuisine'	8 oz	280	33.0	4.0
and noodles, homestyle	10 oz	290	21.0	13.0
and vegetables, w/vermicelli 'Lean Cuisine'	11.75 oz	240	30.0	5.0
breaded, baked, w/parsleyed potatoes and vegetables, 'Lean Cuisine'	8 oz	200	21.0	5.0
breast, baked, in gravy, w/potato, homestyle	8 7/8 oz	250	18.0	10.0
breast, fried, and whipped potatoes, homestyle	7 1/8 oz	350	30.0	18.0
breast, grilled, in barbecue sauce, homestyle	7 5/8 oz	210	14.0	7.0
breast, Marsala, w/vegetables, 'Lean Cuisine'	8 1/8 oz	180	13.0	4.0
breast, Parmesan, w/rib meat, 'Lean Cuisine'	10 7/8 oz	260	25.0	7.0
cacciatore, w/vermicelli, 'Lean Cuisine'	10 7/8 oz	280	31.0	7.0
chow mein, w/rice	10.75 oz	250	39.0	5.0
chow mein, w/rice, 'Lean Cuisine'	9 oz	240	34.0	5.0
creamed	6.5 oz	300	8.0	21.0
divan	8 oz	220	11.0	10.0
escalloped, and noodles	10 oz	420	30.0	24.0
fettuccini, 'Lean Cuisine'	9 oz	280	33.0	6.0
fettuccini, w/vegetable medley, homestyle	9.5 oz	350	27.0	17.0
fiesta, 'Lean Cuisine'	8.5 oz	240	30.0	5.0
glazed, w/vegetable rice, 'Lean Cuisine'	8.5 oz	250	24.0	7.0
honey mustard, 'Lean Cuisine'	7.5 oz	230	30.0	4.0
in barbecue sauce, w/rice pilaf, 'Lean Cuisine'	8.75 oz	260	32.0	6.0
Italiano, w/fettuccini 'Lean Cuisine'	9 oz	270	33.0	6.0

Food Name	Serv. Size	Total Cal.	Carbs GMS	Fat GMS
Oriental, w/vermicelli, 'Lean Cuisine'	9 oz	280	31.0	7.0
parmigiana and pasta Alfredo, homestyle	9 7/8 oz	360	24.0	15.0
pie	10 oz	440	32.0	27.0
sweet-n-sour, w/rice, 'Lean Cuisine'	9 oz	280	39.0	6.0
tenderloins in herb sauce, 'Lean Cuisine'	9.5 oz	240	19.0	5.0
tenderloins in peanut sauce, 'Lean Cuisine'	9 oz	290	33.0	7.0
tenders, breaded, w/potatoes, homestyle	8 3/8 oz	430	46.0	18.0
(Swanson)				
boneless 'Hungry Man'	17.75 oz	700	65.0	28.0
cacciatore 'Homestyle Recipe'	10.95 oz	260	33.0	8.0
fried, barbecue flavored	10 oz	540	61.0	22.0
fried, dark meat	9.75 oz	560	55.0	28.0
fried, dark meat 'Hungry Man'	1 pkg	860	77.0	45.0
fried, white meat	10.25 oz	550	60.0	25.0
fried, white meat 'Hungry Man'	1 pkg	870	80.0	46.0
grilled, white meat in garlic sauce, almonds	10 oz	310	39.0	9.0
nibbles 'Homestyle Recipe'	4.25 oz	340	29.0	20.0
nibbles 'Plump & Juicy'	3.25 oz	300	19.0	19.0
nuggets	8.75 oz	470	47.0	23.0
nuggets 'Plump & Juicy'	3 oz	230	14.0	14.0
parmigiana 'Budget'	10 oz	300	35.0	15.0
pie 'Homestyle Recipe'	8 oz	410	41.0	21.0
pie 'Hungry Man'	16 oz	630	57.0	35.0
thighs/drumsticks 'Plump & Juicy'	3.25 oz	290	17.0	18.0
(Swift)				
cordon bleu 'International'	6 oz	360	23.0	17.0
Kiev 'International'	6 oz	420	22.0	24.0
(Tyson)				
a l'orange 'Gourmet Selection'	9.5 oz	300	36.0	8.0
and beef luau 'Gourmet Selection'	10.5 oz	330	42.0	10.0
'Barbecue Chicken Meal'	12.5 oz	400	56.0	8.0
breast, boneless, barbecue marinated	3.75 oz	120	5.0	3.0
breast, boneless, butter garlic marinated	3.75 oz	160	3.0	7.0
breast, boneless, Italian marinated	3.75 oz	130	6.0	2.0
breast, boneless, lemon pepper marinated	3.75 oz	120	4.0	2.0
breast, boneless, teriyaki marinated	3.75 oz	130	6.0	2.0
breast strips, Oriental, boneless	2.75 oz	110	6.0	3.0
'Chick'n Cheddar' *(Tyson)*	2.6 oz	220	11.0	15.0
'Chick'n Chunks'	2.6 oz	220	11.0	15.0
'Chick'n Chunks' Southern fried	2.6 oz	220	11.0	15.0
'Chicken Marinara Meal'	13.75 oz	340	37.0	7.0
'Classic Colonial' wholesale club item	3.5 oz	180	11.0	9.0
'Cordon Bleu' wholesale club item	7 oz	480	28.0	22.0

Food Name	Serv. Size	Total Cal.	Carbs GMS	Fat GMS
'Cordon Bleu' wholesale club item	5 oz	340	20.0	16.0
Dijon 'Gourmet Selection'	8.5 oz	310	22.0	17.0
Français 'Gourmet Selection'	9.5 oz	280	20.0	14.0
glazed, w/sauce 'Gourmet Selections'	9.25 oz	240	29.0	4.0
grilled, 'Gourmet Selections'	7.75 oz	220	22.0	3.0
grilled, Italian 'Gourmet Selections'	9 oz	210	19.0	3.0
'Herb Chicken Meal'	13.75 oz	340	43.0	4.0
'Honey Mustard Chicken Meal'	13.75 oz	390	52.0	6.0
honey roasted 'Gourmet Selections'	9 oz	220	23.0	4.0
'Italian Style Chicken Meal'	13.75 oz	310	38.0	4.0
Kiev 'Gourmet Selection'	9.25 oz	520	40.0	33.0
'Looney Tunes Bugs Bunny' chunks	7.7 oz	290	31.0	11.0
'Looney Tunes Road Runner'	6.7 oz	300	42.0	11.0
'Looney Tunes Tazmanian Devil' drummettes	8 oz	310	31.0	14.0
'Looney Tunes Yosemite Sam' barbecue glazed	7.38 oz	230	28.0	8.0
Marsala 'Gourmet Selection'	10.5 oz	300	26.0	13.0
mesquite breast tenders, boneless	2.75 oz	110	4.0	3.0
'Mesquite Chicken Meal'	13.25 oz	330	38.0	5.0
mesquite 'Gourmet Selections'	9 oz	320	39.0	8.0
'Mini Cordon Bleu' wholesale club item	1 piece	90	5.0	4.0
nuggets 'Microwave'	3.5 oz	220	11.0	15.0
Oriental 'Gourmet Selection'	10.25 oz	270	32.0	7.0
parmigiana 'Gourmet Selection'	11.25 oz	380	37.0	17.0
piccata 'Gourmet Selection'	9 oz	240	19.0	10.0
pie, premium	9 oz	390	36.0	20.0
pie, white meat, premium	9 oz	400	33.0	20.0
roasted 'Gourmet Selections'	9 oz	200	21.0	2.0
'Salsa Chicken Meal'	13.75 oz	370	52.0	6.0
'Sesame Chicken Meal'	13.5 oz	400	59.0	6.0
sesame 'Healthy Portions'	13.5 oz	390	58.0	5.0
stir fry w/vegetables, wholesale club item	3.5 oz	130	13.0	5.0
supreme 'Gourmet Selections'	9 oz	230	23.0	6.0
sweet and sour 'Gourmet Selection'	11 oz	420	50.0	15.0
tenders 'Microwave'	3.5 oz	230	19.0	11.0
'Wings of Fire' wholesale club item	3.5 oz	220	2.0	12.0
(Ultimate 200)				
barbecue, glazed, w/vegetables	7 oz	200	22.0	6.0
cordon bleu, w/vegetables	7.7 oz	170	15.0	5.0
grilled, glazed	7.5 oz	150	17.0	2.0
imperial	8.5 oz	200	25.0	3.0
Kiev, w/vegetables and rice	7 oz	190	22.0	5.0
patty, Southern baked, w/vegetables	6.3 oz	170	10.0	7.0
teriyaki	7.6 oz	150	7.0	4.0

Food Name	Serv. Size	Total Cal.	Carbs GMS	Fat GMS
(Weaver)				
batter-dipped, assorted pieces	3.6 oz	290	16.0	18.0
crispy, light, skinless	2.9 oz	170	9.0	9.0
'Crispy Dutch Frye' assorted pieces	3.6 oz	290	16.0	18.0
'Crispy Dutch Frye' breast	4.5 oz	350	17.0	22.0
crispy mini drums	3 oz	210	13.0	12.0
croquettes	2 pieces	280	22.0	16.0
mini drums, herb and spice	3 oz	200	13.0	11.0
'Rondolet, Cheese'	2.6 oz	190	12.0	11.0
'Rondolet, Italian'	2.6 oz	190	11.0	11.0
'Rondolet, Original'	3 oz	190	13.0	10.0
'Tenders, Honey Batter'	3 oz	220	14.0	12.0
'Tenders, Premium'	3 oz	170	11.0	9.0
(Weight Watchers)				
fettuccini, w/Parmesan sauce	8.25 oz	280	25.0	9.0
ginger, w/vegetable, Hunan 'Stir Fry'	9 oz	160	21.0	2.0
grilled, Suiza, w/Spanish rice 'Mexican Style'	8.6 oz	220	18.0	7.0
orange glazed, w/rice 'Stir Fry'	9 oz	170	25.0	2.0
Polynesian 'Stir Fry'	9 oz	190	34.0	1.0
sesame, w/lo mein noodles 'Stir Fry'	9 oz	200	23.0	4.0
teriyaki, w/spring vegetables 'Stir Fry'	9 oz	140	16.0	3.0
'Tex Mex' w/Spanish rice 'Mexican Style'	8.3 oz	250	33.0	5.0
CHICKEN DINNER/ENTRÉE, PACKAGED				
(Chicken By George)				
Cajun	5 oz	180	4.0	8.0
Caribbean grill	5 oz	200	10.0	6.0
Italian blue cheese	5 oz	180	2.0	8.0
lemon herb	5 oz	170	6.0	6.0
lemon oregano	5 oz	160	4.0	4.0
mesquite barbecue	5 oz	170	6.0	6.0
mustard dill	5 oz	180	3.0	7.0
roasted	5 oz	150	2.0	4.0
teriyaki	5 oz	180	9.0	5.0
tomato herb, w/basil	5 oz	190	7.0	7.0
(Chicken Helper) 'Skillet Dinner'				
cheesy broccoli, dry	1/5 pkg	160	32.0	2.0
cheesy broccoli, prepared	7 oz	310	34.0	9.0
creamy chicken, dry	1/5 pkg	170	26.0	5.0
creamy chicken, prepared	8.25 oz	330	29.0	13.0
creamy mushroom, dry	1/5 pkg	170	28.0	4.0
creamy mushroom, prepared	8 oz	320	31.0	11.0
fettuccini Alfredo, dry	1/5 pkg	160	25.0	4.0
fettuccini Alfredo, prepared	7.5 oz	320	27.0	12.0

Food Name	Serv. Size	Total Cal.	Carbs GMS	Fat GMS
stir fry, dry	1/5 pkg	170	36.0	<1.0
stir fry, prepared	7 oz	370	36.0	14.0
(Dinty Moore) and dumplings, microwave cup	7.5 oz	190	20.0	6.0
(LaChoy)				
sweet and sour, 'Dinner Classics' prepared	3/4 cup	310	30.0	6.0
sweet and sour, w/noodles	9.383 oz	256	49.4	3.1
(Libby's)				
chow mein 'Diner' microwave cup	7.75 oz	130	19.0	4.0
w/pasta spirals 'Diner' microwave cup	7.75 oz	120	16.0	3.0
(Lipton) 'Microeasy'				
barbecue style, dry	1/4 pkg	110	24.0	<1.0
barbecue style, prepared	1/4 pkg	220	24.0	6.0
country style, dry	1/4 pkg	80	15.0	<1.0
country style, prepared	1/4 pkg	190	15.0	6.0
(Lunch Bucket)				
and dumplings, microwave cup	7.5 oz	140	25.0	2.0
w/beans and rice 'Light'n Healthy' micro cup	7.5 oz	170	28.0	3.0
(Top Shelf)				
à la king	10 oz	360	49.0	10.0
Acapulco	1 serving	390	41.0	13.0
breast, glazed	10 oz	170	19.0	2.0
breast, w/Spanish rice	10 oz	400	38.0	15.0
'Cacciatore'	10 oz	210	25.0	3.0
sweet and sour	1 serving	270	41.0	1.0
(Ultra Slim Fast)				
and vegetables	12 oz	290	45.0	3.0
chow mein	12 oz	320	43.0	6.0
fettuccini	12 oz	390	38.0	12.0
mesquite	12 oz	350	61.0	1.0
roasted, in mushroom sauce	12 oz	280	30.0	6.0
sweet and sour	12 oz	330	57.0	2.0
CHICKEN ENTRÉE, ALTERNATIVE				
(Worthington) pie, frozen	8 oz	380	43.0	20.0
CHICKEN FAT				
	1 cup	1846	0.0	204.6
	1 oz	178	0.0	19.3
	1 tbsp	115	0.0	12.8
CHICKEN FRYING MIX, dry mix (Golden Dipt)	1 oz	90	20.0	0.0
CHICKEN GIBLETS				
fried	1 cup	402	6.3	19.5
simmered	1 cup	228	1.4	6.9
CHICKEN GIZZARD				
all classes, simmered	1 cup	222	1.6	5.3

Food Name	Serv. Size	Total Cal.	Carbs GMS	Fat GMS
broiler-fryer, raw, approx 1.3 oz	1 med	44	0.2	1.6
broiler-fryer, simmered, approx .8 oz	1 med	34	0.3	0.8
CHICKEN HEART				
all classes, simmered	1 cup	268	0.2	11.5
broiler-fryer, raw, 1 heart	2 oz	9	<.1	0.6
broiler-fryer, simmered	4 oz	210	0.1	9.0
CHICKEN LIVER				
all classes, simmered	1 cup	220	1.2	7.6
broiler-fryer, chopped, simmered	1 cup	219	1.2	7.6
broiler-fryer, raw, approx 1.1 oz	1 liver	40	1.1	1.2
broiler-fryer, simmered	4 oz	178	1.0	6.2
CHICKEN POT PIE (Swanson), frozen	7 oz	380	35.0	22.0
CHICKEN SALAD				
(Longacre)	1 oz	64	3.0	5.0
(Longacre) 'Saladfest'	1 oz	47	1.0	3.0
CHICKEN SALAD SPREAD, 'Spreadables' (Libby's)	1.9 oz	90	5.0	6.0
CHICKEN SEASONING MIX				
(Featherweight) dry mix	1/4 pkg	18	8.0	0.0
(Schilling) 'Bag 'n Season'	1 pkg	134	19.0	5.0
(Schilling) dry mix, for fried chicken	1/4 tsp	1	0.2	<.1
CHICKEN SPREAD, CANNED				
(Hormel)	.5 oz	30	0.0	2.0
(Underwood) chunky	2 1/8 oz	150	2.0	9.0
(Underwood) 'Light'	2 1/8 oz	80	2.0	3.0
(Underwood) smoky	2 1/8 oz	150	10.0	8.0
CHICKEN STEW				
(Dinty Moore) canned	7.5 oz	260	15.0	18.0
(Dinty Moore) microwave cup	7.5 oz	260	15.0	18.0
(Featherweight) w/wild rice, canned	7.5 oz	140	23.0	1.0
(Heinz) w/dumplings, canned	7.5 oz	210	22.0	9.0
(Mountain House) freeze-dried, prepared	1 cup	230	30.0	8.0
(Swanson) canned	7 5/8 oz	160	15.0	7.0
CHICORY, WITLOOF				
raw	1/2 cup	8	1.8	0.0
raw, approx 2.1 oz	1 head	9	2.1	0.1
trimmed	1 oz	4	0.9	<.1
untrimmed	1 lb	61	12.9	0.4
CHICORY GREENS				
trimmed	1 oz	7	1.3	0.1
trimmed, chopped	1/2 cup	21	4.2	0.3
untrimmed	1 lb	87	17.5	1.1
CHICORY ROOT				
raw, approx 2.6 oz	1 root	44	10.5	0.1

Food Name	Serv. Size	Total Cal.	Carbs GMS	Fat GMS
raw, 1-inch pieces	1/2 cup	33	7.9	0.1
trimmed	1 oz	21	5.0	0.1
untrimmed	1 lb	272	65.1	0.7
CHILI, CANNED				
beef, w/beans (Cimmaron)	7.5 oz	230	21.0	9.0
chicken, w/beans (Cimmaron)	7.5 oz	180	22.0	5.0
chicken, w/beans (Stagg)	7.5 oz	200	21.0	6.0
'Chili Con Carne' (Heinz)	7.75 oz	350	27.0	21.0
'Chili Mac' (Chef Boyardee)	7.5 oz	230	26.0	11.0
'Chili Mac' (Heinz)	7.5 oz	250	26.0	12.0
country, w/beans (Stagg)	7.5 oz	270	25.0	12.0
plain (Gebhardt)	1 cup	530	20.0	41.0
vegetarian (Gebhardt)	4 oz	219	6.9	17.1
vegetarian (Worthington)	2/3 cup	190	15.0	10.0
vegetarian, plain (Gebhardt)	4.339 oz	232	11.1	18.5
vegetarian, plain (Open Range)	4.409 oz	176	9.4	12.8
vegetarian, spicy (Hain)	7.5 oz	160	29.0	1.0
vegetarian, spicy (Hain) 'Reduced Sodium'	7.5 oz	170	31.0	1.0
vegetarian, spicy (Natural Touch)	2/3 cup	230	19.0	12.0
vegetarian, 3-bean, mild, fat-free (Health Valley)	5 oz	90	12.0	0.0
vegetarian, w/beans (Gebhardt)	4.444 oz	195	18.3	12.0
vegetarian, w/beans (Just Rite)	4.55 oz	190	15.3	13.3
vegetarian, w/beans (Open Range)	4.5 oz	136	12.6	8.0
vegetarian, w/beans, 'Longhorn' (Gebhardt)	4.55 oz	225	16.0	15.7
vegetarian, w/beans, mild (Health Valley)	4 oz	130	16.0	3.0
vegetarian, w/beans, mild (Health Valley) 'No Salt Added'	4 oz	130	16.0	3.0
vegetarian, w/beans, spicy (Health Valley)	4 oz	130	16.0	3.0
vegetarian, w/beans, spicy (Health Valley) 'No Salt Added'	4 oz	130	16.0	3.0
vegetarian, w/black beans, mild, fat-free (Health Valley)	5 oz	140	23.0	0.0
vegetarian, w/black beans, spicy, fat-free (Health Valley)	5 oz	70	9.0	0.0
vegetarian, w/lentils, mild (Health Valley)	4 oz	130	16.0	3.0
vegetarian, w/lentils, mild (Health Valley) 'No Salt Added'	4 oz	130	16.0	3.0
vegetarian, w/tempeh, spicy (Hain)	7.5 oz	160	24.0	4.0
w/beans	1/2 cup	143	15.2	7.0
w/beans (Armour)	6 oz	320	21.0	22.0
w/beans (Armour)	7.5 oz	390	27.0	26.0
w/beans (Estee)	7.5 oz	370	27.0	20.0
w/beans (Featherweight)	7.5 oz	280	29.0	10.0
w/beans (Gebhardt)	1 cup	495	47.0	28.0
w/beans (Just Rite)	4 oz	200	16.0	11.0
w/beans (Nalley's)	7.5 oz	260	27.0	9.0
w/beans (Van Camp's)	1 cup	352	20.9	23.2
w/beans (Wolf Brand)	8 oz	345	21.8	22.0

Food Name	Serv. Size	Total Cal.	Carbs GMS	Fat GMS
w/beans '15-oz' (Dennison's)	7.5 oz	310	27.0	15.0
w/beans '15-oz' (Hormel)	7.5 oz	310	23.0	17.0
w/beans '15-oz' (Libby's)	7.5 oz	270	25.0	13.0
w/beans, 9.2 oz (Quincy's)	1 serving	346	32.0	16.0
w/beans '24-oz' (Libby's)	8 oz	290	27.0	14.0
w/beans '25-oz' (Hormel)	8 1/3 oz	350	26.0	20.0
w/beans '30-oz' (Dennison's)	7.5 oz	310	28.0	15.0
w/beans '40-oz' (Dennison's)	8 oz	340	29.0	17.0
w/beans '40-oz' (Hormel)	8 oz	320	25.0	17.0
w/beans, beef (Chef Boyardee)	7.5 oz	330	30.0	17.0
w/beans, chunky (Dennison's)	7.5 oz	310	28.0	14.0
w/beans, chunky (Hormel)	7.5 oz	290	25.0	14.0
w/beans 'Cook-Off' (Dennison's)	7.5 oz	340	25.0	19.0
w/beans, extra spicy (Wolf Brand)	7.75 oz	324	20.6	20.6
w/beans, hot (Armour)	7.5 oz	390	27.0	26.0
w/beans, hot (Gebhardt)	1 cup	470	47.0	27.0
w/beans, hot (Gebhardt)	4 oz	189	9.2	14.2
w/beans, hot (Heinz)	7.75 oz	330	30.0	16.0
w/beans, hot (Just Rite)	4 oz	195	16.0	10.0
w/beans, hot (Nalley's)	7.5 oz	280	30.0	10.0
w/beans, hot '15 oz' (Hormel)	7.5 oz	310	24.0	16.0
w/beans, hot '15 oz' (Dennison's)	7.5 oz	310	26.0	16.0
w/beans, hot '40 oz' (Dennison's)	8 oz	350	29.0	19.0
w/beans, hot, jalapeño (Nalley's)	7.5 oz	260	29.0	10.0
w/beans 'Laredo' (Stagg)	7.5 oz	260	22.0	12.0
w/beans 'Micro-Cup' (Hormel)	7.5 oz	250	23.0	11.0
w/beans 'Premium Lite' (Armour)	7.5 oz	260	27.0	10.0
w/beans 'Thick' (Nalley's)	7.5 oz	260	29.0	9.0
w/chicken, spicy (Hain)	7.5 oz	130	19.0	2.0
w/o beans (Armour)	7.5 oz	390	14.0	31.0
w/o beans (Hormel)	10.5 oz	540	19.0	41.0
w/o beans (Just Rite)	4 oz	180	9.0	11.0
w/o beans (Libby's)	7.5 oz	390	11.0	30.0
w/o beans (Van Camp's)	1 cup	412	12.1	33.5
w/o beans (Wolf Brand)	8 oz	387	16.2	26.6
w/o beans 'Big Chunk' (Nalley's)	7.5 oz	270	14.0	16.0
w/o beans 'Chili-Mac' (Wolf Brand)	7.75 oz	317	22.9	19.9
w/o beans '15 oz' (Dennison's)	7.5 oz	300	15.0	19.0
w/o beans '15 oz' (Hormel)	7.5 oz	370	12.0	28.0
w/o beans, 15 oz (Libby's)	7.5 oz	390	11.0	30.0
w/o beans '19 oz' (Dennison's)	9.5 oz	380	18.0	24.0
w/o beans 'Steak House' (Stagg)	7.5 oz	300	17.0	19.0
w/o beans '25 oz' (Hormel)	8 1/3 oz	430	13.0	33.0

Food Name	Serv. Size	Total Cal.	Carbs GMS	Fat GMS
w/o beans, extra spicy *(Wolf Brand)*	7.5 oz	363	15.3	24.9
w/o beans, hot '15 oz' *(Hormel)*	7.5 oz	370	12.0	28.0
w/o beans, w/franks 'Chilee Weenee' *(Van Camp's)*	1 cup	309	27.6	15.7
CHILI, FREEZE-DRIED				
w/beans, prepared *(Mountain House)*	1 cup	390	38.0	16.0
w/beef 'Chili Mac' prepared *(Mountain House)*	1 cup	250	31.0	8.0
CHILI, FROZEN				
con carne 'Homestyle Recipe' *(Swanson)*	8.25 oz	270	26.0	10.0
con carne, w/beans *(Stouffer's)*	8.75 oz	260	24.0	10.0
vegetarian *(Right Course)*	9.75 oz	280	45.0	7.0
CHILI, MICROWAVE				
'Chili Mac' micro cup *(Hormel)*	7.5 oz	192	18.0	9.0
w/beans *(Armour)*	7.5 oz	300	26.0	14.0
w/beans, 'Diner' microwave cup *(Libby's)*	7.75 oz	280	29.0	12.0
w/beans, hot, micro cup *(Hormel)*	7.38 oz	250	24.0	11.0
w/beans, microwave cup *(Lunch Bucket)*	7.5 oz	300	26.0	14.0
w/o beans, micro cup *(Hormel)*	7.38 oz	290	15.0	17.0
CHILI BEAN, CANNED. See also KIDNEY BEAN, CANNED; PINTO BEAN.				
(Gebhardt)	4.586 oz	134	30.7	1.0
(Hunt's)	4 oz	102	18.1	0.0
(Hunt's)	4.48 oz	87	17.1	1.0
(S&W)	1/2 cup	130	23.0	1.0
baked style, hot *(Campbell's)*	7.75 oz	180	38.0	4.0
caliente style *(Green Giant)*	1/2 cup	100	20.0	1.0
caliente style *(Joan of Arc)*	1/2 cup	100	20.0	1.0
extra spicy *(Green Giant)*	1/2 cup	100	21.0	1.0
extra spicy *(Joan of Arc)*	1/2 cup	100	21.0	1.0
50% less salt *(Green Giant)*	1/2 cup	100	21.0	1.0
50% less salt *(Joan of Arc)*	1/2 cup	100	21.0	1.0
hot *(A&P)*	1/2 cup	140	24.0	1.0
hot *(Allens)*	1/2 cup	90	17.0	<1.0
hot *(Bush's Best)*	1/2 cup	70	20.0	0.0
in chili gravy *(Dennison's)*	7.5 oz	180	30.0	1.0
in sauce *(Hormel)*	5 oz	130	19.0	3.0
Mexican style *(Allens)*	1/2 cup	135	24.0	<1.0
Mexican style *(Van Camp's)*	1 cup	210	39.0	2.4
spiced *(Gebhardt)*	4 oz	113	19.7	1.1
spicy 'Dry Beans in Sauce' *(Green Giant)*	1/2 cup	100	21.0	1.0
spicy 'Dry Beans in Sauce' *(Joan of Arc)*	1/2 cup	100	21.0	1.0
CHILI MIX				
'Chili Quick' dry *(Gebhardt)*	1.5-oz pkt	82	16.8	1.1
'Chili con Carne' prepared *(Old El Paso)*	1 cup	162	8.0	7.0
'Homestyle Chili Fixins' *(Hunt's)*	4.656 oz	84	18.5	1.2

Food Name	Serv. Size	Total Cal.	Carbs GMS	Fat GMS
vegetarian, w/beans, prepared *(Fantastic Foods)*	1/2 cup	104	19.0	0.8
w/beans, prepared *(Old El Paso)*	1 cup	217	17.0	10.0
CHILI POWDER				
(Durkee)	1 tsp	11	0.0	0.01
(Laurel Leaf)	1 tsp	11	0.0	0.01
CHILI SAUCE. See SAUCE.				
CHILI SEASONING				
(Gebhardt)	1 tsp	6	1.0	0.0
(Gebhardt)	.0106 oz	1	0.1	0.0
(Gebhardt) mix 'Chili Quick'	1 tsp	10	2.0	<1.0
(Hain) hot	1/4 pkg	30	5.0	1.0
(Hain) medium	1/4 pkg	30	5.0	1.0
(Hain) mild	1/2 pkg	30	5.0	1.0
(Lawry's) 'Seasoning Blends'	1 pkg	143	26.6	1.8
(Old El Paso)	1/5 pkg	21	4.0	1.0
(Schilling)	1/4 pkg	27	4.5	0.5
(Tio Sancho)	1.23 oz	109	6.0	2.2
CHIMICHANGA				
beef 'Primera' *(Marquez)*	1 chimichanga	380	42.0	17.0
CHIMICHANGA DINNER, FROZEN				
bean and cheese *(Old El Paso)*	1 pkg	380	40.0	19.0
beef *(Old El Paso)*	1 piece	370	34.0	21.0
beef and cheese 'Festive Dinners' *(Old El Paso)*	11 oz	510	53.0	23.0
beef and pork *(Old El Paso)*	1 pkg	340	35.0	16.0
beef 'Festive Dinners' *(Old El Paso)*	11 oz	540	65.0	21.0
chicken *(Old El Paso)*	1 piece	360	33.0	20.0
CHINESE APPLE. See POMEGRANATE.				
CHINESE CABBAGE. See CABBAGE, NAPA.				
CHINESE DATE				
dried	1 oz	81	20.1	0.3
raw, seeded	1 oz	22	5.7	0.1
raw, w/seeds	1 lb	331	85.3	0.8
CHINESE FUNGUS/Jew's ear				
approx .2 oz	1 piece	2	0.4	(tr)
sliced	1/2 cup	13	3.3	(tr)
trimmed	1 oz	7	1.9	na
untrimmed	1 lb	111	30.0	0.2
CHINESE GOOSEBERRY. See KIWI FRUIT.				
CHINESE NOODLE. See NOODLE, CHINESE.				
CHINESE PARSLEY. See CORIANDER.				
CHINESE PARSLEY LEAF. See CORIANDER LEAF.				
CHINESE PARSLEY SEED. See CORIANDER SEED.				

Food Name	Serv. Size	Total Cal.	Carbs GMS	Fat GMS
CHINESE RADISH				
boiled, drained	4 oz	19	3.9	0.3
boiled, drained, sliced	1/2 cup	13	2.5	0.2
dried	1/2 cup	157	36.8	0.4
dried	1 oz	77	18.0	0.2
raw, 7 inches long, 2 1/4 inches diam, approx 15.1 oz	1 med	62	13.9	0.3
raw, trimmed	1 oz	5	1.2	<.1
raw, trimmed (Frieda's)	1 lb	86	19.1	0.5
raw, trimmed (Frieda's)	1 oz	5	1.2	<.1
raw, trimmed, sliced	1/2 cup	8	1.8	<.1
raw, untrimmed	1 lb	65	14.7	0.4
CHINESE WATERMELON				
boiled, drained	4 oz	15	3.4	0.2
boiled, drained, cubes	1/2 cup	11	2.6	0.2
raw, cubes	1 cup	17	4.0	0.3
raw, trimmed	1 oz	4	0.9	0.1
raw, untrimmed	1 lb	42	9.7	0.6
CHINESE YAM. See JICAMA.				
CHIVES				
	1 oz	7	1.1	0.2
freeze-dried	1 tbsp	1	0.1	0.0
freeze-dried	1/4 cup	2	0.5	0.0
raw, chopped	1 tbsp	1	0.1	0.0
raw, chopped	1 tsp	0	0.0	0.0
CHOCOLATE, BAKING				
Bar				
semi-sweet (Baker's)	1 oz	140	17.0	9.0
semi-sweet (Nestlé)	1 oz	160	16.0	9.0
semi-sweet 'Premium' (Hershey's)	1 oz	140	16.0	8.0
sweet 'German' (Baker's)	1 oz	140	17.0	10.0
unsweetened (Baker's)	1 oz	140	9.0	15.0
unsweetened (Hershey's)	1 oz	190	7.0	16.0
unsweetened (Nestlé)	1 oz	180	9.0	14.0
unsweetened 'Premium' (Hershey's)	1 oz	190	7.0	16.0
white 'Premier' (Nestlé)	1 oz	150	18.0	9.0
Chips				
milk chocolate (Baker's)	1 oz	140	18.0	8.0
milk chocolate (Hershey's)	1/4 cup	220	27.0	12.0
milk chocolate (Hershey's)	1 oz	150	27.0	12.0
milk chocolate 'Big Chips' (Baker's)	1/4 cup	240	30.0	13.0
mint chocolate (Hershey's)	1.5 oz	230	28.0	12.0
semi-sweet (Baker's)	1/4 cup	200	30.0	9.0
semi-sweet 'Big Chips' (Baker's)	1/4 cup	220	31.0	13.0

Food Name	Serv. Size	Total Cal.	Carbs GMS	Fat GMS
semi-sweet, mini, approx 1/4 cup (Hershey's)	1.5 oz	220	26.0	12.0
semi-sweet, real chocolate (Baker's)	1/4 cup	200	28.0	11.0
semi-sweet, regular (Hershey's)	1.5 oz	220	27.0	12.0
vanilla 'White' milk (Hershey's)	1.5 oz	240	25.0	14.0
Chunks				
milk chocolate, 12 pieces (Hershey's)	1 oz	160	16.0	9.0
semi-sweet (Hershey's)	1 oz	140	15.0	8.0
white 'Premier Treasures' (Nestlé)	1 oz	160	15.0	10.0
Grated, bitter	1 cup	667	38.2	70.0
Powder				
cocoa, 100% (Nestlé)	1 oz	80	5.0	5.0
cocoa 'Premium' (Saco Foods)	1 tbsp	15	3.6	0.9
Premelted, unsweetened 'Choco Bake' (Nestlé)	1 oz	190	7.0	16.0
Squares				
unsweetened, grated	1 cup	689	37.4	73.0
unsweetened, 1 oz	1 square	148	8.0	15.7
CHOCOLATE FLAVOR DRINK. See also DIET DRINK.				
Canned				
(Frostee)	8 oz	200	30.0	8.0
Dutch 'Lite' (Sego)	10 oz	150	20.0	3.0
liquid food, nutritionally complete (Sustacal)	8 oz	240	33.0	5.5
liquid nutrition (Ensure)	8 oz	250	33.8	8.8
liquid nutrition 'Plus' (Ensure)	8 oz	355	46.8	12.6
liquid nutrition, w/fiber (Ensure)	8 oz	260	37.8	8.8
'Lite' (Sego)	10 oz	150	20.0	3.0
malt 'Very Chocolate' (Sego)	10 oz	225	43.0	1.0
'Very Chocolate' (Sego)	10 oz	225	43.0	1.0
Mix/powder				
approx 2-3 heaping tsp	.8 oz	75	19.5	0.7
approx 2-3 heaping tsp, prepared w/1 cup 1% milk	1 cup	177	31.2	3.3
approx 2-3 heaping tsp, prepared w/1 cup 2% milk	1 cup	196	31.2	5.4
approx 2-3 heaping tsp, prepared w/1 cup skim milk	1 cup	161	31.4	1.1
'Chocolate Milk Maker' (Swiss Miss)	.6702 oz	73	17.1	0.3
classic chocolate chip (Nestlé)	1.13 oz	90	12.0	2.0
classic chocolate chip, prepared (Nestlé)	8 oz	180	24.0	2.0
creamy milk chocolate (Nestlé)	1.13 oz	90	12.0	2.0
creamy milk chocolate, prepared (Nestlé)	8 oz	180	24.0	2.0
dairy, reduced calorie, w/aspartame	.75-oz pkt	63	10.7	0.6
'Hershey's Chocolate Milk Mix' (Hershey's)	3 heaping tsp	90	22.0	<1.0
protein powder, prepared w/lowfat milk (Turbo Nutrition)	8 oz	330	34.0	6.0
'Quik' (Nestlé)	1 heaping tsp	90	20.0	1.0
'Quik' prepared w/skim milk (Nestlé)	1 cup	170	31.0	1.0
'Quik' prepared w/2% milk (Nestlé)	1 cup	210	31.0	5.0

Food Name	Serv. Size	Total Cal.	Carbs GMS	Fat GMS
'Quik' prepared w/whole milk *(Nestlé)*	1 cup	230	31.0	9.0
'Quik' sugar-free, approx 1 heaping tsp *(Nestlé)*	.2 oz	18	3.0	<1.0
'Quik' sugar-free, prepared w/2% milk *(Nestlé)*	1 cup	140	15.0	5.0
weight gain protein powder, *(Turbo Nutrition)*	2 oz	210	22.0	1.0
Refrigerated				
'Hershey's Genuine' *(Hershey's)*	8 oz	150	28.0	2.0
(Yoo-Hoo)	9 oz	140	27.0	1.0
CHOCOLATE MILK				
whole	1 cup	208	25.8	8.5
whole	1 oz	26	3.2	1.1
whole *(Hershey's)*	1 cup	210	28.0	9.0
whole *(Nestlé Quik)*	1 cup	230	31.0	9.0
3.5% fat *(Hershey's)*	1 cup	210	28.0	8.0
2% fat	1 cup	179	26.0	5.0
2% fat *(Darigold)*	1 cup	190	28.0	5.0
2% fat *(Lucerne)*	1 cup	200	29.0	5.0
2% fat *(Hershey's)*	1 cup	190	29.0	5.0
2% fat 'Dutch Brand' *(Borden)*	1 cup	180	25.0	5.0
1% fat	1 cup	158	26.1	2.5
CHOCOLATE SAUCE. See SAUCE.				
CHOCOLATE SYRUP				
chocolate-flavored *(Hershey's)*	2 tbsp	103	23.9	.4
'Choco-Syp' *(Estee)*	1 tbsp	20	5.0	0.0
fudge-type	1 cup	1176	200.3	45.6
fudge type	1 oz	124	20.3	5.1
fudge-type	1 tbsp	73	12.4	2.8
'Quik' *(Nestlé)*	1.22 oz	100	22.0	1.0
unsweetened, 1 oz	1 pkt	134	9.6	13.5
w/added nutrients	1 cup	735	197.4	3.9
w/added nutrients	1 oz	92	24.7	0.5
w/added nutrients	1 tbsp	46	12.4	0.2
w/o added nutrients	1 cup	654	176.7	2.7
w/o added nutrients	1 oz	82	22.1	0.3
CHOCOLATE TOPPING				
(Kraft)	1 tbsp	50	11.0	0.0
(Mrs. Richardson's) dark chocolate fudge	2 tbsp	130	19.0	6.0
(Mrs. Richardson's) dark, fudge, microwavable	2 tbsp	130	19.0	6.0
(Nestlé) milk chocolate, w/almonds 'Candytops'	1.25 oz	230	14.0	18.0
(Nestlé) milk chocolate, w/crisps 'Crunch Candytops'	2 tbsp	220	16.0	17.0
(Nestlé) white chocolate, w/almonds 'Candytops'	1.25 oz	230	12.0	19.0
(Smucker's) chocolate fudge 'Magic Shell'	2 tbsp	190	16.0	15.0
(Smucker's) dark chocolate 'Special Recipe'	2 tbsp	130	31.0	1.0
(Smucker's) flavored syrup	2 tbsp	130	27.0	2.0

Food Name	Serv. Size	Total Cal.	Carbs GMS	Fat GMS
(Smucker's) 'Magic Shell'	2 tbsp	190	16.0	15.0
(Smucker's) milk chocolate fudge, Swiss	2 tbsp	140	31.0	1.0
(Smucker's) nut 'Magic Shell'	2 tbsp	200	25.0	16.0
CHORIZO				
	1 oz	129	0.5	10.9
4 inches	1 link	273	1.1	23.0
(Carmelita) beef	2.5 oz	250	5.0	23.0
(Carmelita) pork	2.5 oz	250	3.0	23.0
CHOW MEIN				
chicken, w/o noodles, can	1 cup	95	17.7	0.3
vegetarian, Mandarin, prepared w/tofu (Tofu Classics)	1/2 cup	110	14.0	6.0
CHOW MEIN NOODLE				
with almonds (Chun King)	1/3 cup	140	15.0	7.0
with sesame bits (Chun King)	1/3 cup	140	16.0	7.0
CHRYSANTHEMUM GARLAND				
boiled, drained	4 oz	23	4.9	0.1
boiled, drained, 1-inch pieces	1/2 cup	10	2.2	0.1
raw, 1 stem, 8.75 inches long	.5 oz	2	0.6	<.1
raw, 1-inch pieces	1 cup	4	1.1	0.0
raw, 8.75 inches long	1 stem	2	0.6	0.0
raw, trimmed	1 oz	5	1.2	<.1
raw, untrimmed	1 lb	76	19.0	0.8
CHUB/cisco				
raw	1 lb	446	0.0	8.7
raw	1 oz	28	0.0	0.5
smoked	1 oz	50	0.0	3.3
smoked	1 oz	50	0.0	3.3
CILANTRO				
approx .8 oz	9 plants	4	0.5	0.1
trimmed	1 oz	6	0.7	0.2
trimmed	1/4 cup	1	0.1	<.1
untrimmed	1 lb	77	10.0	2.3
CILANTRO LEAF				
dried	1 oz	79	14.8	1.3
dried	1 tbsp	5	0.9	0.1
dried	1 tsp	2	0.3	<.1
CILANTRO SEED				
whole	1 oz	84	15.6	5.0
whole	1 tbsp	15	2.8	0.9
whole	1 tsp	5	1.0	0.3
whole (Spice Islands)	1 tsp	6	0.8	0.3
CINNAMON				
ground	1 oz	74	22.6	0.9

Food Name	Serv. Size	Total Cal.	Carbs GMS	Fat GMS
ground	1 tbsp	18	5.4	0.2
ground	1 tsp	6	1.8	0.1
ground *(Durkee)*	1 tsp	8	0.0	tr
ground *(Laurel Leaf)*	1 tsp	8	0.0	tr
ground *(Spice Islands)*	1 tsp	6	1.4	<.1
CISCO. See CHUB.				
CITRON, candied	1 oz	88	22.5	0.1
CITRUS COOLER DRINK *(Gatorade)* 'Thirst Quencher'	8 oz	50	14.0	0.0
CITRUS DRINK				
(Five Alive) chilled	6 oz	90	22.0	0.0
(Fruitopia) 'Citrus Consciousness' real fruit	8 oz	120	30.0	0.0
CITRUS DRINK MIX				
(Crystal Light) blend, sugar-free, w/NutraSweet	8 oz	4	0.0	0.0
(Five Alive) frozen, diluted	6 oz	90	22.0	0.0
CITRUS FRUIT JUICE DRINK				
frozen concentrate	12-oz can	685	170.5	0.4
frozen concentrate, diluted	1 cup	114	28.5	0.0
(Five Alive) aseptic box	8.45 oz	123	30.7	0.0
(Five Alive) chilled or frozen, berry, diluted	6 oz	88	22.1	0.1
(Five Alive) chilled or frozen, diluted	6 oz	87	21.8	0.0
(Five Alive) chilled or frozen, tropical, diluted	6 oz	85	21.3	0.1
(Hi-C) 'Citrus Cooler'	6 oz	95	23.3	<.1
CITRUS GRILL MARINADE *(Lawry's)*	2 tbsp	34	3.4	0.4
CITRUS JUICE *(Santa Cruz Natural)* organic 'Cruz'	8 oz	125	29.0	<1.0
CITRUS PUNCH				
(Minute Maid) can or bottle 'Juices To Go'	6 oz	90	23.0	0.0
(Minute Maid) chilled	6 oz	90	23.0	0.0
(Tampico) 2% orange, tangerine, and lemon juice	8 oz	120	30.0	0.0
CITRUS PUNCH DRINK				
(Sunny Delight) 'California Style'	8 oz	100	23.0	0.0
(Sunny Delight) 'Florida Citrus Punch'	8 oz	120	27.0	<1.0
(Sunny Delight) 'Florida Citrus Punch' plus calcium	8 oz	130	32.0	<1.0
CITRUS PUNCH MIX *(Minute Maid)* frozen, concentrate	6 oz	90	22.0	0.0
CITRUS SALAD *(Florigold)*	8 oz	120	27.2	0.0
CLAM, CANNED				
chopped *(Gorton's)*	3.25 oz	40	2.0	<1.0
chopped *(Progresso)*	1/2 cup	70	2.0	<1.0
chopped, w/liquid *(Doxsee)*	6.5 oz	100	8.0	<1.0
chopped, w/liquid *(Orleans)*	6.5 oz	100	8.0	<1.0
minced *(Gorton's)*	3.25 oz	40	2.0	<1.0
minced *(Progresso)*	1/2 cup	70	2.0	<1.0
minced, w/liquid *(Doxsee)*	6.5 oz	100	8.0	<1.0
minced, w/liquid *(Orleans)*	6.5 oz	100	8.0	<1.0

Food Name	Serv. Size	Total Cal.	Carbs GMS	Fat GMS
mixed species, drained	1 cup	237	8.2	3.1
mixed species, drained	4 oz	168	5.8	2.2
mixed species, drained	3 oz	126	4.4	1.7
mixed species, liquid only	1 cup	5	0.2	0.1
mixed species, liquid only	3 oz	2	0.1	0.0
CLAM, MIXED SPECIES				
boiled	4 oz	168	5.8	2.2
breaded and fried	20 small	380	19.4	21.0
breaded and fried	4 oz	229	11.7	12.6
breaded and fried	3 oz	172	8.8	9.5
moist-heat cooked	20 small	133	4.6	1.8
moist-heat cooked	3 oz	126	4.4	1.7
poached	4 oz	168	5.8	2.2
raw	1 lb	335	11.6	4.4
raw		21	0.7	0.3
raw	20 small	133	4.6	1.8
raw	9 large	133	4.6	1.8
raw	3 oz	63	2.2	0.8
steamed	4 oz	168	5.8	2.2
CLAM, STUFFED, New England style *(Matlaw's)*	2 clams	180	21.0	8.0
CLAM JUICE				
(Doxsee)	3 oz	4	0.0	0.0
(Snow's)	3 oz	4	0.0	0.0
CLAM SAUCE. See SAUCE.				
CLAM TOMATO JUICE, canned	5.5 oz	76	18.1	0.2
CLARIFIED BUTTER. See GHEE.				
CLEARMALT. See ALCOHOLIC BEVERAGES.				
CLOVES				
ground	1 tbsp	21	4.0	1.3
ground	1 tsp	7	1.3	0.4
ground *(Durkee)*	1 tsp	9	0.0	<0.1
ground *(Laurel Leaf)*	1 tsp	9	0.0	<0.1
ground *(Spice Islands)*	1 tsp	7	1.2	0.2
CLUB SODA. See SOFT DRINKS AND MIXERS.				
COATING MIX. See SEASONING AND COATING MIX.				
COBBLER				
Fresh				
apple *(Stilwell)*	4 oz	200	4.0	4.0
apple, deep dish *(Awrey's)*	1/8 pie	320	48.0	14.0
blueberry, deep dish *(Awrey's)*	1/8 pie	310	45.0	14.0
Frozen				
apple, 4.33 oz *(Pet-Ritz)*	1/6 pkg	290	50.0	9.0
blackberry *(Stilwell)*	**4 oz**	**280**	**50.0**	**8.0**

Food Name	Serv. Size	Total Cal.	Carbs GMS	Fat GMS
blackberry, 4.33 oz *(Pet-Ritz)*	1/6 pkg	250	39.0	10.0
blueberry, 4.33 oz *(Pet-Ritz)*	1/6 pkg	370	50.0	12.0
cherry *(Stilwell)*	4 oz	250	46.0	6.0
cherry, 4.33 oz *(Pet-Ritz)*	1/6 pkg	280	46.0	10.0
peach *(Stilwell)*	4 oz	270	55.0	5.0
peach, 4.33 oz *(Pet-Ritz)*	1/6 pkg	260	46.0	10.0
strawberry, 4.33 oz *(Pet-Ritz)*	1/6 pkg	290	50.0	9.0

COBNUT, SHELLED. See HAZELNUT, SHELLED.

COCKTAIL ONION. See ONION, COCKTAIL.

COCKTAIL SAUCE. See SAUCE.

COCOA BUTTER OIL

Food Name	Serv. Size	Total Cal.	Carbs GMS	Fat GMS
	1 cup	1927	0.0	218.0
	1 oz	251	0.0	28.4
	1 tbsp	120	0.0	13.6

COCOA MIX

Food Name	Serv. Size	Total Cal.	Carbs GMS	Fat GMS
Amaretto creme flavor *(Swiss Miss)*	1.25 oz	150	29.0	3.0
Bavarian chocolate, hot cocoa *(Swiss Miss)*	1 oz	110	20.0	3.0
chocolate, w/marshmallows *(Carnation)*	1 oz	110	24.0	1.2
chocolate almond mocha *(Swiss Miss)*	1.235 oz	144	28.0	2.7
chocolate and mint 'Cocoa Classics' *(Land O'Lakes)*	1 envelope	160	24.0	5.0
chocolate and raspberry 'Cocoa Classics' *(Land O'Lakes)*	1 envelope	160	25.0	5.0
chocolate Bavarian mint *(Swiss Miss)*	1.235 oz	142	28.3	2.3
chocolate English toffee *(Swiss Miss)*	1.235 oz	142	28.5	2.3
chocolate flavor *(Pathmark)*	1 oz	110	24.0	1.0
chocolate flavor *(Swiss Miss)*	1 oz	110	24.0	1.0
chocolate flavor 'Sugar-free' *(Swiss Miss)*	.5 oz	50	9.0	1.0
chocolate fudge flavor *(Carnation)*	1-oz pkt	110	24.0	1.3
chocolate praline and creme *(Swiss Miss)*	1.235 oz	142	28.5	2.3
chocolate raspberry truffle *(Swiss Miss)*	1.235 oz	144	27.8	2.8
chocolate supreme 'Cocoa Classics' *(Land O'Lakes)*	1 envelope	160	25.0	5.0
dark chocolate truffle *(Swiss Miss)*	1.235 oz	142	27.9	2.5
diet *(Swiss Miss)*	.26 oz	20	3.0	<1.0
diet 'Hot Cocoa Mix' *(Swiss Miss)*	.26 oz	22	3.8	0.2
double rich chocolate flavor *(Swiss Miss)*	1 oz	110	24.0	1.0
fat-free 'Hot Cocoa Mix' *(Swiss Miss)*	.5 oz	50	9.0	0.3
lite *(Swiss Miss)*	.75 oz	70	17.0	<1.0
lite 'Hot Cocoa Mix' *(Swiss Miss)*	.7407 oz	74	17.1	0.5
marshmallow lovers 'Hot Cocoa Mix' *(Swiss Miss)*	1.199 oz	132	23.6	1.5
milk chocolate flavor *(Alba '66)*	.68 oz	60	10.0	0.0
milk chocolate flavor *(Saco Foods)*	1 oz	110	24.0	1.0
milk chocolate flavor *(Swiss Miss)*	1-oz pkt	110	20.0	3.0
milk chocolate flavor 'Sugar-free' *(Swiss Miss)*	.5 oz	60	10.0	0.0
milk chocolate flavor, w/marshmallows *(Alba '66)*	.68 oz	60	10.0	0.0

Food Name	Serv. Size	Total Cal.	Carbs GMS	Fat GMS
milk chocolate 'Hot Cocoa Mix' (Swiss Miss)	1.199 oz	133	28.9	1.5
milk chocolate 'Hot Cocoa Mix' (Swiss Miss)	1 oz	110	23.9	1.3
milk chocolate w/mini marshmallows 'Hot Cocoa Mix' (Swiss Miss)	1.199 oz	132	28.5	1.5
milk chocolate w/mini marshmallows 'Hot Cocoa Mix' (Swiss Miss)	1 oz	109	23.5	1.3
milk flavor (Carnation)	1-oz pkt	110	24.0	1.1
mini (Pathmark)	1 oz	110	24.0	1.0
mint flavor (Featherweight)	.44 oz	50	8.0	1.0
mocha flavor 'Sugar-free' (Carnation)	1 pkt	50	9.0	0.3
reduced calorie, aspartame sweetened	1 oz	8	1.4	0.1
regular (Finast)	6 oz	110	24.0	1.0
rich, sugar-free 'Hot Cocoa Mix' (Swiss Miss)	.5 oz	50	10.0	0.3
rich chocolate 'Hot Cocoa Mix' (Swiss Miss)	1 oz	110	23.5	1.2
rich milk flavor (Carnation)	1-oz pkt	110	24.0	1.1
rich milk flavor 'Sugar-free' (Carnation)	1 pkt	50	8.0	0.4
rich milk flavor, w/marshmallows (Weight Watchers)	1 pkt	60	10.0	0.0
'70-Calorie' (Carnation)	1 pkt	70	16.0	0.3
'Sugar-free' (Hills Bros)	3 tbsp	60	9.0	2.0
sugar-free 'Hot Cocoa Mix' (Swiss Miss)	.7055 oz	67	13.6	0.8
sugar-free 'Hot Cocoa Mix' (Swiss Miss)	.5 oz	49	10.0	0.2
sugar-free, sweetened w/NutraSweet (Saco Foods)	1 pkt	50	9.0	1.0
sugar-free, w/mini marshmallows 'Hot Cocoa Mix' (Swiss Miss)	.7055 oz	68	13.9	0.8
sugar-free, w/mini marshmallows 'Hot Cocoa Mix' (Swiss Miss)	.5 oz	51	10.5	0.6
vending 'Hot Cocoa Mix' (Swiss Miss)	1.34 oz	146	31.7	1.7
white chocolate 'Hot Cocoa Mix' (Swiss Miss)	1 oz	111	21.4	1.4
w/added nutrients	1-oz pkt	120	24.0	3.0
w/added nutrients, prepared	1 pkt	119	24.0	2.9
w/aspartame	.53-oz pkt	48	8.4	0.4
w/aspartame, w/added calcium and potassium	.53-oz pkt	48	8.5	0.5
w/aspartame, w/added sodium and vitamin A	.53-oz pkt	48	8.5	0.5
w/marshmallows (Carnation)	1-oz pkt	110	24.0	1.0
w/mini marshmallows (Finast)	6 oz	110	24.0	1.0
w/mini marshmallows (Swiss Miss)	1 oz	110	23.0	1.0
w/mini marshmallows 'Sugar-free' (Swiss Miss)	.5-oz pkt	50	9.0	<1.0
w/o added nutrients	1-oz pkt	103	22.5	1.1
w/o added nutrients, prepared	3-4 heaping tsp	103	22.5	1.2

COCOA POWDER. See also CHOCOLATE, BAKING.

Food Name	Serv. Size	Total Cal.	Carbs GMS	Fat GMS
(Bensdorp)	1 oz	130	8.0	7.0
(Hershey's) approx 1/3 cup	1 oz	120	13.0	4.0
(Hershey's) 'European'	1 oz	90	8.0	3.0

Food Name	Serv. Size	Total Cal.	Carbs GMS	Fat GMS
(Hershey's) unsweetened, European style	1 cup	170	48.8	8.3
(Hershey's) unsweetened, European style	1 tbsp	10	2.8	0.5
(Nestlé)	1.5 oz	180	21.0	6.0
COCONUT				
mature kernel, in shell	1 lb	834	35.9	79.0
mature kernel, shelled	1 oz	100	4.3	9.5
mature kernel, shelled, grated, packed	1 cup	460	19.8	43.5
meat, raw, 2 x 2 x 1/2 inch	1 piece	159	6.8	15.1
meat, raw, shredded	1 cup	283	12.2	26.8
COCONUT, DRIED				
creamed	1 oz	194	6.1	19.6
sweetened, flaked, canned	4 oz	505	46.6	36.1
sweetened, flaked, canned	1 cup	341	31.5	24.4
sweetened, flaked, canned	1 oz	126	11.6	9.0
sweetened, flaked, canned 'Angel Flake' (Baker's)	1/3 cup	110	10.0	9.0
sweetened, flaked, packaged	7-oz pkg	943	94.7	64.0
sweetened, flaked, packaged	1 cup	351	35.2	23.8
sweetened, flaked, packaged	1 oz	134	13.5	9.1
sweetened, flaked, packaged 'Angel Flake' (Baker's)	1/3 cup	120	10.0	8.0
sweetened, flaked, packaged 'Snowflake' (Finast)	1 oz	137	12.0	9.0
sweetened, flaked, packaged, toasted (Baker's)	1/3 cup	200	17.0	17.0
sweetened, shredded	7-oz pkg	997	94.9	70.6
sweetened, shredded	1 cup	466	44.3	33.0
sweetened, shredded	1 oz	142	13.5	10.1
sweetened, shredded 'Premium Shred' (Baker's)	1/3 cup	140	12.0	9.0
sweetened, shredded, toasted	1 oz	168	12.6	13.4
sweetened, shredded, toasted 'Angel Flake' (Baker's)	1/3 cup	200	17.0	17.0
unsweetened	1 oz	187	6.7	18.3
COCONUT CREAM				
Canned				
liquid expressed from grated meat	1 cup	568	24.7	52.5
liquid expressed from grated meat	1 tbsp	36	1.6	3.4
sweetened	1 oz	54	2.4	5.0
sweetened (Coco Lopez)	2 tbsp	120	20.0	5.0
sweetened (Holland House)	1 oz	81	18.0	(mq)
Raw				
liquid expressed from grated meat	1 cup	792	16.0	83.2
liquid expressed from grated meat	1 tbsp	49	1.0	5.2
liquid expressed from grated meat	1 oz	94	1.9	9.8
COCONUT MILK				
canned	1 cup	445	6.3	48.2
canned	1 oz	56	0.8	6.0
canned	1 tbsp	30	0.4	3.2

Food Name	Serv. Size	Total Cal.	Carbs GMS	Fat GMS
frozen	1 cup	485	13.4	49.9
frozen	1 oz	57	1.6	5.9
frozen	1 tbsp	30	0.8	3.1
raw	1 cup	552	13.3	57.2
raw	1 oz	65	1.6	6.8
raw	1 tbsp	35	0.8	3.6
COCONUT NECTAR *(Knudsen & Sons)*	8 oz	150	29.0	0.0
COCONUT OIL				
	1/2 cup	964	0.0	109.0
	1 oz	251	0.0	28.4
	1 tbsp	120	0.0	13.6
(Hain)	1 tbsp	120	0.0	14.0
COCONUT PINEAPPLE NECTAR, can or bottle *(Kern's)*	6 oz	140	26.0	4.0
COCONUT VEGETABLE OIL				
	1 cup	1879	0.0	218.0
	1 tbsp	117	0.0	13.6
COCONUT WATER				
	1 cup	46	8.9	0.5
	1 oz	5	1.1	0.1
	1 tbsp	3	0.6	0.0
COD, ALASKAN				
raw	1 oz	55	0.0	4.3
raw, 6.8 oz	1/2 fillet	377	0.0	29.5
smoked	4 oz	291	0.0	22.8
COD, ATLANTIC				
baked	4 oz	119	0.0	1.0
broiled	4 oz	119	0.0	1.0
dried and salted	3 oz	247	0.0	2.0
dried and salted	1 oz	81	0.0	0.7
dry-heat cooked	3 oz	89	0.0	0.7
microwaved	4 oz	119	0.0	1.0
raw	1 lb	372	0.0	3.1
raw	3 oz	70	0.0	0.6
raw	1 oz	23	0.0	0.2
COD, BLACK				
raw	1 lb	886	0.0	69.4
raw	1 oz	55	0.0	4.3
smoked	1 oz	73	0.0	5.7
COD, FROZEN				
breaded 'Light' *(Mrs. Paul's)*	1 piece	240	22.0	11.0
breaded 'Light' *(Van de Kamp's)*	1 piece	250	20.0	11.0
breaded, lemon thyme crumb 'Select' *(Gorton's)*	1 fillet	90	5.0	2.0
fillet *(Booth)*	4 oz	89	0.0	1.0

Food Name	Serv. Size	Total Cal.	Carbs GMS	Fat GMS
fillet *(Finast)*	4 oz	80	0.0	1.0
fillet *(SeaPak)*	4 oz	90	0.0	1.0
fillet 'Fishmarket Fresh' *(Gorton's)*	5 oz	110	0.0	1.0
fillet 'Individually Wrapped' *(Booth)*	4 oz	90	0.0	1.0
fillet, light *(Van de Kamp's)*	1 piece	250	20.0	11.0
fillet, natural *(Van de Kamp's)*	4 oz	90	0.0	1.0
natural *(Van de Kamp's)*	4 oz	90	0.0	1.0
COD, PACIFIC				
dry-heat cooked	3 oz	89	0.0	0.7
fillets, raw *(Peter Pan Seafoods)*	3.5 oz	80	na	0.6
raw	1 lb	372	0.0	2.9
raw	3 oz	70	0.0	0.5
raw	1 oz	23	0.0	0.2
COD CAKE, CANNED, 2 cakes *(Gorton's)*	4 oz	100	16.0	<1.0
COD ENTRÉE, FROZEN				
fillet, au gratin *(Booth)*	9.5 oz	280	18.0	11.0
fillet, Florentine *(Booth)*	9.5 oz	244	29.0	6.0
fillet, w/lemon butter sauce and rice *(Booth)*	9.5 oz	567	27.0	38.0
fillet, w/mushroom sauce and rice *(Booth)*	9.5 oz	280	19.0	11.0
COD LIVER OIL				
cherry *(Hain)*	1 tbsp	120	0.0	14.0
mint *(Hain)*	1 tbsp	120	0.0	14.0
regular	1 cup	1966	0.0	218.0
regular	1 tbsp	123	0.0	13.6
regular *(Hain)*	1 tbsp	120	0.0	14.0
COD NUGGETS, FROZEN				
minced, crunchy 'Bunch O'Crunch' 4 oz *(Frionor)*	8 pieces	320	19.0	21.0
COFFEE				
brewed	6 oz	4	0.7	0.0
brewed 'Regular' *(Chock Full o'Nuts)*	6 oz	2	(mq)	0.0
freeze-dried, prepared, dark roast 'Maragor' *(Taster's Choice)*	8 oz	4	1.0	<1.0
freeze-dried, prepared 'Colombian Select' *(Taster's Choice)*	8 oz	4	1.0	<1.0
freeze-dried, prepared 'Original' *(Taster's Choice)*	8 oz	4	1.0	<1.0
COFFEE, ALTERNATIVE				
cereal grain beverage, powder *(Pero)*	1 serving	4	<1.0	0.0
cereal grain beverage, powder *(Pionier)*	1 serving	6	1.4	0.0
cereal grain beverage, powder, dry	1 tsp	9	1.9	0.1
cereal grain beverage, powder, 'Instant,' prepared *(Postum)*	6 oz	12	3.0	0.0
cereal grain beverage, prepared w/water	1 tsp	9	1.8	0.0
cereal grain beverage, prepared w/skim milk	6 oz	74	10.8	0.4
cereal grain beverage, prepared w/1% milk	6 oz	86	10.6	2.0
cereal grain beverage, prepared w/2% milk	6 oz	100	10.7	3.6
cereal grain beverage, prepared w/whole milk	6 oz	120	10.4	6.1

Food Name	Serv. Size	Total Cal.	Carbs GMS	Fat GMS
cereal grain beverage, w/o added ingredients (Kaffree Roma)	8 oz	6	1.0	0.0
COFFEE, DECAFFEINATED				
(Chock Full o'Nuts)	6 oz	2	(mq)	0.0
freeze-dried, prepared, dark roast 'Maragor' (Taster's Choice)	8 oz	4	1.0	<1.0
freeze-dried, prepared 'Original' (Taster's Choice)	8 oz	4	1.0	<1.0
instant, powder	1 round tsp	4	0.8	0.0
instant, powder, prepared	6 oz	4	0.7	0.0
instant, prepared 'Decaf' (Nescafé)	8 oz	4	1.0	<1.0
instant, w/chicory, prepared (Mountain Blend)	8 oz	6	1.0	<1.0
'Suisse Mocha International' (General Foods)	6 oz	50	7.0	3.0
'Suisse Mocha International' sugar-free (General Foods)	6 oz	30	3.0	2.0
COFFEE, FLAVORED				
'Cafe Amaretto International' prepared (General Foods)	6 oz	50	7.0	2.0
'Cafe Français International' prepared (General Foods)	6 oz	60	6.0	3.0
'Cafe Français International' sugar-free prepared (General Foods)	6 oz	35	3.0	2.0
'Cafe Irish Creme International' prepared (General Foods)	6 oz	50	8.0	2.0
cafe Vienna 'Cafe Coffees' prepared (Hills Bros)	6 oz	60	9.0	2.0
'Cafe Vienna International' prepared (General Foods)	6 oz	60	10.0	2.0
'Cafe Vienna International' sugar-free, prepared (General Foods)	6 oz	30	3.0	2.0
'Cappio Cinnamon Iced Cappuccino' (Maxwell House)	8 oz	130	25.0	3.0
'Cappio Coffee Iced Cappuccino' (Maxwell House)	8 oz	120	23.0	3.0
'Cappio Mocha Iced Cappuccino' (Maxwell House)	8 oz	130	25.0	2.0
'Cinnamon Hot Cappuccino' (Maxwell House)	6 oz	60	11.0	1.0
'Coffee Hot Cappuccino' (Maxwell House)	6 oz	60	12.0	1.0
'Double Dutch Chocolate International' prepared (General Foods)	6 oz	50	8.0	2.0
'Dutch Chocolate Mint International' prepared (General Foods)	6 oz	50	8.0	2.0
'French Vanilla Cafe International' prepared (General Foods)	6 oz	60	9.0	3.0
'Hazelnut Belgian Cafe International' prepared (General Foods)	6 oz	60	10.0	2.0
mocha, banana nut 'Sugar-free' prepared (MJB)	6 oz	39	4.9	1.8
mocha, cherry, prepared (MJB)	6 oz	53	9.7	1.4
mocha, fudge 'Sugar-free' prepared (MJB)	6 oz	39	4.5	1.8
mocha, mint, prepared (MJB)	6 oz	53	9.9	1.3
mocha, mint 'Sugar-free' prepared (MJB)	6 oz	37	5.6	1.3
mocha, prepared (MJB)	6 oz	52	9.5	1.3
mocha, Swiss 'Cafe Coffees' prepared (Hills Bros)	6 oz	60	8.0	2.0
mocha, Swiss 'Cafe Coffees Sugar-free' prepared (Hills Bros)	6 oz	40	5.0	2.0
mocha, vanilla 'Sugar-free' prepared (MJB)	6 oz	39	5.2	1.7
'Mocha Hot Cappuccino' (Maxwell House)	6 oz	70	12.0	2.0
orange, Capri 'Cafe Coffees' prepared (Hills Bros)	6 oz	60	9.0	2.0
'Orange Cappuccino International' prepared (General Foods)	6 oz	60	10.0	2.0

Food Name	Serv. Size	Total Cal.	Carbs GMS	Fat GMS
'Orange Cappuccino International sugar-free, prepared				
(General Foods)	6 oz	30	3.0	2.0
'Suisse Mocha International' prepared (General Foods)	6 oz	50	7.0	3.0
'Suisse Mocha International' sugar-free, prepared				
(General Foods)	6 oz	30	3.0	2.0
'Viennese Chocolate Cafe International' prepared				
(General Foods)	6 oz	50	8.0	2.0
COFFEE, INSTANT				
'Brava' prepared (Nescafé)	8 oz	4	1.0	<1.0
Classic' prepared '(Nescafé)	8 oz	4	1.0	<1.0
powder (Kava)	1 tsp	2	1.0	0.0
prepared (Nescafé)	8 oz	4	1.0	<1.0
regular powder	1 oz	68	11.7	0.1
regular, powder	1 round tsp	4	0.7	0.0
regular, prepared	6 oz	4	0.7	0.0
'Silka' prepared (Nescafé)	8 oz	4	1.0	<1.0
w/chicory, powder	1 round tsp	6	1.3	0.0
w/chicory, prepared	6 oz	7	1.3	0.0
w/chicory, prepared (Sunrise)	8 oz	6	1.0	<1.0
w/chicory 'Mountain Blend' prepared (Nescafé)	8 oz	6	1.0	<1.0
w/sugar, cappuccino flavor, powder	2 round tsp	62	10.7	2.1
w/sugar, cappuccino flavor, prepared	6 oz	61	10.8	2.1
w/sugar, French flavor, powder	2 round tsp	57	6.6	3.4
w/sugar, French flavor, prepared	6 oz	57	6.6	3.4
w/sugar, mocha flavor, powder	2 round tsp	51	8.4	1.9
w/sugar, mocha flavor, prepared	6 oz	51	8.5	1.9
COFFEE FLAVOR DRINK, canned, liquid nutrition (Ensure)	8 oz	250	34.3	8.8
COFFEE LIQUEUR. See ALCOHOLIC BEVERAGES.				
COLA BEVERAGE. See SOFT DRINKS AND MIXERS.				
COLD CUTS. See LUNCHEON MEATS.				
COLE. See KALE.				
COLESLAW				
fresh	4 oz	78	14.1	3.0
fresh	1/2 cup	41	7.4	1.6
fresh	1 tbsp	6	1.0	0.2
COLESLAW DRESSING				
(Kraft)	1 tbsp	70	4.0	6.0
(Kraft) 'Miracle Whip'	1 tbsp	70	3.0	6.0
(Litehouse) refrigerated	1 tbsp	80	2.0	8.0
(T. Marzetti) light	1 tbsp	50	6.0	3.0
(T. Marzetti) original	1 tbsp	79	3.0	7.0
(T. Marzetti) 'South Recipe'	1 tbsp	66	6.0	5.0
COLEWORT. See KALE.				

Food Name	Serv. Size	Total Cal.	Carbs GMS	Fat GMS
COLLARDS				
boiled, drained	4 oz	31	7.0	0.2
boiled, drained, chopped	1/2 cup	17	3.9	0.1
raw, chopped	1/2 cup	6	1.3	0.0
raw, trimmed	1 oz	9	2.0	0.1
raw, untrimmed	1 lb	80	18.4	0.6
Canned				
chopped *(Allens)*	1/2 cup	20	2.0	<1.0
chopped, greens *(Bush's Best)*	1/2 cup	30	5.0	0.0
chopped, w/pork *(Luck's)*	7.5 oz	90	7.0	7.0
Frozen				
boiled, drained	4 oz	41	8.1	0.5
chopped *(Seabrook)*	3.3 oz	25	4.0	0.0
chopped *(Southern)*	3.5 oz	30	4.6	0.4
chopped, boiled, drained	1/2 cup	31	6.0	0.4
chopped, unprepared	10-oz pkg	94	18.3	1.0
COLORADO PINYON PINE NUT. See PINE NUT.				
CONCORD PUNCH, 'Juices To Go' *(Minute Maid)*	6 oz	90	23.0	0.0
CONDIMENTS. See individual listings.				
COOKIE				
ALMOND				
(Health Valley) date 'Fruit Jumbos'	1 cookie	70	10.0	3.0
(Mother's) shortbread	2 cookies	120	13.0	7.0
(Natures Warehouse) butter, approx 1 oz	2 cookies	122	19.2	4.1
(Stella D'oro) 'Breakfast Treats'	1 cookie	101	15.4	3.6
(Stella D'oro) 'Chinese Dessert'	1 cookie	169	19.5	8.9
(Stella D'oro) toast 'Mandel'	1 cookie	58	10.2	1.4
AMARANTH *(Health Valley)*	1 cookie	90	12.0	3.0
ANGEL WINGS *(Stella D'oro)*	1 cookie	74	7.0	4.7
ANIMAL CRACKERS				
(FFV)	1.25-oz pkg	160	26.0	6.0
(Finast) 15 pieces	1 oz	120	22.0	3.0
(Grandma's) candied, 5 cookies	1 oz	140	20.0	6.0
(Keebler) approx .5 oz	5 cookies	70	11.0	3.0
(Mother's) circus animal	4 cookies	110	14.0	6.0
(Nabisco) 'Barnum's Animals' 5 1/2 pieces	.5 oz	60	11.0	2.0
(Sunshine)	13 cookies	130	21.0	4.0
ANISE				
(Stella D'oro) 'Anisette Sponge'	1 cookie	51	9.9	0.8
(Stella D'oro) 'Anisette Toast'	1 cookie	46	9.3	0.6
(Stella D'oro) 'Anisette Toast Jumbo'	1 cookie	109	23.0	1.0
APPLE				
(Archway) n' raisin	1 cookie	120	20.0	3.0

Food Name	Serv. Size	Total Cal.	Carbs GMS	Fat GMS
(Bakery Wagon) cinnamon	1 cookie	100	17.0	3.0
(Bakery Wagon) filled oatmeal	1 cookie	90	14.0	4.0
(Bakery Wagon) walnut raisin	1 cookie	100	17.0	3.0
(Break Cake) sandwich	1 cookie	90	15.0	3.0
(Estee) cinnamon 'Snack Crisps' new blue pkg	.66 oz	80	15.0	2.0
(Frookie) cinnamon oat bran	1 cookie	45	6.5	2.0
(Frookie) 'Fruitins'	1 cookie	60	12.0	1.0
(Frookie) spice, fat-free	1 cookie	50	11.0	0.0
(Great Cakes)	4.5 oz	260	40.0	6.0
(Health Valley) cinnamon 'Mini Fruit Centers' fat-free	3 cookies	75	17.0	0.0
(Health Valley) 'Fruit Centers' fat-free	1 cookie	80	17.0	0.0
(Health Valley) raisin 'Fruit Chunks'	3 cookies	85	19.0	0.0
(Health Valley) raisin 'Jumbos' fat-free	1 cookie	80	17.0	0.0
(Health Valley) spice, fat-free	3 cookies	80	18.0	0.0
(Healthy Times) 'Hugga Bears' organic	1 oz	120	17.0	3.0
(Nabisco) 'Newtons' 1.25 oz	1 cookie	120	24.0	3.0
(Nabisco) 'Newtons' .75 oz	1 cookie	70	15.0	2.0
(Nabisco) 'Newtons' fat-free, .75 oz	1 cookie	70	16.0	0.0
(Stella D'oro) bar, Dutch	1 cookie	112	18.9	3.3
(Stella D'oro) pastry, dietetic	1 cookie	86	13.0	3.3
(Weight Watchers) fruit filled	1 cookie	80	21.0	<1.0
(Weight Watchers) raisin bar	1 cookie	100	18.0	3.0
APRICOT				
(Health Valley) almond 'Fancy Fruit Chunks'	2 cookies	90	14.0	4.0
(Health Valley) apple 'Fruit Chunks'	3 cookies	85	19.0	0.0
(Health Valley) delight, fat-free	3 cookies	80	18.0	0.0
(Health Valley) 'Fruit Centers' fat-free	1 cookie	80	17.0	0.0
(Pepperidge Farm) raspberry 'Fruit Cookies'	2 cookies	100	15.0	4.0
(Pepperidge Farm) raspberry 'Zurich'	1 cookie	60	10.0	2.0
ARROWROOT (Nabisco) 'National Arrowroot Biscuit' 6 pieces	1 oz	130	21.0	4.0
ASSORTED				
(Archway) 'Select Assortment'	1 cookie	50	7.0	2.0
(Fifty 50) wafers, creme filled, w/o sugar	1 wafer	35	4.0	2.0
(Stella D'oro) 'Hostess'	1 cookie	42	5.5	2.0
(Stella D'oro) 'Lady Stella'	1 cookie	42	5.5	2.0
BANANA				
(Break Cake) creme	1 cookie	240	37.0	9.0
(Frookie) fat-free	1 cookie	45	10.0	0.0
(Health Valley) spice 'Fruit Chunks'	3 cookies	85	19.0	0.0
(Natures Warehouse) wheat-free, fat-free	1 oz	90	20.5	0.7
BLUEBERRY (Great Cakes)	4.5 oz	260	40.0	6.0
BROWNIE				
(Break Cake) creme	1 cookie	240	38.0	8.0

Food Name	Serv. Size	Total Cal.	Carbs GMS	Fat GMS
(Pepperidge Farm) chocolate nut 'Old Fashioned'	2 pieces	110	11.0	7.0
(Pepperidge Farm) cream sandwich 'Capri'	1 cookie	80	10.0	5.0
BUTTER				
(Barbara's Bakery) pecan bites 'Small Indulgences'	1 oz	140	16.0	8.0
(Delicious) frosted, made w/Land O'Lakes butter	1 cookie	88	11.0	5.0
(Fifty 50) fructose sweetened, low sodium	1 cookie	40	5.0	2.0
(Keebler) flavor, chocolate coated 'Baby Bear' .5 oz	3 cookies	70	10.0	2.0
(Keebler) flavor, chocolate coated 'E.L. Fudge' .5 oz	2 cookies	80	10.0	4.0
(Lu) 'Little Schoolboy'	1 cookie	70	8.0	4.0
(Lu) 'Petite Beurre'	1 cookie	40	7.0	1.0
(Mother's) flavored	5 cookies	140	20.0	6.0
(Pepperidge Farm) flavor 'Chessmen'	2 cookies	90	12.0	4.0
(Stella D'oro) 'Como Delight'	1 cookie	145	17.9	7.2
CANDY *(Oven Lovin')*	1 cookie	70	10.0	3.0
CARAMEL				
(FFV) patties, approx 1 oz	2 cookies	150	20.0	7.0
(Keebler) apple oatmeal 'Elfin Delights'	1 cookie	65	12.0	2.0
(Natures Warehouse) crisp, wheat-free, fat-free	1 oz	90	20.5	0.7
CAROB				
(Health Valley) 'Healthy Chips' fat-free	3 cookies	80	18.0	0.0
(Natures Warehouse) fudge, approx 1 oz	2 cookies	116	20.5	3.1
(Westbrae) 'Rice Malt Snap'	1 oz	140	18.0	7.0
CARROT WALNUT 'Wholesome Choice' *(Pepperidge Farm)*	1 piece	60	11.0	1.0
CHERRY				
(Great Cakes) carob	4.5 oz	280	40.0	8.0
(Natures Warehouse) wheat-free, fat-free	1 oz	90	20.5	0.7
CHIPS AND CREME				
(Break Cake)	1 cookie	140	21.0	6.0
(Frookie) and vanilla sandwich 'Frookwich'	1 cookie	50	7.0	2.0
CHOCOLATE				
(Barbara's Bakery) raspberry 'Cookies & Creme'	2 cookies	120	18.0	5.0
(Barbara's Bakery) vanilla 'Cookies & Creme'	2 cookies	120	18.0	5.0
(Betty Crocker) w/peanut butter creme 'Dunkaroos'	1 tray	140	15.0	8.0
(Drake's) approx 1 oz	2 cookies	130	19.0	5.0
(Estee) 'Snack Crisps'	.66 oz	80	15.0	2.0
(Featherweight) creme wafer	1 cookie	20	3.0	1.0
(Frookie) 'Animal Frackers'	6 cookies	60	9.0	2.0
(Frookie) 'Funky Monkeys'	8 cookies	60	10.0	2.0
(Grandma's) 'Chocolate Cookie Bits' 8 cookies	1 oz	140	19.0	6.0
(Lu) 'Chocolatiers'	2 cookies	85	10.0	4.0
(Lu) 'Chocolatiers' dipped	2 cookies	105	12.0	6.0
(Nabisco) 'Chocolate Snap' 4 pieces	.5 oz	70	10.0	2.0
(Nabisco) 'Pure Chocolate Middles'	.5 oz cookie	80	9.0	5.0

Food Name	Serv. Size	Total Cal.	Carbs GMS	Fat GMS
(Pepperidge Farm) walnut 'Beacon Hill'	1 cookie	120	14.0	7.0
(Stella D'oro) 'Castelets'	1 cookie	64	9.0	2.8
(Stella D'oro) 'Margherite'	1 cookie	72	10.2	3.1
(Tastykake) 'Soft 'n Chewy'	1.4 oz	171	26.2	7.0
(Weight Watchers)	3 cookies	80	13.0	3.0
CHOCOLATE CHIP				
(Almost Home)	.5 oz	60	8.0	3.0
(Archway)	1 cookie	50	7.0	3.0
(Barbara's Bakery)	1 oz	130	16.0	6.0
(Barbara's Bakery) crisp 'Small Indulgences'	1 oz	140	18.0	7.0
(Break Cake) approx 1 oz	5 cookies	140	20.0	6.0
(Chips Ahoy!)	.5 oz	50	7.0	2.0
(Chips Ahoy!) 'Chewy'	.5 oz	60	7.0	3.0
(Chips Ahoy!) 'Mini'	.5 oz	70	9.0	3.0
(Chips Ahoy!) pecan 'Selections'	.5 oz	100	10.0	6.0
(Chips Ahoy!) 'Rockers'	1 cookie	60	8.0	3.0
(Chips Ahoy!) 'Sprinkled'	.5 oz	60	8.0	3.0
(Chips Ahoy!) 'Striped'	.5 oz	90	10.0	5.0
(Chips Ahoy!) walnut 'Selections'	.5 oz	100	9.0	6.0
(Chips Ahoy!) white fudge chunk	1 cookie	90	11.0	5.0
(Drake's) approx 1 oz	2 cookies	140	18.0	6.0
(Duncan Hines)	2 cookies	110	15.0	5.0
(Entenmann's)	3 cookies	140	19.0	7.0
(Estee)	3 cookies	110	13.0	5.0
(Featherweight)	1 cookie	45	6.0	2.0
(Fifty 50) fructose sweetened	1 cookie	35	4.0	2.0
(Finast)	1 oz	90	18.0	7.0
(Frookie)	1 cookie	45	6.5	2.0
(Frookie) Mandarin	1 cookie	45	6.5	2.0
(Frookie) mint	1 cookie	45	6.5	2.0
(Grandma's) 'Big Cookies' 2.75 oz	2 cookies	370	50.0	17.0
(Grandma's) 'Rich'N Chewy' 3 cookies	1 oz	140	20.0	6.0
(Keebler) bakery crisp 'Chips Deluxe'	1 cookie	60	7.0	3.0
(Keebler) chewy 'Elfin Delights'	1 cookie	65	11.0	2.0
(Keebler) 'Chips Deluxe' approx .5 oz	1 cookie	80	10.0	4.0
(Keebler) 'Coconut Chocolate Drop'	1 cookie	80	10.0	5.0
(Keebler) deluxe 'Bakery Crisp'	1 cookie	60	7.0	3.0
(Keebler) 'Rainbow Chips Deluxe' .5 oz	1 cookie	80	11.0	3.0
(Keebler) 'Soft Batch' approx .5 oz	1 cookie	80	10.0	4.0
(Mother's)	1 cookie	70	10.0	3.0
(Mother's) angel	2 cookies	120	14.0	8.0
(Nabisco) bite size 'Snack Wells'	.5 oz	60	11.0	1.0
(Nabisco) 'Chocolate Chip Snaps' 3 pieces	.5 oz	70	11.0	2.0

Food Name	Serv. Size	Total Cal.	Carbs GMS	Fat GMS
(Oven Lovin')	1 cookie	70	9.0	3.0
(Pepperidge Farm) 'Family Request'	2 cookies	90	15.0	5.0
(Pepperidge Farm) 'Old Fashioned'	2 cookies	100	12.0	5.0
(Pepperidge Farm) w/macadamia nuts 'Big, Soft and Chewy'	1 cookie	130	16.0	7.0
(Pepperidge Farm) w/macadamia nuts 'Sausalito'	1 cookie	120	14.0	7.0
(Tastykake) bar, 1.5 oz	1 cookie	193	28.3	8.4
(Tastykake) 'Soft 'n Chewy'	1.4 oz	174	25.5	7.3
(Weight Watchers)	2 cookies	90	18.0	2.0
CHOCOLATE CHOCOLATE CHIP				
(Barbara's Bakery(	1oz	125	17.0	5.0
(Natures Warehouse) approx 1 oz	2 cookies	130	16.4	6.1
(Pepperidge Farm) walnut, big, soft & chewy	1 cookie	130	17.0	6.0
(Pillsbury's Best)	1 cookie	70	9.0	3.0
CHOCOLATE CHUNK				
(Chips Ahoy!) 'Chunky'	1 cookie	80	11.0	4.0
(Chips Ahoy!) 'Selections'	.5 oz	90	10.0	5.0
(Dunkin' Donuts) 1.5 oz	1 cookie	200	25.0	10.0
(Dunkin' Donuts) w/nuts, 1.5 oz	1 cookie	210	23.0	11.0
(Pepperidge Farm) 'Big, Soft and Chewy'	1 cookie	130	17.0	6.0
CHOCOLATE-FILLED SANDWICH				
(Keebler) 'E.L. Fudge'	1 cookie	60	8.0	3.0
(Pepperidge Farm) 'Brussels'	2 cookies	110	13.0	5.0
(Pepperidge Farm) 'Brussels Mint'	2 cookies	130	17.0	7.0
(Pepperidge Farm) 'Double Chocolate Milano'	2 cookies	150	18.0	8.0
(Pepperidge Farm) 'Hazelnut Milano'	2 cookies	130	15.0	8.0
(Pepperidge Farm) 'Lido'	1 cookie	90	10.0	5.0
(Pepperidge Farm) 'Milano'	2 cookies	120	15.0	6.0
(Pepperidge Farm) 'Mint Milano'	2 cookies	150	17.0	7.0
(Pepperidge Farm) 'Orange Milano'	2 cookies	150	17.0	7.0
(Pepperidge Farm) 'Orleans'	2 cookies	120	14.0	8.0
CHOCOLATE GRAHAM				
(Keebler) 'Thin Bits' approx .5 oz	12 cookies	70	9.0	3.0
(Nabisco) approx .5 oz	11 cookies	60	10.0	2.0
(Nabisco) 'Bugs Bunny'	.5 oz	60	10.0	2.0
(Nabisco) 'Chocolate Grahams'	.5 oz	150	17.0	2.0
(Teddy Grahams) 'Bearwichs'	.5 oz	70	10.0	3.0
(Teddy Grahams) w/vanilla creme 'Bearwichs'	4 cookies	70	10.0	3.0
CHOCOLATE SANDWICH				
(Estee)	1 cookie	50	7.0	2.0
(Frookie) 'Frookwich'	1 cookie	50	7.0	2.0
(Keebler) 'Chocolate Creme Sandwich'	.5 oz	80	12.0	4.0
(Keebler) 'E.L. Fudge'	1 cookie	70	9.0	3.0

Food Name	Serv. Size	Total Cal.	Carbs GMS	Fat GMS
(Keebler) fudge creme 'Elfin Delights'	1 cookie	55	10.0	2.0
(Keebler) peanut butter 'E.L. Fudge'	1 cookie	50	7.0	3.0
(Little Debbie)	1.8 oz	250	35.0	12.0
(Oreo) 'Big Stuf'	.25 oz	200	27.0	9.0
(Oreo) 'Double Stuf' 2 cookies	1 oz	70	9.0	4.0
(Oreo) fudge covered	.75 oz	110	13.0	6.0
(Oreo) 'Halloween Treats' 1 oz	2 cookies	140	20.0	7.0
(Oreo) 2 1/2 cookies	1 oz	140	20.0	6.0
(Oreo) white fudge covered	.75 oz	110	14.0	6.0
(Weight Watchers)	2 cookies	90	15.0	3.0
CHUNK				
(Pepperidge Farm) 'Nantucket'	1 cookie	120	15.0	6.0
(Pepperidge Farm) pecan 'Chesapeake'	1 cookie	120	14.0	7.0
(Pepperidge Farm) pecan 'Special Collection'	1 cookie	70	8.0	4.0
CINNAMON				
(Frookie) 'Animal Frackers'	6 cookies	60	9.0	2.0
(Mother's) dinosaur, mini	7 cookies	70	9.0	2.0
(Mother's) dinosaur grahams	1 cookie	80	12.0	3.0
CINNAMON GRAHAM				
(Honey Maid) approx .5 oz	2 cookies	60	12.0	1.0
(Keebler) 'Alpha Grahams'	6 cookies	70	10.0	2.0
(Keebler) 'Cinnamon Crisp' .5 oz	4 cookies	70	11.0	2.0
(Keebler) fudge covered 'Deluxe' .5 oz	2 cookies	90	11.0	4.0
(Keebler) 'Thin Bits' approx .5 oz	12 cookies	70	10.0	3.0
(Nabisco) 'Bugs Bunny'	.5 oz	60	11.0	2.0
(Nabisco) fat-free 'Snack Wells'	.5 oz	50	12.0	0.0
(Nabisco) w/fudge 'Cookies'N Fudge'	1 cookie	45	6.0	2.0
(Natures Warehouse) approx 1 oz	2 cookies	113	18.8	3.6
(Pepperidge Farm) sugar 'Family Request'	2 cookies	80	12.0	4.0
(Sunshine)	1 cookie	70	11.0	3.0
(Teddy Grahams) 'Bearwichs'	.5 oz	70	10.0	3.0
COCOA				
(Westbrae) chip 'Rice Malt Snap'	1 oz	130	18.0	7.0
(Westbrae) 'Rice Malt Snap'	1 oz	140	17.0	7.0
COCONUT				
(Break Cake) macaroons	2 cookies	270	34.0	14.0
(Drake's) approx 1 oz	2 cookies	130	20.0	5.0
(Estee)	3 cookies	110	14.0	5.0
(Glenny's) almonds, raisins 'Nookie Bar'	1.15 oz	138	18.0	3.0
(Mother's) cocadas	4 cookies	120	17.0	6.0
(Mother's) macaroons	1 cookie	80	8.0	5.0
(Natures Warehouse) approx 1 oz	2 cookies	130	13.9	7.6
(Pepperidge Farm) chocolate-filled 'Tahiti'	1 cookie	90	9.0	6.0

Food Name	Serv. Size	Total Cal.	Carbs GMS	Fat GMS
(Stella D'oro) dietetic	1 cookie	52	6.8	2.4
(Stella D'oro) macaroon	1 cookie	60	6.6	3.4
COFFEE				
(Barbara's Bakery) coffee cake crunch 'Small Indulgences'	1 oz	130	18.0	6.0
(Pepperidge Farm)	1 cookie	50	6.0	3.0
CRANBERRY				
(Frookie) orange, fat-free	1 cookie	45	10.0	0.0
(Nabisco) 'Newtons' fat-free	1 cookie	70	16.0	0.0
(Pepperidge Farm) honey, soft 'Wholesome Choice'	1 cookie	60	11.0	2.0
CROKINE *(Lu)*	2 cookies	35	7.0	0.0
DATE				
(Bakery Wagon) filled oatmeal	1 cookie	90	15.0	3.0
(Break Cake) creme	1 cookie	140	21.0	5.0
(Health Valley) delight, fat-free	3 cookies	80	18.0	0.0
(Health Valley) 'Fruit Centers' fat-free	1 cookie	70	16.0	0.0
(Health Valley) pecan 'Fancy Fruit Chunks'	2 cookies	90	15.0	4.0
(Pepperidge Farm) pecan 'Kitchen Hearth'	2 cookies	110	15.0	5.0
DEVIL'S FOOD				
(Break Cake) creme	1 cookie	130	20.0	5.0
(FFV) 'Trolley Cakes' 2 oz	2 cookies	120	25.0	2.0
(Nabisco) cakes	1 cookie	70	15.0	1.0
DUPLEX SANDWICH *(Mother's)*	2 cookies	105	15.0	5.0
EGG BISCUIT				
(Estee) 'Original Sandwich'	1 cookie	45	6.0	2.0
(FFV) 'Kreem Pilot Bread'	1 cookie	60	9.0	2.0
(FFV) 'Royal Dainty' .7 oz	2 cookies	120	14.0	6.0
(FFV) 'T.C. Rounds' approx 1 oz	2 cookies	160	20.0	8.0
(FFV) 'Tango' 1.2 oz	2 cookies	160	26.0	5.0
(Stella D'oro)	1 cookie	43	6.7	1.1
(Stella D'oro) 'Anginetti'	1 cookie	31	4.9	1.0
(Stella D'oro) dietetic	1 cookie	43	6.5	1.1
(Stella D'oro) dietetic 'Kitchen'	1 cookie	8	0.7	0.5
(Stella D'oro) 'Jumbo'	1 cookie	47	9.1	0.7
(Stella D'oro) 'Roman'	1 cookie	137	20.4	5.0
(Stella D'oro) sugared	1 cookie	75	14.3	1.4
ENGLISH TEA *(Mother's)* sandwich	1 cookie	100	14.0	4.0
FIG				
(Estee) bar	2 cookies	90	21.0	1.0
(FFV) bar, vanilla	1 cookie	70	12.0	1.0
(FFV) bar, whole wheat	1 cookie	70	11.0	2.0
(Frookie) 'Fruitins'	1 cookie	60	12.0	1.0
(Frookie) 'Fruitins' fat-free	2 cookies	90	21.0	0.0
(Keebler) bar	1 cookie	60	11.0	2.0

Food Name	Serv. Size	Total Cal.	Carbs GMS	Fat GMS
(Mother's) bar	2 cookies	110	23.0	2.0
(Mother's) whole wheat	2 cookies	120	25.0	2.0
(Nabisco) 'Newtons'	.5 oz	60	11.0	1.0
(Nabisco) 'Newtons'	1.25 oz	120	24.0	3.0
(Nabisco) 'Newtons Cookie Variety'	1 oz	120	24.0	3.0
(Nabisco) 'Newtons' fat-free, 1 piece	.75 oz	70	15.0	0.0
(Natures Warehouse) bar, apple cinnamon, wheat-free	1 oz	98	19.0	2.0
(Natures Warehouse) bar, raspberry, wheat-free	1 oz	98	19.0	2.0
(Natures Warehouse) bar, wheat-free	1 oz	98	19.0	2.0
(Natures Warehouse) bar, whole wheat	1 oz	98	19.0	2.0
(Stella D'oro) pastry, dietetic	1 cookie	89	13.0	3.7
FORTUNE				
(LaChoy)	1 oz	112	26.3	0.2
(LaChoy)	1 cookie	15	4.0	<1.0
FRUIT				
(Barbara's Bakery) and nut	1 oz	140	18.0	6.0
(Health Valley) 'Fruit & Fitness'	5 cookies	200	40.0	6.0
(Health Valley) Hawaiian, fat-free	3 cookies	80	18.0	0.0
(Health Valley) tropical 'Fancy Fruit Chunks'	2 cookies	80	13.0	3.0
(Health Valley) tropical 'Fruit Centers' fat-free	1 cookie	80	17.0	0.0
(Health Valley) tropical 'Fruit Jumbos'	1 cookie	70	10.0	2.0
(Stella D'oro) slices	1 cookie	60	8.7	2.2
FUDGE				
(Almost Home)	.5 oz	70	9.0	3.0
(Almost Home) chocolate chip	.5 oz	70	9.0	3.0
(Chips Ahoy!) mini bites 'Little Fudgies'	1 oz	230	27.0	12.0
(Estee)	1 cookie	30	4.0	1.0
(Fifty 50) brownie, fructose sweetened	1 cookie	35	5.0	2.0
(Grandma's) 'Big Cookies' 2.75 oz	2 cookies	350	54.0	13.0
(Keebler) mint 'Grasshopper' approx .5 oz	2 cookies	70	10.0	3.0
(M&M/Mars) 'Twix'	1 bar	100	11.0	6.0
(Mother's) double fudge sandwich	2 cookies	100	15.0	4.0
(Mother's) wafer 'Flaky Flix'	2 cookies	130	14.0	9.0
(Nabisco) caramel, peanut 'Heyday Bars' 1 piece	.75 oz	110	13.0	6.0
(Nabisco) middles	.5 oz	80	9.0	5.0
(Nabisco) wafer 'Famous Wafers' 2-1/2 pieces	.5 oz	70	11.0	2.0
(Nabisco) snaps, approx .5 oz	4 cookies	70	11.0	2.0
(Stella D'oro) 'Swiss Fudge Cookie'	1 cookie	68	8.5	3.4
(Tastykake) bar	1.8 oz	205	35.0	6.8
GINGER				
(FFV) boys	1.25-oz pkg	150	26.0	5.0
(Frookie) spice	1 cookie	45	6.5	2.0
(Pepperidge Farm) 'Gingerman'	2 cookies	70	10.0	3.0

Food Name	Serv. Size	Total Cal.	Carbs GMS	Fat GMS
(Westbrae) 'Rice Malt Snap'	1 oz	130	20.0	5.0
GINGERSNAPS				
(Archway) '80/pkg'	1 cookie	25	4.0	<1.0
(Archway) '54/pkg'	1 cookie	35	6.0	1.0
(Break Cake) approx 1 oz	5 cookies	130	0.0	5.0
(Delicious)	.5 oz	64	11.3	1.7
(FFV) approx 1 oz	5 cookies	130	22.0	4.0
(Nabisco) 'Old Fashioned'	.25 oz	30	6.0	1.0
(Sunshine)	5 cookies	100	16.0	3.0
GRAHAM. See also HONEY GRAHAM.				
(Betty Crocker) w/chocolate frosting 'Dunkaroos'	1 tray	130	19.0	5.0
(Betty Crocker) w/vanilla frosting 'Dunkaroos'	1 tray	130	21.0	5.0
(Keebler) chocolate 'Selects'	4 cookies	60	9.0	3.0
(Keebler) honey nut 'Selects'	4 cookies	60	9.0	3.0
(Mother's) dinosaur, original	1 cookie	70	12.0	2.0
(Mother's) dinosaur, mini	7 cookies	60	9.0	1.0
(Nabisco) 'Bugs Bunny' 5 pieces	.5 oz	60	11.0	2.0
(Pepperidge Farm) cinnamon 'Goldfish'	1 oz	130	19.0	7.0
(Pepperidge Farm) 'Goldfish'	1 oz	140	18.0	7.0
(Teddy Grahams) snacks, chocolate	.5-oz	60	10.0	2.0
(Teddy Grahams) snacks, cinnamon	.75-oz bag	100	16.0	3.0
(Teddy Grahams) snacks, honey, 11 pieces	.5 oz	60	11.0	2.0
(Teddy Grahams) vanilla honey 'Bearwichs'	4 cookies	70	10.0	3.0
GRANOLA				
(Betty Crocker) chocolate filling 'Incredibites'	1 pouch	170	24.0	7.0
(Betty Crocker) peanut butter 'Incredibites'	1 pouch	170	23.0	8.0
(Betty Crocker) vanilla creme 'Incredibites'	1 pouch	170	24.0	7.0
(Health Valley) 'Healthy'	3 cookies	75	17.0	0.0
'HERMIT' *(Break Cake)*	1 cookie	230	38.0	7.0
'HOB-NOBS' *(Carr's)*	1 cookie	72	9.6	3.2
HONEY				
(Bakery Wagon) fruit bar	1 cookie	100	16.0	3.0
(Health Valley) cinnamon, crisp 'Honey Jumbos'	1 cookie	70	10.0	2.0
(Health Valley) oat bran, fancy 'Honey Jumbos'	1 cookie	70	10.0	2.0
(Health Valley) peanut butter, crisp 'Honey Jumbos'	1 cookie	70	10.0	2.0
(Stella D'oro) 'Royal Nuggets'	2	0.1	0.1	
HONEY GRAHAM				
(Carafection) 'Original' carob coated	1 oz	139	17.0	7.0
(Carr's) wheat 'Home Wheat Graham'	1 cookie	74	10.9	3.3
(Health Valley) 'Fancy'	7 cookies	130	21.0	5.0
(Health Valley) oat bran	7 cookies	130	25.0	2.0
(Honey Maid) .5 oz	2 pieces	60	11.0	1.0
(Honey Maid) honey'n oat bran 'Graham Bites'	.5 oz	60	11.0	2.0

Food Name	Serv. Size	Total Cal.	Carbs GMS	Fat GMS
(Keebler) approx .5 oz	4 cookies	70	12.0	2.0
(Nabisco) vanilla, approx .5 oz	11 cookies	60	10.0	2.0
(Pepperidge Farm) hazelnut 'Old Fashioned'	2 cookies	110	15.0	6.0
(Sunshine)	1 piece	60	10.0	2.0
JELLY				
(Delicious) top	.8 oz	112	14.3	5.3
(FFV) tarts	1 cookie	60	11.0	2.0
LEMON				
(Barbara's Bakery) almond delights 'Small Indulgences'	1 oz	140	18.0	6.0
(Delicious) sugar wafer	1 wafer	35	4.0	2.0
(Estee)	3 cookies	100	14.0	5.0
(Estee) 'Snack Crisps'	.66 oz	80	15.0	2.0
(Featherweight)	1 cookie	45	6.0	2.0
(Frookie) sandwich 'Frookwich'	1 cookie	50	7.0	2.0
(Pepperidge Farm) nut crunch 'Old Fashioned'	2 cookies	110	13.0	7.0
(Westbrae) 'Rice Malt Snap'	1 oz	130	20.0	6.0
MARSHMALLOW				
(Nabisco) cake 'Mallomars'	1 cookie	60	8.0	3.0
(Nabisco) fudge cake 'Puffs'	.75 oz	90	14.0	4.0
(Nabisco) fudge cake 'Twirls'	1 oz	140	20.0	6.0
(Nabisco) fudge graham 'Suddenly S'Mores'	.75 oz	100	15.0	4.0
(Nabisco) 'Pinwheels'	1 cookie	130	20.0	5.0
(Pinwheels) chocolate cake	1 oz	130	20.0	5.0
MINI-CREME *(Delicious)*	1 wafer	24	3.0	1.0
MINT				
(Carafection) honey graham, carob coated	1 oz	139	17.0	7.0
(FFV) sandwich, approx 1.1 oz	2 cookies	160	22.0	7.0
(Girl Scout Cookies) thin mints	4 cookies	160	20.0	9.0
(Keebler) 'Soft Batch'	1 cookie	80	10.0	4.0
(Nabisco) sandwich 'Mystic Mint'	.5 oz	90	11.0	4.0
MOLASSES				
(Archway)	1 cookie	100	18.0	2.0
(Bakery Wagon) iced	1 cookie	100	17.0	4.0
(Grandma's) 'Old Time Big Cookies'	2 cookies	320	58.0	9.0
(Nabisco) 'Pantry'	.5 oz	80	13.0	3.0
(Pepperidge Farm) crisps 'Old Fashioned'	2 cookies	70	8.0	3.0
MUESLI *(Carr's)*	1 cookie	84	10.8	4.1
OAT BRAN				
(Awrey's) raisin	1 cookie	100	14.0	4.0
(Frookie) muffin	1 cookie	45	6.5	2.0
(Health Valley) animal cookies	7 cookies	110	20.0	4.0
(Health Valley) fruit and nut	2 cookies	110	17.0	4.0
(Health Valley) fruit 'Oat Bran Fruit Jumbos'	1 cookie	70	10.0	2.0

Food Name	Serv. Size	Total Cal.	Carbs GMS	Fat GMS
(Health Valley) raisin 'Fancy Fruit Chunks'	2 cookies	90	15.0	3.0
(Natures Warehouse) chocolate chip, approx 1 oz	2 cookies	139	16.6	6.0
(Natures Warehouse) wheat-free, approx 1 oz	2 cookies	129	16.0	6.2
OATMEAL				
(Almost Home) raisin	.5 oz	70	10.0	3.0
(Archway)	1 cookie	110	19.0	3.0
(Archway) apple filled	1 cookie	90	18.0	1.0
(Archway) date filled	1 cookie	100	18.0	2.0
(Archway) iced	1 cookie	140	22.0	5.0
(Archway) 'Ruth's Golden'	1 cookie	120	20.0	4.0
(Bakers Bonus)	.5 oz	80	12.0	3.0
(Bakery Wagon) chocolate chunk	1 cookie	100	17.0	3.0
(Bakery Wagon) soft	1 cookie	100	15.0	5.0
(Bakery Wagon) walnut raisin	1 cookie	100	16.0	4.0
(Barbara's Bakery) raisin	1 oz	100	19.0	2.0
(Break Cake) approx 1 oz	5 cookies	140	20.0	6.0
(Chips Ahoy!) chocolate chip 'Selections'	.5 oz	90	10.0	5.0
(Drake's) approx 1 oz	2 cookies	120	19.0	4.0
(Dunkin' Donuts) pecan, raisin	1 cookie	200	28.0	9.0
(Duncan Hines) raisin	2 cookies	110	15.0	5.0
(Entemann's) chocolatey chip 'Fat-Free Cholesterol-Free'	2 cookies	80	19.0	0.0
(Entenmann's) raisin	2 cookies	30	17.0	0.0
(Estee) raisin	3 cookies	100	14.0	4.0
(FFV) approx 1 oz	5 cookies	130	20.0	4.0
(Fifty 50) hearty oatmeal, fructose sweetened	1 cookie	35	5.0	1.0
(Frookie) raisin	1 cookie	45	6.5	2.0
(Frookie) raisin, fat-free	1 cookie	50	11.0	0.0
(Frookie) 7-grain oatmeal	1 cookie	45	6.5	2.0
(Glenny's) wheat-free 'Noah 'N Friends Animal'	.5 oz	65	10.0	2.0
(Grandma's) apple spice 'Big Cookies' 2.75 oz	2 cookies	330	51.0	12.0
(Health Valley) raisin cinnamon 'Fruit Chunks'	3 cookies	85	19.0	0.0
(Keebler) 'Old Fashion' approx .5 oz	1 cookie	80	12.0	3.0
(Keebler) w/chocolate 'Magic Middles' .5 oz	1 cookie	80	8.0	5.0
(Keebler) w/raisins, chewy 'Raisin Ruckus'	1 cookie	70	10.0	3.0
(Little Debbie)	2.75 oz	340	52.0	12.0
(Mother's)	1 cookie	60	8.0	3.0
(Mother's) chocolate chip	1 cookie	70	10.0	3.0
(Mother's) iced	1 cookie	70	10.0	3.0
(Mother's) walnut chocolate chip	1 cookie	70	9.0	3.0
(Nabisco) raisin, 'Snack Wells'	1 cookie	60	10.0	1.0
(Natures Warehouse) raisin, approx 1 oz	2 cookies	135	17.3	6.4
(Pepperidge Farm) chocolate chunk 'Dakota'	1 cookie	110	15.0	6.0
(Pepperidge Farm) 'Family Request'	2 cookies	90	13.0	4.0

Food Name	Serv. Size	Total Cal.	Carbs GMS	Fat GMS
(Pepperidge Farm) Irish 'Old Fashioned'	2 cookies	90	13.0	5.0
(Pepperidge Farm) raisin, soft, low-fat 'Wholesome Choice'	1 cookie	60	11.0	1.0
(Weight Watchers) raisin	2 cookies	90	20.0	<1.0
(Weight Watchers) spice	3 cookies	80	13.0	2.0
(Westbrae) 'Rice Malt Snap'	1 oz	130	19.0	5.0
ORANGE-PINEAPPLE				
(Health Valley) 'Mini Fruit Centers' fat-free	3 cookies	75	17.0	0.0
peach (Great Cakes)	4.5 oz	260	40.0	6.0
PEACH-APRICOT				
(FFV) bar, vanilla	1 cookie	70	14.0	1.0
(FFV) bar, whole wheat	1 cookie	70	11.0	2.0
(Health Valley) 'Mini Fruit Centers' fat-free	3 cookies	75	17.0	0.0
(Stella D'oro) pastry	1 cookie	93	13.6	3.8
(Stella D'oro) pastry, dietetic	1 cookie	87	12.3	3.7
PEANUT (Health Valley) 'Fancy Peanut Chunks'	2 cookies	100	14.0	3.0
PEANUT BUTTER				
(Bakery Wagon) oatmeal	1 cookie	110	12.0	7.0
(Break Cake)	1 cookie	140	18.0	7.0
(Break Cake) wafer	1 wafer	180	24.0	9.0
(Delicious) and jelly sandwich 'Skippy & Welchs'	1 cookie	120	15.0	6.0
(Delicious) made w/Skippy peanut butter	1 cookie	80	7.0	5.0
(Estee) sandwich	1 cookie	50	5.0	3.0
(Featherweight)	1 cookie	40	5.0	2.0
(Featherweight) creme wafer	1 cookie	25	3.0	1.0
(FFV) sandwich, approx 1.1 oz	2 cookies	170	21.0	8.0
(Fifty 50) fructose sweetened	1 cookie	40	5.0	2.0
(Frookie) sandwich 'Frookwich'	1 cookie	50	7.0	2.0
(Glenny's) 'Noah 'N Friends Animal Cookies'	.5 oz	65	9.0	3.0
(Grandma's) 'Big Cookies' 2.75 oz	2 cookies	410	43.0	30.0
(Grandma's) cookie bits, 8 cookies	1 oz	140	19.0	6.0
(Great Cakes) and jelly	4.5 oz	280	40.0	8.0
(Keebler) chocolate chip 'Soft Batch' .5 oz	1 cookie	80	9.0	5.0
(Keebler) nut 'Soft Batch' approx .5 oz	1 cookie	80	9.0	4.0
(Mother's) sandwich 'Gaucho'	1 cookie	90	12.0	5.0
(Nabisco) 'Ideal Bars'	.5 oz cookie	90	10.0	5.0
(Nabisco) 'Nutter Butter Peanut Sandwich'	.5 oz	70	9.0	3.0
(Natures Warehouse) approx 1 oz	2 cookies	128	18.2	6.1
(Natures Warehouse) chocolate chip, approx 1 oz	2 cookies	139	13.9	8.5
(Pepperidge Farm) chocolate chunk 'Cheyenne'	1 cookie	110	13.0	6.0
(Pepperidge Farm) chocolate filled 'Nassau'	1 cookie	80	9.0	5.0
(Pepperidge Farm) 'Family Request'	2 cookies	80	10.0	5.0
(Pitter Patter) cream filled, approx .5 oz	1 cookie	90	12.0	4.0
(Planters) crispy cookie 'P.B. Crisps'	1 oz	140	17.0	7.0

Food Name	Serv. Size	Total Cal.	Carbs GMS	Fat GMS
PEANUT CREME *(Nabisco)* 'Nutter Butter Patties'	.5 oz	80	8.0	4.0
PECAN				
(Archway) crunch	1 cookie	60	8.0	3.0
(Dunkin' Donuts) raisin cookie, 1.6 oz	1 cookie	200	28.0	9.0
PRALINE PECAN *(FFV)*	1 cookie	40	10.0	2.0
PRUNE, pastry, dietetic *(Stella D'oro)*	1 cookie	95	15.0	3.4
RAISIN				
(Almost Home)	.5 oz	70	10.0	3.0
(Archway)	1 cookie	100	18.0	3.0
(Archway) bran	1 cookie	100	18.0	3.0
(Archway) oatmeal	1 cookie	50	7.0	2.0
(Break Cake) creme	1 cookie	140	22.0	5.0
(Entenmann's)	2 cookies	80	17.0	0.0
(Featherweight)	1 cookie	45	6.0	2.0
(Grandma's) soft 'Big Cookies' approx 2.75 oz	2 cookies	320	54.0	10.0
(Health Valley) apple 'Fruit Centers' fat-free	1 cookie	70	16.0	0.0
(Health Valley) 'Jumbos' fat-free	1 cookie	80	17.0	0.0
(Health Valley) nut 'Fruit Jumbos'	1 cookie	70	10.0	3.0
(Health Valley) oatmeal, fat-free	3 cookies	80	18.0	0.0
(Keebler) bar, iced	1 cookie	80	11.0	4.0
(Keebler) 'Soft Batch' approx .5 oz	1 cookie	70	10.0	3.0
(Mother's) iced	1 cookie	80	11.0	4.0
(Nabisco) nut 'Newtons'	.5 oz	60	11.0	2.0
(Pepperidge Farm) bran 'Kitchen Hearth'	2 cookies	110	13.0	5.0
(Pepperidge Farm) 'Old Fashioned'	2 cookies	110	15.0	5.0
(Pepperidge Farm) 'Santa Fe'	1 cookie	100	16.0	4.0
(Stella D'oro) 'Golden Bars'	1 cookie	109	16.0	4.3
(Sunshine)	2 cookies	110	16.0	5.0
(Tastykake) bar	1.8 oz	212	31.8	8.3
(Tastykake) 'Soft'n Chewy'	1.4 oz	161	26.8	5.4
(Weight Watchers) spice	3 cookies	80	13.0	2.0
RASPBERRY				
(Bakery Wagon) filled	1 cookie	90	16.0	3.0
(Frookie) 'Fruitins' fat-free	2 cookies	90	21.0	0.0
(Great Cakes)	4.5 oz	260	40.0	6.0
(Health Valley) apple 'Fruit Chunks'	3 cookies	85	19.0	0.0
(Health Valley) apple 'Mini Fruit Centers' fat-free	3 cookies	75	17.0	0.0
(Health Valley) 'Fruit Centers' fat-free	1 cookie	80	17.0	0.0
(Health Valley) 'Jumbos' fat-free	1 cookie	80	17.0	0.0
(Lu) 'Pims'	2 cookies	95	18.0	2.0
(Nabisco) 'Newtons' .75 oz	1 cookie	80	15.0	2.0
(Nabisco) 'Newtons' fat-free	1 cookie	60	16.0	0.0
(Natural Nectar) swirl 'Incredible Edible Novelties'	1 cookie	220	33.0	8.0

Food Name	Serv. Size	Total Cal.	Carbs GMS	Fat GMS
(Natures Warehouse) wheat-free, fat-free	1 oz	90	20.5	0.7
(Pepperidge Farm) filled 'Chantilly'	1 cookie	80	14.0	2.0
(Pepperidge Farm) filled, chocolate 'Chantilly'	1 cookie	90	14.0	3.0
(Pepperidge Farm) filled 'Linzer'	1 cookie	120	20.0	4.0
(Pepperidge Farm) tart, low fat 'Wholesome Choice'	1 cookie	60	11.0	1.0
(Weight Watchers) fruit filled	1 cookie	80	22.0	<1.0
REESE'S PIECES *(Oven Lovin')*	1 cookie	70	9.0	3.0
SESAME				
(Glenny's) 'Nookie' bite size	.5 oz	60	6.0	4.0
(Stella D'oro) dietetic 'Regina'	1 cookie	41	5.1	2.0
(Stella D'oro) 'Regina'	1 cookie	48	6.1	2.2
SHORTBREAD				
(Break Cake) approx 1 oz	5 cookies	140	19.0	6.0
(Estee)	3 cookies	100	16.0	3.0
(FFV) country	1 cookie	70	9.0	4.0
(Keebler) covered 'Fudge'n Caramel'	1 cookie	60	8.0	3.0
(Keebler) fudge covered 'Toffee Toppers'	2 cookies	60	10.0	4.0
(Keebler) fudge striped 'Fudge Stripes' .5 oz	1 cookie	50	7.0	3.0
(Keebler) 'Pecan Sandies' approx .5 oz	1 cookie	80	9.0	5.0
(Keebler) 'Pecan Sandies' bite size	4 cookies	90	9.0	5.0
(Keebler) w/chocolate center 'Magic Middles' .5 oz	1 cookie	80	9.0	5.0
(Keebler) w/toffee pieces 'Toffee Sandies'	1 cookie	70	8.0	4.0
(Lorna Doone) .5 oz	3 cookies	70	9.0	4.0
(Mother's) striped	2 cookies	100	14.0	5.0
(Nabisco) fudge striped 'Cookies 'n Fudge'	.5 oz	60	7.0	3.0
(Nabisco) pecan supreme, low cholesterol	1 cookie	80	9.0	5.0
(Pepperidge Farm) 'Old Fashioned'	2 cookies	150	17.0	8.0
(Pepperidge Farm) pecan 'Old Fashioned'	1 cookie	70	7.0	5.0
(Weight Watchers)	3 cookies	80	13.0	2.0
SNACK, for weight control *(Spicer's)*	1 oz	100	12.0	4.0
SPICE *(Stella D'oro)* 'Pfeffernusse'	1 piece	35	6.7	0.8
STRAWBERRY				
(Healthy Times) 'Hugga Bears' organic	1 oz	120	17.0	3.0
(Health Valley) 'Mini Fruit Centers' fat-free	3 cookies	75	17.0	0.0
(Nabisco) 'Newtons'	1.25 oz	120	24.0	3.0
(Nabisco) 'Newtons' .75 oz	1 cookie	70	15.0	2.0
(Nabisco) 'Newtons' fat-free	1 cookie	60	16.0	0.0
(Nabisco) 'Suddenly S'Mores'	.75 oz	100	15.0	4.0
(Natural Nectar) swirl 'Incredible Edible Novelties'	1 cookie	220	33.0	8.0
(Pepperidge Farm) 'Fruit Cookies'	2 cookies	100	15.0	5.0
SUGAR				
(Almost Home)	.5 oz	70	10.0	3.0
(Almost Home) 'Old Fashioned'	.5 oz	70	10.0	3.0

Food Name	Serv. Size	Total Cal.	Carbs GMS	Fat GMS
(Mother's)	1 cookie	70	8.0	4.0
(Pepperidge Farm) 'Old Fashioned'	2 cookies	100	13.0	5.0
(Stella D'oro) 'Holiday Trinkets'	1 cookie	38	4.6	1.9
TAFFY *(Mother's)* sandwich	1 cookie	100	12.0	6.0
TEA BISCUIT *(Nabisco)* 'Social Tea Biscuit' 3 pieces	.5 oz	60	11.0	2.0
TOFFEE				
(Chips Ahoy!) chunk, Heath 'Selections'	1 cookie	90	5.0	5.0
(Delicious) w/Heath English toffee	1 cookie	90	10.0	5.0
(Pepperidge Farm) 'Old Fashioned'	2 cookies	100	12.0	5.0
TOFU *(Health Valley)* 'The Great Tofu Cookie'	2 cookies	90	16.0	3.0
VANILLA				
(Barbara's Bakery) animal cookies	1 oz	145	18.0	7.0
(Barbara's Bakery) 'Cookies & Creme'	2 cookies	120	18.0	5.0
(Barbara's Bakery) raspberry 'Cookies & Creme'	2 cookies	120	18.0	5.0
(Estee)	3 cookies	100	14.0	5.0
(Estee) sandwich	2 cookies	110	17.0	4.0
(Featherweight)	1 cookie	45	6.0	2.0
(Frookie) 'Funky Monkeys'	8 cookies	60	10.0	2.0
(Frookie) sandwich 'Frookwich'	1 cookie	50	7.0	2.0
(Frookie) 'Trolls'	11 cookies	60	10.0	2.0
(Glenny's) 'Noah 'N Friends Animal Cookies'	.5 oz	65	10.0	2.0
(Grandma's) cookie bits, artificially flavored	1 oz	140	20.0	6.0
(Keebler) creme sandwich 'French' .5 oz	1 cookie	80	12.0	4.0
(Lu) 'Marie Lu'	1 cookie	50	8.0	2.0
(Lu) 'Marie Lu' mini	5 cookies	50	8.0	2.0
(Nabisco) creme sandwich 'Cameo'	.5 oz	70	10.0	3.0
(Nabisco) creme sandwich 'Cookie Break'	1 cookie	50	7.0	2.0
(Nabisco) creme sandwich 'Giggles' 2 pieces	1 oz	60	8.0	3.0
(Nabisco) reduced fat 'Snack Wells'	.5 oz	50	10.0	1.0
(Pepperidge Farm) 'Bordeaux'	2 cookies	70	11.0	3.0
(Pepperidge Farm) chocolate coated 'Orleans'	3 cookies	90	11.0	6.0
(Pepperidge Farm) chocolate laced 'Pirouettes'	2 cookies	70	8.0	4.0
(Pepperidge Farm) chocolate nut coated 'Geneva'	2 cookies	130	14.0	6.0
(Pepperidge Farm) 'Goldfish'	1 oz	140	19.0	7.0
(Pepperidge Farm) 'Pirouettes'	2 cookies	70	9.0	4.0
(Stella D'oro) 'Angelica Goodies'	1 cookie	106	15.7	4.0
(Stella D'oro) 'Castelets'	1 cookie	72	10.0	3.1
(Stella D'oro) 'Margherite'	1 cookie	72	10.8	2.8
(Tastykake) creme sandwich, shortbread	.4 oz	55	6.4	3.0
(Weight Watchers) sandwich	2 cookies	90	15.0	3.0
WAFER				
(Archway) vanilla	1 wafer	30	6.0	<1.0
(Biscos) sugar, 4 pieces	.5 oz	70	10.0	3.0

Food Name	Serv. Size	Total Cal.	Carbs GMS	Fat GMS
(Biscos) waffle creme	1 wafers	45	6.0	2.0
(Break Cake) chocolate, sugar	4 wafers	200	30.0	9.0
(Break Cake) strawberry, sugar	4 wafers	220	28.0	11.0
(Break Cake) 'Striper Wafer'	1 wafer	.190	23.0	10.0
(Break Cake) vanilla, sugar	4 wafers	220	28.0	11.0
(Delicious) chocolate strawberry, sugar	1 wafer	35	3.0	2.0
(Delicious) chocolate, sugar	1 wafer	34	2.0	2.0
(Delicious) strawberry, sugar	1 wafer	35	4.0	2.0
(Delicious) sugar, assorted	.25 oz	38	4.0	2.0
(Delicious) vanilla	.5 oz	70	10.5	2.2
(Delicious) vanilla, sugar	.25 oz	37	4.0	2.0
(Delicious) vanilla, sugar	1 wafer	35	4.0	2.0
(Estee) chocolate creme	4 wafers	90	11.0	5.0
(Estee) strawberry	3 wafers	100	14.0	5.0
(Estee) vanilla	3 wafers	100	14.0	5.0
(Estee) vanilla creme	4 wafers	90	12.0	4.0
(Featherweight) strawberry creme	1 wafer	20	3.0	1.0
(Featherweight) vanilla creme	1 wafers	20	3.0	1.0
(FFV) vanilla, approx 1 oz	8 wafers	130	19.0	5.0
(Fifty 50) chocolate creme filled, w/o sugar	1 wafer	35	4.0	2.0
(Fifty 50) vanilla, creme filled, w/o sugar	1 wafer	35	4.0	2.0
(Keebler) vanilla, golden	4 wafers	80	10.0	3.0
(Lu) cream	3 cookies	110	11.0	7.0
(Mother's) checkerboard	5 wafers	85	13.0	4.0
(Mother's) vanilla, 'Flaky Flix'	2 wafers	115	18.0	5.0
(Nabisco) 'Brown Edge Wafers' 2 1/2 wafers	.5 oz	70	10.0	3.0
(Nabisco) 'Famous Chocolate Wafers' 2 1/2 wafers	.5 oz	60	11.0	2.0
(Nabisco) striped wafer 'Cookies 'N Fudge'	1 wafer	70	8.0	4.0
(Nabisco) vanilla, cinnamon 'Nilla Wafers' .5 oz	3 1/2 wafers	60	11.0	2.0
(Nabisco) vanilla, 'Nilla Wafers' approx .5 oz	3 1/2 wafers	60	11.0	2.0
(Tastykake) vanilla, sugar	10 wafers	34	4.1	1.9
(Weider) 'Victory Explosive Workout'	6 wafers	30	6.0	0.0
(Westbrae) 5-spice	4 1/2 wafers	40	8.0	0.0
WALNUT				
(Keebler) 'Soft Batch' approx .5 oz	1 cookie	80	10.0	4.0
(Lu) whole wheat and cinnamon 'Marie Lu'	1 cookie	45	8.0	1.0
(Mother's) fudge	1 cookie	70	8.0	4.0
COOKIE DOUGH, PREPARED				
chocolate chip	1 oz	126	17.4	5.8
chocolate chip	1 cookie	71	9.8	3.3
chocolate chip *(Pillsbury)*	1 cookie	70	9.0	3.0
chocolate chip, baked	1 oz	139	19.3	6.4
chocolate chip, baked	1 cookie	59	8.2	2.7

Food Name	Serv. Size	Total Cal.	Carbs GMS	Fat GMS
chocolate chip 'Ready To Bake' *(Toll House)*	1.2 oz	150	20.0	7.0
chocolate chip 'Ready To Bake' w/nuts *(Toll House)*	1.2 oz	160	19.0	8.0
double chocolate chip 'Ready To Bake' 1.2 oz *(Toll House)*	2 cookies	150	19.0	7.0
oatmeal	1 oz	120	16.7	5.4
oatmeal	1 cookie	68	9.5	3.0
oatmeal, baked	1 oz	134	18.6	5.9
oatmeal, baked	1 cookie	57	7.9	2.5
oatmeal raisin *(Pillsbury)*	1 cookie	60	9.0	3.0
oatmeal raisin 'Ready To Bake' 2 cookies *(Toll House)*	1.2 oz	130	21.0	5.0
peanut butter *(Pillsbury)*	1 cookie	70	9.0	3.0
sugar	1 oz	124	16.7	5.9
sugar	1 cookie	70	9.4	3.3
sugar *(Pillsbury)*	1 cookie	70	9.0	3.0
sugar, baked	1 oz	137	18.6	6.6

COOKIE MIX

Food Name	Serv. Size	Total Cal.	Carbs GMS	Fat GMS
chocolate chip *(Duncan Hines)*	2 cookies	130	20.0	5.0
chocolate chip *(Finast)*	2 cookies	110	16.0	5.0
chocolate chip, 2-inch diam each *(Estee)*	2 cookies	90	13.0	4.0
chocolate chip 'Big Batch' *(Betty Crocker)*	2 cookies	120	16.0	6.0
'Deluxe' 2-inch diam *(Krusteaz)*	1 cookie	120	16.0	5.0
golden sugar *(Duncan Hines)*	2 cookies	130	17.0	6.0
oatmeal raisin *(Duncan Hines)*	2 cookies	130	18.0	6.0
peanut butter *(Duncan Hines)*	2 cookies	140	15.0	7.0

COOKING SPRAY

Food Name	Serv. Size	Total Cal.	Carbs GMS	Fat GMS
(Mazola) corn oil 'No Stick'	2.5-sec spray	6	0.0	1.0
(Pam) for 1/3 of 10-inch skillet	1 spray	2	0.0	1.0
(Weight Watchers) 'Buttery Spray' butter flavor	1-sec spray	2	0.0	<1.0
(Weight Watchers) canola oil spray	.33 grams	2	0.0	<1.0
(Weight Watchers) 'Cooking Spray'	1-sec spray	2	0.0	1.0
(Wesson) lite	.27 grams	<1	0.0	<1.0
(Wesson) no-stick	.25 gram	2	0.0	0.3

COOL WHIP. See CREAM TOPPING, NONDAIRY.

CORIANDER/Chinese parsley

Food Name	Serv. Size	Total Cal.	Carbs GMS	Fat GMS
raw	1 tbsp	5	0.9	0.1
raw	1 tsp	2	0.3	0.0
raw, approx .8 oz	9 plants	4	0.5	0.1
trimmed	1 oz	6	0.7	0.2
untrimmed	1 lb	77	10.0	2.3

CORIANDER LEAF/Chinese parsley leaf

Food Name	Serv. Size	Total Cal.	Carbs GMS	Fat GMS
dried	1 oz	79	14.8	1.3
dried	1 tbsp	5	0.9	0.1
dried	1 tsp	2	0.3	<.1

Food Name	Serv. Size	Total Cal.	Carbs GMS	Fat GMS
CORIANDER SEED/Chinese parsley seed				
whole	1 oz	84	15.6	5.0
whole	1 tbsp	15	2.8	0.9
whole	1 tsp	5	1.0	0.3
whole *(Durkee)*	1 tsp	8	0.0	<.1
whole *(Laurel Leaf)*	1 tsp	8	0.0	<.1
whole *(Spice Islands)*	1 tsp	6	0.8	0.3
CORN				
cooked	1/2 cup	88	19.5	0.5
dry	1 cup	375	83.2	2.2
dry	2 oz	203	45.2	1.2
sweet, boiled, drained	4 oz	122	28.5	1.5
sweet, raw, trimmed	1 oz	24	5.4	0.3
sweet, raw, untrimmed	1 lb	140	31.1	1.9
sweet, white, boiled, drained, cut	1/2 cup	89	20.6	1.0
sweet, white, kernels, boiled, drained	1 ear	83	19.3	1.0
sweet, white, kernels from cob, raw	1 ear	77	17.1	1.1
sweet, white, raw, cut	1/2 cup	66	14.7	0.9
sweet, yellow, boiled, drained, cut	1/2 cup	89	20.6	1.0
sweet, yellow, kernels, boiled, drained	1 ear	83	19.3	1.0
sweet, yellow, kernels from cob, raw	1 ear	77	17.1	1.1
sweet, yellow, raw, cut	1/2 cup	66	14.7	0.9
white	1/2 cup	303	61.6	3.9
yellow	1/2 cup	303	61.6	3.9
CORN, CANNED				
cream style	1/2 cup	93	23.2	0.5
cream style	4 oz	82	20.6	0.5
cream style *(A&P)*	1/2 cup	100	25.0	1.0
cream style *(Finast)*	1/2 cup	105	25.0	1.0
cream style *(Green Giant)*	1/2 cup	100	24.0	<1.0
cream style *(S&W Nutradiet)*	1/2 cup	100	21.0	1.0
cream style, golden *(Del Monte)*	1/2 cup	80	18.0	1.0
cream style, golden *(Pathmark)*	1/2 cup	100	25.0	1.0
cream style, golden *(Stokely)*	1/2 cup	100	23.0	0.0
cream style, golden, low-sodium	4 oz	82	20.6	0.5
cream style, golden 'No Salt Added' *(Del Monte)*	1/2 cup	80	20.0	1.0
cream style, golden, white *(Stokely)*	1/2 cup	100	23.0	0.0
cream style 'No Frills' *(Pathmark)*	1 cup	210	51.0	1.0
cream style 'Premium Homestyle No Starch Added' *(S&W)*	1/2 cup	120	24.0	1.0
cream style 'Premium Homestyle Starch Added' *(S&W)*	1/2 cup	105	25.0	1.0
cream style, white *(Del Monte)*	1/2 cup	90	21.0	0.0
'Crisp 'N Sweet' vacuum packed *(Freshlike)*	1/2 cup	80	18.0	1.0
'Delicorn' *(Green Giant)*	1/2 cup	80	19.0	<1.0

Food Name	Serv. Size	Total Cal.	Carbs GMS	Fat GMS
golden (Pathmark)	1/2 cup	90	19.0	1.0
golden (Stokely)	1/2 cup	90	20.0	0.0
golden, cream style (Freshlike)	1/2 cup	110	25.0	1.0
golden, cream style (Veg•All)	1/2 cup	110	25.0	1.0
golden, cream style, no salt added (Freshlike)	1/2 cup	110	25.0	1.0
golden, 50% less salt (Green Giant)	1/2 cup	70	16.0	<1.0
golden 'No Salt Added' (Del Monte)	1/2 cup	80	18.0	1.0
golden 'No Salt or Sugar Added' (Green Giant)	1/2 cup	80	18.0	<1.0
golden 'No Salt or Sugar Added' (Stokely)	1/2 cup	80	16.0	0.0
golden 'Pantry Express' (Green Giant)	1/2 cup	80	18.0	<1.0
golden, sweet (IGA)	1/2 cup	70	16.0	1.0
golden, vacuum pack (Green Giant)	1/2 cup	80	20.0	0.0
golden, vacuum pack (Stokely)	1/2 cup	90	22.0	0.0
golden, whole kernel (Veg•All)	1/2 cup	80	19.0	1.0
golden, whole kernel, vacuum packed (Freshlike)	1/2 cup	100	22.0	1.0
golden, whole kernel, vacuum packed (Veg•All)	1/2 cup	100	22.0	1.0
golden, whole kernel, water packed, w/o salt (Freshlike)	1/2 cup	80	19.0	1.0
golden, whole kernel, water packed, w/o sugar and salt (Freshlike)	1/2 cup	80	19.0	1.0
golden, w/liquid (Del Monte)	1/2 cup	70	17.0	1.0
in brine, w/liquid (Green Giant)	1/2 cup	70	18.0	0.0
kernel, w/liquid	4 oz	69	16.8	0.5
kernel, w/liquid (A&P)	1/2 cup	80	20.0	1.0
kernel, w/liquid (Featherweight)	1/2 cup	80	16.0	1.0
kernel, w/liquid (Finast)	1/2 cup	90	20.0	1.0
kernel, w/liquid (Green Giant)	1/2 cup	80	18.0	0.0
kernel, w/liquid (S&W Nutradiet)	1/2 cup	80	15.0	1.0
kernel, w/liquid, drained	4 oz	92	21.1	1.1
kernel, w/liquid, 50% less salt, no sugar (Green Giant)	1/2 cup	50	11.0	1.0
kernel, w/liquid, low-sodium	4 oz	69	16.8	0.5
kernel, w/liquid 'No Frills' (Pathmark)	1 cup	160	38.0	1.0
kernel, w/liquid 'No Salt Added' (A&P)	1/2 cup	80	18.0	<1.0
kernel, w/liquid 'No Salt Added' (Finast)	1/2 cup	80	19.0	1.0
kernel, w/liquid 'No Salt Added' (Pathmark)	1/2 cup	70	16.0	1.0
niblets (Green Giant)	1/2 cup	80	20.0	0.0
niblets, no salt, no sugar added (Green Giant)	1/2 cup	80	18.0	<1.0
sweet, select (Green Giant)	1/2 cup	60	15.0	<1.0
sweet, white, brine pack, drained solids	1/2 cup	66	15.2	0.8
sweet, white, brine pack, regular, w/liquid	1/2 cup	78	19.0	0.6
sweet, white, brine pack, dietary, w/liquid	1/2 cup	78	19.0	0.6
sweet, white, cream style, regular pack	1/2 cup	92	23.2	0.5
sweet, white, cream style, special dietary pack	1/2 cup	92	23.2	0.5
sweet, white, vacuum pack, regular pack	1/2 cup	83	20.4	0.5

Food Name	Serv. Size	Total Cal.	Carbs GMS	Fat GMS
sweet, white, vacuum pack, special dietary pack	1/2 cup	83	20.4	0.5
sweet, yellow, brine pack, drained solids	1/2 cup	66	15.2	0.8
sweet, yellow, brine pack, regular, w/liquid	1/2 cup	78	19.0	0.6
sweet, yellow, brine pack, dietary, w/liquid	1/2 cup	78	19.0	0.6
sweet, yellow, cream style, regular pack	1/2 cup	92	23.2	0.5
sweet, yellow, cream style, special dietary pack	1/2 cup	92	23.2	0.5
sweet, yellow, vacuum pack, regular pack	1/2 cup	83	20.4	0.5
sweet, yellow, vacuum pack, special dietary pack	1/2 cup	83	20.4	0.5
vacuum pack, w/liquid (Del Monte)	1/2 cup	90	22.0	1.0
vacuum pack, w/liquid 'No Salt Added' (Del Monte)	1/2 cup	90	22.0	1.0
white (Green Giant)	1/2 cup	80	20.0	0.0
white (Stokely)	1/2 cup	90	21.0	0.0
white, vacuum pack (A&P)	1/2 cup	100	25.0	1.0
white, vacuum pack (Finast)	4 oz	90	20.0	1.0
white, vacuum pack (Green Giant)	1/2 cup	80	20.0	0.0
white, vacuum pack (Pathmark)	1/2 cup	120	25.0	1.0
white, vacuum pack 'Niblets' (Green Giant)	1/2 cup	80	16.0	1.0
white, w/liquid (Del Monte)	1/2 cup	70	16.0	0.0
white, young, tender 'Premium' (S&W)	1/2 cup	90	20.0	1.0
whole kernel, golden, sweet (Green Giant)	1/2 cup	70	18.0	0.0
whole kernel, golden, sweet,50% less salt (Green Giant)	1/2 cup	70	16.0	<1.0
w/peppers 'Mexicorn' (Green Giant)	1/2 cup	80	19.0	<1.0
CORN, FROZEN				
(Health Valley)	1/2 cup	76	17.0	0.0
cream style (Green Giant)	1/2 cup	110	25.0	1.0
freeze-dried, prepared (Mountain House)	1/2 cup	90	18.0	1.0
golden, in butter sauce (Green Giant)	1/2 cup	100	19.0	2.0
in butter sauce (Finast)	1/2 cup	170	30.0	4.0
in butter sauce 'Niblets' (Green Giant)	1/2 cup	100	18.0	2.0
in butter sauce 'Niblets One Serving' (Green Giant)	4.5 oz	120	24.0	2.0
in butter sauce 'Side Dish' (Budget Gourmet)	5.5 oz	190	31.0	6.0
in butter sauce 'Singles' (Stokely)	4 oz	110	23.0	1.0
in sauce, country style 'Side Dish' (Budget Gourmet)	5.75 oz	140	19.0	5.0
kernel (A&P)	3.3 oz	80	18.0	<1.0
kernel (Finast)	3.3 oz	80	20.0	1.0
kernel, cut (Frosty Acres)	3.3 oz	80	20.0	1.0
kernel, cut (Seabrook)	3.3 oz	80	20.0	1.0
kernel, cut (Southern)	3.5 oz	98	21.3	0.7
kernel, cut, petite 'Deluxe' (Birds Eye)	2.6 oz	70	16.0	1.0
kernel, cut 'Portion Pack' (Birds Eye)	3 oz	70	18.0	1.0
kernel, cut 'Singles' (Stokely)	3 oz	75	18.0	1.0
kernel 'Harvest Fresh Niblets' (Green Giant)	1/2 cup	80	17.0	1.0
kernel 'Niblets' (Green Giant)	1/2 cup	90	19.0	<1.0

Food Name	Serv. Size	Total Cal.	Carbs GMS	Fat GMS
kernel 'Niblets Supersweet' (Green Giant)	1/2 cup	60	13.0	1.0
kernel 'Sweet' (Birds Eye)	3.3 oz	80	20.0	1.0
kernel 'Tender Sweet Deluxe' (Birds Eye)	3.3 oz	80	20.0	1.0
niblets 'Butter Sauce' (Green Giant)	1/2 cup	100	19.0	2.0
niblets 'Plain Polybag' (Green Giant)	1/2 cup	90	19.0	<1.0
on the cob (A&P)	1 ear	120	28.0	1.0
on the cob (Birds Eye)	1 ear	120	29.0	1.0
on the cob (Frosty Acres)	1 ear	120	29.0	1.0
on the cob (Seabrook)	5-inch ear	120	29.0	1.0
on the cob (Southern)	5-inch ear	140	30.0	1.0
on the cob, baby 'Deluxe' (Birds Eye)	2.6 oz	25	4.0	0.0
on the cob 'Big Ears' (Birds Eye)	1 ear	160	37.0	1.0
on the cob, boiled, drained, kernels from ear	4 oz	59	14.1	0.5
on the cob 'Cob Treats' (A&P)	2 ears	130	28.0	1.0
on the cob, 5.3 oz edible portion (Ore-Ida)	1 ear	180	39.0	2.0
on the cob, in butter sauce 'Singles' (Stokely)	1 ear	70	16.0	1.0
on the cob, kernels from ear	8 oz	123	29.4	1.0
on the cob 'Little Ears' (Birds Eye)	2 ears	130	30.0	1.0
on the cob, miniature 'Mini-Gold' (Ore-Ida)	2 ears	180	39.0	2.0
on the cob 'Nibblers, 6-ear pkg' (Green Giant)	2 ears	120	27.0	1.0
on the cob 'Nibblers Supersweet' (Green Giant)	2 ears	90	19.0	2.0
on the cob 'Niblet Ears' (Green Giant)	1 ear	120	27.0	1.0
on the cob 'Niblet Ears Supersweet' (Green Giant)	1 ear	90	19.0	2.0
on the cob 'One Serving' (Green Giant)	2 half ears	120	26.0	1.0
on the cob 'Sweet Select' (Green Giant)	1 ear	90	19.0	2.0
on the cob 'Sweet Select' half ears (Green Giant)	2 half ears	90	19.0	2.0
sweet (Birds Eye)	3.3 oz	80	20.0	1.0
sweet, select 'Plain Polybag' (Green Giant)	1/2 cup	60	13.0	1.0
sweet, tender 'Butter Sauce Combination' (Birds Eye)	3.3 oz	90	17.0	2.0
sweet, tender 'Deluxe' (Birds Eye)	3.3 oz	80	20.0	1.0
sweet, white, kernels, boiled, drained	1 ear	59	14.1	0.5
sweet, white, kernels, boiled, drained	1/2 cup	76	18.3	0.6
sweet, white, kernels, unprepared	1/2 cup	72	17.1	0.6
sweet, yellow, kernels, boiled, drained	1 ear	59	14.1	0.5
sweet, yellow, kernels, boiled, drained	1/2 cup	76	18.3	0.6
sweet, yellow, kernels, unprepared	1/2 cup	72	17.1	0.6
white (Green Giant)	1/2 cup	90	19.0	1.0
white (Seabrook)	3.3 oz	80	19.0	1.0
white, in butter sauce (Green Giant)	1/2 cup	100	20.0	2.0
white, shoepeg 'Butter Sauce' (Green Giant)	1/2 cup	100	20.0	2.0
white, shoepeg 'Harvest Fresh' (Green Giant)	1/2 cup	90	19.0	1.0
white, shoepeg 'Select' (Green Giant)	1/2 cup	90	19.0	<1.0
whole kernel, 'Portion Pack' (Birds Eye)	3 oz	70	18.0	1.0

Food Name	Serv. Size	Total Cal.	Carbs GMS	Fat GMS
CORN AND PEPPERS, CANNED				
red and green peppers, solid and liquid	1/2 cup	86	20.7	0.6
vacuum packed *(Freshlike)*	1/2 cup	90	23.0	1.0
vacuum packed *(Veg•All)*	1/2 cup	90	23.0	1.0
CORN BRAN				
crude	1 cup	170	65.1	0.7
crude	1 oz	64	24.3	0.3
CORN CAKE				
apple cinnamon flavor *(Roman Meal)*	1 cake	49	10.5	<1.0
caramel, fat-free *(Quaker)*	1 cake	50	12.0	0.0
caramel flavor, fat free *(Roman Meal)*	1 cake	50	11.0	0.0
cheddar flavor *(Roman Meal)*	1 cake	43	9.0	<1.0
natural butter flavor, fat free *(Roman Meal)*	1 cake	40	8.0	0.0
plain	1 cake	35	7.5	0.2
popcorn	1 cake	38	8.0	0.3
popcorn, butter flavor *(Chico-San)*	1 cake	40	8.0	0.0
popcorn, caramel *(Chico-San)*	1 cake	50	10.0	0.0
popcorn, lightly salted *(Chico-San)*	1 cake	40	8.0	0.0
popcorn, white cheddar cheese *(Chico-San)*	1 cake	50	9.0	1.0
popped, butter flavor *(Quaker)*	1 cake	35	7.0	0.0
popped, white cheddar flavor *(Quaker)*	1 cake	40	8.0	0.0
very low sodium	1 cake	24	6.3	0.0
white cheddar flavor, fat free *(Roman Meal)*	1 cake	45	9.0	0.0
CORN CHIPS AND SNACKS. See also TORTILLA CHIPS.				
barbecue *(Bachman)*	1 oz	150	17.0	9.0
barbecue 'Rowdy Rustlers' 34 chips *(Fritos)*	1 oz	150	17.0	9.0
'Bar-B-Q Fritos' 34 pieces *(Fritos)*	1 oz	150	16.0	9.0
bare bean 'Garden Vegetable Chips' *(Harry's)*	1 oz	144	17.0	7.0
bare bean 'Offbeat Originals' *(Peddlers)*	1 oz	144	17.0	7.0
beet garlic 'Garden Vegetable Chips' *(Harry's)*	1 oz	134	20.0	5.0
beet garlic 'Offbeat Originals' *(Peddlers)*	1 oz	134	20.0	5.0
bell pepper 'Garden Vegetable Chips' *(Harry's)*	1 oz	140	19.0	6.0
bell pepper 'Offbeat Originals' *(Peddlers)*	1 oz	140	19.0	6.0
blue corn 'Corn Curls' *(Arrowhead Mills)*	1 oz	120	22.0	2.0
blue corn 'Corn Curls Unsalted' *(Arrowhead Mills)*	1 oz	120	22.0	2.0
blue corn, no salt added *(Barbara's Bakery)*	1 oz	140	18.0	7.0
blue corn, regular *(Barbara's Bakery)*	1 oz	140	18.0	7.0
blue garlic 'Garden Vegetable Chips' *(Harry's)*	1 oz	129	21.0	4.0
blue garlic 'Offbeat Originals' *(Peddlers)*	1 oz	129	21.0	4.0
caramel corn puffs, apple cinnamon, fat-free *(Health Valley)*	1 oz	100	21.0	0.0
caramel corn puffs, original style, fat-free *(Health Valley)*	1 oz	100	21.0	0.0
caramel corn puffs, peanut flavor, fat-free *(Health Valley)*	1 oz	100	21.0	0.0
carrot caraway 'Garden Vegetable Chips' *(Harry's)*	1 oz	131	20.0	4.0

Food Name	Serv. Size	Total Cal.	Carbs GMS	Fat GMS
carrot caraway 'Offbeat Originals' (Peddlers)	1 oz	131	20.0	4.0
cheddar cheese (Health Valley)	1 oz	160	15.0	10.0
cheese 'Baked' (Jax)	1 oz	140	17.0	7.0
cheese 'Baked, Corn Puffs' (Cheez Doodles)	1 oz	150	17.0	8.0
cheese 'Cheese Curls Low Salt' (Featherweight)	1 oz	150	16.0	9.0
cheese 'Crunchy' (Jax)	1 oz	160	14.0	11.0
cheese curls 'Great Tasting' (Ultra Slim Fast)	1 oz	110	20.0	3.0
cheese 'Fried Corn Puffs' (Cheez Doodles)	1 oz	160	15.0	10.0
chili cheese, 34 chips (Fritos)	1 oz	160	15.0	10.0
cones, nacho-flavor	1 oz	152	16.2	9.0
cones, plain	1 oz	145	17.8	7.6
cool ranch (Doritos)	1 oz	140	18.0	7.0
corn chips (Wise)	1 oz	160	15.0	10.0
corn crunchies (Wise)	1 oz	160	15.0	10.0
corn nuggets, toasted (Fritos)	1.38 oz	170	29.0	5.0
corn ridgies (Wise)	1 oz	160	15.0	10.0
corn spirals, toasted (Wise)	1 oz	160	15.0	10.0
corn twists, crispy (Wise)	1 oz	160	15.0	10.0
'Crisp 'N Thin' 18 chips (Fritos)	1 oz	160	16.0	10.0
curls, barbecue flavored (Weight Watchers)	.5 oz	60	10.0	2.0
curls, pizza flavored (Weight Watchers)	.5 oz	60	10.0	2.0
curls, ranch flavored (Weight Watchers)	.5 oz	60	9.0	2.0
'Dip Size Fritos' 13 pieces (Fritos)	1 oz	150	17.0	9.0
'Fritos' 34 pieces (Fritos)	1 oz	150	16.0	9.0
'Low Salt' (Featherweight)	1 oz	170	15.0	11.0
mild bean 'Garden Vegetable Chips' (Harry's)	1 oz	144	17.0	7.0
mild bean 'Offbeat Originals' (Peddlers)	1 oz	144	17.0	7.0
nacho cheese (Bugles)	1 oz	160	17.0	9.0
nacho cheese (Corn Snackers)	.5-oz pkg	60	10.0	2.0
nacho cheese flavor (Doritos)	1 oz	140	18.0	7.0
nacho cheese 'Non-Stop' 34 chips (Fritos)	1 oz	150	16.0	9.0
'No Salt Added' (Health Valley)	1 oz	160	13.0	11.0
onion-flavor	1 oz	142	18.5	6.4
'Pinta Blues' picante (Barbara's Bakery)	1 oz	130	18.0	6.0
'Pinta Blues' regular (Barbara's Bakery)	1 oz	140	20.0	6.0
'Pinta Puffs' salsa (Barbara's Bakery)	1 oz	70	10.0	6.0
'Pinta' regular (Barbara's Bakery)	1 oz	138	18.0	6.0
plain	1 oz	153	16.1	9.5
plain (Bachman)	1 oz	160	15.0	10.0
plain (Bugles)	1 oz	150	18.0	8.0
plain (Corn Snackers)	.5-oz pkg	60	10.0	2.0
plain (Health Valley)	1 oz	160	13.0	11.0
plain (Planters)	1 oz	160	15.0	10.0

Food Name	Serv. Size	Total Cal.	Carbs GMS	Fat GMS
plain *(Snyder's)*	1 oz	160	14.0	11.0
'Potilla' chipotle chili *(Barbara's Bakery)*	1 oz	140	18.0	8.0
'Potilla' regular *(Barbara's Bakery)*	1 oz	140	18.0	8.0
puffs, cheese-flavor	1 oz	157	15.2	9.8
puffs, cheese-flavor, enriched	1 oz	110	23.6	0.7
ranch *(Bugles)*	1 oz	150	16.0	9.0
'Rippled Corn Chips' *(Dipsy Doodles)*	1 oz	160	15.0	10.0
toasted corn, crunchy, barbecue *(Cornuts)*	2 oz	247	40.7	8.1
toasted corn, crunchy, barbecue *(Cornuts)*	1 oz	124	20.3	4.1
toasted corn, crunchy, chili picante *(Cornuts)*	1 oz	120	22.0	4.0
toasted corn, crunchy, nacho *(Cornuts)*	2 oz	248	40.6	8.1
toasted corn, crunchy, nacho *(Cornuts)*	1 oz	124	20.3	4.0
toasted corn, crunchy, original *(Cornuts)*	2 oz	249	41.6	8.0
toasted corn, crunchy, original *(Cornuts)*	1 oz	124	20.8	4.0
toasted corn, crunchy, ranch *(Cornuts)*	1 oz	120	20.0	4.0
toasted corn, crunchy, unsalted *(Cornuts)*	1 oz	120	19.0	4.0
'Unsalted' *(Azteca)*	1 oz	140	18.0	7.0
veggie 'Garden Vegetable Chips' *(Harry's)*	1 oz	141	18.0	7.0
veggie 'Offbeat Originals' *(Peddlers)*	1 oz	141	18.0	7.0
wild bean 'Garden Vegetable Chips' *(Harry's)*	1 oz	141	17.8	6.0
wild bean 'Offbeat Originals' *(Peddlers)*	1 oz	141	17.8	6.0
'Wild 'N Mild' 32 chips *(Fritos)*	1 oz	160	16.0	9.0
yellow 'Corn Chips' *(Arrowhead Mills)*	.75 oz	90	18.0	1.0
yellow, w/cheese 'Corn Chips' *(Arrowhead Mills)*	.75 oz	90	15.0	2.0
CORN FLAKE CRUMBS *(Kellogg's)*	1 oz	100	24.0	0.0
CORN FLOUR				
masa	1 oz	103	21.6	1.1
masa, enriched, white	1 cup	416	86.9	4.3
masa, enriched, yellow	1 cup	416	86.9	4.3
'Masa Harina De Maiz' approx 1/3 cup *(Quaker)*	1.3 oz	137	27.4	1.5
'Masa Trigo' approx 1/3 cup *(Quaker)*	1.3 oz	149	24.7	4.0
whole-grain	1 oz	102	21.8	1.1
whole-grain, white	1/2 cup	209	44.6	2.2
whole-grain, yellow	1/2 cup	209	44.6	2.2
CORN FRITTER, frozen *(Mrs. Paul's)*	2 pieces	240	35.0	9.0
CORN GRITS: See GRITS.				
CORN NUGGETS, FROZEN				
breaded, fried 'Quickkrisp' *(Stilwell)*	3 oz	210	30.0	8.0
CORN OIL				
	1/2 cup	964	0.0	109.0
	1 oz	251	0.0	28.4
	1 tbsp	120	0.0	13.6
(Crisco)	1 tbsp	120	0.0	14.0

Food Name	Serv. Size	Total Cal.	Carbs GMS	Fat GMS
(Crisco) 'Puritan'	1 tbsp	120	0.0	14.0
(Hain)	1 tbsp	120	0.0	14.0
(Kroger)	1 tbsp	122	0.0	13.6
(Mazola)	1 tbsp	120	0.0	14.0
(Pathmark)	1 tbsp	130	0.0	14.0
(Pathmark) 'No Frills'	1 tbsp	130	0.0	14.0
(Spectrum Naturals)	1 tbsp	120	0.0	14.0
(Wesson)	1 tbsp	120	0.0	14.0
CORN OIL SPRAY. See COOKING SPRAY.				
CORN OIL SPREAD				
(Fleischmann's) 60% oil 'Light'	1 tbsp	80	0.0	8.0
(Fleischmann's) 40% oil 'Extra Light'	1 tbsp	50	0.0	6.0
CORN SALAD, raw	1/2 cup	6	1.0	0.1
CORN SOUFFLÉ, FROZEN, 1 pkg (Stouffer's)	6 oz	240	27.0	11.0
CORN SYRUP				
dark	1 cup	925	251.3	0.0
dark	1 tbsp	56	15.3	0.0
dark (Karo)	1 tbsp	60	15.0	0.0
high-fructose	1 cup	871	235.6	0.0
high-fructose	1 tbsp	53	14.4	0.0
light	1 cup	925	251.3	0.0
light	1 tbsp	56	15.3	0.0
light (Karo)	1 tbsp	60	15.0	0.0
table blends, refiner, and sugar	1 cup	1008	265.1	0.0
table blends, refiner, and sugar	1 tbsp	64	16.8	0.0
CORNBREAD. See BREAD.				
CORNMEAL				
	1 cup	605	123.3	7.9
	1 oz	103	21.1	1.3
blue, whole-grain (Arrowhead Mills)	2 oz	210	41.0	3.0
degermed	1 oz	104	22.0	0.5
degermed, enriched, white	1 cup	505	107.2	2.3
degermed, enriched, yellow	1 cup	505	107.2	2.3
degermed, unenriched, white	1 cup	505	107.2	2.3
degermed, unenriched, yellow	1 cup	505	107.2	2.3
white, bolted (Aunt Jemima)	1 oz	99	20.8	0.7
white, bolted, enriched (Aunt Jemima)	1 oz	99	20.4	0.9
white, dry (Albers)	1 oz	100	22.0	1.0
white, enriched, approx 3 tbsp (Aunt Jemima)	1 oz	102	22.2	0.5
white, whole-grain	1 cup	442	93.8	4.4
whole-grain	1 oz	103	21.8	1.0
whole-grain, hi-lysine (Arrowhead Mills)	2 oz	210	43.0	2.0
yellow, dry (Albers)	1 oz	100	22.0	1.0

Food Name	Serv. Size	Total Cal.	Carbs GMS	Fat GMS
yellow, enriched (Aunt Jemima)	1 oz	102	22.2	0.5
yellow, whole-grain	1 cup	442	93.8	4.4
yellow, whole-grain (Arrowhead Mills)	2 oz	210	43.0	2.0
CORNMEAL, SELF-RISING				
bolted	1 oz	95	19.9	1.0
bolted, w/wheat flour	1 oz	99	20.8	0.8
degermed	1 oz	101	21.2	0.5
white (Aunt Jemima)	1 oz	98	21.1	0.5
white, bolted (Aunt Jemima)	1 oz	98	21.1	0.5
white, bolted, enriched (Aunt Jemima)	1 oz	99	20.4	0.9
white, bolted, plain, enriched	1 cup	407	85.7	4.2
white, bolted, wheat flour added, enriched	1 cup	592	124.8	4.8
white, buttermilk (Aunt Jemima)	3 tbsp	101	20.2	1.1
white, degermed, enriched	1 cup	490	103.2	2.4
yellow (Aunt Jemima)	3 tbsp	100	21.0	1.0
yellow, bolted, plain, enriched	1 cup	407	85.7	4.2
yellow, bolted, wheat flour added, enriched	1 cup	592	124.8	4.8
yellow, degermed, enriched	1 cup	490	103.2	2.4
CORNED BEEF. See BEEF, CORNED.				
CORNISH GAME HEN				
frozen (Tyson)	3.5 oz	240	0.0	14.0
frozen, w/skin (Tyson)	3.5 oz	250	1.0	15.0
w/wild rice, wholesale club item (Tyson)	3.5 oz	190	6.0	11.0
CORNSTARCH				
	1 cup	488	116.8	0.1
	1 oz	108	25.9	<.1
	1 tbsp	30	7.3	tr
(Argo)	1 tbsp	30	7.0	0.0
(Cream)	1 tbsp	29	7.0	tr
(Kingsford)	1 tbsp	30	7.0	0.0
COTTAGE CHEESE. See CHEESE.				
COTTONSEED FLOUR				
lowfat	1 oz	94	10.2	0.4
partially defatted	1 cup	337	38.1	5.8
partially defatted	1 oz	102	11.5	1.8
partially defatted	1 tbsp	18	2.0	0.3
COTTONSEED KERNELS				
roasted	1 cup	754	32.6	54.1
roasted	1 oz	143	6.2	10.3
roasted	1 tbsp	51	2.2	3.6
COTTONSEED MEAL, partially defatted	1 oz	104	10.9	1.4
COTTONSEED OIL				
	1 cup	1927	0.0	218.0

Food Name	Serv. Size	Total Cal.	Carbs GMS	Fat GMS
....	1/2 cup	964	0.0	109.0
....	1 tbsp	120	0.0	13.6
(Wesson)	1 tbsp	122	0.0	13.6
COUSCOUS				
cooked	1/2 cup	101	20.8	.1
cooked	4 oz	127	26.3	0.2
dry	1/2 cup	346	71.2	0.6
dry	1 oz	107	22.0	0.2
mix, dry *(Near East)*	1.25 oz	120	26.0	0.0
mix, prepared w/2 tbsp salted butter *(Fantastic Foods)*	1/2 cup	122	22.0	3.0
mix, prepared w/o added ingredients *(Fantastic Foods)* ...	1/2 cup	105	22.0	0.0
mix, whole-wheat *(Fantastic Foods)*	1/2 cup	94	20.0	0.0
mix, whole-wheat, prepared w/2 tbsp salted butter				
(Fantastic Foods)	1/2 cup	111	20.0	2.0
COUSCOUS PILAF MIX				
(Casbah) dry	1 oz	100	20.0	0.0
(Casbah) prepared w/o added ingredients	1/2 cup	100	20.0	0.0
(Quick Pilaf) savory, prepared w/2 tbsp salted butter	1/2 cup	124	19.0	3.0
(Quick Pilaf) savory, prepared w/o added ingredients	1/2 cup	94	19.0	0.0
COWPEA. See BLACK-EYED PEAS.				
CRAB				
ALASKAN KING				
boiled	4 oz	110	0.0	1.7
boiled, approx 4.7 oz	1 leg	129	0.0	1.7
moist-heat cooked	3 oz	82	0.0	1.3
poached	4 oz	110	0.0	1.7
poached, approx 4.7 oz	1 leg	129	0.0	1.7
raw	1 lb	379	0.0	2.7
raw	3 oz	71	0.0	0.5
raw	1 oz	24	0.0	0.2
steamed	4 oz	110	0.0	1.7
steamed, approx 4.7 oz	1 leg	129	0.0	1.7
BLUE				
boiled	4 oz	116	0.0	2.0
boiled, approx 4.75 oz	1 cup	138	0.0	2.4
cake, fried	4 oz	176	0.5	8.5
cake, fried, approx 2.1 oz	1 med	93	0.3	4.5
canned	1 cup	134	0.0	1.7
canned	4 oz	112	0.0	1.4
canned	3 oz	84	0.0	1.0
moist-heat cooked	1 cup	138	0.0	2.4
moist-heat cooked	3 oz	87	0.0	1.5
poached	4 oz	116	0.0	2.0

Food Name	Serv. Size	Total Cal.	Carbs GMS	Fat GMS
poached, approx 4.75 oz	1 cup	138	0.0	2.4
raw	1 lb	395	0.2	4.9
raw	3 oz	74	0.0	0.9
raw	1 oz	25	<.1	0.3
steamed	4 oz	116	0.0	2.0
steamed, approx 4.75 oz	1 cup	138	0.0	2.4
DUNGENESS				
canned (S&W)	3.25 oz	81	1.0	2.0
moist-heat cooked	3 oz	94	0.8	1.0
raw	1 lb	391	3.3	4.4
raw	3 oz	73	0.6	0.8
raw	1 oz	24	0.2	0.3
IMPERIAL	1 cup	323	8.6	16.7
QUEEN				
moist-heat cooked	100 gm	115	0.0	1.5
moist-heat cooked	3 oz	98	0.0	1.3
raw	1 lb	407	0.0	5.4
raw	3 oz	77	0.0	1.0
raw	1 oz	26	0.0	0.3
SNOW				
frozen (Wakefield)	3 oz	60	0.0	1.0
raw, Opilio, clusters (Peter Pan Seafoods)	3.5 oz	91	na	1.2
raw, Opilio, 'Snap 'n' Eat' scored (Peter Pan Seafoods)	3.5 oz	91	na	1.2
SOFTSHELL				
boiled	4 oz	116	0.0	2.0
boiled, approx 4.75 oz	1 cup	138	0.0	2.4
cake, fried	4 oz	176	0.5	8.5
cake, fried, approx 2.1 oz	1 med	93	0.3	4.5
poached	4 oz	116	0.0	2.0
poached, approx 4.75 oz	1 cup	138	0.0	2.4
raw	1 lb	395	0.2	4.9
raw	1 oz	25	<.1	0.3
raw, approx .7 oz	1 crab	18	<.1	0.2
steamed	4 oz	116	0.0	2.0
steamed, approx 4.75 oz	1 cup	138	0.0	2.4
CRAB, ALTERNATIVE				
	1 lb	463	46.4	5.9
	1 oz	29	3.0	0.4
Alaskan King, made from surimi	3 oz	87	8.7	1.1
(Icicle Brand)	3.5 oz	99	11.0	0.1
CRAB, DEVILED				
	1 cup	451	31.9	22.6
breaded, frozen, cake (Mrs. Paul's)	3 oz	180	18.0	9.0

Food Name	Serv. Size	Total Cal.	Carbs GMS	Fat GMS
breaded, frozen, miniature (Mrs. Paul's)	3.5 oz	240	25.0	12.0
CRAB AND SHRIMP, frozen (Wakefield)	3 oz	60	0.0	1.0
CRAB CAKE				
	100 gm	147	3.9	2.1
	1 cake	88	2.3	1.3
blue crab	1 cake	93	0.3	4.5
CRABAPPLE				
raw	100 gm	76	20.0	0.3
raw, slices, w/skin	1 cup	84	21.9	0.3
trimmed, w/skin	1 oz	22	5.7	0.1
trimmed, w/skin, sliced	1/2 cup	42	11.0	0.2
untrimmed	1 lb	316	83.2	1.3
CRABAPPLE, CANNED				
spiced (Lucky Leaf)	4 oz	110	28.0	0.0
spiced (Musselman's)	4 oz	110	28.0	0.0
CRACKER				
apple cinnamon, 'Orchard Crisps' (Nabisco)	.5 oz	60	11.0	2.0
bacon flavor (Delicious)	.5 oz	70	10.0	3.0
bacon flavor 'Bacon Flavored Thins' .5 oz (Nabisco)	7 crackers	70	9.0	4.0
bacon flavor 'Toasteds' approx .5 oz (Keebler)	4 crackers	60	8.0	3.0
banana walnut 'Orchard Crisps' (Nabisco)	.5 oz	60	11.0	2.0
barbecue wheat, for weight control (Spicer's)	1 oz	100	12.0	5.0
bar-b-que, tater crisps (Mr. Phipps)	.5 oz	60	10.0	2.0
bite size (Delicious)	.5 oz	70	9.0	3.0
bite size, low sodium (Delicious)	.5 oz	70	9.0	3.0
'Bits' approx .5 oz (Triscuit)	15 crackers	60	10.0	3.0
bran (FiberRich)	1 cracker	18	6.0	<1.0
bran, toasted 'Bran Thins' (Nabisco)	7 crackers	60	9.0	3.0
butter, country flavor (McCrakens)	1 oz	140	18.0	8.0
butter flavor (Ritz)	4 crackers	70	9.0	4.0
butter flavor, approx .5 oz (Escort)	3 crackers	70	9.0	4.0
butter flavor 'Club Low Salt' approx .5 oz (Keebler)	4 crackers	60	9.0	3.0
butter flavor, dairy, .5 oz (American Classic)	4 crackers	70	9.0	4.0
butter flavor 'Flutters' (Pepperidge Farm)	.75 oz	100	15.0	4.0
butter flavor 'Ritz Bits' 22 pieces (Ritz)	.5 oz	70	9.0	4.0
butter flavor 'Ritz Bits Low Salt' 22 pieces (Ritz)	.5 oz	70	9.0	4.0
butter flavor 'Ritz Low Salt' approx .5 oz (Ritz)	4 crackers	70	9.0	4.0
butter flavor 'Ritz' approx .5 oz (Ritz)	4 crackers	70	9.0	4.0
butter flavor 'Toasteds Buttercrisp' .5 oz (Keebler)	4 crackers	60	8.0	3.0
butter flavor 'Town House Low Salt' .5 oz (Keebler)	4 crackers	70	8.0	4.0
butter flavor 'Town House' approx .5 oz (Keebler)	4 crackers	70	8.0	4.0
butter flavor, thins 'Distinctive' (Pepperidge Farm)	4 crackers	70	10.0	3.0
cheese (Combos)	1.8 oz	240	34.0	10.0

Food Name	Serv. Size	Total Cal.	Carbs GMS	Fat GMS
cheese *(Delicious)*	.5 oz	70	9.0	3.0
cheese 'Better Cheddars' *(Nabisco)*	.5 oz	70	8.0	4.0
cheese 'Better Cheddars' low salt *(Nabisco)*	.5 oz	70	8.0	4.0
cheese, bite size *(Delicious)*	.5 oz	70	9.0	3.0
cheese, cheddar, approx 13-16 crackers *(Frito-Lay's)*	.5 oz	70	8.0	4.0
cheese, cheddar, baked, cracker chips 'Zings' *(Nabisco)*	.5 oz	70	9.0	3.0
cheese, cheddar 'Crackups' *(Nabisco)*	.5 oz	70	10.0	3.0
cheese, cheddar 'Goldfish' *(Pepperidge Farm)*	1 oz	120	19.0	4.0
cheese, cheddar 'Goldfish Thins' *(Pepperidge Farm)*	4 crackers	50	8.0	2.0
cheese, cheddar 'Guppies' 12 pieces *(Pepperidge Farm)*	.5 oz	40	5.0	2.0
cheese, cheddar 'Original Goldfish' *(Pepperidge Farm)*	1 oz	130	18.0	5.0
cheese, cheddar 'Snorkels' *(Nabisco)*	.5 oz	70	9.0	2.0
cheese, cheddar, tangy *(McCrakens)*	1 oz	140	18.0	8.0
cheese, cheddar 'Town House Jrs.' 8 pieces *(Keebler)*	.5 oz	80	8.0	4.0
cheese 'Cheddar Wedges' 31 pieces *(Nabisco)*	.5 oz	70	9.0	3.0
cheese 'Cheese Nips' 13 pieces *(Nabisco)*	.5 oz	70	9.0	3.0
cheese 'Cheese Peanut Butter Sandwich' 4 pieces *(Nabisco)*	1 oz	130	15.0	7.0
cheese 'Cheese Ritz Bits Mini Ritz' 22 pieces *(Ritz)*	.5 oz	70	8.0	4.0
cheese 'Cheez-Its' *(Sunshine)*	12 crackers	70	7.0	4.0
cheese 'Cheez-Its Low Salt' *(Sunshine)*	12 crackers	70	7.0	4.0
cheese, Parmesan 'Goldfish' *(Pepperidge Farm)*	1 oz	120	19.0	4.0
cheese, reduced fat 'Snack Wells' 18 pieces *(Nabisco)*	.5 oz	60	11.0	1.0
cheese 'Ritz Bits Sandwiches' approx .5 oz *(Ritz)*	6 crackers	80	7.0	5.0
cheese, sandwich-type w/peanut butter filling	.5 oz	68	8.1	3.3
cheese, Swiss 'Naturally Flavored' .5 oz *(Nabisco)*	7 crackers	70	9.0	3.0
cheese 'Tid-Bits' 15 pieces *(Nabisco)*	.5 oz	70	8.0	4.0
cheese, white cheddar 'Cheez-Its' *(Sunshine)*	.5 oz	76	9.0	4.0
cheese flavor *(Hain)*	1 oz	130	17.0	6.0
cheese flavor, organic, fat-free *(Health Valley)*	.5 oz	40	9.0	0.0
cheese flavor, 25 pieces *(Rokeach)*	1 oz	140	16.0	8.0
cheese sandwich, and cheese 'Handi-Snacks' *(Kraft)*	1 pkg	120	9.0	8.0
cheese sandwich, and peanut butter, .5 oz *(Keebler)*	2 crackers	70	9.0	3.0
cheese sandwich, cheddar 'Town House' .5 oz *(Keebler)*	1 cracker	70	6.0	4.0
cheese sandwich, wheat and American cheese, .5 oz *(Keebler)*	1 cracker	70	7.0	4.0
cheese-filled, 6 crackers *(Frito-Lay's)*	1.5 oz	210	24.0	10.0
chicken flavor 'Chicken in a Biskit' 7 pieces *(Nabisco)*	.5 oz	80	8.0	5.0
cinnamon graham *(Delicious)*	.5 oz	60	11.0	2.0
cinnamon graham, fat-free 'Snack Wells' *(Nabisco)*	.5 oz	50	12.0	0.0
cracked pepper, fat-free 'Snack Wells' *(Nabisco)*	.5 oz	60	12.0	0.0
cracked pepper 'Gourmet' fat-free *(Frookie)*	4 crackers	35	7.0	0.0
cracked wheat, approx .5 oz *(American Classic)*	4 crackers	70	8.0	4.0
cracked wheat 'Distinctive' *(Pepperidge Farm)*	3 crackers	100	14.0	4.0

Food Name	Serv. Size	Total Cal.	Carbs GMS	Fat GMS
cracked wheat 'Wafers' (Hickory Farms)	8 crackers	100	17.0	3.0
'Crackerbread' (Crisp & Light)	1 slice	17	3.0	<1.0
'Crackerbread Salt Free' (Crisp & Light)	1 slice	17	3.0	<1.0
'Crackerdiles' (Delicious)	.5 oz	70	9.0	3.0
crispbread (Dar-Vida)	1 cracker	20	4.0	<1.0
crispbread 'Breakfast' (Wasa)	1 cracker	50	8.0	1.0
crispbread, dark (Finn Crisp)	2 crackers	38	9.0	<1.0
crispbread 'Extra Crisp' (Wasa)	1 cracker	25	5.0	0.0
crispbread 'Fiber Plus' (Wasa)	1 cracker	35	5.0	1.0
crispbread, garlic flavor (Weight Watchers)	2 crackers	30	7.0	0.0
crispbread, high fiber 'Crisp Bread' (Ryvita)	1 cracker	23	4.0	<1.0
crispbread, high fiber 'Snackbread' (Ryvita)	1 cracker	14	3.0	<1.0
crispbread, regular (Finn Crisp)	2 crackers	38	9.0	<1.0
crispbread, thick (Kavli Norwegian)	1 slice	35	7.5	0.3
crispbread, thin (Kavli Norwegian)	2 slices	40	8.0	0.3
crispbread, w/caraway (Finn Crisp)	2 slices	38	9.0	<1.0
5-spice wafer (Westbrae)	4.5 wafers	40	8.0	1.0
garlic 'Discos' (Delicious)	.5 oz	78	6.0	5.0
garlic 'Garlic Tams' (Manischewitz)	10 crackers	153	19.0	8.0
garlic and herb 'Gourmet' fat-free (Frookie)	8 crackers	70	16.0	0.0
graham, chocolate 'Selects' (Keebler)	4 crackers	60	9.0	3.0
graham, honey nut 'Selects' (Keebler)	4 crackers	60	9.0	3.0
graham cracker 'Amaranth Graham Crackers' (Health Valley)	7 crackers	110	25.0	3.0
graham cracker, apple cinnamon 'Graham Bites' (Honey Maid)	11 crackers	60	11.0	2.0
graham cracker, approx .5 oz (Keebler)	4 crackers	70	12.0	2.0
graham cracker, approx 1 oz (Regal)	2 crackers	140	19.0	7.0
graham cracker, approx 1 oz (Rokeach)	8 crackers	120	21.0	3.0
graham cracker, brown sugar 'Graham Bites' .5 oz (Honey Maid)	11 crackers	60	11.0	2.0
graham cracker 'Grahamy Bears' (Sunshine)	9 crackers	130	21.0	5.0
graham cracker, 2 pieces (Nabisco)	.5 oz	60	11.0	1.0
grain, 6 pieces (Harvest Crisps)	.5 oz	60	10.0	2.0
hearty wheat 'Distinctive' (Pepperidge Farm)	4 crackers	100	13.0	5.0
herb, garden 'Flutters' (Pepperidge Farm)	.75 oz	100	14.0	4.0
herb, organic, fat-free (Health Valley)	.5 oz	40	9.0	0.0
herb 'Stoned Wheat' (Health Valley)	13 crackers	120	17.0	6.0
herb 'Stoned Wheat No Salt Added' (Health Valley)	13 crackers	120	17.0	6.0
honey graham (Delicious)	.5 oz	60	11.0	2.0
hot and spicy 'Cheez-Its' approx 12 crackers (Sunshine)	.5 oz	70	8.0	4.0
'Low Salt' (Featherweight)	2 crackers	30	5.0	1.0
matzo, American board (Manischewitz)	1 oz	115	22.0	1.9

Food Name	Serv. Size	Total Cal.	Carbs GMS	Fat GMS
matzo 'Daily Unsalted' board (Manischewitz)	1 oz	110	24.0	0.3
matzo, dietetic, thin board (Manischewitz)	.8 oz	91	19.0	0.4
matzo, egg	.5 oz	55	11.1	0.3
matzo, egg, 1 oz	1 matzo	111	22.3	0.6
matzo, egg, miniature 'Passover' approx 1 oz (Manischewitz)	10 crackers	108	20.0	2.0
matzo, egg 'Passover' board (Manischewitz)	1.2 oz	132	27.0	2.0
matzo, egg and onion	.5 oz	55	10.9	0.6
matzo, egg and onion, 1 oz	1 matzo	111	21.9	1.1
matzo, egg n' onion, board (Manischewitz)	1 oz	112	23.0	1.0
matzo, miniature (Manischewitz)	10 crackers	90	20.0	<1.0
matzo 'Passover' board (Manischewitz)	1.1 oz	129	27.0	0.4
matzo, plain	.5 oz	56	11.9	0.2
matzo, plain, 1 oz	1 matzo	112	23.7	0.4
matzo, tea 'Daily' thin board (Manischewitz)	.9 oz	103	22.0	0.3
matzo, thin board (Manischewitz)	.9 oz	100	21.0	0.3
matzo, whole-wheat	.5 oz	50	11.2	0.2
matzo, whole-wheat, 1 oz	1 matzo	100	22.4	0.4
matzo, whole wheat, w/bran, board (Manischewitz)	1 oz	110	21.0	0.6
melba toast, bacon 'Rounds' (Old London)	.5 oz	53	10.1	1.0
melba toast, garlic 'Rounds' (Old London)	.5 oz	56	9.9	1.2
melba toast, honey bran (Devonsheer)	1 cracker	16	3.0	0.4
melba toast, honey bran 'Rounds' (Devonsheer)	.5 oz	52	10.2	0.9
melba toast, oat, .5 oz (Harvest Crisps)	6 crackers	60	10.0	2.0
melba toast, onion 'Rounds' (Devonsheer)	.5 oz	51	10.7	0.6
melba toast, onion 'Rounds' (Old London)	.5 oz	52	10.2	0.8
melba toast, plain	.5 oz	55	10.9	0.5
melba toast, plain (Devonsheer)	1 cracker	16	3.0	0.4
melba toast, plain 'Rounds' (Devonsheer)	.5 oz	53	11.0	0.6
melba toast, plain 'Unsalted' (Devonsheer)	1 cracker	16	3.0	0.4
melba toast, plain 'Unsalted Rounds' (Devonsheer)	.5 oz	52	10.9	0.6
melba toast, plain, w/o salt	.5 oz	55	10.9	0.5
melba toast, pumpernickel (Old London)	.5 oz	54	11.0	0.6
melba toast, rye	.5 oz	55	11.0	0.5
melba toast, rye (Devonsheer)	1 cracker	16	3.0	0.4
melba toast, rye (Old London)	.5 oz	52	10.9	0.7
melba toast, rye, .5 oz (Devonsheer)	1 cracker	16	3.0	0.4
melba toast, rye 'Rounds' (Devonsheer)	.5 oz	53	10.7	0.6
melba toast, rye 'Rounds' (Old London)	.5 oz	52	10.8	0.7
melba toast, rye 'Unsalted' (Devonsheer)	1 cracker	16	3.0	0.4
melba toast, sesame (Devonsheer)	1 cracker	16	3.0	0.5
melba toast, sesame (Old London)	.5 oz	55	8.9	1.8
melba toast, sesame 'Rounds' (Devonsheer)	.5 oz	57	9.0	1.8

Food Name	Serv. Size	Total Cal.	Carbs GMS	Fat GMS
melba toast, sesame 'Rounds' (Old London)	.5 oz	56	8.9	1.8
melba toast, sesame 'Unsalted' (Old London)	.5 oz	55	8.9	1.8
melba toast, vegetable (Devonsheer)	1 cracker	16	3.0	0.4
melba toast, wheat	.5 oz	53	10.8	0.3
melba toast, wheat (Old London)	.5 oz	51	10.5	0.7
melba toast, wheat '6-calorie' (Estee)	1 cracker	6	1.0	<1.0
melba toast, wheat 'Snax' (Estee)	1 oz	100	22.0	<1.0
melba toast, white (Old London)	.5 oz	51	10.4	0.6
melba toast, white 'Rounds' (Old London)	.5 oz	48	9.8	0.6
melba toast, white 'Unsalted' (Old London)	.5 oz	51	10.7	0.6
melba toast, whole grain (Old London)	.5 oz	52	10.1	0.9
melba toast, whole grain 'Rounds' (Old London)	.5 oz	54	9.9	1.2
melba toast, whole grain 'Unsalted' (Old London)	.5 oz	53	10.0	1.0
melba toast, whole wheat (Devonsheer)	1 cracker	16	3.0	0.4
melba toast, whole wheat 'Unsalted' (Devonsheer)	1 cracker	16	3.0	0.4
milk	.5 oz	65	9.9	2.2
multi-grain (Premium)	.5 oz	60	10.0	2.0
multi-grain 'Wheat Thins' (Nabisco)	.5 oz	60	10.0	2.0
nacho cheese flavor (Delicious)	.5 oz	89	8.0	5.0
natural, for weight control (Spicer's)	1 oz	100	11.0	4.0
nutty wheat 'Wheat Thins' approx .5 oz (Nabisco)	7 crackers	70	9.0	4.0
oat 'Oat Krisp' (Ralston)	.5 oz	50	7.0	2.0
oat 'Oat Thins' approx .5 oz (Nabisco)	8 crackers	70	10.0	3.0
oat, .5 oz (Harvest Crisps)	6 crackers	60	10.0	2.0
oat bran 'Oat Bran Krisps' (Ralston)	.5 oz	60	9.0	3.0
'Old Fashioned' (Hickory Farms)	10 crackers	90	16.0	3.0
onion (Delicious)	.5 oz	70	10.0	3.0
onion 'Discos' (Delicious)	.5 oz	76	7.0	5.0
onion, minced, approx .5 oz (American Classic)	4 crackers	70	10.0	3.0
onion, organic, fat-free (Health Valley)	.5 oz	40	9.0	0.0
onion flavor (Hain)	1 oz	130	17.0	6.0
onion flavor 'No Salt Added' (Hain)	1 oz	130	17.0	6.0
onion flavor 'Onion Tams' (Manischewitz)	10 crackers	150	18.0	8.0
onion flavor 'Toasteds' approx .5 oz (Keebler)	4 crackers	60	9.0	3.0
onion garlic wafer (Westbrae)	4.5 crackers	40	8.0	0.0
oyster	.5 oz	62	10.1	1.7
oyster (OTC)	1 cracker	25	4.0	1.0
oyster (Premium)	20 crackers	60	10.0	1.0
oyster (Sunshine)	16 crackers	60	11.0	1.0
oyster, approx .5 oz (Dandy)	20 crackers	60	10.0	2.0
oyster, low salt	.5 oz	62	10.1	1.7
oyster 'Oysterettes' approx .5 oz (Nabisco)	18 crackers	60	10.0	1.0
oyster, unsalted tops	.5 oz	62	10.1	1.7

Food Name	Serv. Size	Total Cal.	Carbs GMS	Fat GMS
peanut butter *(Combos)*	1.8 oz	240	30.0	10.0
peanut butter, cheese *(Little Debbie)*	1.4 oz	190	23.0	9.0
peanut butter, cheese *(Little Debbie)*	.93 oz	130	14.0	6.0
peanut butter, cheese sandwich *(Handi-Snacks)*	1 pkg	190	11.0	14.0
peanut butter 'Ritz Bits Sandwiches' 1 oz *(Ritz)*	12 crackers	80	8.0	4.0
peanut butter, toast, approx .5 oz *(Keebler)*	2 crackers	70	9.0	3.0
peanut butter 'Toast Sandwich' 4 pieces *(Nabisco)*	1 oz	130	15.0	7.0
peanut butter, toasty *(Little Debbie)*	1.4 oz	200	21.0	12.0
peanut butter, toasty *(Little Debbie)*	.93 oz	140	14.0	7.0
peanut butter bar *(Frito-Lay's)*	1.75 oz	270	30.0	16.0
peanut butter-filled, 6 crackers *(Frito-Lay's)*	1.5 oz	210	24.0	10.0
pizza 'Goldfish' *(Pepperidge Farm)*	1 oz	130	19.0	5.0
poppy, toasted, approx .5 oz *(American Classic)*	4 crackers	70	9.0	3.0
pumpernickel *(Delicious)*	.5 oz	70	9.0	3.0
pumpernickel 'Snack Sticks' *(Pepperidge Farm)*	8 crackers	140	20.0	6.0
ranch, baked, cracker chips 'Zings' *(Nabisco)*	.5 oz	70	9.0	3.0
ranch 'Snack Crisps' *(Estee)*	.66 oz	80	13.0	2.0
'Regency' *(Delicious)*	.5 oz	70	9.0	<3.0
rice, approx .5 oz *(Harvest Crisps)*	6 crackers	60	11.0	2.0
rice, harvest 'Crispbread' *(Weight Watchers)*	2 crackers	30	7.0	0.0
rice bran *(Health Valley)*	7 crackers	130	19.0	4.0
'Rich' *(Hain)*	1 oz	130	18.0	5.0
'Rich, No Salt Added' *(Hain)*	1 oz	130	18.0	5.0
'Royal Lunch Milk Crackers' .5 oz *(Nabisco)*	1 cracker	60	10.0	2.0
rusk toast	.5 oz	58	10.2	1.0
rye	.5 oz	52	11.6	0.2
rye *(Hain)*	1 oz	120	19.0	4.0
rye, BBQ 'Rounds O' Rye' *(Hickory Farms)*	1 oz	153	13.0	10.6
rye, dark 'Crisp Bread' *(Ryvita)*	1 cracker	26	6.0	<1.0
rye, garlic 'Rounds O' Rye' *(Hickory Farms)*	1 oz	147	14.5	8.9
rye, golden 'Crispbread' *(Wasa)*	1 cracker	35	7.0	0.0
rye, hearty 'Crispbread' *(Wasa)*	1 cracker	45	9.0	0.0
rye, light 'Crisp Bread' *(Ryvita)*	1 cracker	26	6.0	<1.0
rye, light 'Crispbread Lite' *(Wasa)*	1 cracker	25	5.0	0.0
rye, light 'Hi-Fiber' *(Finn Crisp)*	1 cracker	35	8.0	1.0
rye, natural 'Rounds O' Rye' *(Hickory Farms)*	1 oz	156	12.2	10.9
rye 'No Salt Added' *(Hain)*	1 oz	120	19.0	4.0
rye, original 'Hi-Fiber' *(Finn Crisp)*	1 cracker	40	10.0	1.0
rye 'RyKrisp' *(Ralston)*	.5 oz	40	11.0	0.0
rye 'Rykrisp Twindividuals' 2 triple pieces *(Ralston)*	.5 oz	45	11.0	1.0
rye 'Salt Free' *(Hickory Farms)*	8 crackers	90	18.0	1.0
rye, sandwich-type w/cheese filling	.5 oz	68	8.6	3.2
rye, seasoned 'Rykrisp' *(Ralston)*	.5 oz	45	11.0	1.0

Food Name	Serv. Size	Total Cal.	Carbs GMS	Fat GMS
rye, sesame 'Rykrisp' 2 triple pieces *(Ralston)*	.5 oz	50	10.0	2.0
rye, sesame, toasted 'Crisp Bread' *(Ryvita)*	1 cracker	31	5.0	<1.0
rye, sour cream 'Rounds O'Rye' *(Hickory Farms)*	1 oz	155	12.6	10.7
rye 'Toasteds' approx .5 oz *(Keebler)*	4 crackers	60	8.0	3.0
rye 'Wafers' *(Hickory Farms)*	8 crackers	90	17.0	2.0
rye wafers, plain	.5 oz	47	11.4	0.1
rye wafers, seasoned	.5 oz	54	10.5	1.3
salsa 'Crackups' *(Nabisco)*	.5 oz	70	9.0	3.0
salt sticks, Vienna bread type, 6.5 inches long	1 stick	106	20.3	1.1
saltine, approx .5 oz *(Zesta)*	5 crackers	60	10.0	2.0
saltine 'Bits Mini Saltine Crackers' .5 oz *(Premium)*	16 crackers	70	9.0	3.0
saltine, crumbs, not packed	1 cup	303	50.0	8.4
saltine 'Fat-Free' .5 oz *(Premium)*	4 crackers	50	12.0	0.0
saltine 'Krispy' *(Sunshine)*	5 crackers	60	11.0	1.0
saltine 'Krispy Unsalted Tops' *(Sunshine)*	5 crackers	60	11.0	1.0
saltine, low salt	.5 oz	62	10.1	1.7
saltine 'Low Salt' approx .5 oz *(Premium)*	5 crackers	60	10.0	2.0
saltine 'Low Salt' approx .5 oz *(Zesta)*	5 crackers	60	10.0	2.0
saltine, mild cheddar 'Krispy' *(Sunshine)*	5 crackers	60	10.0	2.0
saltine, 1 7/8-inch square	10 crackers	123	20.3	3.4
saltine, original, .5 oz *(Premium)*	5 crackers	60	10.0	2.0
saltine, 10 pieces *(Rokeach)*	1 oz	120	20.0	3.0
saltine, unsalted tops	.5 oz	62	10.1	1.7
saltine 'Unsalted' *(Estee)*	4 crackers	60	9.0	2.0
saltine 'Unsalted Tops' approx .5 oz *(Premium)*	5 crackers	60	10.0	2.0
saltine 'Unsalted Tops' approx .5 oz *(Zesta)*	5 crackers	60	10.0	2.0
saltine, wheat, approx .5 oz *(Zesta)*	5 crackers	60	10.0	2.0
saltine, wheat 'Whole Wheat Premium Plus' .5 oz *(Premium)*	4 crackers	60	10.0	2.0
sandwich, peanut-cheese, 6 sandwiches	1 pkt	206	23.6	10.0
sandwich, peanut-cheese, 4 sandwiches	1 pkt	137	15.7	6.7
sandwich, w/cheese filling	.5 oz	68	8.8	3.0
sandwich, w/peanut butter filling	.5 oz	69	8.3	3.4
'Schooners' 33 pieces *(FFV)*	.5 oz	60	10.0	2.0
sesame *(Hain)*	1 oz	140	16.0	7.0
sesame, bread wafer, approx .5 oz *(Meal Mates)*	3 crackers	70	9.0	3.0
sesame 'Crisp' *(FFV)*	1 cracker	60	10.0	2.0
sesame 'Crispbread' *(Dar-Vida)*	1 cracker	22	4.0	1.0
sesame 'Distinctive' *(Pepperidge Farm)*	4 crackers	80	12.0	4.0
sesame, golden *(American Classic)*	4 crackers	70	9.0	3.0
sesame, golden, .5 oz *(American Classic)*	4 crackers	70	9.0	3.0
sesame, golden 'Flutters' *(Pepperidge Farm)*	.75 oz	110	13.0	5.0
sesame 'No Salt Added' *(Hain)*	1 oz	140	16.0	7.0

Food Name	Serv. Size	Total Cal.	Carbs GMS	Fat GMS
sesame 'RyKrisp' (Ralston)	.5 oz	50	10.0	2.0
sesame, savory 'Crispbread' (Wasa)	1 cracker	30	4.0	1.0
sesame 'Snack Sticks' (Pepperidge Farm)	8 crackers	140	19.0	5.0
sesame 'Toasteds' approx .5 oz (Keebler)	4 crackers	60	8.0	3.0
sesame, wafer 'Crisp' approx .5 oz (FFV)	4 crackers	60	9.0	2.0
sesame and cheese 'Twigs Snack Sticks' .5 oz (Nabisco)	5 crackers	70	8.0	4.0
sesame chips (Flavor Tree)	1/4 cup	163	10.6	9.2
sesame wafer (Westbrae)	4.5 crackers	40	8.0	0.0
sesame wheat (Delicious)	.5 oz	80	9.0	4.0
sesame wheat 'Crispbread' (Wasa)	1 cracker	50	8.0	2.0
sesame wheat 'Stoned Wheat' (Health Valley)	13 crackers	130	16.0	6.0
sesame wheat 'Stoned Wheat No Salt Added' (Health Valley)	13 crackers	130	17.0	6.0
seven grain 'Stoned Wheat' (Health Valley)	13 crackers	120	17.0	5.0
seven grain 'Stoned Wheat No Salt Added' (Health Valley)	13 crackers	120	17.0	5.0
seven-grain vegetable, organic, fat-free (Health Valley)	.5 oz	40	9.0	0.0
seven-grain vegetable, organic, no salt added (Health Valley)	.5 oz	40	9.0	0.0
snack, approx .5 oz (Finast)	12 crackers	70	9.0	3.0
snack, approx .5 oz (Rokeach)	9 crackers	130	19.0	5.0
'Snack N' Cracker' (Delicious)	.5 oz	70	10.0	3.0
'Snackers' (Delicious)	.5 oz	70	9.0	3.0
'Sociables' approx .5 oz (Nabisco)	6 crackers	70	9.0	4.0
soda (Sailor Boy Pilot)	1 cracker	100	17.0	3.0
soda 'Distinctive English Water Biscuit' (Pepperidge Farm)	4 crackers	70	13.0	1.0
soda 'English' (North Castles)	1 cracker	10	3.0	0.0
soda, .5 oz (Crown Pilot)	1 cracker	70	11.0	2.0
soda, low salt	.5 oz	62	10.1	1.7
soda, 'Lunch' 1 cracker (Royal)	.5 oz	60	17.0	3.0
soda 'Ocean Crisps' (FFV)	1 cracker	60	10.0	2.0
soda, unsalted tops	.5 oz	62	10.1	1.7
soup, low salt	.5 oz	62	10.1	1.7
soup, unsalted tops	.5 oz	62	10.1	1.7
sour cream and chive (Hain)	1 oz	130	15.0	6.0
sour cream and chive 'No Salt Added' (Hain)	1 oz	130	15.0	6.0
sour cream and chive flavor (McCrakens)	1 oz	140	18.0	8.0
sour cream and onion 'Discos' (Delicious)	.5 oz	79	6.0	5.0
sour cream and onion, for weight control (Spicer's)	1 oz	100	12.0	4.0
sour cream and onion 'Mr. Phipp's Tater Crisps' (Nabisco)	.5 oz	60	10.0	2.0
sourdough (Delicious)	.5 oz	70	9.0	3.0
sourdough (Hain)	.5 oz	65	9.0	3.0

Food Name	Serv. Size	Total Cal.	Carbs GMS	Fat GMS
sourdough 'Low Salt' (Hain)	1 oz	130	18.0	5.0
sticks 'Snack Sticks' (Pepperidge Farm)	8 crackers	130	19.0	5.0
'Tam Tams' (Manischewitz)	10 crackers	147	17.0	8.0
'Tam Tams No Salt' (Manischewitz)	10 crackers	138	18.0	7.0
tamari wafer (Westbrae)	4.5 crackers	40	8.0	0.0
'Uneeda Biscuits Unsalted Tops' approx .5 oz (Nabisco)	2 crackers	60	10.0	2.0
vegetable (Hain)	1 oz	130	10.0	5.0
vegetable, garden (Delicious)	.5 oz	70	10.0	3.0
vegetable 'Garden Crisps' (Nabisco)	.5 oz	60	11.0	2.0
vegetable 'No Salt Added' (Hain)	1 oz	130	10.0	5.0
'Vegetable Thins' (Nabisco)	7 crackers	70	8.0	4.0
wafer, no salt (Westbrae)	4.5 wafers	40	8.0	0.0
water (Sailor Boy Pilot)	1 cracker	100	17.0	3.0
water 'Distinctive English Water Biscuit' (Pepperidge Farm)	4 crackers	70	13.0	1.0
water 'English' (North Castles)	1 cracker	10	3.0	0.0
water, .5 oz (Crown Pilot)	1 cracker	70	11.0	2.0
water 'Gourmet' fat-free (Frookie)	4 crackers	35	7.0	0.0
water, 'Lunch' 1 cracker (Royal)	.5 oz	60	17.0	3.0
water 'Ocean Crisps' (FFV)	1 cracker	60	10.0	2.0
water 'Table Water, Bite Size' (Carr's)	2 crackers	25	5.0	1.0
'Waverly Crackers' approx .5 oz (Nabisco)	4 crackers	70	10.0	3.0
'Waverly Crackers Low Salt' approx .5 oz (Nabisco)	4 crackers	70	10.0	3.0
'Waverly Wafer' approx .5 oz (Nabisco)	4 crackers	70	10.0	3.0
wheat (Delicious)	.5 oz	70	9.0	3.0
wheat, approx .5 oz (Sociables)	6 crackers	70	9.0	3.0
wheat 'Bits' approx .5 oz (Triscuit)	8 crackers	60	10.0	2.0
wheat 'Crispy Wafer' approx .5 oz (FFV)	6 crackers	70	9.0	3.0
wheat, low salt	.5 oz	67	9.2	2.9
wheat 'Low Salt' approx .5 oz (Triscuit)	3 crackers	60	10.0	2.0
'Wheat On' (Delicious)	.5 oz	68	8.0	3.0
wheat 'Original Snackbread' (Ryvita)	1 cracker	20	4.0	<1.0
wheat 'Original Wheat Thins' approx .5 oz (Nabisco)	8 crackers	70	9.0	3.0
wheat, regular	.5 oz	67	9.2	2.9
wheat, sandwich, w/cheese filling	.5 oz	70	8.3	3.5
wheat, sandwich, w/peanut butter filling	.5 oz	70	7.6	3.8
wheat 'Snack Wells' (Nabisco)	.5 oz	50	11.0	0.0
wheat 'Snacks' approx .5 oz (Finast)	7 crackers	70	9.0	3.0
wheat 'Stone Ground' approx .5 oz (Wheatsworth)	4 crackers	70	9.0	3.0
wheat 'Stoned Wheat' (Health Valley)	13 crackers	120	17.0	6.0
wheat 'Stoned Wheat No Salt Added' (Health Valley)	13 crackers	120	17.0	6.0
wheat 'Stoned Wheat Wafer' approx .5 oz (FFV)	4 crackers	60	10.0	2.0
wheat 'Stoned Wheat Wafers Salt Free' (Hickory Farms)	8 crackers	100	18.0	2.0
wheat toasted (McCrakens)	1 oz	140	18.0	8.0

Food Name	Serv. Size	Total Cal.	Carbs GMS	Fat GMS
wheat, toasted 'Distinctive' (Pepperidge Farm)	4 crackers	80	12.0	3.0
wheat, toasted 'Flutters' (Pepperidge Farm)	.75 oz	110	13.0	5.0
wheat 'Wheat Krisp' (Ralston)	.5 oz	50	11.0	1.0
wheat 'Wheat Mill Wafers Salt Free' (Hickory Farms)	4 crackers	50	9.0	1.0
wheat 'Wheat Tams' (Manischewitz)	10 crackers	150	18.0	8.0
wheat 'Wheat Thins' (Nabisco)	8 crackers	70	9.0	3.0
wheat 'Wheat Thins Low Salt' approx .5 oz (Nabisco)	8 crackers	70	9.0	3.0
wheat 'Wheats' (Sunshine)	8 crackers	70	9.0	4.0
wheat 'Whole Wheat'N Bran Wafers' (Triscuit)	3 crackers	60	10.0	2.0
'Wheatine' bits (Barbara's Bakery)	.5 oz	60	9.0	2.0
'Wheatines' cracked pepper (Barbara's Bakery)	.5 oz	60	9.0	2.0
'Wheatines' lightly salted tops (Barbara's Bakery)	.5 oz	60	9.0	2.0
'Wheatines' sesame (Barbara's Bakery)	.5 oz	60	9.0	2.0
'Wheatines' unsalted tops (Barbara's Bakery)	.5 oz	60	9.0	2.0
wheatstone (Delicious)	.5 oz	70	9.0	3.0
whole grain 'Crispbread' approx .35 oz (Wasa)	1 slice	30	4.0	1.0
whole grain 'Harvest Wheats' approx .5 oz (Keebler)	4 crackers	60	8.0	3.0
whole wheat	.5 oz	63	9.7	2.4
whole wheat (Carr's)	2 crackers	70	12.0	1.0
whole wheat (Manischewitz)	10 crackers	90	18.0	1.0
whole wheat, approx .5 oz (Ritz)	5 crackers	70	9.0	3.0
whole wheat 'Gourmet' fat-free (Frookie)	4 crackers	35	7.0	0.0
whole wheat, low salt	.5 oz	63	9.7	2.4
whole wheat, organic, fat-free (Health Valley)	.5 oz	40	9.0	0.0
whole wheat 'Wheatables' approx .5 oz (Keebler)	12 crackers	70	9.0	3.0
w/bacon and cheese (Handi-Snacks)	1 pkg	130	8.0	9.0
zesty Italian, approx 13-16 crackers (Frito-Lay's)	.5 oz	70	9.0	3.0
zwieback	1 oz	121	21.0	2.8
'Zwieback Teething Toast' approx .5 oz (Nabisco)	2 crackers	60	10.0	1.0

CRACKER CRUMBS AND MEAL

Food Name	Serv. Size	Total Cal.	Carbs GMS	Fat GMS
meal	1 cup	440	93.0	2.0
meal	1 oz	109	22.9	0.5
(Golden Dipt) meal	1 oz	100	22.0	0.5
(Manischewitz) matzo 'Farfel'	1 cup	280	60.0	0.8
(Manischewitz) matzo meal 'Daily'	1 cup	514	109.0	1.4
(Nabisco) meal	1/4 cup	110	24.0	0.0
(Premium) fat-free	2 tbsp	50	11.0	0.0

CRANBERRY

Food Name	Serv. Size	Total Cal.	Carbs GMS	Fat GMS
raw (Ocean Spray) approx 2 oz	1/2 cup	25	6.0	0.0
raw, chopped	1 cup	54	14.0	0.2
raw, whole	1 cup	47	12.0	0.2
trimmed	1 oz	14	3.6	0.1
trimmed, chopped	1/2 cup	27	7.0	0.1

Food Name	Serv. Size	Total Cal.	Carbs GMS	Fat GMS
trimmed, whole	1/2 cup	23	6.0	0.1
w/stems	1 lb	210	54.6	0.9
CRANBERRY APPLE COCKTAIL				
(Minute Maid) 'Juices To Go'	6 oz	120	30.0	0.0
(Welch's) frozen, diluted	6 oz	120	30.0	0.0
CRANBERRY APPLE DRINK				
	6 oz	123	31.5	0.0
(A&P)	6 oz	130	32.0	(tr)
(Ocean Spray) 'Cran•Apple'	6 oz	120	31.0	0.0
(Ocean Spray) 'Cran•Apple Low Calorie'	6 oz	35	9.0	0.0
(P&Q)	6 oz	130	32.0	(tr)
(Pathmark)	6 oz	130	32.0	0.0
CRANBERRY APPLESAUCE, 'Cran•Fruit' *(Ocean Spray)*	2 oz	100	23.0	0.0
CRANBERRY APRICOT DRINK				
	6 oz	118	29.8	0.0
'Cranicot' *(Ocean Spray)*	6 oz	120	29.0	0.0
CRANBERRY BEAN/borlotti/Roman bean/rose coco				
boiled	1 cup	241	43.3	0.8
boiled	1/2 cup	120	21.5	0.4
boiled	4 oz	154	27.7	0.5
raw	1 cup	653	117.1	2.4
raw	1/2 cup	328	58.9	1.2
raw	1 oz	95	17.0	0.3
CRANBERRY BEAN, CANNED				
	1 cup	216	39.3	0.7
(Progresso)	1/2 cup	110	18.0	<1.0
w/liquid	1/2 cup	108	19.7	0.4
w/liquid	4 oz	94	17.1	0.3
CRANBERRY BLUEBERRY JUICE *(Knudsen & Sons)*	8 oz	115	36.0	0.0
CRANBERRY COCKTAIL JUICE				
(J. Hungerford)	9.03 oz	141	35.5	0.0
(J. Hungerford) 50% juice	9.03 oz	134	34.8	0.1
(J. Hungerford) 100% juice	9.03 oz	133	33.0	0.0
CRANBERRY DRINK				
(Ocean Spray) citrus 'Refreshers'	6 oz	100	26.0	0.0
(Ocean Spray) 'Cran•Blueberry'	6 oz	120	31.0	0.0
(Ocean Spray) 'Cran•Raspberry'	6 oz	110	27.0	0.0
(Ocean Spray) 'Cran•Raspberry Low Calorie'	6 oz	40	9.0	0.0
(Ocean Spray) 'Cran•Strawberry'	6 oz	110	27.0	0.0
(Tropicana) 'Cranberry Orchard Juice Sparkler'	8 oz	120	30.0	0.0
CRANBERRY GRAPE COCKTAIL				
frozen, prepared *(Welch's)*	6 oz	110	27.0	0.0

Food Name	Serv. Size	Total Cal.	Carbs GMS	Fat GMS
CRANBERRY GRAPE DRINK				
(Finast)	6 oz	103	26.0	0.0
(Ocean Spray) 'Cran•Grape'	6 oz	120	31.0	0.0
(Pathmark)	6 oz	103	26.0	0.0
CRANBERRY JUICE				
(Knudsen & Sons) 'Just Cranberry'	8 oz	40	10.0	0.0
(Knudsen & Sons) 'Yankee'	8 oz	125	31.0	0.0
(Lucky Leaf)	6 oz	110	26.0	0.0
(Ocean Spray) 'Cran•tastic'	6 oz	100	26.0	0.0
(Santa Cruz Natural) organic 'Sparkling'	8 oz	90	22.0	<1.0
(Snapple) 'Cranberry Royale'	8 oz	150	37.0	0.0
CRANBERRY JUICE COCKTAIL				
	1 cup	144	36.4	0.3
	6 oz	108	27.4	0.2
(A&P)	6 oz	100	26.0	<1.0
(Ocean Spray)	6 oz	110	26.0	0.0
(Ocean Spray) 'Low Calorie'	6 oz	40	9.0	0.0
(P&Q)	6 oz	100	24.0	<1.0
(Pathmark)	6 oz	100	26.0	0.0
(Pathmark) 'No Frills'	6 oz	100	26.0	0.0
(Sunkist)	6 oz	110	28.2	0.1
(Sunkist) frozen, prepared	6 oz	110	28.2	0.1
(Veryfine)	8 oz	160	40.0	0.0
(Welch's) frozen 'No Sugar Added' prepared	6 oz	40	10.0	0.0
(Welch's) frozen, prepared	6 oz	100	26.0	0.0
(Welch's) frozen, w/blueberry, prepared	6 oz	110	27.0	0.0
(Welch's) frozen, w/raspberry, prepared	6 oz	110	28.0	0.0
CRANBERRY JUICE DRINK				
citrus 'Refreshers' (Ocean Spray)	6 oz	100	26.0	0.0
CRANBERRY LEMONADE				
(Knudsen & Sons)	8 oz	115	29.0	0.0
(Santa Cruz Natural) organic	8 oz	100	24.0	<1.0
CRANBERRY NECTAR				
(Knudsen & Sons)	8 oz	110	28.0	0.0
(Santa Cruz Natural) organic	8 oz	110	28.0	<1.0
CRANBERRY RASPBERRY DRINK				
(Tropicana) w/strawberry 'Twister'	6 oz	110	27.0	<1.0
(Tropicana) w/strawberry 'Twister Light' w/NutraSweet	6 oz	30	7.0	<1.0
CRANBERRY RASPBERRY JUICE (Knudsen & Sons)	8 oz	100	25.0	0.0
CRANBERRY RASPBERRY SAUCE				
'Cran•Fruit' (Ocean Spray)	2 oz	100	23.0	0.0
CRANBERRY SAUCE				
canned (A&P)	2 oz	100	25.0	<1.0

Food Name	Serv. Size	Total Cal.	Carbs GMS	Fat GMS
canned *(Knudsen & Sons)*	1 oz	30	8.0	<1.0
canned, sweetened	1 cup	418	107.7	0.4
canned, sweetened	4 oz	171	44.1	0.2
jellied *(Finast)*	2 oz	90	22.0	0.0
jellied *(Ocean Spray)*	2 oz	80	22.0	0.0
jellied *(Pathmark)*	2 oz	90	22.0	0.0
jellied 'Old Fashioned' *(S&W)*	1/2 cup	90	22.0	0.0
whole berry *(Finast)*	2 oz	90	22.0	0.0
whole berry *(Ocean Spray)*	2 oz	80	21.0	0.0
whole berry 'Old Fashioned' *(S&W)*	1/2 cup	90	22.0	0.0

CRANBERRY STRAWBERRY SAUCE

Food Name	Serv. Size	Total Cal.	Carbs GMS	Fat GMS
crushed, for chicken 'Cran Fruit' *(Ocean Spray)*	2 oz	90	22.0	0.0

CRAPPIE. See SUNFISH.

CRAWFISH ENTRÉE, frozen, étouffée *(Cajun Cookin')*

	Serv. Size	Total Cal.	Carbs GMS	Fat GMS
	12 oz	390	51.0	10.0

CRAYFISH, MIXED SPECIES

Food Name	Serv. Size	Total Cal.	Carbs GMS	Fat GMS
farmed, moist-heat cooked	100 gm	87	0.0	1.3
farmed, moist-heat cooked	3 oz	74	0.0	1.1
farmed, raw	3 oz	61	0.0	0.8
farmed, raw	8 crayfish	19	0.0	0.3
wild, moist-heat cooked	100 gm	88	0.0	1.2
wild, moist-heat cooked	3 oz	75	0.0	1.0
wild, raw	3 oz	65	0.0	0.8
wild, raw	8 crayfish	21	0.0	0.3

CREAM

Food Name	Serv. Size	Total Cal.	Carbs GMS	Fat GMS
half and half	1 cup	315	10.4	27.8
half and half	1 oz	37	1.2	3.3
half and half	1 tbsp	20	0.7	1.7
half and half *(Crowley)*	1 oz	35	1.0	3.0
half and half *(Darigold)*	8 oz	310	11.0	27.0
half and half *(Knudsen)*	4 oz	150	5.0	13.0
half and half *(Rockview)*	2 tbsp	35	0.0	3.0
heavy, whipping	1 cup	821	6.6	88.1
heavy, whipping	1 tbsp	52	0.4	5.6
light, whipping	1 cup	699	7.1	73.9
light, whipping	1 tbsp	44	0.4	4.6
light, coffee or table	1 cup	469	8.8	46.3
light, coffee or table	1 oz	55	1.0	5.5
light, coffee or table	1 tbsp	29	0.6	2.9
medium, 25% fat	1 cup	583	8.3	59.7
medium, 25% fat	1 oz	69	1.0	7.1
medium, 25% fat	1 tbsp	37	0.5	3.8

CREAM CHEESE. See CHEESE.

CREAM NUT. See BRAZIL NUT.

Food Name	Serv. Size	Total Cal.	Carbs GMS	Fat GMS
CREAM OF TARTAR	1 tsp	8	1.8	0.0
CREAM SODA. See SOFT DRINKS AND MIXERS.				
CREAM TOPPING				
creamy white 'Dolci Frutta Crema Bianca' *(Saco Foods)*	1 box	900	98.4	50.1
dark chocolate 'Dolci Frutta Con Cioccolatta' *(Saco Foods)*	1 box	886	110.5	52.8
frozen, whipped *(La Creme)*	1 tbsp	16	1.0	1.0
frozen, whipped 'Real Cream' *(Kraft)*	1/4 cup	30	2.0	2.0
pressurized can, whipped	1 cup	154	7.5	13.3
pressurized can, whipped	1 oz	73	3.5	6.3
pressurized can, whipped	1 tbsp	8	0.4	0.7
pressurized can, whipped *(Crowley)*	1 tbsp	20	<1.0	1.0
whipping, heavy	1 oz	98	0.8	10.5
whipping, heavy *(Crowley)*	1 oz	110	1.0	11.0
whipping, heavy *(Darigold)*	1 cup	790	8.0	81.0
whipping, heavy 'Classic' *(Darigold)*	1 cup	858	6.9	90.0
whipping, heavy 'UHT' *(Darigold)*	1 cup	790	8.0	81.0
whipping, heavy, whipped	2 cups	821	6.6	90.0
whipping, heavy, whipped	2 tbsp	52	0.4	5.6
whipping, light	1 oz	83	0.8	8.8
whipping, light, whipped	2 cups	699	7.1	5.6
whipping, light, whipped	2 tbsp	44	0.4	8.8
CREAM TOPPING, NONDAIRY				
frozen	1 cup	239	17.3	19.0
frozen	1 oz	90	6.5	7.2
frozen	1 tbsp	13	0.9	1.0
frozen, chocolate 'Cool Whip' *(Birds Eye)*	1 tbsp	12	1.0	1.0
frozen 'Cool Whip' *(Birds Eye)*	1 tbsp	12	1.0	1.0
frozen 'Cool Whip Lite' *(Birds Eye)*	1 tbsp	8	1.0	<1.0
frozen, extra creamy 'Cool Whip Dairy Recipe' *(Birds Eye)*	1 tbsp	14	1.0	1.0
frozen, semisolid	1 cup	239	17.3	19.0
frozen, semisolid	1 tbsp	13	0.9	1.0
frozen 'Whip' *(Pet)*	1 tbsp	14	1.0	1.0
frozen 'Whipped Topping' *(Kraft)*	1/4 cup	35	2.0	3.0
mix, dry	1.5 oz	245	22.3	17.0
mix, prepared *(D-Zerta)*	1 tbsp	8	0.0	1.0
mix, prepared *(Featherweight)*	1 tbsp	4	0.0	0.0
mix, prepared *(Dream Whip)*	1 tbsp	10	1.0	0.0
pressurized can	1 cup	184	11.3	15.6
pressurized can	1 oz	75	4.6	6.3
pressurized can	1 tbsp	11	0.6	0.9
pressurized can 'Richwhip' *(Rich's)*	.25 oz	20	1.0	2.0

Food Name	Serv. Size	Total Cal.	Carbs GMS	Fat GMS
prewhipped *(Estee)*	1 tbsp	4	<1.0	<1.0
prewhipped 'Richwhip' *(Rich's)*	1 tbsp	12	1.0	1.0
reduced calorie *(D-Zerta)*	1 tbsp	8	0.0	1.0
unwhipped 'Richwhip' *(Rich's)*	.25 oz	20	1.0	2.0

CREAMER, NONDAIRY

Liquid

Food Name	Serv. Size	Total Cal.	Carbs GMS	Fat GMS
frozen	1/2 cup	164	13.7	12.0
frozen	1 oz	39	3.2	2.8
frozen	1 tbsp	20	1.7	1.5
w/hydrogenated vegetable oil and soy protein	1/2 cup	163	13.7	12.0
w/hydrogenated vegetable oil and soy protein	1/2 oz	20	1.7	1.5
w/lauric acid oil and sodium caseinate	1/2 cup	164	13.7	12.0
w/lauric acid oil and sodium caseinate	1/2 oz	20	1.7	1.5
(Coffee-Mate)	1 tbsp	16	2.0	1.0
(Coffee-Mate) 'Amaretto'	1 tbsp	40	5.0	2.0
(Coffee-Mate) 'Cinnamon Creme'	1 tbsp	40	5.0	2.0
(Coffee-Mate) fat-free	1 tbsp	10	2.0	0.0
(Coffee-Mate) 'Hazelnut'	1 tbsp	40	5.0	2.0
(Coffee-Mate) 'Irish Creme'	1 tbsp	40	5.0	2.0
(Crowley)	.5 oz	16	1.0	1.0
(Diehl)	1 tsp	10	1.0	<1.0
(Finast) frozen	.5 oz	20	2.0	2.0
(IGA)	1 tsp	10	2.0	<1.0
(N-Rich)	1 tsp	10	2.0	0.6
(Pathmark) 'No Frills'	1 tsp	10	1.0	0.0
(Rich's) frozen 'Coffee Rich'	.5 oz	20	2.0	2.0
(Rich's) frozen 'Farm Rich'	.5 oz	20	1.0	2.0
(Rich's) frozen 'Poly Rich'	.5 oz	20	2.0	1.0
(Saco Foods) 'kwik kream'	1 tbsp	10	2.0	<1.0
(Westbrae)	1 tbsp	10	2.0	<1.0

Powder

Food Name	Serv. Size	Total Cal.	Carbs GMS	Fat GMS
	1/2 cup	257	16.7	25.8
	1 oz	155	15.6	10.1
	1 tsp	11	1.1	0.7
(Coffee-Mate)	1 tsp	10	1.0	<1.0
(Coffee-Mate) 'Amaretto'	2 tsp	60	9.0	3.0
(Coffee-Mate) 'Hazelnut'	2 tsp	60	0.0	3.0
(Coffee-Mate) 'Irish Creme'	2 tsp	60	9.0	3.0
(Coffee-Mate) 'Lite'	1 tsp	8	2.0	<1.0
(Cremora)	1 tsp	10	1.0	<1.0

CREME DE MENTHE. See ALCOHOLIC BEVERAGES.

CRÊPE MIX, 7-inch crêpes *(Krusteaz)* . . . 2 crêpes | 80 | 14.0 | 1.0

Food Name	Serv. Size	Total Cal.	Carbs GMS	Fat GMS
CRESS, GARDEN				
boiled, drained	4 oz	26	4.3	0.7
boiled, drained	1/2 cup	16	2.6	0.4
raw	1/2 cup	8	1.4	0.2
raw, trimmed	1 oz	9	1.6	0.2
raw, untrimmed	1 lb	103	17.7	2.3
CROAKER, ATLANTIC				
raw	1 lb	474	0.0	14.4
raw	3 oz	88	0.0	2.7
raw	1 oz	29	0.0	0.9
raw, approx 2.8 oz	1 fillet	82	0.0	2.5
CROISSANT				
almond, 3.7 oz *(Dunkin' Donuts)*	1 croissant	420	38.0	27.0
butter *(Awrey's)*	3 oz	300	32.0	17.0
butter *(Awrey's)*	2 oz	200	21.0	11.0
butter *(Awrey's)*	1 oz	100	10.0	6.0
frozen, butter, 1.5 oz *(Sara Lee)*	1 croissant	170	19.0	9.0
frozen, butter, petite *(Pepperidge Farm)*	1 croissant	140	13.0	7.0
frozen, butter, petite 1 oz *(Sara Lee)*	1 croissant	120	13.0	6.0
margarine *(Awrey's)*	2.5 oz	250	26.0	14.0
margarine *(Awrey's)*	1.25 oz	120	13.0	7.0
plain, 2.5 oz *(Dunkin' Donuts)*	1 croissant	310	27.0	19.0
'Sandwich Quartet' *(Pepperidge Farm)*	1 croissant	170	22.0	7.0
wheat *(Awrey's)*	2.5 oz	240	24.0	14.0
CROOKNECK SQUASH. See SQUASH, CROOKNECK.				
CROUTONS				
Caesar salad *(Brownberry)*	.5 oz	62	8.0	2.6
Caesar salad *(Reese)*	.5 oz	60	9.0	2.0
cheddar and Romano cheese *(Pepperidge Farm)*	.5 oz	60	10.0	2.0
cheddar cheese *(Brownberry)*	.5 oz	63	8.3	2.8
cheese and garlic *(Pepperidge Farm)*	.5 oz	70	9.0	3.0
onion and garlic *(Brownberry)*	.5 oz	60	8.8	2.2
onion and garlic *(Pepperidge Farm)*	.5 oz	70	9.0	3.0
plain	1 cup	122	22.0	2.0
plain	.5 oz	58	10.4	0.9
seasoned	1 cup	186	25.4	7.3
seasoned	.5 oz	66	9.0	2.6
seasoned *(Brownberry)*	.5 oz	59	8.5	2.2
seasoned *(Pepperidge Farm)*	.5 oz	70	9.0	3.0
seasoned *(Weight Watchers)*	1 pouch	30	5.0	0.0
sour cream and chive *(Pepperidge Farm)*	.5 oz	70	9.0	3.0
toasted *(Brownberry)*	.5 oz	56	9.7	1.4

Food Name	Serv. Size	Total Cal.	Carbs GMS	Fat GMS
CRUMPET				
blueberry, low-fat, cholestrol-free *(Wolferman's)*	1 crumpet	90	21.0	<1.0
brown sugar cinnamon, low-fat *(Wolferman's)*	1 crumpet	110	21.0	2.0
raspberry, low-fat, cholestrol-free *(Wolferman's)*	1 crumpet	90	20.0	1.0
CUCUMBER				
raw, approx 10.9 oz	1 med	39	8.3	0.4
raw, slices	1/2 cup	7	1.4	0.1
raw, w/peel, trimmed	1 oz	4	0.8	<.1
raw, w/peel, untrimmed	1 lb	56	12.8	0.6
CUMIN SEED				
whole	1 oz	106	12.5	6.3
whole	1 tbsp	22	2.7	1.3
whole	1 tsp	8	0.9	0.5
whole *(Durkee)*	1 tsp	10	0.0	<0.1
whole *(Laurel Leaf)*	1 tsp	10	0.0	<0.1
whole *(Spice Islands)*	1 tsp	7	0.7	0.4
CUPU ASSU OIL				
	1/2 cup	964	0.0	109.0
	1 oz	251	0.0	28.4
	1 tbsp	120	0.0	13.6
CUPU ASSU PUNCH, 'Rain Forest' *(Knudsen & Sons)*	8 oz	110	25.0	0.0
CURRANT, BLACK/European currant				
raw	1 cup	71	17.2	0.5
trimmed	1 oz	18	4.4	0.1
untrimmed	1 lb	282	68.4	1.8
CURRANT, RED				
raw	1 cup	63	15.5	0.2
trimmed	1 oz	16	3.9	0.1
untrimmed	1 lb	249	61.3	0.9
CURRANT, WHITE				
raw	1 cup	63	15.5	0.2
trimmed	1/2 cup	31	7.7	0.1
trimmed	1 oz	16	3.9	0.1
untrimmed	1 lb	249	61.3	0.9
CURRANT, ZANTE				
dried	1 lb	1282	336.0	1.2
dried	1 cup	408	106.7	0.4
dried	1 oz	80	21.0	0.1
dried *(Del Monte)*	1/2 cup	200	53.0	0.0
CURRY POWDER				
ground	1 oz	92	16.5	3.9
ground	1 tbsp	20	3.7	0.9
ground	1 tsp	7	1.2	0.3

Food Name	Serv. Size	Total Cal.	Carbs GMS	Fat GMS
CUSK/torsk/tusk				
dry-heat cooked	3 oz	95	0.0	0.8
raw	1 lb	396	0.0	3.1
raw	3 oz	74	0.0	0.6
raw	1 oz	25	0.0	0.2
raw, approx 4.3 oz	1 fillet	106	0.0	0.8
CUSTARD. See PUDDING MIX; PUDDING/PIE FILLING, MIX.				
CUSTARD APPLE/bullock's heart/cherimoya				
raw	100 gm	101	25.2	0.6
trimmed	1 oz	29	7.1	0.2
untrimmed	1 lb	267	66.3	1.6
CUTTLEFISH, MIXED SPECIES				
moist-heat cooked	100 gm	158	1.6	1.4
moist-heat cooked	3 oz	134	1.4	1.2
raw	1 lb	359	3.7	3.2
raw	3 oz	67	0.7	0.6
raw	1 oz	22	0.2	0.2
CYMLING. See SQUASH, SCALLOP.				

D

Food Name	Serv. Size	Total Cal.	Carbs GMS	Fat GMS
DAIKON/mullangi/Oriental radish				
boiled, drained	4 oz	19	3.9	0.3
boiled, drained, sliced	1/2 cup	13	2.5	0.2
dried	1/2 cup	157	36.8	0.4
dried	1 oz	77	18.0	0.2
raw, trimmed	1 oz	5	1.2	<.1
raw, trimmed (Frieda's)	1 lb	86	19.1	0.5
raw, trimmed (Frieda's)	1 oz	5	1.2	<.1
raw, trimmed, sliced	1/2 cup	8	1.8	<.1
raw, untrimmed	1 lb	65	14.7	0.4
DAIQUIRI. See ALCOHOLIC BEVERAGES.				
DANDELION GREENS				
boiled, drained	4 oz	37	7.3	0.7
boiled, drained, chopped	1 cup	35	6.7	0.6
raw, chopped	1 oz	13	2.6	0.2
raw, trimmed	1 lb	204	41.7	3.2
DANISH CABBAGE. See CABBAGE, DANISH.				

Food Name	Serv. Size	Total Cal.	Carbs GMS	Fat GMS
DANISH PASTRY				
APPLE				
(Awrey's)				
filled, 'Miniature' 1.7 oz	1 piece	160	21.0	8.0
filled 'Round' 4.5 oz	1 piece	390	50.0	20.0
filled 'Round' 2.75 oz	1 piece	270	34.0	14.0
filled 'Square' 3 oz	1 piece	220	34.0	8.0
(Pepperidge Farm) frozen, 2.25 oz	1 piece	220	35.0	8.0
(Sara Lee)				
frozen 'Free & Light'	1/8 pkg	130	30.0	0.0
frozen 'Individual' 1.3 oz	1 piece	120	15.0	6.0
frozen twist	1/8 pkg	190	22.0	10.0
CARAMEL *(Pillsbury)* w/nuts, refrigerated	1 piece	160	19.0	8.0
CHEESE				
(Awrey's)				
filled, 'Miniature' 1.7 oz	1 piece	170	21.0	9.0
filled 'Round' 4.5 oz	1 piece	420	52.0	22.0
filled 'Round' 2.75 oz	1 piece	280	34.0	15.0
filled 'Square' 2.5 oz	1 piece	210	25.0	11.0
(Pepperidge Farm) frozen, 2.25 oz	1 piece	240	25.0	14.0
(Sara Lee) frozen, 'Individual' 1.3 oz	1 piece	130	13.0	8.0
CINNAMON *(Sara Lee)* twist, frozen	1/8 pkg	200	21.0	12.0
CINNAMON-RAISIN				
(Awrey's)				
filled 'Square' 3 oz	1 piece	290	41.0	12.0
filled 'Miniature' 1.5 oz	1 piece	160	21.0	8.0
(Pepperidge Farm) frozen, 2.25 oz	1 piece	250	35.0	11.0
(Pillsbury) w/icing, refrigerated	1 piece	150	20.0	7.0
(Sara Lee) frozen, 'Individual' 1.3 oz	1 piece	150	17.0	8.0
CINNAMON-WALNUT *(Awrey's)* 'Round' 2.75 oz	1 piece	300	31.0	18.0
LEMON *(Entenmann's)* twist	1.2 oz	140	17.0	7.0
ORANGE *(Pillsbury)* w/icing, refrigerated	1 piece	150	19.0	7.0
PECAN RING *(Entenmann's)*	1.5 oz	190	19.0	12.0
PINEAPPLE *(Awrey's)* filled, 'Miniature' 1.7 oz	1 piece	157	21.0	8.0
RASPBERRY				
(Awrey's) filled 'Square' 3 oz	1 piece	260	45.0	8.0
(Entenmann's) twist	1.2 oz	140	18.0	7.0
(Pepperidge Farm) frozen, 2.25 oz	1 piece	220	31.0	9.0
(Sara Lee) twist, frozen	1/8 pkg	200	25.0	9.0
RING *(Entenmann's)*	1.5 oz	180	18.0	10.0
STRAWBERRY				
(Awrey's)				
filled 'Miniature' 1.7 oz	1 piece	160	21.0	8.0

Food Name	Serv. Size	Total Cal.	Carbs GMS	Fat GMS
filled 'Round' 4.5 oz	1 piece	400	53.0	20.0
filled 'Round' 2.75 oz	1 piece	270	34.0	14.0
WALNUT RING *(Entenmann's)*	1.5 oz	190	19.0	12.0
DASHEEN				
cooked	4 oz	161	39.2	0.1
cooked, sliced	1/2 cup	94	22.8	0.1
raw, sliced	1/2 cup	56	13.8	0.1
raw, trimmed	1 oz	30	7.5	0.1
raw, untrimmed	1 lb	419	103.2	0.8
DASHEEN LEAF				
raw	1/2 cup	6	0.9	0.1
raw, trimmed	1 oz	12	1.9	0.2
raw, untrimmed	1 lb	115	18.3	2.0
steamed	1/2 cup	18	3.0	0.3
steamed	4 oz	27	4.6	0.5
DASHEEN SHOOTS				
cooked	4 oz	16	3.6	0.1
cooked, sliced	1/2 cup	10	2.2	0.1
raw, sliced	1/2 cup	5	1.0	<.1
raw, trimmed	1 oz	3	0.7	<.1
raw, untrimmed	1 lb	45	9.3	0.4
DATE				
Domestic, natural and dry				
chopped	1/2 cup	245	65.4	0.4
w/pits	1 lb	1123	300.1	1.8
w/o pits	1 oz	78	20.8	0.1
w/o pits, 2.9 oz	10 dates	228	61.0	0.4
w/o pits *(Dole)*	1/2 cup	280	62.0	0.0
Imported, pitted				
(Amport Foods) chopped	1.5 oz	135	36.0	0.0
(Amport Foods) whole	1.5 oz	135	36.0	0.0
(Bordo)	2 oz	204	47.2	1.2
(Bordo) diced	2 oz	203	47.5	1.1
(Dromedary) approx 1 oz	5 dates	100	23.0	0.0
(Dromedary) chopped	1/4 cup	130	31.0	0.0
DEER				
raw	1 lb	544	0.0	11.0
raw	1 oz	34	0.0	0.7
roasted	3 oz	134	0.0	2.7
DIET BAR. See also SNACK BAR.				
(Figurines)				
chocolate	1 bar	100	11.0	5.0
chocolate caramel	1 bar	100	11.0	6.0

Food Name	Serv. Size	Total Cal.	Carbs GMS	Fat GMS
chocolate caramel '100'	1 bar	100	10.0	6.0
chocolate peanut butter	1 bar	100	10.0	6.0
'S'mores'	1 bar	100	11.0	5.0
vanilla	1 bar	100	11.0	6.0
(Nestlé)				
chewy chocolate brownie 'Sweet Success'	1 bar	120	18.0	4.0
chewy chocolate chip 'Sweet Success'	1 bar	120	18.0	4.0
chewy chocolate peanut butter 'Sweet Success'	1 bar	120	18.0	4.0
(Ultra Slim Fast) chocolate chip crunch	1 bar	120	19.0	4.0
DIET DRINK				
(Nestlé)				
chocolate mocha, ready to drink, 'Sweet Success'	10 oz	200	32.0	3.0
chocolate raspberry truffle, powder, 'Sweet Success'	1.13 oz	90	11.0	2.0
chocolate raspberry truffle, prepared, 'Sweet Success'	8 oz	180	23.0	2.0
creamy milk chocolate, canned, 'Sweet Success'	10 oz	200	32.0	3.0
dark chocolate fudge, canned, 'Sweet Success'	10 oz	200	32.0	3.0
dark chocolate fudge, powder, 'Sweet Success'	1.13 oz	90	11.0	2.0
dark chocolate fudge, prepared, 'Sweet Success'	8 oz	180	23.0	2.0
rich chocolate almond, powder, 'Sweet Success'	1.13 oz	90	12.0	2.0
rich chocolate almond, prepared, 'Sweet Success'	8 oz	180	24.0	2.0
(Ultra Slim Fast)				
cafe mocha powder	1 scoop	100	24.0	<1.0
cafe mocha powder, prepared w/skim milk	8 oz	200	38.0	1.0
chocolate fantasy 'Plus' powder	1 scoop	120	33.0	1.0
chocolate fantasy 'Plus' powder, prepared w/skim milk	12 oz	250	50.0	2.0
French vanilla powder	1 scoop	100	24.0	<1.0
French vanilla powder, prepared w/skim milk	8 oz	190	36.0	1.0
'French Vanilla' canned	12 oz	220	38.0	1.0
piña colada 'Plus' powder	1 scoop	90	24.0	<1.0
piña colada 'Plus' powder, prepared w/skim milk	8 oz	190	38.0	<1.0
strawberry jubilee 'Plus' powder	1 scoop	110	32.0	1.0
strawbery jubilee 'Plus' powder, prepared w/skim milk	12 oz	240	50.0	2.0
DILL SEASONING, 'Parsley Patch It's a Dilly' *(Schilling)*	1 tsp	11	2.0	0.4
DILL SEED				
whole	1 oz	86	15.6	4.1
whole	1 tbsp	20	3.6	1.0
whole	1 tsp	6	1.2	0.3
whole *(Durkee)*	1 tsp	9	0.0	<0.1
whole *(Laurel Leaf)*	1 tsp	9	0.0	<0.1
whole *(Spice Islands)*	1 tsp	9	1.2	0.4
DILL WEED				
dried	1 oz	72	15.8	1.2
dried	1 tbsp	8	1.7	0.1

Food Name	Serv. Size	Total Cal.	Carbs GMS	Fat GMS
dried	1 tsp	3	0.6	0.0
fresh, sprigs	1 cup	4	0.6	0.1
DIP				
ACAPULCO *(Ortega)*	1 oz	8	2.0	0.0
AVOCADO *(Kraft)*	2 tbsp	50	3.0	4.0
BACON AND HORSERADISH				
(Breakstone's)	2 tbsp	70	2.0	6.0
(Kraft)	2 tbsp	60	3.0	5.0
(Kraft) 'Premium'	2 tbsp	50	2.0	5.0
(Sealtest)	2 tbsp	70	2.0	6.0
BACON AND ONION				
(Breakstone's) 'Gourmet'	2 tbsp	70	2.0	6.0
(Kraft) 'Premium'	2 tbsp	60	2.0	5.0
BEAN				
(Chi-Chi's) 'Fiesta'	1 oz	30	4.0	1.0
(Hain) hot	4 tbsp	70	10.0	1.0
BLACK BEAN				
(Guiltless Gourmet) barbeque, mild	1 oz	23	4.0	0.0
(Guiltless Gourmet) barbeque, spicy	1 oz	23	4.0	0.0
(Guiltless Gourmet) mild	1 oz	23	4.0	0.0
(Guiltless Gourmet) spicy	1 oz	23	4.0	0.0
(Tostitos) fat free, medium	2 tbsp	30	6.0	0.0
BLUE CHEESE				
(Kraft) 'Premium'	2 tbsp	50	2.0	4.0
(Litehouse) 'Lite' and dressing, refrigerated	1 tbsp	33	1.0	3.0
(Litehouse) 'Original' and dressing, refrigerated	1 tbsp	77	0.0	8.0
CAESAR *(Litehouse)* and dressing, refrigerated	1 tbsp	57	0.0	6.0
CHEDDAR CHEESE				
(Frito-Lay's)	1 oz	45	3.0	3.0
(Guiltless Gourmet) queso, mild	1 oz	20	5.0	0.0
(Guiltless Gourmet) queso, spicy	1 oz	20	5.0	0.0
CHEESE *(Chi-Chi's)* 'Fiesta'	1 oz	41	3.0	3.0
CHILI *(La Victoria)*	1 tbsp	6	1.0	<1.0
CLAM				
(Breakstone's)	2 tbsp	50	2.0	4.0
(Breakstone's) 'Gourmet Chesapeake'	2 tbsp	50	2.0	4.0
(Kraft)	2 tbsp	60	3.0	4.0
(Kraft) 'Premium'	2 tbsp	45	2.0	4.0
(Sealtest)	2 tbsp	50	2.0	4.0
COUNTRY BLUE CHEESE				
(Litehouse) and dressing, refrigerated	1 tbsp	76	0.0	8.0
COUNTRY RANCH *(Litehouse)* and dressing, refrigerated	1 tbsp	61	1.0	7.0
CUCUMBER *(Kraft)* creamy 'Premium'	2 tbsp	50	2.0	4.0

Food Name	Serv. Size	Total Cal.	Carbs GMS	Fat GMS
CUCUMBER AND ONION				
(Breakstone's)	2 tbsp	50	2.0	4.0
(Sealtest)	2 tbsp	50	2.0	4.0
DILL (Nasoya) creamy 'Vegi-Dip'	1 oz	60	4.0	4.0
FRENCH ONION				
(Bison)	1 oz	60	2.0	5.0
(Breakstone's)	2 tbsp	50	2.0	5.0
(Frito-Lay's)	1 oz	50	3.0	3.0
(Heluva Good) real sour cream	2 tbsp	50	2.0	5.0
(Kraft)	2 tbsp	60	3.0	4.0
(Kraft) 'Premium'	2 tbsp	45	2.0	4.0
(Lucerne)	2 tbsp	70	2.0	6.0
(Nasoya) 'Vegi-Dip'	1 oz	50	4.0	3.0
(Sealtest)	2 tbsp	50	2.0	5.0
GARLIC (Life) and dressing, w/tofu 'All Natural'	1 tbsp	70	1.4	7.1
GARLIC AND HERB (Nasoya) 'Vegi-Dip'	1 oz	50	6.0	2.0
GUACAMOLE				
(Kraft)	2 tbsp	50	3.0	4.0
(Lucerne)	2 tbsp	80	1.0	8.0
HONEY MUSTARD (Litehouse) and dressing, refrigerated	1 tbsp	67	2.0	7.0
HUMMUS (Fantastic Foods)	2 oz	111	9.5	6.5
ITALIAN (Litehouse) and dressing, creamy, refrigerated	1 tbsp	60	0.0	6.0
JALAPEÑO				
(Breakstone's) cheddar 'Gourmet'	2 tbsp	70	2.0	6.0
(Frito-Lay's)	1 oz	30	4.0	1.0
(Hain) medium	4 tbsp	70	10.0	1.0
(Kraft)	2 tbsp	50	3.0	4.0
(Kraft) cheese 'Premium'	2 tbsp	50	3.0	4.0
(Litehouse) ranch, and dressing, refrigerated	1 tbsp	60	1.0	6.0
(Old El Paso)	1 tbsp	14	2.0	0.0
(Price's) nacho	1 oz	80	2.0	7.1
(Wise)	2 tbsp	25	5.0	0.0
MEXICAN BEAN (Hain)	4 tbsp	60	9.0	1.0
MUSHROOM AND HERB (Breakstone's) 'Gourmet'	2 tbsp	50	2.0	4.0
NACHO CHEESE				
(Kraft) 'Premium'	2 tbsp	55	2.0	4.0
(Tio Sancho) 'Microwave Snacks' cheese sauce mix	3.5 oz	247	2.3	20.0
ONION				
(Breakstone's) toasted 'Gourmet'	2 tbsp	50	2.0	5.0
(Hain) bean	4 tbsp	70	10.0	1.0
(Kraft) creamy 'Premium'	2 tbsp	45	2.0	4.0
(Kraft) green	2 tbsp	60	3.0	4.0
PEPPERCORN (Litehouse) and dressing, refrigerated	1 tbsp	67	0.0	7.0

Food Name	Serv. Size	Total Cal.	Carbs GMS	Fat GMS
PICANTE SAUCE				
(Frito-Lay's)	1 oz	10	3.0	0.0
(Wise)	2 tbsp	12	3.0	0.0
PINTO BEAN				
(Guiltless Gourmet) barbecue, mild	1 oz	27	5.0	0.0
(Guiltless Gourmet) barbecue, spicy	1 oz	27	5.0	0.0
(Guiltless Gourmet) mild	1 oz	27	5.0	0.0
(Guiltless Gourmet) spicy	1 oz	27	5.0	0.0
POPPYSEED (Litehouse) and dressing, refrigerated	1 tbsp	65	3.0	6.0
RANCH				
(Heluva Good) real sour cream	2 tbsp	60	2.0	5.0
(Litehouse) and dressing, refrigerated	1 tbsp	59	1.0	6.0
(Litehouse) 'Lite' and dressing, refrigerated	1 tbsp	35	1.0	3.0
(Litehouse) 'Vegi-Dip' refrigerated	1 tbsp	60	1.0	7.0
(Lucerne)	2 tbsp	110	2.0	11.0
SALSA				
(Pace) 'Chunky' medium	2 tbsp	4	<1.0	<1.0
(Pace) 'Chunky' mild	2 tbsp	4	<1.0	<1.0
SOUR CREAM AND CHIVES				
(Litehouse) vinaigrette, and dressing, refrigerated	1 tbsp	63	1.0	7.0
TACO				
(Hain) and sauce	4 tbsp	25	5.0	1.0
(Wise)	2 tbsp	12	3.0	0.0
THOUSAND ISLAND (Litehouse) and dressing, refrigerated	1 tbsp	65	1.0	7.0
VEGETABLE (T. Marzetti) and dressing	1 tbsp	88	1.0	10.0
DISHCLOTH GOURD. See GOURD, DISHCLOTH.				
DOCK				
boiled, drained	4 oz	23	3.3	0.7
boiled, drained	100 gm	20	2.9	0.6
raw, chopped	1/2 cup	15	2.1	0.5
raw, trimmed	1 oz	6	0.9	0.2
raw, untrimmed	1 lb	70	10.2	2.2
DOLLARFISH				
raw	1 lb	663	0.0	36.4
raw	1 oz	41	0.0	2.3
DOLPHIN FISH. See MAHI MAHI.				
DONUT				
(Awrey's)				
crunch	1 donut	600	65.0	34.0
plain	1 donut	490	48.0	30.0
sugared	1 donut	610	68.0	35.0
(Break Cake)				
chocolate, 1 oz	1 donut	130	14.0	8.0

Food Name	Serv. Size	Total Cal.	Carbs GMS	Fat GMS
chocolate, gem, .5 oz	1 donut	70	7.0	4.0
chocolate, gem, .5 oz	6 donuts	400	42.0	24.0
cinnamon, 1 oz	1 donut	120	15.0	6.0
cinnamon, gem, .5 oz	1 donut	60	8.0	3.0
dunkin stix, .5 oz	2 stix	420	43.0	27.0
powdered, 1 oz	1 donut	120	16.0	5.0
powdered, gem, .5 oz	1 donut	60	8.0	3.0
powdered, gem, .5 oz	6 donuts	350	47.0	16.0
(Dunkin' Donuts)				
apple filled, w/cinnamon sugar, 2.8 oz	1 donut	250	33.0	11.0
Bavarian filled, w/chocolate frosting, 2.8 oz	1 donut	240	32.0	11.0
blueberry filled, 2.4 oz	1 donut	210	29.0	8.0
'Boston Kreme'	1 donut	240	30.0	11.0
cinnamon, apple filled	1 donut	190	25.0	9.0
coffee roll, glazed, 2.9 oz	1 donut	280	37.0	12.0
cruller, French, glazed, 1.3 oz	1 donut	140	16.0	8.0
cruller, honey dipped	1 donut	260	36.0	11.0
jelly filled, 2.4 oz	1 donut	220	31.0	9.0
lemon filled, 2.8 oz	1 donut	260	33.0	12.0
plain, cake w/handle	1 donut	240	26.0	14.0
ring, buttermilk, glazed, 2.6 oz	1 donut	290	37.0	14.0
ring, chocolate, glazed, 2.5 oz	1 donut	324	34.0	21.0
ring, plain, cake	1 donut	262	23.0	18.0
ring, plain, cake, 2.2 oz	1 donut	270	25.0	17.0
ring, powdered, cake	1 donut	270	28.0	16.0
ring, whole wheat, glazed, 2.9 oz	1 donut	330	39.0	18.0
ring, yeast, chocolate frosted, 1.9 oz	1 donut	200	25.0	10.0
ring, yeast, glazed, 1.9 oz	1 donut	200	26.0	9.0
(Entenmann's)				
crumb topped	1 donut	260	34.0	12.0
devil's food crumb	1 donut	250	34.0	12.0
rich, frosted	1 donut	280	27.0	18.0
(Hostess)				
cinnamon, 'Donette Gems'	1 donut	60	7.0	3.0
cinnamon, 'Family Pack'	1 donut	120	14.0	6.0
crumb	1 donut	160	16.0	10.0
crumb, 'Donette Gems'	1 donut	80	8.0	5.0
frosted, 1.5 oz	1 donut	190	20.0	12.0
frosted, 'Donette Gems'	1 donut	80	8.0	5.0
glazed, 'Old Fashioned'	1 donut	250	33.0	12.0
glazed whirl	1 donut	190	27.0	7.0
honey wheat	1 donut	250	32.0	12.0
plain, 'Old Fashioned'	1 donut	170	21.0	9.0

Food Name	Serv. Size	Total Cal.	Carbs GMS	Fat GMS
(Little Debbie) stick 1.67 oz	1 stick	230	26.0	13.0
(Rich's)				
frozen, glazed 'Ever Fresh' 1.2 oz	1 donut	141	17.2	7.0
frozen, jelly 'Ever Fresh' 2.17 oz	1 donut	213	26.0	9.5
(Tastykake)				
cinnamon, 'Assorted' 1.6 oz	1 donut	179	24.5	8.2
cinnamon, mini	1 donut	48	6.4	2.4
frosted, rich, 2 oz	1 donut	258	28.2	16.0
frosted, rich, mini	1 donut	61	7.7	3.2
honey wheat, 2 oz	1 donut	209	33.3	7.5
honey wheat, mini	1 donut	40	7.2	1.2
orange glazed, 2 oz	1 donut	219	32.1	9.1
plain, 'Assorted' 1.6 oz	1 donut	185	21.6	10.1
powdered sugar, 'Assorted' 1.6 oz	1 donut	188	24.4	8.6
powdered sugar, mini	1 donut	42	6.9	1.3
DRAGON'S EYE				
dried	1 oz	81	21.0	0.1
raw, approx .2 oz	1 med	2	0.5	tr
raw, shelled and seeded	1 oz	17	4.3	<.1
raw, untrimmed	1 lb	144	36.4	0.2
DREAM WHIP. See CREAM TOPPING, NONDAIRY.				
DRESSING. See SALAD DRESSING.				
DRINKS. See ALCOHOL-FREE BEVERAGES; ALCOHOLIC BEVERAGES; COFFEE; DIET DRINK; MILK; SOFT DRINKS AND MIXERS; SPORTS DRINK; TEA; WATER; and individual listings.				
DRINK MIX. See individual drink mix flavors.				
DRUM, FRESHWATER				
dry-heat cooked	3 oz	130	0.0	5.4
raw	1 lb	541	0.0	22.4
raw	3 oz	101	0.0	4.2
raw	1 oz	34	0.0	1.4
DUCK, DOMESTICATED				
Meat and skin				
raw	1 oz	115	0.0	11.2
roasted	4 oz	382	0.0	32.1
Meat only				
raw	1 oz	37	0.0	1.7
roasted	4 oz	228	0.0	12.7
DUCK, WILD				
Breast meat, raw	1 oz	35	0.0	1.2
Meat and skin, raw	1 oz	60	0.0	4.3
DUCK FAT				
	1 cup	1846	0.0	204.6
	1 oz	255	0.0	28.3

Food Name	Serv. Size	Total Cal.	Carbs GMS	Fat GMS
....	1 tbsp	115	0.0	12.8
DUCK LIVER, domesticated, raw	1 oz	39	1.0	1.3
DULSE, raw	100 gm	0	0.0	3.2

E

Food Name	Serv. Size	Total Cal.	Carbs GMS	Fat GMS
EEL, MIXED SPECIES				
broiled	4 oz	268	0.0	17.0
dry-heat cooked	3 oz	201	0.0	12.7
raw	1 lb	834	0.0	52.9
raw	1 oz	52	0.0	3.3
EGG, ALTERNATIVE				
Frozen				
(Fleischmann's) 'Egg Beaters' cheese omelet	1/2 cup	110	2.0	5.0
(Fleischmann's) 'Egg Beaters' vegetable omelet	1/2 cup	50	5.0	0.0
(Morningstar Farms) 'Scramblers'	1/4 cup	60	3.0	3.0
(Tofutti) 'Egg Watchers'	2 oz	50	2.0	2.0
Refrigerated				
(Featherweight)	2 eggs	120	2.0	8.0
(Fleischmann's) 'Egg Beaters'	1/4 cup	25	1.0	0.0
Mix				
(Healthy Choice) 'Cholesterol Free Egg Product' ....1.9-oz serving		30	1.0	<1.0
(Tofu Scrambler) prepared w/tofu	1/2 cup	98	7.0	5.0
EGG, CHICKEN. See also EGG WHITE, CHICKEN; EGG YOLK, CHICKEN.				
Cooked				
fried	1 large	91	0.6	6.9
hard-boiled	1 oz	44	0.3	3.0
hard-boiled, chopped	1 cup	211	1.5	14.4
poached	1 large	74	0.6	5.0
poached	1 oz	42	0.3	2.8
scrambled	1 cup	365	4.8	26.9
scrambled	1 large	100	1.3	7.3
Dried				
....	1 oz	168	1.4	11.9
....	1 tbsp	30	0.2	2.1
sifted	1 cup	505	4.1	35.5
stabilized, glucose reduced	1 oz	174	0.7	12.5
stabilized, glucose reduced	1 tbsp	31	0.1	2.2
stabilized, glucose reduced, sifted	1 cup	523	2.0	37.4
Pickled *(Penrose)*	1 large	80	1.0	5.0

Food Name	Serv. Size	Total Cal.	Carbs GMS	Fat GMS
Raw				
fresh or frozen	1 cup	363	3.0	24.3
fresh or frozen	1 large	75	0.6	5.0
fresh or frozen	1 oz	42	0.3	2.8
EGG, DUCK				
raw	1 large	130	1.0	9.6
raw	1 oz	52	0.4	3.9
EGG, GOOSE				
raw	1 large	267	1.9	19.1
raw	1 oz	52	0.4	3.8
EGG, QUAIL				
raw	1 oz	45	0.1	3.1
raw	1 large	14	0.0	1.0
EGG, TURKEY				
raw	1 large	135	0.9	9.4
raw	1 oz	48	0.3	3.4
EGG BREAKFAST, ALTERNATIVE, FROZEN				
vegetarian, w/hash browns and links 'Scramblers'				
(Morningstar Farms)	7 oz	360	22.0	23.0
vegetarian, w/pancakes and links 'Scramblers'				
(Morningstar Farms)	6.8 oz	380	33.0	19.0
EGG BREAKFAST, FREEZE-DRIED				
(Mountain House)				
cheese omelet, prepared	1/2 pkg	180	8.0	9.0
w/bacon, prepared	1/2 pkg	170	7.0	10.0
w/butter, prepared	1/2 pkg	160	8.0	8.0
EGG BREAKFAST, SCRAMBLED, FROZEN				
w/bacon and home fried potatoes (Swanson)	5.6 oz	340	16.0	26.0
w/cheddar cheese and fried potatoes (Aunt Jemima)	5.9 oz	250	22.0	13.0
w/ham and hash browns (Downyflake)	6.25 oz	360	17.0	26.0
w/ham and pecan twirl (Downyflake)	6.25 oz	470	40.0	28.0
w/hash browns and sausage link (Downyflake)	6.25 oz	420	17.0	34.0
w/home fried potatoes 'Great Starts' Budget Breakfast				
(Swanson)	4.6 oz	260	14.0	19.0
w/sausages and hash browns (Aunt Jemima)	5.7 oz	290	14.0	20.0
w/sausages and hash browns (Swanson)	6.5 oz	430	19.0	34.0
w/sausages and pancakes (Aunt Jemima)	5.2 oz	270	21.0	14.0
w/sausages and pecan twirl (Downyflake)	6.25 oz	510	39.0	33.0
EGG FOO YUNG				
(LaChoy) mix, prepared	8.8 oz	164	19.2	7.0
(LaChoy) packaged 'Dinner Classics' prepared	2 patties	170	20.0	7.0
EGG NOODLE. See NOODLE, EGG.				

Food Name	Serv. Size	Total Cal.	Carbs GMS	Fat GMS
EGG ROLL				
Frozen				
(Chun King)				
chicken	3.6 oz	220	32.0	8.0
meat and shrimp	3.6 oz	220	31.0	8.0
pork 'Restaurant Style'	3 oz	180	23.0	6.0
shrimp	3.6 oz	200	31.0	6.0
(Jeno's)				
chicken 'Snacks' approx 6 rolls	3 oz	190	21.0	9.0
meat and shrimp 'Snacks' approx 6 rolls	3 oz	200	21.0	11.0
shrimp and cheese 'Snacks' approx 6 rolls	3 oz	190	22.0	8.0
(LaChoy)				
almond chicken	3 oz	120	19.0	3.0
chicken 'Snack'	1.45 oz	90	12.0	3.0
lobster 'Snack'	1.45 oz	75	12.0	2.0
meat and shrimp 'Snack'	1.45 oz	80	11.0	3.0
pork 'Restaurant Style'	3 oz	150	20.0	5.0
shrimp 'Restaurant Style'	3 oz	130	19.0	4.0
shrimp 'Snack'	1.45 oz	75	12.0	2.0
sweet and sour chicken	3 oz	150	24.0	4.0
(Worthington) vegetarian roll, frozen	3 oz	160	20.0	6.0
Refrigerated				
(Chung's)				
chicken, white meat	3 oz	150	21.0	6.0
pork	3 oz	190	20.0	10.0
shrimp	3 oz	170	22.0	7.0
vegetable	3 oz	180	23.0	8.0
EGG ROLL WRAPPER				
(Azumaya Pasta)	2 pieces	130	26.0	0.0
(Nasoya)	1 piece	23	4.5	0.0
EGG WHITE, CHICKEN				
Dried				
stabilized, glucose reduced, flakes	1 oz	100	1.2	<.1
stabilized, glucose reduced, powder	1 cup	402	4.8	<.1
stabilized, glucose reduced, powder	1 oz	107	1.3	<.1
Raw				
fresh or frozen	1 cup	122	2.5	0.0
fresh or frozen	1 large	17	0.3	0.0
fresh or frozen	1 oz	14	0.3	0.0
EGG WHITE STABILIZER *(Tone's)*	1 tsp	12	3.0	(tr)
EGG YOLK, CHICKEN				
Dried				
sifted	1 cup	460	0.3	41.1

Food Name	Serv. Size	Total Cal.	Carbs GMS	Fat GMS
sifted	1 oz	195	0.1	17.4
sifted	1 tbsp	27	0.0	2.5
Raw				
fresh	1 cup	870	4.3	75.0
fresh	1 oz	101	0.5	8.8
fresh	1 large	59	0.3	5.1
frozen, salted	100 gm	278	1.5	23.4
frozen, sugared	100 gm	317	11.5	23.4
frozen, sugared	1 oz	92	2.7	7.2
EGGNOG, NON-ALCOHOLIC				
Canned *(Borden)*	1/2 cup	160	16.0	9.0
Chilled				
(Crowley)	6 oz	270	34.0	13.0
(Darigold)	8 oz	350	43.0	17.0
(Darigold) 'Classic'	8 oz	390	48.0	17.0
(Ensure) liquid nutrition	8 oz	250	34.3	8.8
EGGNOG MIX				
dry, 2 heaping tsp	1 oz	111	27.7	0.3
1 oz powder, prepared w/whole milk	1 cup	261	38.9	8.4
1 oz powder, prepared w/2% milk	1 cup	232	39.4	5.0
1 oz powder, prepared w/1% milk	1 cup	213	39.4	2.9
1 oz powder, prepared w/skim milk	1 cup	197	39.6	0.7
EGGPLANT/aubergine				
boiled, drained	4 oz	32	7.5	0.3
boiled, drained, 1-inch cubes	1 cup	27	6.4	0.2
raw, 1-inch pieces	1/2 cup	11	2.5	0.1
raw, peeled, approx 1 lb	1 eggplant	119	27.8	0.8
raw, trimmed	1 oz	7	1.8	<.1
raw, untrimmed	1 lb	95	23.0	0.4
EGGPLANT APPETIZER, 'Caponata' *(Progresso)*	1/2 can	70	4.0	4.0
EGGPLANT ENTRÉE, FROZEN				
(Celentano)				
parmigiana	10 oz	350	29.0	19.0
parmigiana	8 oz	280	23.0	15.0
parmigiana	6.25 oz	260	36.0	10.0
rollettes	11 oz	320	36.0	14.0
(Mrs. Paul's) parmigiana	5 oz	240	18.0	16.0
ELBOW MACARONI. See PASTA.				
ELDERBERRY				
fresh	1 lb	329	83.5	2.3
fresh	1 oz	21	5.2	0.1
fresh	1 cup	106	26.7	0.7

Food Name	Serv. Size	Total Cal.	Carbs GMS	Fat GMS
ELK				
raw	1 lb	504	0.0	6.6
raw	1 oz	31	0.0	0.4
roasted	3 oz	124	0.0	1.6
roasted	4 oz	166	0.0	2.2
roasted, diced, approx 4.9 oz	1 cup	204	0.0	2.7
ENCHILADA (Gebhardt)	2 enchiladas	310	20.0	24.0
ENCHILADA DINNER, FROZEN. See also ENCHILADA ENTRÉE, FROZEN.				
BEEF				
(Banquet)	12 oz	500	72.0	15.0
(Banquet) chili and gravy 'Family Entrées'	7 oz	270	28.0	13.0
(Healthy Choice)	13.4 oz	370	66.0	5.0
(Old El Paso) 'Festive Dinners'	11 oz	390	56.0	8.0
(Patio)	13.25 oz	520	59.0	24.0
(Swanson)	13.75 oz	480	55.0	21.0
(Van de Kamp's) 'Mexican Dinner'	1/2 pkg	200	27.0	7.0
CHEESE				
(Banquet)	12 oz	550	71.0	19.0
(Patio)	12.25 oz	380	59.0	10.0
(Old El Paso) 'Festive Dinners'	11 oz	590	51.0	31.0
(Van de Kamp's) 'Mexican Dinner'	1/2 pkg	220	26.0	9.0
CHICKEN				
(Healthy Choice)	13.4 oz	340	61.0	5.0
(Healthy Choice)	9.5 oz	310	44.0	9.0
(Old El Paso) 'Festive Dinners'	11 oz	460	54.0	18.0
(Weight Watchers) nacho grande 'Mexican Style'	9 oz	280	38.0	8.0
ENCHILADA DINNER, MIX				
(Old El Paso) prepared	1 enchilada	145	11.0	8.0
(Tio Sancho) 'Dinner Kit'	1 shell	80	10.8	3.5
(Tio Sancho) 'Dinner Kit' and sauce mix	3 oz	278	62.0	1.5
ENCHILADA ENTRÉE, FROZEN. See also ENCHILADA DINNER, FROZEN.				
BEEF				
(Hormel)	1 enchilada	140	17.0	5.0
(Old El Paso)	1 pkg	210	16.0	13.0
(Ultimate 200) Ranchero	9.12 oz	190	18.0	5.0
(Van de Kamp's) 'Mexican Entrées'	1 pkg	270	30.0	12.0
(Van de Kamp's) 'Mexican Entrées Family Pack'	1/4 pkg	150	19.0	5.0
(Van de Kamp's) shredded, 'Mexican Entrées'	1 pkg	360	40.0	14.0
BLACK BEAN-VEGETABLE (Amy's Kitchen)	4.75 oz	135	20.0	4.0
CHEESE				
(Amy's Kitchen) organic	4.75 oz	210	16.0	9.0
(Hormel)	1 enchilada	151	18.0	6.0
(Old El Paso)	1 pkg	250	24.0	12.0

Food Name	Serv. Size	Total Cal.	Carbs GMS	Fat GMS
(Stouffer's)	9.75 oz	490	33.0	29.0
(Van de Kamp's) 'Mexican Entrées'	1 pkg	300	31.0	15.0
(Van de Kamp's) 'Mexican Entrées Family Pack'	1/4 pkg	200	19.0	10.0
CHICKEN				
(Le Menu) 'Light Style'	8 oz	280	32.0	8.0
(Old El Paso)	1 pkg	220	20.0	12.0
(Old El Paso) w/sour cream sauce	1 pkg	280	18.0	19.0
(Stouffer's)	10 oz	490	31.0	31.0
(Van de Kamp's) 'Mexican Entrées'	1 pkg	260	27.0	11.0
RANCHERO *(Van de Kamp's)* 'Mexican Entrées'	1/2 pkg	260	26.0	12.0
SUIZA				
(Van de Kamp's) 'Mexican Entrées'	1 pkg	230	23.0	10.0
(Weight Watchers)	9 oz	230	25.0	7.0
VEGETABLE *(Legume)* w/tofu and sauce	11 oz	270	36.0	8.0
ENCHILADA SEASONING MIX				
(Old El Paso)	1/8 pkg	6	1.0	0.0
(Lawry's) 'Seasoning Blends'	1 pkg	152	29.9	1.2
ENDIVE				
approx 1.3 lb	1 head	87	17.2	1.0
chopped	1/2 cup	4	0.8	0.1
trimmed	1 oz	5	0.9	0.1
untrimmed	1 lb	65	13.1	0.8
ENGLISH MUFFIN				
(Earth Grains)				
oat bran, 12-oz pkg	1 muffin	120	24.0	1.0
plain, 12.5-oz pkg	1 muffin	130	26.0	1.0
plain, 12-oz pkg	1 muffin	120	25.0	1.0
raisin, 14-oz pkg	1 muffin	160	33.0	2.0
raisin, 'Sun Maid' 15-oz pkg	1 muffin	160	34.0	1.0
sourdough, 12.5-oz pkg	1 muffin	130	26.0	1.0
sourdough, 12-oz pkg	1 muffin	120	25.0	1.0
whole wheat, 15-oz pkg	1 muffin	140	28.0	2.0
whole wheat, 14-oz pkg	1 muffin	130	26.0	1.0
(Hi Fiber)				
cinnamon raisin	1 muffin	110	21.0	1.0
multigrain	1 muffin	120	23.0	1.0
plain	1 muffin	110	21.0	1.0
(Oatmeal Goodness)				
cinnamon and raisin oatmeal	1 muffin	140	26.0	2.0
honey and oatmeal	1 muffin	140	26.0	2.0
(Oroweat)				
extra crisp	1 muffin	130	26.0	1.0
health nut	1 muffin	170	29.0	4.0

Food Name	Serv. Size	Total Cal.	Carbs GMS	Fat GMS
sourdough	1 muffin	140	27.0	1.0
(Pepperidge Farm)				
cinnamon apple	1 muffin	140	27.0	1.0
cinnamon chip	1 muffin	160	28.0	3.0
cinnamon raisin	1 muffin	150	29.0	2.0
plain	1 muffin	140	27.0	1.0
sourdough	1 muffin	135	27.0	1.0
(Roman Meal)				
honey nut and oat bran, refrigerated	1/2 muffin	81	14.7	1.3
plain, 'Original'	1 muffin	146	28.5	1.8
wheatberry, 14-oz pkg	1 muffin	140	28.0	1.0
(Thomas')				
honey wheat	1 muffin	129	24.0	1.1
oat bran	1 muffin	116	26.0	1.2
plain	1 muffin	130	25.4	1.3
raisin	1 muffin	153	30.4	1.5
rye	1 muffin	120	27.0	1.0
(Wonder) plain	1 muffin	130	26.0	1.0

ENSURE NUTRITION DRINK. See individual flavors.

ENTRÉES. See individual entrées.

EPPAW, raw	1/2 cup	75	15.8	0.9

EQUAL. See SUGAR SUBSTITUTE.

EUCHALON. See CANDLEFISH.

F

Food Name	Serv. Size	Total Cal.	Carbs GMS	Fat GMS
FAJITA ENTRÉE, refrigerated *(Chicken By George)*	5 oz	170	2.0	6.0
FAJITA ENTRÉE, FROZEN				
beef *(Healthy Choice)*	7 oz	210	26.0	4.0
chicken *(Healthy Choice)*	7 oz	200	25.0	3.0
FAJITA ENTRÉE KIT				
(Tyson)	4 oz	80	2.0	2.0
(Tyson) Wholesale Club Item	3.5 oz	160	18.0	5.0
FAJITA MARINADE *(Old El Paso)*	1/8 jar	14	3.0	0.0
FAJITA SAUCE. See SAUCE.				
FAJITA SEASONING MIX, 'Seasoning Blends' *(Lawry's)*	1 pkg	63	14.0	0.4
FALAFEL				
(Casbah) mix, dry	1 oz	103	15.0	2.0
(Fantastic Foods) mix 'Falafil' prepared	3 oz	129	20.0	2.0
(Near East) mix, prepared	3 patties	270	22.0	15.0
FARINA. See CEREAL, HOT.				

Food Name	Serv. Size	Total Cal.	Carbs GMS	Fat GMS
FAT, ALTERNATIVE, 'Neutral Nyafat' *(Rokeach)*	1 tbsp	99	0.0	11.0
FATHEAD. See SHEEPSHEAD.				
FAVA BEAN/horse bean/jack bean				
boiled, drained	4 oz	64	11.5	0.6
mature seeds, boiled	1/2 cup	94	16.7	0.3
mature seeds, raw	1/2 cup	256	43.7	1.1
raw, trimmed	1/2 cup	40	6.4	0.4
raw, trimmed	1 oz	20	3.3	0.2
raw, untrimmed	1 lb	317	51.5	2.6
Canned				
mature seeds	1/2 cup	91	15.9	0.3
mature seeds, w/liquid	4 oz	81	14.1	0.2
Dried				
mature seeds, boiled	4 oz	125	22.3	0.5
mature seeds, boiled	1/2 cup	93	16.7	0.3
mature seeds, raw	1/2 cup	256	43.7	1.2
mature seeds, raw	1 oz	97	16.5	0.4
FEIJAO				
raw	1 fruit	25	5.3	0.4
raw, purée	1 cup	119	25.8	1.9
FENNEL/finocchio				
(Frieda's)	1 lb	68	11.8	0.5
(Frieda's)	1 oz	4	0.7	<.1
raw, bulb	1 bulb	73	17.1	0.5
raw, leaves	100 gm	28	5.1	0.4
raw, sliced	1 cup	27	6.3	0.2
FENNEL SEED				
whole	1 oz	98	14.8	4.2
whole	1 tbsp	20	3.0	0.9
whole	1 tsp	7	1.0	0.3
whole *(Durkee)*	1 tsp	7	0.0	tr
whole *(Laurel Leaf)*	1 tsp	7	0.0	tr
whole *(Spice Islands)*	1 tsp	8	1.3	0.2
FENUGREEK SEED				
whole	1 oz	92	16.5	1.8
whole	1 tbsp	36	6.5	0.7
whole	1 tsp	12	2.2	0.2
FETTUCCINE ENTRÉE, FROZEN				
Alfredo *(Healthy Choice)*	8 oz	240	36.0	7.0
Alfredo *(Lean Cuisine)*	9 oz	280	41.0	7.0
Alfredo *(Weight Watchers)*	8 oz	230	28.0	7.0
Alfredo, 10-oz pkg *(Stouffer's)*	5 oz	245	22.0	14.0
Alfredo, w/broccoli 'Lowfat' *(Weight Watchers)*	8 oz	230	28.0	7.0

Food Name	Serv. Size	Total Cal.	Carbs GMS	Fat GMS
chicken (Healthy Choice)	8.5 oz	240	29.0	4.0
primavera (Green Giant)	1 pkg	230	26.0	8.0
primavera (Lean Cuisine)	10 oz	260	32.0	8.0
primavera 'Microwave Garden Gourmet' (Green Giant)	1 pkg	260	25.0	13.0
w/broccoli (Dining Lite)	9 oz	290	33.0	12.0
w/meat sauce (Budget Gourmet)	10 oz	290	34.0	10.0
FETTUCCINE ENTRÉE, MIX				
Alfredo 'Pasta & Cheese' prepared (Kraft)	1/2 cup	180	19.0	9.0
Alfredo 'Pasta & Sauce' (Hain)	1/4 pkg	180	27.0	4.0
FETTUCCINE LUNCH, FROZEN, Alfredo sauce 'Lunch Express' w/chicken (Lean Cuisine)	10.25 oz	240	31.0	6.0
FIELD PEAS, CANNED				
'Fresh' (Allens)	1/2 cup	100	18.0	<1.0
'Fresh' w/snaps (Allens)	1/2 cup	100	20.0	<1.0
tiny, 'Fresh' w/snaps (Allens)	1/2 cup	70	13.0	<1.0
w/snaps (Bush's Best)	1/2 cup	80	16.0	0.0
FIG				
candied	100 gm	299	73.7	0.2
raw, w/o stem	1 large	47	12.3	0.2
raw, w/o stem	1 med	37	9.6	0.2
trimmed	1 oz	21	5.4	0.1
w/stems	1 lb	333	86.1	1.4
Canned				
in extra heavy syrup	4 oz	121	31.6	0.1
in extra heavy syrup, solid and liquid	1 cup	279	72.7	0.3
in extra heavy syrup, w/1.75 tbsp liquid	3 fruits	91	23.7	0.1
in heavy syrup	4 oz	100	26.0	0.1
in heavy syrup, solid and liquid	1 cup	228	59.3	0.3
in heavy syrup, whole (Del Monte)	1/2 cup	100	28.0	0.0
in heavy syrup, whole, Kadota 'Fancy' (S&W)	1/2 cup	100	28.0	0.0
in heavy syrup, w/1.75 tbsp liquid	3 fruits	75	19.5	0.1
in light syrup	1/2 cup	87	22.6	0.1
in light syrup	4 oz	78	20.4	0.1
in light syrup, solid and liquid	1 cup	174	45.2	0.3
in light syrup, w/1.75 tbsp liquid	3 fruits	59	15.3	0.1
in water	1/2 cup	65	17.3	0.1
in water	4 oz	60	15.9	0.1
in water, solid and liquid	1 cup	131	34.7	0.3
in water, w/1.75 tbsp liquid	3 fruits	42	11.2	0.1
Dried				
cooked	4 oz	122	31.3	0.6
stewed	1/2 cup	140	35.8	0.6
uncooked	1 cup	507	130.1	2.3

Food Name	Serv. Size	Total Cal.	Carbs GMS	Fat GMS
uncooked	4 oz	289	74.1	1.3
uncooked, Calimyrna *(Blue Ribbon)*	1/2 cup	250	58.0	2.0
uncooked, Calimyrna *(Sun•Maid)*	1/2 cup	250	58.0	2.0
uncooked, Mission *(Blue Ribbon)*	1/2 cup	210	1.0	(mq)
uncooked, Mission *(Sun•Maid)*	1/2 cup	210	1.0	(mq)
uncooked, trimmed	10 fruits	477	122.2	2.2

FILBERT, SHELLED. See HAZELNUT, SHELLED.

FILBERT BUTTER, roasted *(Maranatha Natural)* | 2 tbsp | 180 | 6.0 | 16.0

FILO DOUGH. See PHYLLO DOUGH.

FINNAN HADDIE, smoked | 4 oz | 132 | 0.0 | 1.1

FINOCCHIO. See FENNEL.

FISH. See individual listings.

FISH CAKE

fried	1 cake	103	5.6	4.8
fried, bite size	5 cakes	103	5.6	4.8
frozen *(Mrs. Paul's)*	2 pieces	190	24.0	7.0

FISH DINNER, FROZEN

(Healthy Choice) lemon pepper, 10.7 oz	1 serving	300	52.0	5.0
(Kid Cuisine) nuggets	7 oz	320	33.0	15.0
(Morton)	9.75 oz	370	46.0	13.0
(Swanson) n' chips	10 oz	500	60.0	21.0

FISH ENTRÉE

Canned, Dijon 'Light' *(Mrs. Paul's)*	8.75 oz	200	17.0	5.0
Frozen				
fillet of, divan *(Lean Cuisine)*	10 3/8 oz	210	13.0	5.0
fillet of, Florentine *(Lean Cuisine)*	9 5/8 oz	220	13.0	7.0
fillet of, Florentine 'Light' *(Mrs. Paul's)*	8 oz	220	10.0	8.0
fish 'n fries 'Home Style Recipe' *(Swanson)*	6.5 oz	340	37.0	16.0
gems, fancy style *(Wakefield)*	4 oz	80	11.0	1.0
gems, salad style *(Wakefield)*	3 oz	70	8.0	1.0
in herb sauce *(Gorton's)*	1 pkg	190	3.0	8.0
Mornay 'Light' *(Mrs. Paul's)*	9 oz	230	12.0	10.0
oven baked, w/vegetable medley *(Ultimate 200)*	6.64 oz	120	10.0	2.0
'Platters' *(Banquet)*	8.75 oz	450	33.0	22.0
salmon, Keta *(Libby's)*	3.7 oz	130	0.0	6.0
sticks 'Looney Tunes Sylvester' *(Tyson)*	7.5 oz	290	36.0	11.0

FISH FILLET, ALTERNATIVE

vegetarian, frozen *(Worthington)* 1.5-oz pieces	2 pieces	180	9.0	9.0

FISH FILLET, FROZEN

battered *(Mrs. Paul's)*	2 pieces	330	28.0	17.0
battered *(Van de Kamp's)*	1 piece	170	13.0	10.0
battered 'Crispy Batter' *(Gorton's)*	2 pieces	290	18.0	19.0
battered 'Crispy Batter' large *(Gorton's)*	1 piece	320	20.0	21.0

Food Name	Serv. Size	Total Cal.	Carbs GMS	Fat GMS
battered 'Crunchy' (Gorton's)	2 pieces	230	16.0	13.0
battered 'Crunchy' (Mrs. Paul's)	2 pieces	280	26.0	14.0
battered 'Crunchy Microwave' (Gorton's)	2 pieces	340	17.0	26.0
battered 'Crunchy Microwave' large (Gorton's)	1 piece	320	20.0	22.0
battered, minced 'Portions' (Mrs. Paul's)	2 pieces	300	21.0	19.0
battered 'Potato Crisp' (Gorton's)	2 pieces	300	18.0	20.0
battered, tempura 'Light Recipe' (Gorton's)	1 piece	200	8.0	14.0
battered 'Value Pack Portions' (Gorton's)	1 piece	180	13.0	11.0
breaded (Van de Kamp's)	2 pieces	280	18.0	18.0
breaded 'Crisp and Healthy' baked (Van de Kamp's)	2 pieces	150	18.0	3.0
breaded 'Crispy Crunchy' (Mrs. Paul's)	2 pieces	220	23.0	9.0
breaded, crispy 'Microwave' (Van de Kamp's)	1 piece	140	9.0	9.0
breaded, crispy 'Microwave' large (Van de Kamp's)	1 piece	290	21.0	17.0
breaded, 8 fillets (Healthy Choice)	2.5 oz	120	11.0	4.0
breaded, 4 fillets (Healthy Choice)	3 oz	140	14.0	4.0
breaded 'Light Recipe' (Gorton's)	1 piece	180	16.0	8.0
breaded, minced 'Crispy Crunchy Portions' (Mrs. Paul's)	2 pieces	230	14.0	15.0
breaded, reheated, 2 oz	1 piece	155	13.5	7.0
breaded 'Snack Pack' (Van de Kamp's)	2 pieces	220	13.0	10.0
breaded, 2 fillets (Healthy Choice)	3.5 oz	160	16.0	5.0
coated, ranch 'Specialty Microwave' (Gorton's)	1 piece	330	24.0	21.0
crispy, microwave (Van de Kamp's)	1 piece	140	9.0	9.0
crispy, microwave large (Van de Kamp's)	1 piece	290	21.0	17.0
in butter sauce 'Light' (Mrs. Paul's)	1 piece	140	1.0	6.0
marinated, Cajun style, catfish 'Select' (Gorton's)	1 fillet	220	3.0	13.0
FISH LOAF, cooked	1 loaf	1507	88.7	45.0
FISH NUGGET, FROZEN, battered (Van de Kamp's)	4 pieces	130	8.0	9.0
FISH OIL				
herring	1 cup	1966	0.0	218.0
herring	1 tbsp	123	0.0	13.6
menhaden	1 cup	1966	0.0	218.0
menhaden	1 tbsp	123	0.0	13.6
menhaden, fully hydrogenated	1 cup	1849	0.0	205.0
menhaden, fully hydrogenated	1 tbsp	113	0.0	12.5
salmon	1 cup	1966	0.0	218.0
salmon	1 tbsp	123	0.0	13.6
sardine	1 cup	1966	0.0	218.0
sardine	1 tbsp	123	0.0	13.6
FISH PASTE CAKE				
Japanese, block, steamed 'Kamoboko'	4 oz	111	11.0	1.0
Japanese, stick, grilled 'Chikuwa'	4 oz	143	15.3	2.4

FISH SEASONING MIX. See SEAFOOD SEASONING MIX.

Food Name	Serv. Size	Total Cal.	Carbs GMS	Fat GMS
FISH STICKS, FROZEN				
battered *(Mrs. Paul's)*	4 pieces	210	15.0	12.0
battered *(Van de Kamp's)*	4 pieces	160	12.0	9.0
battered 'Crispy Batter' *(Gorton's)*	4 pieces	260	16.0	18.0
battered 'Crunchy' *(Gorton's)*	4 pieces	210	15.0	13.0
battered, minced *(Mrs. Paul's)*	4 pieces	220	20.0	13.0
battered 'Potato Crisp' *(Gorton's)*	4 pieces	260	21.0	16.0
battered 'Value Pack' *(Gorton's)*	4 pieces	190	17.0	9.0
breaded *(Healthy Choice)*	2.4 oz	120	14.0	4.0
breaded *(Van de Kamp's)*	4 pieces	200	15.0	12.0
breaded 'Bunch o' Crunch' approx 2.7 oz *(Frionor)*	4 pieces	210	13.0	14.0
breaded 'Crisp and Healthy' baked *(Van de Kamp's)*	4 pieces	120	17.0	2.0
breaded 'Crispy Crunchy' *(Mrs. Paul's)*	4 pieces	140	14.0	6.0
breaded, crispy 'Microwave' *(Van de Kamp's)*	3 pieces	130	11.0	7.0
breaded, minced 'Crispy Crunchy' *(Mrs. Paul's)*	4 pieces	190	18.0	8.0
breaded 'Snack Pack' *(Van de Kamp's)*	4 pieces	170	13.0	10.0
breaded 'Value Pack' *(Van de Kamp's)*	4 pieces	170	13.0	10.0
breaded w/whole wheat 'Microwave' *(Booth)*	2 oz	150	14.0	8.0
FIVE-SPICE, Oriental spice *(Tone's)*	1 tsp	9	1.9	0.3
FLAN. See PUDDING MIX.				
FLATFISH. See FLOUNDER; HALIBUT; SOLE.				
FLAX OIL				
(Spectrum Naturals) organic 'Veg-Omega 3'	1 tbsp	120	0.0	14.0
(Spectrum Naturals) organic 'Veg-Omega 3' cinnamon flavored	1 tbsp	120	0.0	14.0
FLAXSEED *(Arrowhead Mills)*	1 oz	140	11.0	10.0
FLOUNDER				
dry-heat cooked	3 oz	99	0.0	1.3
raw	3 oz	77	0.0	1.0
FLOUNDER, FROZEN				
(Booth) Atlantic	4 oz	90	0.0	1.0
(Finast)	4 oz	90	0.0	1.0
(Gorton's) crunch breaded, fillet 'Select' approx. 2.9 oz	1 fillet	190	17.0	9.0
(Gorton's) 'Fishmarket Fresh'	5 oz	110	1.0	1.0
(Mrs. Paul's) battered, fillets 'Crunchy'	2 pieces	220	23.0	9.0
(Mrs. Paul's) breaded, fillets 'Light'	1 piece	240	20.0	10.0
(SeaPak)	4 oz	90	0.0	1.0
(Van de Kamp's) breaded fillets 'Light'	1 piece	260	21.0	12.0
(Van de Kamp's) fillet 'Light'	1 piece	260	21.0	12.0
(Van de Kamp's) 'Natural'	4 oz	100	0.0	2.0
FLOUNDER ENTRÉE, FROZEN				
stuffed 'Microwave Entrees' *(Gorton's)*	1 pkg	350	21.0	18.0

Food Name	Serv. Size	Total Cal.	Carbs GMS	Fat GMS
FLOUR. See also individual listings.				
all-purpose, 4 oz *(Gold Medal)*	1 cup	400	87.0	1.0
all-purpose, 4 oz *(Red Band)*	1 cup	290	85.0	1.0
all-purpose, 4 oz *(Robin Hood)*	1 cup	400	85.0	1.0
'Better for Bread' 4 oz *(Gold Medal)*	1 cup	400	83.0	1.0
'Drifted Snow' 4 oz *(Red Band)*	1 cup	400	87.0	1.0
'La Piña' 4 oz *(Red Band)*	1 cup	400	87.0	1.0
self-rising, 4 oz *(Gold Medal)*	1 cup	380	83.0	1.0
self-rising, 4 oz *(Red Band)*	1 cup	380	83.0	1.0
self-rising, 4 oz *(Robin Hood)*	1 cup	380	83.0	1.0
'Softasilk' 1 oz *(Red Band)*	1/4 cup	100	23.0	0.0
unbleached, 4 oz *(Gold Medal)*	1 cup	400	87.0	1.0
unbleached, 4 oz *(Robin Hood)*	1 cup	400	85.0	1.0
'Wondra' 4 oz *(Red Band)*	1 cup	400	87.0	1.0
FLYING FISH				
raw	1 lb	413	0.0	0.9
raw	1 oz	26	0.0	<.1
FON GOOT YAM. See JICAMA.				
FONDANT. See CANDY.				
FORMULA, INFANT. See BABY FOOD.				
FRANKFURTER				
beef and pork, 1 oz	1 frank	91	0.7	8.3
cheesefurter/cheese smokie, 1 oz	1 frank	93	0.4	8.2
cheesefurter/cheese smokie, approx 1.5 oz	1 frank	141	0.6	12.5
chicken, 1 oz	1 frank	73	1.9	5.5
raw, beef and pork, 2 oz	1 frank	182	1.5	16.6
raw, w/nonfat dry milk and cereal, 2 oz	1 frank	156	0.0	12.4
turkey, 1 oz	1 frank	64	0.4	5.0
(Ball Park)				
beef 'Lite'	1 frank	140	1.0	12.0
beef, pork and chicken 'Lite'	1 frank	140	1.0	12.0
(Boar's Head)				
beef, 1 oz	1 frank	80	<1.0	7.0
pork and beef, 1 oz	1 frank	80	<1.0	7.0
(Butterball) turkey	1 frank	140	2.0	11.0
(Eckrich)				
beef 'Jumbo'	1 frank	190	2.0	17.0
beef '1-lb pkg'	1 frank	150	2.0	14.0
'Bunsize'	1 frank	190	2.0	17.0
cheesefurter/cheese smokie	1 frank	180	2.0	16.0
'Jumbo Lean Supreme'	1 frank	140	2.0	12.0
'1-lb pkg'	1 frank	160	2.0	14.0

Food Name	Serv. Size	Total Cal.	Carbs GMS	Fat GMS
(Health Valley)				
chicken 'Weiners'	1 frank	96	1.0	8.0
turkey 'Weiners'	1 frank	96	1.0	8.0
(Healthy Choice) turkey, pork, and beef 'Jumbo' lowfat	1 frank	70	5.0	2.0
(Healthy Favorites) w/turkey, 2 oz	1 frank	57	2.1	1.6
(Hebrew National) beef, 1.7 oz	1 frank	149	<1.0	14.0
(Hillshire Farm)				
beef 'Bun Size Wieners' 2 oz	1 frank	180	2.0	16.0
beef 'Hot Links' 2 oz	1 frank	190	1.0	17.0
cheesefurter/cheese smokie 'Bun Size Wieners' 2 oz	1 frank	180	2.0	16.0
'Hot Links' 2 oz	1 frank	190	2.0	16.0
natural casing 'Wieners' 2 oz	1 frank	180	2.0	17.0
(Hormel)				
batter-wrapped, frozen 'Corn Dogs'	1 frank	220	21.0	12.0
batter-wrapped, frozen 'Tater Dogs'	1 frank	210	15.0	14.0
beef '1-lb pkg'	1 frank	140	1.0	13.0
beef '12-oz pkg'	1 frank	100	1.0	10.0
chili 'Frank 'n Stuff'	1 frank	165	2.0	15.0
'Light & Lean 97' 1.6 oz	1 frank	45	2.0	1.0
'Mexicali Dogs' 5 oz	1 frank	400	41.0	21.0
'1-lb pkg'	1 frank	140	1.0	13.0
smoked, beef 'Wranglers'	1 frank	170	2.0	15.0
smoked 'Range Brand Wranglers'	1 frank	170	1.0	16.0
smoked, w/cheese 'Wranglers'	1 frank	180	1.0	16.0
'12-oz pkg'	1 frank	110	1.0	10.0
(Hygrade) chicken 'Grillmaster'	1 frank	130	3.0	11.0
(JM)				
beef, 1.2 oz	1 frank	100	1.0	9.0
beef 'Jumbo' 2 oz	1 frank	180	2.0	16.0
beef '10 per lb pkg' 1.6 oz	1 frank	140	1.0	13.0
cheesefurter/cheese smokie 'Cheese Franks' 1.6 oz	1 frank	140	2.0	13.0
'German Brand' 2 oz	1 frank	160	1.0	14.0
1.2 oz	1 frank	110	1.0	10.0
'10 per lb' 1.6 oz	1 frank	140	1.0	13.0
w/cheese 'German Brand' 2 oz	1 frank	160	2.0	14.0
(Kahn's)				
beef	1 frank	140	2.0	13.0
beef 'Bun Size Franks'	1 frank	190	3.0	17.0
beef 'Jumbo'	1 frank	190	3.0	18.0
beef w/cheddar 'Beef n' Cheddar'	1 frank	180	2.0	16.0
cheesefurter/cheese smokie 'Cheese Wiener'	1 frank	150	1.0	13.0
smoked, beef 'Bun Size Beef Smokey'	1 frank	190	2.0	17.0
smoked 'Big Red Smokey'	1 frank	170	2.0	14.0

Food Name	Serv. Size	Total Cal.	Carbs GMS	Fat GMS
smoked 'Bun Size Smokey'	1 frank	180	2.0	15.0
'Wieners'	1 frank	140	1.0	13.0
(King Kold) beef, 2 oz	1 frank	173	1.0	16.3
(Longacre)				
chicken	1 frank	63	1.0	5.0
turkey	1 frank	66	0.0	6.0
(Louis Rich)				
turkey 'Bun Length' 2 oz	1 frank	128	1.5	10.4
turkey, cheese, 1.6 oz	1 frank	109	1.3	8.9
turkey, 1.6 oz	1 frank	101	1.2	8.2
(Mr. Turkey)				
turkey, 1.6 oz	1 frank	106	0.9	8.9
turkey, cheese, 1.6 oz	1 frank	109	0.9	9.1
(OHSE)				
beef, 1 oz	1 frank	85	1.0	8.0
chicken, beef, and pork, 1 oz	1 frank	85	1.0	8.0
'Wieners' 1 oz	1 frank	90	1.0	8.0
(Oscar Mayer)				
bacon and cheddar cheese 'Hot Dogs' 1.6 oz	1 frank	137	1.0	12.0
beef 'Bun-Length Franks' 2 oz	1 frank	182	1.4	16.8
beef, deli 'Big & Juicy' 2.7 oz	1 frank	249	0.5	23.5
beef 'Franks' 2 oz	1 frank	181	1.4	16.7
beef, garlic 'Big & Juicy' 2.7 oz	1 frank	239	0.2	22.5
beef 'Light Franks' 2 oz	1 frank	131	0.9	11.1
beef, quarter lb, bun length 'Big & Juicy' 4 oz	1 frank	359	1.6	33.5
beef w/cheddar 'Franks' 2 oz	1 frank	163	1.1	14.3
'Bun-Length Wieners' 2 oz	1 frank	184	1.4	16.9
cheesefurter/cheese smokie 'Hot Dogs' 1.6 oz	1 frank	143	1.1	12.9
cocktail 'Little Wieners' .3 oz	1 frank	28	0.2	2.6
hot and spicy 'Big & Juicy' 2.7 oz	1 frank	224	0.6	20.4
'Hot Dogs' 1.6 oz	1 frank	137	1.0	12.0
'Light Wieners' 2 oz	1 frank	127	0.3	10.8
97% fat-free, turkey, beef 'Healthy Favorites'	1 frank	60	2.0	1.5
original 'Big & Juicy' 2.7 oz	1 frank	244	0.0	23.2
'Wieners' 2 oz	1 frank	181	1.4	16.9
(Pilgrim's Pride)				
'1-lb pkg' 2-oz frank	1 frank	118	1.1	8.8
'12-oz pkg' 1.5-oz frank	1 frank	88	0.8	6.6
(Quick Meal) w/chili, and cheese, 4.5 oz	1 frank	340	25.0	20.0
(State Fair) beef, batter-wrapped, on stick 'Corn Dogs' 2.67 oz	1 frank	210	24.0	10.0
(Tyson)				
chicken	1 frank	115	1.0	10.0
chicken, batter-wrapped 'Corn Dogs' 3.5 oz	1 frank	280	28.0	14.0

Food Name	Serv. Size	Total Cal.	Carbs GMS	Fat GMS
w/cheese	1 frank	145	1.0	11.0
FRANKFURTER, ALTERNATIVE				
(Smart Dog) 'Lightlife' fat-free, 1.5 oz	1 frank	40	1.1	0.0
(White Wave Soyfood) 'Healthy' 1.5 oz	1 frank	120	5.0	8.0
(Worthington)				
canned 'Super-Links' 1.7 oz	1 frank	100	3.0	7.0
canned 'Veja-Links'	2 franks	140	4.0	10.0
frozen 'Leanies' 1.4 oz	1 frank	100	2.0	6.0
frozen, on a stick 'Dixie Dogs' 2.5 oz	1 frank	200	21.0	10.0
FRENCH ARTICHOKE. See ARTICHOKES, FRENCH.				
FRENCH BEAN				
boiled	4 oz	146	27.2	0.9
dried, boiled	1/2 cup	111	20.7	0.7
raw	1/2 cup	316	59.0	1.9
raw, dried	1 oz	97	18.2	0.6
FRENCH TOAST, FROZEN				
(Aunt Jemima) cinnamon swirl	3 oz	171	27.5	4.3
(Aunt Jemima) 'Original'	3 oz	166	26.5	4.4
(Aunt Jemima) sticks, and syrup 'Homestyle'	5.2 oz	400	48.0	20.0
(Aunt Jemima) wedges, and sausages 'Homestyle'	5.3 oz	360	40.0	17.0
(Downyflake)	2 slices	270	34.0	12.0
(Downyflake) 'Extra Thick'	1 slice	150	11.0	9.0
(Downyflake) Texas style, and sausage	4.25 oz	400	37.0	24.0
(Krusteaz) cinnamon swirl	2 slices	270	46.0	5.0
(Krusteaz) regular	2 slices	250	38.0	6.0
(Morningstar Farms) vegetarian, cinnamon swirl, w/patties . .	6.5 oz	380	37.0	15.0
(Swanson) cinnamon swirl, w/sausages 'Great Starts'	5.5 oz	390	37.0	21.0
(Swanson) mini, w/sausage 'Great Starts'	2.5 oz	190	22.0	9.0
(Swanson) oatmeal, w/lite links 'Great Starts'	4.65 oz	310	35.0	13.0
(Swanson) w/sausages 'Great Starts'	5.5 oz	380	35.0	21.0
FRENCH TOAST, STICKS				
apple cinnamon *(Farm Rich)*	3 oz	310	39.0	15.0
blueberry *(Farm Rich)*	3 oz	310	37.0	14.0
original *(Farm Rich)*	3 oz	300	37.0	15.0
FRENCH FRY SEASONING *(Tone's)*	1 tsp	5	1.0	0.1
FROG'S LEGS				
raw	100 gm	73	0.0	0.3
raw	1 oz	21	0.0	<1.0
FROGFISH. See MONKFISH.				
FROSTING MIX				
(Betty Crocker)				
cherry 'Creamy' prepared w/margarine	1/12 pkg	180	31.0	6.0
chocolate fudge 'Creamy' dry	1/12 pkg	140	30.0	2.0

Food Name	Serv. Size	Total Cal.	Carbs GMS	Fat GMS
chocolate fudge 'Creamy' prepared w/butter	1/12 pkg	180	30.0	6.0
chocolate fudge 'Creamy' prepared w/margarine	1/12 pkg	180	30.0	6.0
coconut pecan 'Creamy' dry	1/12 pkg	110	19.0	4.0
coconut pecan 'Creamy' prepared w/butter, 2% milk	1/12 pkg	150	19.0	8.0
coconut pecan 'Creamy' prepared w/margarine, skim milk	1/12 pkg	150	19.0	8.0
milk chocolate 'Creamy' prepared w/margarine	1/12 pkg	170	29.0	5.0
rainbow chip 'Creamy' prepared w/margarine	1/12 pkg	190	32.0	7.0
sour cream, chocolate fudge 'Creamy' prepared w/margarine	1/12 pkg	180	30.0	6.0
sour cream, white 'Creamy' prepared w/margarine	1/12 pkg	170	31.0	5.0
vanilla 'Creamy' dry	1/12 pkg	150	32.0	2.0
vanilla 'Creamy' prepared w/butter	1/12 pkg	170	32.0	5.0
vanilla 'Creamy' prepared w/margarine	1/12 pkg	170	32.0	5.0
white 'Fluffy'	1/12 pkg	70	16.0	0.0
(Estee)	1 tbsp	65	13.0	1.5

FROSTING, READY-TO-SPREAD
(Betty Crocker)

Food Name	Serv. Size	Total Cal.	Carbs GMS	Fat GMS
amaretto almond 'Creamy Deluxe'	1/12 tub	160	27.0	6.0
butter pecan 'Creamy Deluxe'	1/12 tub	170	26.0	7.0
cherry 'Creamy Deluxe'	1/12 tub	160	27.0	6.0
chocolate 'Creamy Deluxe'	1/12 tub	160	24.0	7.0
chocolate 'Creamy Deluxe Light'	1/12 tub	130	28.0	2.0
chocolate chip 'Creamy Deluxe'	1/12 tub	170	27.0	7.0
chocolate chip, coated 'Creamy Deluxe Party'	1/12 tub	160	24.0	7.0
chocolate chip, double 'Creamy Deluxe'	1/12 tub	170	24.0	8.0
chocolate coconut almond 'Creamy Deluxe'	1/12 tub	160	21.0	8.0
chocolate w/dinosaurs 'Creamy Deluxe Party'	1/12 tub	160	24.0	7.0
chocolate w/red gel 'Creamy Deluxe Party'	1/12 tub	160	24.0	7.0
chocolate w/turbo racers 'Creamy Deluxe Party'	1/12 tub	160	24.0	7.0
coconut pecan 'Creamy Deluxe'	1/12 tub	160	20.0	9.0
cream cheese 'Creamy Deluxe'	1/12 tub	170	26.0	7.0
dark Dutch fudge 'Creamy Deluxe'	1/12 tub	160	22.0	7.0
lemon 'Creamy Deluxe'	1/12 tub	170	28.0	6.0
milk chocolate 'Creamy Deluxe'	1/12 tub	160	25.0	6.0
milk chocolate 'Creamy Deluxe Light'	1/12 tub	140	29.0	2.0
rainbow chip 'Creamy Deluxe'	1/12 tub	170	27.0	7.0
rocky road 'Creamy Deluxe'	1/12 tub	150	20.0	8.0
sour cream chocolate 'Creamy Deluxe'	1/12 tub	160	23.0	7.0
sour cream white 'Creamy Deluxe'	1/12 tub	160	27.0	6.0
vanilla 'Creamy Deluxe'	1/12 tub	160	27.0	6.0
vanilla 'Creamy Deluxe Light'	1/12 tub	140	30.0	2.0
vanilla w/blue gel 'Creamy Deluxe Party'	1/12 tub	160	27.0	6.0
vanilla w/teddy bears 'Creamy Deluxe Party'	1/12 tub	160	27.0	6.0

Food Name	Serv. Size	Total Cal.	Carbs GMS	Fat GMS
(Duncan Hines)				
chocolate	1/12 tub	160	24.0	7.0
cream cheese	1/12 tub	160	24.0	8.0
cream cheese 'Homestyle'	1/12 tub	160	26.0	6.0
dark chocolate 'Homestyle'	1/12 tub	160	25.0	6.0
Dutch fudge	1/12 tub	160	24.0	7.0
lemon	1/12 tub	120	18.0	6.0
milk chocolate	1/12 tub	160	24.0	7.0
milk chocolate 'Homestyle'	1/12 tub	160	25.0	6.0
vanilla	1/12 tub	160	24.0	7.0
vanilla 'Homestyle'	1/12 tub	160	26.0	6.0
(Finast) milk chocolate	1/12 tub	160	25.0	6.0
(Lovin' Lites)				
chocolate fudge	1/12 tub	130	28.0	2.0
milk chocolate	1/12 tub	130	28.0	2.0
vanilla	1/12 tub	130	29.0	2.0
(Pathmark)				
chocolate, creamy	1/12 tub	160	25.0	6.0
fudge, creamy	1/12 tub	160	25.0	7.0
white, creamy	1/12 tub	160	25.0	6.0
(Pillsbury)				
butter fudge 'Frosting Supreme'	1/12 tub	140	22.0	6.0
caramel pecan 'Frosting Supreme'	1/12 tub	150	20.0	8.0
chocolate chip 'Frosting Supreme'	1/12 tub	150	27.0	5.0
chocolate fudge 'Frosting Supreme'	1/12 tub	150	22.0	6.0
chocolate fudge 'Funfetti'	1/12 tub	140	23.0	6.0
chocolate, double Dutch 'Frosting Supreme'	1/12 tub	140	22.0	6.0
coconut almond 'Frosting Supreme'	1/12 tub	150	17.0	9.0
coconut pecan 'Frosting Supreme'	1/12 tub	160	17.0	10.0
cream cheese 'Frosting Supreme'	1/12 tub	160	26.0	6.0
decorator, all flavors except chocolate	1 tbsp	70	12.0	2.0
decorator, chocolate	1 tbsp	60	11.0	2.0
double Dutch 'Frosting Supreme'	1/12 tub	140	22.0	6.0
fudge 'Frosting Supreme'	1/12 tub	150	24.0	6.0
lemon 'Frosting Supreme'	1/12 tub	160	26.0	6.0
milk chocolate 'Frosting Supreme'	1/12 tub	150	23.0	6.0
milk chocolate w/fudge swirl 'Frosting Supreme'	1/12 tub	150	23.0	6.0
mint 'Frosting Supreme'	1/12 tub	150	24.0	7.0
mocha 'Frosting Supreme'	1/12 tub	150	24.0	6.0
sour cream vanilla 'Frosting Supreme'	1/12 tub	160	27.0	6.0
strawberry 'Frosting Supreme'	1/12 tub	160	26.0	6.0
vanilla 'Frosting Supreme'	1/12 tub	160	26.0	6.0
vanilla 'Funfetti'	1/12 tub	150	25.0	6.0

Food Name	Serv. Size	Total Cal.	Carbs GMS	Fat GMS
vanilla 'Funfetti Sunshine'	1/12 tub	150	25.0	6.0
vanilla, pink and white 'Funfetti'	1/12 tub	150	24.0	6.0
vanilla w/fudge swirl 'Frosting Supreme'	1/12 tub	150	25.0	6.0
white, fluffy	1/12 tub	60	15.0	0.0
FRUCTOSE				
(Estee)	1 tsp	16	4.0	0.0
(Estee) packet	1 pkt	12	3.0	0.0
(Featherweight)	1 tsp	12	3.0	0.0
FRUIT. See individual listings.				
FRUIT, MIXED				
Canned				
(A&P) in light syrup	1/2 cup	75	20.0	<1.0
(Del Monte) chunky	1/2 cup	80	23.0	0.0
(Del Monte) chunky 'Lite'	1/2 cup	50	14.0	0.0
(Del Monte) 'Fruit Cup'	5 oz	100	27.0	0.0
(Del Monte) tropical	1/2 cup	90	26.0	0.0
(Dole) pineapple and Mandarin orange segments	1/2 cup	80	19.0	<1.0
(Dole) tropical fruit salad	1/2 cup	70	17.0	0.0
(Finast) in heavy syrup, chunky	1/2 cup	70	18.0	0.0
(Kraft) salad 'Pure'	1/2 cup	80	18.0	0.0
(Libby's) in juice, chunky 'Lite'	1/2 cup	50	14.0	0.0
(Pathmark) in juice, chunky	1/2 cup	50	14.0	0.0
(Pathmark) in light syrup 'No Frills'	1 cup	150	39.0	0.0
(S&W) in juice, chunky, sweetened, clarified	1/2 cup	90	21.0	0.0
(S&W Nutradiet) chunky	1/2 cup	40	10.0	0.0
(Sun Fresh) jar, chilled, in light syrup 'Tropical Salad'	3.5 oz	88	18.7	0.9
Dried				
(Del Monte)	2 oz	130	34.0	0.0
(SunSweet)	2 oz	150	39.0	0.0
(SunSweet) bits	2 oz	150	40.0	<1.0
(Sun•Maid)	2 oz	150	39.0	0.0
(Sun•Maid) bits	2 oz	150	40.0	<1.0
Frozen (Birds Eye) in syrup 'Quick Thaw pouch'	5 oz	120	31.0	0.0
FRUIT AND NUT MIX				
(Estee)	14 pieces	70	6.0	5.0
(Estee)	4 pieces	35	3.0	2.0
(Planters) 'Caribbean Crunch'	1 oz	150	14.0	10.0
(Planters) 'Fruit 'n Nut'	1 oz	150	13.0	9.0
FRUIT BAR, FROZEN. See also ICE BARS AND DESSERTS; SHERBET; SORBET.				
all flavors 'Fruit Juicee' (Minute Maid)	1 bar	60	14.0	0.0
blueberry and cream 'Fruit & Cream' (Dole)	1 bar	90	19.4	1.4
cherry 'Fresh Lites' (Dole)	1 bar	25	6.0	<1.0
cherry and yogurt 'Fruit & Yogurt' (Dole)	1 bar	80	17.0	<1.0

Food Name	Serv. Size	Total Cal.	Carbs GMS	Fat GMS
chocolate/banana and cream 'Fruit & Cream' (Dole)	1 bar	175	22.0	9.0
chocolate/strawberry and cream 'Fruit & Cream' (Dole)	1 bar	140	23.0	8.0
coconut (Sunkist)	1 bar	170	15.0	10.0
grape 'SunTops' (Dole)	1 bar	40	9.0	<1.0
lemon 'Fresh Lites' (Dole)	1 bar	25	6.0	<1.0
lemonade (Sunkist)	1 bar	90	24.0	0.0
lemonade 'SunTops' (Dole)	1 bar	40	9.0	<1.0
orange 'Juice Bar' (Sunkist)	1 bar	100	25.0	0.0
orange, tropical 'SunTops' (Dole)	1 bar	40	9.0	<1.0
peach and cream 'Fruit & Cream' (Dole)	1 bar	90	19.4	1.4
pineapple 'Fruit 'n Juice' (Dole)	1 bar	70	17.0	<.1
pineapple-orange 'Fresh Lites' (Dole)	1 bar	25	6.0	<1.0
piña colada 'Fruit 'n Juice' (Dole)	1 bar	90	16.0	3.0
punch 'SunTops' (Dole)	1 bar	40	9.0	<1.0
raspberry 'Fresh Lites' (Dole)	1 bar	25	6.0	<1.0
raspberry 'Fruit 'n Juice' (Dole)	1 bar	70	16.0	<.1
raspberry and cream 'Fruit & Cream' (Dole)	1 bar	90	20.0	1.4
strawberry and cream (Sunkist)	1 bar	90	19.0	1.0
strawberry and cream 'Fruit & Cream' (Dole)	1 bar	90	19.3	1.4
raspberry and yogurt 'Fruit & Yogurt' (Dole)	1 bar	70	17.0	<1.0
strawberry and yogurt 'Fruit & Yogurt' (Dole)	1 bar	70	17.0	<1.0
strawberry 'Fruit 'n Juice' (Dole)	1 bar	70	16.0	<.1
wildberry (Sunkist)	1 bar	140	33.0	0.0
FRUIT COCKTAIL, CANNED				
(Del Monte)	1/2 cup	80	23.0	0.0
(Hunt's)	4 oz	90	23.0	<1.0
fruit for salad (Del Monte)	1/2 cup	90	22.0	0.0
in extra heavy syrup	4 oz	98	26.0	0.1
in extra heavy syrup, solid and liquid	1/2 cup	114	29.8	0.1
in extra light syrup	4 oz	51	13.2	0.1
in extra light syrup, solid and liquid	1/2 cup	55	14.3	0.1
in heavy syrup	4 oz	83	21.4	0.1
in heavy syrup (A&P)	1/2 cup	90	24.0	<1.0
in heavy syrup (Finast)	1/2 cup	90	24.0	0.0
in heavy syrup (Pathmark)	1 cup	180	48.0	0.0
in heavy syrup (S&W)	1/2 cup	90	24.0	0.0
in heavy syrup, solid and liquid	1/2 cup	93	24.2	0.1
in juice	4 oz	52	13.4	<.1
in juice (Featherweight)	1/2 cup	50	14.0	0.0
in juice (IGA)	1/2 cup	60	15.0	0.0
in juice (S&W)	1/2 cup	90	21.0	0.0
in juice 'Lite' (Libby's)	1/2 cup	50	13.0	0.0
in juice, solid and liquid	1/2 cup	57	14.7	0.0

Food Name	Serv. Size	Total Cal.	Carbs GMS	Fat GMS
in light syrup	4 oz	65	16.9	0.1
in light syrup, solid and liquid	1/2 cup	72	18.8	0.1
in pear juice (A&P)	1/2 cup	50	14.0	<1.0
in water	4 oz	36	9.7	0.1
in water, solid and liquid	1/2 cup	39	10.4	0.1
'Lite' (Del Monte)	1/2 cup	50	15.0	0.0
'No Sugar Added' (Finast)	1/2 cup	50	14.0	0.0
'Regular Unsweetened' (S&W Nutradiet)	1/2 cup	40	10.0	0.0
FRUIT DRINK				
(Finast)	8 oz	80	21.0	0.0
(Fruitopia) 'Fruit Integration' real fruit	8 oz	120	31.0	0.0
(Hi-C) 'Bubble Gum' aseptic box or chilled	6 oz	90	22.0	0.0
(Hi-C) 'Double Fruit Cooler'	6 oz	93	22.9	<.1
(Hi-C) 'Double Fruit Cooler' aseptic box	6 oz	90	22.0	0.0
(Hi-C) 'Ecto Cooler'	6 oz	95	23.3	<.1
(Hi-C) 'Ecto Cooler' aseptic box	6 oz	90	23.0	0.0
(Hi-C) 'Hula Cooler'	6 oz	97	23.9	<.1
FRUIT JUICE				
(Juicy Juice) bottled	6 oz	100	23.0	0.0
(Juicy Juice) boxed	8.45 oz	140	33.0	0.0
(McCain) mixed fruit, 100% juice 'Junior'	4.2 oz	60	15.0	0.0
FRUIT JUICE COCKTAIL				
'Orchard Harvest Blend' (Welch's)	6 oz	110	27.0	0.0
'Orchard Harvest Blend' 'Cocktails-In-A-Box' (Welch's)	8.45 oz	150	38.0	0.0
'Orchard Harvest Blend' frozen, prepared (Welch's)	6 oz	110	27.0	0.0
FRUIT JUICE DRINK, mixed 'Fruit Box' (Tang)	8.45 oz	140	36.0	0.0
FRUIT JUICE DRINK MIX				
'Mixes w/Fruit Juice' powder (Ultra Slim Fast)	1 scoop	90	17.0	0.0
'Mixes w/Fruit Juice' prepared w/orange juice				
(Ultra Slim Fast)	8 oz	200	43.0	<1.0
FRUIT JUICE PUNCH DRINK				
concentrate, prepared w/water	1 cup	124	30.3	0.5
concentrate, prepared w/water	1 oz	15	3.8	0.1
concentrate, undiluted	12 oz	739	182.1	3.0
(Veryfine) can, bottle, or box '100% Juice Punch'	8 oz	122	30.0	0.0
FRUIT PUNCH				
(Bright & Early) frozen 'Bright & Early Fruit Punch'				
prepared	6 oz	90	22.0	0.0
(Juicy Juice) can, bottle, or box	6 oz	100	23.0	0.0
(Minute Maid) aseptic box, canned, or chilled	6 oz	90	22.0	0.0
(Minute Maid) frozen, concentrate, prepared	6 oz	90	23.0	0.0
(Pathmark) can, bottle, or box	6 oz	90	22.0	0.0
(Snapple)	8 oz	120	29.0	0.0

Food Name	Serv. Size	Total Cal.	Carbs GMS	Fat GMS
FRUIT PUNCH DRINK				
(All Sport) thirst quencher, caffeine-free	8 oz	80	21.0	0.0
(Bama)	8.45 oz	130	32.0	0.0
(Crowley)	8 oz	130	32.0	0.0
(Gatorade) low sodium, no caffeine	8 oz	50	14.0	0.0
(Hawaiian Punch) island fruit	6 oz	90	22.0	0.0
(Hawaiian Punch) red 'Fruit Juicy'	6 oz	90	22.0	0.0
(Hawaiian Punch) red 'Fruit Juicy Lite'	6 oz	60	15.0	0.0
(Hawaiian Punch) tropical	6 oz	90	22.0	0.0
(Hawaiian Punch) tropical, wild fruit	6 oz	90	23.0	0.0
(Hi-C)	6 oz	96	23.7	<.1
(Hi-C) aseptic box or chilled	6 oz	90	23.0	0.0
(Hi-C) 'Hula Punch'	6 oz	87	21.4	<.1
(Hi-C) 'Hula Punch Drink' aseptic box	6 oz	90	23.0	0.0
(J. Hungerford) 20% juice	9.03 oz	43	11.2	0.0
(J. Hungerford) 50% juice	9.03 oz	107	26.6	0.0
(J. Hungerford) 100% juice	9.03 oz	116	29.5	0.0
(Mott's)	10 oz	170	42.0	0.0
(Mott's)	9.5 oz	161	40.0	0.0
(PowerAde) thirst quencher, high energy	8 oz	70	19.0	0.0
(10-K)	8 oz	60	15.0	0.0
(Tropicana)	6 oz	90	21.0	<1.0
(Tropicana) 'Single Serve'	10 oz	148	37.0	0.0
(Welch's) 'Orchard Fruit Harvest Punch'	10 oz	180	45.0	0.0
(Wyler's)	6 oz	84	21.3	0.1
(Wyler's) tropical	6 oz	157	39.3	0.0
(Wyler's) tropical 'Fruit Slush'	4 oz	157	39.3	0.0
FRUIT PUNCH DRINK MIX				
frozen concentrate, prepared	12 oz	677	173.0	0.0
frozen, prepared w/water	1 cup	114	28.9	0.0
frozen, prepared w/water	1 oz	14	3.6	0.0
instant 'Thirst Quencher' prepared (Gatorade)	8 oz	60	15.0	0.0
'No Frills' prepared (Pathmark)	8 oz	90	22.0	0.0
powder, w/added sodium, dry	2 rounded tbsp	97	24.8	0.0
powder, w/added sodium, prepared	8 oz	97	24.9	0.0
powder, w/o added sodium, dry	2 rounded tbsp	97	24.8	0.0
powder, w/o added sodium, prepared	8 oz	97	24.9	0.0
sugar-free, prepared (Crystal Light)	8 oz	4	0.0	0.0
sugar-free, w/NutraSweet, prepared (Crystal Light)	8 oz	4	0.0	0.0
tropical 'Crystals' prepared (Wyler's)	8 oz	85	21.1	0.1

FRUIT ROLL. See FRUIT SNACK.

FRUIT SALAD, CANNED. See FRUIT COCKTAIL, CANNED.

Food Name	Serv. Size	Total Cal.	Carbs GMS	Fat GMS
FRUIT SNACK				
all flavors 'Berry Bears' *(Betty Crocker)*	1 pouch	100	22.0	<1.0
all flavors 'Fruit Roll-Ups Peel-Outs' *(Betty Crocker)*	1 roll	50	12.0	<1.0
all flavors 'Shark Bites' *(Betty Crocker)*	1 pouch	100	22.0	<1.0
apple *(Weight Watchers)*	1 pouch	50	13.0	<1.0
apple chips *(Weight Watchers)*	.75 oz	70	19.0	0.0
apple roll *(Flavor Tree)*	1 piece	75	18.5	0.0
apricot roll *(Flavor Tree)*	1 piece	76	17.7	0.5
assorted flavors, all shapes 'Fun Fruits' *(Sunkist)*	1 pouch	100	21.8	1.4
assorted flavors 'Bugs Bunny and Friends' *(Betty Crocker)*	1 pouch	90	21.0	1.0
assorted flavors 'Chip `N Dale Rescue Rangers' *(Fruit Parade)*	1 pouch	100	22.0	1.0
assorted flavors 'Darkwing Duck' *(Fruit Parade)*	1 pouch	100	22.0	1.0
assorted flavors 'Dinosaurs' *(Farley's)*	1 oz	90	22.0	<1.0
assorted flavors 'Fruit Circus Fruit Bears' *(Flavor Tree)*	1.05 oz	117	25.4	1.6
assorted flavors 'Tale Spin' *(Fruit Parade)*	1 pouch	100	22.0	1.0
assorted flavors 'Tasmanian Devil' *(Betty Crocker)*	1 pouch	90	21.0	1.0
assorted flavors 'Teenage Mutant Ninja Turtles' *(Farley's)*	1 oz	90	22.0	<1.0
assorted flavors 'Trolls' *(Farley's)*	1 oz	90	22.0	<1.0
berry 'Fun Fruits Berry Bunch' *(Sunkist)*	1 pouch	100	21.8	1.4
cherry 'Fruit by the Foot' *(Betty Crocker)*	1 roll	80	17.0	2.0
cherry 'Fruit Roll-Ups' *(Betty Crocker)*	.5-oz roll	50	12.0	<1.0
cherry 'Fun Fruits' *(Sunkist)*	1 pouch	100	21.8	1.4
cherry 'Wild Cherry Gushers' w/juicy centers *(Betty Crocker)*	1 pouch	90	21.0	1.0
cherry roll *(Flavor Tree)*	1 piece	75	18.3	0.1
cinnamon flavor *(Weight Watchers)*	1 pouch	50	13.0	<1.0
compote *(Rokeach)*	4 oz	120	31.0	1.0
crazy colors 'Fruit Roll-Ups' *(Betty Crocker)*	.5-oz roll	50	12.0	<1.0
'Fun Fruits Fantastic Fruit' *(Sunkist)*	1 pouch	100	21.8	1.4
'Garfield and Friends' 'Wild Blue' *(Betty Crocker)*	1 roll	50	12.0	<1.0
grape 'Fruit by the Foot' *(Betty Crocker)*	1 roll	80	17.0	2.0
grape 'Fruit Roll-Ups' *(Betty Crocker)*	.5-oz roll	50	12.0	<1.0
grape 'Fun Fruits' *(Sunkist)*	1 pouch	100	21.8	1.4
grape 'Gushin Grape Gushers' *(Betty Crocker)*	1 pouch	90	21.0	<1.0
grape roll *(Flavor Tree)*	1 piece	76	18.5	0.1
orange 'Fun Fruits' *(Sunkist)*	1 pouch	100	21.8	1.4
peach *(Weight Watchers)*	.5 oz	50	13.0	<1.0
raspberry 'Fruit Roll-Ups' *(Betty Crocker)*	.5-oz roll	50	12.0	<1.0
raspberry roll *(Flavor Tree)*	1 piece	75	18.3	0.1
strawberry *(Weight Watchers)*	1 pouch	50	13.0	<1.0
strawberry 'Fruit by the Foot' *(Betty Crocker)*	1 roll	80	17.0	2.0
strawberry 'Fruit Roll-Ups' *(Betty Crocker)*	.5-oz roll	50	12.0	<1.0

Food Name	Serv. Size	Total Cal.	Carbs GMS	Fat GMS
strawberry 'Fun Fruits' *(Sunkist)*	1 pouch	100	21.8	1.4
strawberry roll *(Flavor Tree)*	1 piece	74	18.0	0.1
strawberry 'Strawberry Splash Gushers' *(Betty Crocker)*	1 pouch	90	21.0	1.0
strawberry, yogurt coated 'Creme Supremes' *(Sunkist)*	1 pouch	114	20.1	3.6

FRUIT SPREAD

Food Name	Serv. Size	Total Cal.	Carbs GMS	Fat GMS
all flavors 'Homestyle' *(Smucker's)*	1 tsp	15	3.0	0.0
all flavors 'Slenderella' *(Smucker's)*	1 tsp	7	2.0	0.0
apple, no sugar added *(Fifty 50)*	1 tsp	2	<1.0	0.0
apricot 'All Fruit Spreadable Fruit' *(Polaner)*	1 tsp	14	4.0	0.0
apricot 'Light' w/NutraSweet *(Smucker's)*	1 tsp	7	2.0	0.0
apricot, low sugar *(Smucker's)*	1 tsp	8	2.0	0.0
apricot 'Simply Fruit' *(Smucker's)*	1 tsp	16	4.0	0.0
apricot-pineapple *(Knott's Berry Farm)*	1 tsp	16	4.0	0.0
apricot-pineapple 'Light' w/NutraSweet *(Knott's Berry Farm)*	1 tsp	8	2.0	0.0
apricot-pineapple, portion pack *(Knott's Berry Farm)*	.5 oz	35	9.0	0.0
black cherry 'All Fruit Spreadable Fruit' *(Polaner)*	1 tsp	14	4.0	0.0
black raspberry 'Simply Fruit' *(Smucker's)*	1 tsp	16	4.0	0.0
blackberry *(Knott's Berry Farm)*	1 tsp	16	4.0	0.0
blackberry 'Light' w/NutraSweet *(Knott's Berry Farm)*	1 tsp	8	2.0	0.0
blackberry, low sugar *(Smucker's)*	1 tsp	8	2.0	0.0
blackberry, portion pack *(Knott's Berry Farm)*	.5 oz	35	9.0	0.0
blackberry 'Simply Fruit' *(Smucker's)*	1 tsp	16	4.0	0.0
blueberry 'All Fruit Spreadable Fruit' *(Polaner)*	1 tsp	14	4.0	0.0
blueberry 'Simply Fruit' *(Smucker's)*	1 tsp	16	4.0	0.0
boysenberry *(Knott's Berry Farm)*	1 tsp	16	4.0	0.0
boysenberry 'Light' w/NutraSweet *(Knott's Berry Farm)*	1 tsp	8	2.0	0.0
boysenberry 'Light' w/NutraSweet *(Smucker's)*	1 tsp	7	2.0	0.0
boysenberry, low sugar *(Smucker's)*	1 tsp	8	2.0	0.0
boysenberry, portion pack *(Knott's Berry Farm)*	.5 oz	35	9.0	0.0
calamansi 'Tropical Rainforest' *(Knudsen & Sons)*	2 tsp	35	8.0	0.0
grape *(Weight Watchers)*	1 tsp	8	2.0	0.0
grape 'All Fruit Spreadable Fruit' *(Polaner)*	1 tsp	14	4.0	0.0
grape, Concord, low sugar *(Smucker's)*	1 tsp	8	2.0	0.0
grape 'Imitation' *(Smucker's)*	1 tsp	2	1.0	0.0
grape, no sugar added *(Fifty 50)*	1 tsp	2	<1.0	0.0
grape 'Simply Fruit' *(Smucker's)*	1 tsp	16	4.0	0.0
guanabana 'Tropical Rainforest' *(Knudsen & Sons)*	2 tsp	35	8.0	0.0
orange 'All Fruit Spreadable Fruit' *(Polaner)*	1 tsp	14	4.0	0.0
orange marmalade *(Knott's Berry Farm)*	1 tsp	16	4.0	0.0
orange marmalade 'Light' w/NutraSweet *(Knott's Berry Farm)*	1 tsp	8	2.0	0.0
orange marmalade 'Light' w/NutraSweet *(Smucker's)*	1 tsp	7	2.0	0.0
orange marmalade, low sugar *(Smucker's)*	1 tsp	8	2.0	0.0
orange marmalade, no sugar added *(Fifty 50)*	1 tsp	2	<1.0	0.0

Food Name	Serv. Size	Total Cal.	Carbs GMS	Fat GMS
orange marmalade, portion pack *(Knott's Berry Farm)*	.5 oz	35	9.0	0.0
orange marmalade 'Simply Fruit' *(Smucker's)*	1 tsp	16	4.0	0.0
peach 'Simply Fruit' *(Smucker's)*	1 tsp	16	4.0	0.0
raspberry *(Weight Watchers)*	1 tsp	8	2.0	0.0
raspberry 'All Fruit Spreadable Fruit' *(Polaner)*	1 tsp	14	4.0	0.0
raspberry 'All Fruit Spreadable Fruit' seedless *(Polaner)*	1 tsp	14	4.0	0.0
raspberry, no sugar added *(Fifty 50)*	1 tsp	2	<1.0	0.0
red raspberry *(Knott's Berry Farm)*	1 tsp	16	4.0	0.0
red raspberry 'Light' w/NutraSweet *(Knott's Berry Farm)*	1 tsp	8	2.0	0.0
red raspberry 'Light' w/NutraSweet *(Smucker's)*	1 tsp	7	2.0	0.0
red raspberry, low sugar *(Smucker's)*	1 tsp	8	2.0	0.0
red raspberry, portion pack *(Knott's Berry Farm)*	.5 oz	35	9.0	0.0
red raspberry 'Simply Fruit' *(Smucker's)*	1 tsp	16	4.0	0.0
strawberry *(Weight Watchers)*	1 tsp	8	2.0	0.0
strawberry 'All Fruit Spreadable Fruit' *(Polaner)*	1 tsp	14	4.0	0.0
strawberry 'Imitation' *(Smucker's)*	1 tsp	2	1.0	0.0
strawberry 'Light' w/NutraSweet *(Knott's Berry Farm)*	1 tsp	8	2.0	0.0
strawberry 'Light' w/NutraSweet *(Smucker's)*	1 tsp	7	2.0	0.0
strawberry, low sugar *(Smucker's)*	1 tsp	8	2.0	0.0
strawberry, no sugar added *(Fifty 50)*	1 tsp	2	<1.0	0.0
strawberry 'Simply Fruit' *(Smucker's)*	1 tsp	16	4.0	0.0
FRUIT SYRUP				
all flavors *(Smucker's)*	2 tbsp	100	26.0	0.0
'Fruit 'n Maple' *(Knudsen & Sons)*	1 oz	105	26.0	<1.0
'Fruit 'n Maple' pourable *(Knudsen & Sons)*	1 oz	105	26.0	0.0
raspberry, pourable *(Knudsen & Sons)*	1 oz	75	18.0	1.0
strawberry, pourable *(Knudsen & Sons)*	1 oz	75	18.0	1.0
FUDGE TOPPING				
(Hershey's)	2 tbsp	100	14.0	4.0
(Kraft) hot	1 tbsp	70	11.0	2.0
(Mrs. Richardson's) hot	2 tbsp	140	20.0	7.0
(Mrs. Richardson's) hot, microwavable	2 tbsp	140	20.0	7.0
(Smucker's)	2 tbsp	130	31.0	1.0
(Smucker's) hot	2 tbsp	110	18.0	4.0
(Smucker's) hot 'Light'	2 tbsp	70	19.0	0.0
(Smucker's) hot 'Special Recipe'	2 tbsp	150	23.0	5.0
(Smucker's) 'Magic Shell'	2 tbsp	190	16.0	15.0

FUKI. See BUTTERBUR.

G

Food Name	Serv. Size	Total Cal.	Carbs GMS	Fat GMS
GARBANZO BEAN/ceci/chick pea				
boiled	4 oz	186	31.1	2.9
boiled	1/2 cup	134	22.5	2.1
raw	1/2 cup	364	60.7	6.0
raw	1 oz	103	17.2	1.7
raw *(Arrowhead Mills)*	2 oz	200	35.0	3.0
Canned				
(A&P)	1/2 cup	100	17.0	1.0
(Allens)	1/2 cup	110	18.0	<1.0
(Bush's Best)	1/2 cup	80	21.0	1.0
(Eden Foods) organic, very low sodium, no salt added	1/2 cup	90	17.0	1.0
(Eden Foods) organic, w/liquid	1/2 cup	110	17.0	2.0
(Finast)	8 oz	210	35.0	3.0
(Green Giant)	1/2 cup	90	18.0	2.0
(Green Giant) 50% less salt	1/2 cup	90	18.0	2.0
(Joan of Arc) 50% less salt	1/2 cup	90	18.0	2.0
(Old El Paso)	1/2 cup	190	16.0	<1.0
(Progresso)	1/2 cup	110	22.0	1.0
(S&W) large, 50% less salt 'Lite'	1/2 cup	110	21.0	1.0
(S&W Nutradiet)	1/2 cup	100	19.0	1.0
GARBANZO FLOUR/chick pea flour				
(Arrowhead Mills)	2 oz	200	35.0	3.0
GARDEN SALAD				
(Joan of Arc) canned	1/2 cup	70	17.0	0.0
(Read) canned	1/2 cup	70	17.0	0.0
(S&W) refrigerated marinated	1/2 cup	60	11.0	0.0
(Trader Joe's) refrigerated fresh vegetables, no-oil vinaigrette	1 container	90	17.0	1.0
(Trader Joe's) refrigerated w/eggless egg salad, no-oil vinaigrette	1 container	140	8.0	7.0
GARLIC				
trimmed	1 oz	42	9.4	0.1
untrimmed	1 lb	587	130.5	2.0
GARLIC BREAD. See BREAD.				
GARLIC BREAD SEASONING				
'Garlic Bread Sprinkle' *(Schilling)*	1/4 tsp	5	0.1	0.4
GARLIC BREAD SPREAD *(Lawry's)*	1/2 tbsp	47	1.0	4.6
GARLIC PEPPER, 'Spice Blends' *(Lawry's)*	1 tsp	11	2.0	<.1
GARLIC POWDER				
dry	1 oz	94	20.6	0.2
dry	1 tbsp	28	6.1	0.1

Food Name	Serv. Size	Total Cal.	Carbs GMS	Fat GMS
dry	1 tsp	9	2.0	0.0
dry *(Durkee)*	1 tsp	10	0.1	tr
dry *(Laurel Leaf)*	1 tsp	10	0.1	tr
dry *(Lawry's)* w/parsley	1 tsp	12	2.3	0.9
dry *(Spice Islands)*	1 tsp	5	1.1	tr
GARLIC SALT				
(Lawry's)	1 tsp	4	0.8	<.1
(Morton)	1 tsp	3	<1.0	<.1
GARLIC SEASONING				
(Gilroy) crushed	1 tsp	8	2.0	0.0
(Gilroy) minced	1 tsp	23	2.0	1.0
(Golden Dipt)	2 grams	8	1.0	0.0
(Schilling) 'Parsley Patch'	1 tsp	13	2.0	0.5
(Schilling) 'Season All'	1/4 tsp	2	0.1	(tr)
GARLIC SPREAD, concentrate *(Lawry's)*	1 tbsp	15	0.2	1.6
GATORADE. See individual flavors.				
GEFILTE FISH				
Hors d'oeuvres *(Rokeach)*	8 balls	60	4.0	1.0
In jelled broth				
(Mother's) 'Old Fashioned' 24-oz jar	1 ball	70	5.0	1.0
(Mother's) 'Old Fashioned' 12-oz jar	1 ball	54	4.0	0.8
(Mother's) 'Old World'	1 ball	70	7.0	1.0
(Mother's) 'Unsalted'	1 ball	45	2.0	1.0
(Rokeach) 'Old Vienna' 31-oz jar	3 oz	81	9.0	1.0
(Rokeach) 'Old Vienna' 24-oz jar	2.6 oz	70	8.0	1.0
(Rokeach) 'Old Vienna' 12-oz jar	2 oz	54	6.0	1.0
(Rokeach) 'Redi-Jelled'	4 oz	92	6.0	2.0
(Rokeach) 'Redi-Jelled'	3 oz	65	5.0	1.0
(Rokeach) 'Redi-Jelled'	2 oz	46	3.0	1.0
In liquid				
(Mother's) 'Old Fashioned' 24- or 31-oz jar	1 ball	70	7.0	1.0
(Mother's) 'Old Fashioned' 12-oz jar	1 ball	54	5.0	0.8
In natural broth				
(Rokeach) 24-oz jar	4 oz	60	4.0	1.0
(Rokeach) 24-oz jar	2.6 oz	50	4.0	1.0
Sweet *(Mother's)* 'Old World'	1 ball	54	5.0	0.8
WHITEFISH				
In jelled broth				
(Mother's) 24- or 31-oz jar	1 ball	60	4.0	1.0
(Mother's) 12-oz jar	1 ball	46	3.0	0.8
In liquid				
(Mother's) 24- or 31-oz jar	1 ball	70	7.0	1.0
(Mother's) 12-oz jar	1 ball	54	5.0	0.8

Food Name	Serv. Size	Total Cal.	Carbs GMS	Fat GMS
WHITEFISH AND PIKE				
In jelled broth				
(Mother's) 24- or 31-oz jar	1 ball	60	4.0	1.0
(Mother's) 12-oz jar	1 ball	46	3.0	0.8
(Mother's) 'Old World'	1 ball	54	5.0	0.8
(Rokeach)	2.6 oz	60	4.0	1.0
(Rokeach)	2 oz	46	3.0	1.0
In liquid (Mother's)	1 ball	70	7.0	1.0
GELATIN, JAPANESE				
raw	1 lb	116	30.6	0.1
raw	1 oz	7	1.9	tr
GELATIN, UNFLAVORED (Knox)	1 pkt	25	0.0	0.0
GELATIN DESSERT				
PREPARED FROM MIX				
(D-Zerta)				
all flavors	1/2 cup	8	0.0	0.0
all flavors, low calorie, w/aspartame	1/2 cup	8	0.0	0.0
(Featherweight) all flavors	1/2 cup	10	1.0	0.0
(Jell-O)				
berry blue	1/2 cup	80	19.0	0.0
black raspberry	1/2 cup	80	19.0	0.0
cherry	1/2 cup	80	19.0	0.0
cherry, sugar-free	1/2 cup	8	0.0	0.0
Concord grape	1/2 cup	80	19.0	0.0
lemon	1/2 cup	80	19.0	0.0
lemon, sugar-free	1/2 cup	8	0.0	0.0
lime	1/2 cup	80	19.0	0.0
lime, sugar-free	1/2 cup	8	0.0	0.0
orange, sugar-free	1/2 cup	8	0.0	0.0
orange-pineapple	1/2 cup	80	19.0	0.0
raspberry, sugar-free	1/2 cup	8	0.0	0.0
strawberry, sugar-free	1/2 cup	8	0.0	0.0
strawberry banana, sugar-free	1/2 cup	8	0.0	0.0
watermelon	1/2 cup	80	20.0	0.0
wild strawberry	1/2 cup	80	19.0	0.0
(Royal)				
apple	1/2 cup	80	19.0	0.0
blackberry	1/2 cup	80	19.0	0.0
cherry	1/2 cup	80	19.0	0.0
cherry, sugar-free	1/2 cup	8	1.0	0.0
Concord grape	1/2 cup	80	19.0	0.0
fruit punch	1/2 cup	80	19.0	0.0
lemon	1/2 cup	80	19.0	0.0

Food Name	Serv. Size	Total Cal.	Carbs GMS	Fat GMS
lemon-lime	1/2 cup	80	19.0	0.0
lime	1/2 cup	80	19.0	0.0
lime, sugar-free	1/2 cup	8	1.0	0.0
mixed berry	1/2 cup	80	19.0	0.0
orange	1/2 cup	80	19.0	0.0
orange, sugar-free	1/2 cup	10	1.0	0.0
peach	1/2 cup	80	19.0	0.0
pineapple	1/2 cup	80	19.0	0.0
raspberry	1/2 cup	80	19.0	0.0
raspberry, sugar-free	1/2 cup	8	1.0	0.0
strawberry	1/2 cup	80	19.0	0.0
strawberry, sugar-free	1/2 cup	8	1.0	0.0
strawberry banana	1/2 cup	80	19.0	0.0
strawberry banana, sugar-free	1/2 cup	8	1.0	0.0
strawberry orange	1/2 cup	80	19.0	0.0
tropical fruit	1/2 cup	80	19.0	0.0
READY TO SERVE				
(Estee)	1/2 cup	8	<1.0	0.0
(Jell-O) berry blue, six pack	3.5 oz	80	18.0	0.0
(Jell-O) cherry, six pack	3.5 oz	80	18.0	0.0
(Jell-O) strawberry, six pack	3.5 oz	80	18.0	0.0
GELATIN DRINK MIX				
orange flavor	1 oz	108	17.1	0.3
orange flavor (Knox)	1 envelope	39	4.0	0.1
GERMAN SAUSAGE. See also individual listings.				
(Hickory Farms)	1 oz	100	1.0	8.0
GHEE/clarified butter	1 oz	249	0.0	28.4
GIN. See ALCOHOLIC BEVERAGES.				
GINGER				
ground	1 oz	98	20.1	1.7
ground	1 tbsp	19	3.8	0.3
ground	1 tsp	6	1.3	0.1
ground (Durkee)	1 tsp	7	0.0	tr
ground (Laurel Leaf)	1 tsp	7	0.0	tr
ground (Spice Islands)	1 tsp	6	1.2	0.1
GINGER, PICKLED, Japanese	1 oz	10	2.1	<.1
GINGER ALE. See SOFT DRINKS AND MIXERS.				
GINGER ROOT				
candied, crystallized	1 lb	1544	395.4	0.9
candied, crystallized	1 oz	95	24.4	0.1
raw, slices, 1-inch diam	1/4 cup	17	3.6	0.2
raw, slices, 1-inch diam	5 slices	8	1.7	0.1
trimmed	1 oz	20	4.3	0.2

Food Name	Serv. Size	Total Cal.	Carbs GMS	Fat GMS
untrimmed	1 lb	291	63.6	3.1
GINGER TERIYAKI MARINADE (Golden Dipt)	1 oz	120	12.0	7.0
GINGERBREAD. See BREAD.				
GINKGO NUT				
canned	1 cup	172	34.3	2.5
canned, approx 9 large, 14 medium, or 22 small	1 oz	32	6.3	0.5
dried	1 oz	99	20.6	0.6
dried, in shell	1 lb	1198	249.8	6.9
raw	1 oz	52	10.7	0.5
raw, in shell	1 lb	628	129.6	5.8
GLOBE ARTICHOKE. See ARTICHOKES, GLOBE.				
GLUTEN. See WHEAT GLUTEN.				
GOA BEAN. See WINGED BEAN.				
GOAT				
raw	1 lb	494	0.0	10.5
raw	1 oz	31	0.0	0.7
roasted	4 oz	162	0.0	3.4
roasted, diced	1 cup	200	0.0	4.2
GOATFISH				
raw	1 lb	435	0.0	4.5
raw	1 oz	27	0.0	0.3
GOBO. See BURDOCK ROOT.				
GOOSE, DOMESTICATED				
meat and skin, raw	1 oz	105	0.0	9.5
meat and skin, roasted	4 oz	346	0.0	24.9
meat only, raw	1 oz	46	0.0	2.0
meat only, roasted	4 oz	270	0.0	14.4
GOOSE FAT				
	1/2 cup	923	0.0	102.3
	1 oz	255	0.0	28.3
	1 tbsp	115	0.0	12.8
GOOSE GIBLETS, raw	100 gm	156	0.6	7.0
GOOSE GIZZARD, raw	100 gm	139	0.0	5.3
GOOSE LIVER, raw	1 lb	15	0.7	0.5
GOOSEBERRY				
whole	1 lb	202	46.2	2.6
whole	1 oz	12	2.9	0.2
whole	1 cup	66	15.3	0.9
GOOSEBERRY, CANNED, in light syrup	4 oz	83	21.3	0.2
GOOSEFISH. See MONKFISH.				
GOURD, BOTTLE/calabash gourd/white-flowered gourd				
boiled, drained	4 oz	17	4.2	<.1
boiled, drained, 1-inch cubes	1/2 cup	11	2.7	<.1

Food Name	Serv. Size	Total Cal.	Carbs GMS	Fat GMS
raw, approx 2.4 lb	1 med	106	26.1	0.2
raw, 1-inch cubes	1/2 cup	8	2.0	<.1
raw, trimmed	1 oz	4	1.0	tr
raw, untrimmed	1 lb	44	10.8	0.1
GOURD, CALABASH. See GOURD, BOTTLE.				
GOURD, DISHCLOTH/loofah gourd/rag gourd/sponge gourd/towel gourd/vegetable sponge				
boiled, drained	4 oz	64	16.3	0.4
boiled, drained, 1-inch slices	1/2 cup	50	12.8	0.3
raw, approx 8.6 oz	1 med	36	7.8	0.4
raw, 1-inch slices	1 cup	19	4.1	0.2
raw, trimmed	1 oz	6	1.2	0.1
raw, untrimmed	1 lb	67	14.4	0.7
GOURD, RAG. See GOURD, DISHCLOTH.				
GOURD, SPONGE. See GOURD, DISHCLOTH.				
GOURD, WAX				
boiled, drained	4 oz	15	3.4	0.2
boiled, drained, cubes	1/2 cup	11	2.6	0.2
raw, cubes	1 cup	17	4.0	0.3
raw, trimmed	1 oz	4	0.9	0.1
raw, untrimmed	1 lb	42	9.7	0.6
GOURD, WHITE/tunka				
boiled, drained	4 oz	15	3.4	0.2
boiled, drained, cubes	1/2 cup	11	2.6	0.2
raw, cubes	1 cup	17	4.0	0.3
raw, trimmed	1 oz	4	0.9	0.1
raw, untrimmed	1 lb	42	9.7	0.6
GOURD, WHITE-FLOWERED. See GOURD, BOTTLE.				
GOVERNOR PLUM, trimmed	1 oz	31	8.4	0.0
GRANADILLA. See PASSION FRUIT.				
GRANOLA. See CEREAL, READY-TO-SERVE.				
GRANOLA AND CEREAL BAR. See also GRANOLA SNACKS.				
(Barbara's Bakery)				
cinnamon and oats, 2 oz	1 bar	281	31.0	15.0
coconut almond, 2 oz	1 bar	306	23.0	20.0
peanut butter, 2 oz	1 bar	275	28.0	15.0
(Bear Valley)				
carob-cocoa, food bar 'Pemmican' 3.75 oz	1 bar	440	68.0	12.0
coconut almond, food bar 'Meal Pack' 3.75 oz	1 bar	400	56.0	12.0
sesame lemon, food bar 'Meal Pack' 3.75 oz	1 bar	410	57.0	13.0
fruit 'n nut, food bar 'Pemmican' 3.75 oz	1 bar	420	59.0	13.0
(Glenny's)				
apple, 'Original Fruit Bar'	1 bar	100	15.0	3.0
'Bee Pollen Sunrise' 1.5 oz	1 bar	190	22.0	8.0

Food Name	Serv. Size	Total Cal.	Carbs GMS	Fat GMS
carob mint w/oat bran 'Brown Rice Treats'	1 bar	180	37.0	2.0
cinnamon and raisin 'Brown Rice Treats' 1.75 oz	1 bar	170	38.0	1.0
coconut amandine 'Moist and Chewy' 1.5 oz	1 bar	190	22.0	10.0
'Ginseng Sunrise' 1.5 oz	1 bar	160	24.0	7.0
oatmeal raisin 'Moist and Chewy' 1.5 oz	1 bar	160	30.0	3.0
peanut and raisin 'Brown Rice Treats' 2 oz	1 bar	210	39.0	5.0
peanut snack 'Moist and Chewy' 1.5 oz	1 bar	180	24.0	7.0
plain and fancy 'Brown Rice Treats' 1.25 oz	1 bar	120	28.0	1.0
raisin bran 'Brown Rice Treats' 1.75 oz	1 bar	170	38.0	1.0
'Spirulina Sunrise' 1.5 oz	1 bar	140	21.0	5.0
sunflower 'Moist and Chewy' 1.5 oz	1 bar	180	24.0	7.0
toasted almond w/oat bran 'Brown Rice Treats'	1 bar	200	34.0	5.0
(Golden Temple)				
cashew almond 'Wha Guru Chew Bar'	1 bar	164	15.0	11.0
peanut cashew 'Wha Guru Chew Bar'	1 bar	167	14.0	11.0
sesame almond 'Wha Guru Chew Bar'	1 bar	160	15.0	10.0
(Health Valley)				
blueberry apple, fat-free	1 bar	140	33.0	0.0
date almond flavor, fat-free	1 bar	140	33.0	0.0
raspberry, fat-free	1 bar	140	33.0	0.0
(Hershey's)				
chocolate chip, chocolate coated, 1.2 oz	1 bar	170	22.0	8.0
cocoa creme, chocolate coated, 1.2 oz	1 bar	180	22.0	9.0
cookies and creme, chocolate coated, 1.2 oz	1 bar	170	22.0	8.0
peanut butter, chocolate coated, 1.2 oz	1 bar	180	19.0	10.0
raspberry filled 'Common Sense Smart Start'	1 bar	170	28.0	6.0
(Kudo's)				
chocolate chip	1 bar	180	21.0	9.0
chocolate chunk 'Simply Kudos'	1 bar	100	13.0	4.0
fudge, nutty	1 bar	190	19.0	11.0
honey nut 'Simply Kudos'	1 bar	100	13.0	4.0
oatmeal raisin 'Simply Kudos'	1 bar	90	13.0	4.0
peanut butter, chocolate coated, 1.3 oz	1 bar	190	18.0	12.0
(Natural Nectar)				
almond, 'Treat Yourself Right'	1 bar	150	22.0	5.0
apple-oatmeal spice, 'Fi-Bar A.M.'	1 bar	150	27.0	3.0
banana nut, 'Fi-Bar A.M.'	1 bar	150	26.0	4.0
cocoa almond, 'Fi-Bar Chewy & Nutty'	1 bar	130	21.0	4.0
cocoa almond crunch, 'Canadian Chewy & Nutty'	1 bar	130	21.0	4.0
cocoa peanut, 'Fi-Bar Chewy & Nutty'	1 bar	130	20.0	1.0
cocoa peanut butter crunch, 'Chewy & Nutty'	1 bar	130	20.0	4.0
coconut	1 bar	120	20.0	4.0
cranberry, w/wild berries 'Original Fruit Bar'	1 bar	120	23.0	2.0

Food Name	Serv. Size	Total Cal.	Carbs GMS	Fat GMS
lemon 'Original Fruit Bar'	1 bar	100	15.0	3.0
Mandarin orange 'Original Fruit Bar'	1 bar	100	15.0	3.0
peanut butter	1 bar	130	20.0	4.0
peanut butter 'Treat Yourself Right'	1 bar	150	18.0	5.0
raisin nut bran, 'Fi-Bar A.M.'	1 bar	150	26.0	4.0
raspberry 'Canadian'	1 bar	120	21.0	3.0
raspberry 'Original Fruit Bar'	1 bar	120	23.0	2.0
strawberry 'Canadian'	1 bar	120	21.0	3.0
strawberry 'Original Fruit Bar'	1 bar	120	23.0	2.0
strawberry-oatmeal w/almonds, 'Fi-Bar A.M.'	1 bar	150	24.0	4.0
vanilla almond, 'Fi-Bar Chewy & Nutty'	1 bar	130	21.0	4.0
vanilla almond crunch, 'Canadian Chewy & Nutty'	1 bar	130	21.0	4.0
vanilla peanut, 'Fi-Bar Chewy & Nutty'	1 bar	130	20.0	4.0
wild cranberry 'Canadian'	1 bar	120	21.0	3.0
(Nature Valley)				
cinnamon, .8 oz	1 bar	120	17.0	5.0
oat bran-honey graham, .8 oz	1 bar	110	16.0	4.0
oats and honey, .8 oz	1 bar	120	17.0	5.0
peanut butter, .8 oz	1 bar	120	15.0	6.0
(Nature's Choice)				
carob chip, .75 oz	1 bar	90	15.0	3.0
cinnamon-raisin, .75 oz	1 bar	90	15.0	3.0
oats 'n honey, .75 oz	1 bar	90	15.0	3.0
peanut butter, .75 oz	1 bar	90	14.0	3.0
(Nutri Grain)				
blueberry 'Smart Start' 1.5 oz	1 bar	180	26.0	8.0
corn flakes, mixed berry-filled 'Smart Start'	1 bar	170	27.0	7.0
raisin bran 'Smart Start' 1.5 oz	1 bar	160	28.0	5.0
rice krispies w/almonds 'Smart Start' 1 oz	1 bar	130	18.0	6.0
strawberry 'Smart Start' 1.5 oz	1 bar	180	26.0	8.0
(Quaker)				
apple berry 'Chewy'	1 bar	120	20.0	4.0
caramel nut 'Granola Dipps' 1 oz	1 bar	148	20.9	6.4
chocolate chip 'Chewy'	1 bar	128	19.3	4.7
chocolate chip 'Granola Dipps' 1 oz	1 bar	139	18.7	6.3
chocolate fudge 'Granola Dipps' 1 oz	1 bar	160	20.0	7.9
chunky nut and raisin 'Chewy' 1 oz	1 bar	131	17.2	5.8
honey and oats 'Chewy', 1 oz	1 bar	125	19.1	4.4
peanut butter 'Chewy' 1 oz	1 bar	128	17.8	4.9
peanut butter, chocolate chip 'Chewy' 1 oz	1 bar	131	17.0	5.7
peanut butter, chocolate chip 'Granola Dipps'	1 bar	174	17.4	10.0
peanut butter 'Granola Dipps' 1 oz	1 bar	170	18.5	9.1
raisin and cinnamon 'Chewy' 1 oz	1 bar	128	18.6	5.0

Food Name	Serv. Size	Total Cal.	Carbs GMS	Fat GMS
S'mores 'Chewy' 1 oz	1 bar	126	19.7	4.4
trail mix 'Chewy' 1 oz	1 bar	130	18.0	5.0
(Sunbelt)				
apple bar, baked 1.31 oz	1 bar	130	28.0	2.0
chocolate chip, chewy, 1.25 oz	1 bar	150	23.0	7.0
chocolate chip, fudge dipped, chewy, 1.63 oz	1 bar	220	29.0	11.0
chocolate chip, fudge dipped, chewy, 1.5 oz	1 bar	210	26.0	10.0
oats and honey, chewy, 1 oz	1 bar	130	18.0	5.0
oats and honey, fudge dipped, chewy, 1.38 oz	1 bar	190	24.0	10.0
w/almonds, chewy, 1 oz	1 bar	120	18.0	6.0
w/chocolate chips, chewy, 1.75 oz	1 bar	220	32.0	9.0
w/peanuts, fudge dipped, chewy, 2.25 oz	1 bar	300	36.0	18.0
w/peanuts, fudge dipped, chewy, 1.38 oz	1 bar	190	24.0	10.0
w/raisins, chewy, 1.25 oz	1 bar	150	24.0	6.0
w/raisins, fudge dipped, chewy, 1.5 oz	1 bar	200	24.0	12.0

GRANOLA SNACKS. See also GRANOLA AND CEREAL BAR.

Food Name	Serv. Size	Total Cal.	Carbs GMS	Fat GMS
(Natural Nectar)				
almond butter crunch 'Nectar Nuggets'	1 cup	120	11.0	7.0
almond cappuccino crunch 'Nectar Nuggets'	1 cup	110	14.0	5.0
coconut almond crunch 'Nectar Nuggets'	1 cup	110	15.0	5.0
peanut butter crunch 'Nectar Nuggets'	1 cup	120	11.0	7.0
(Nature Valley)				
apple-cinnamon 'Granola Bites'	1 pkg	170	25.0	7.0
honey nut 'Granola Bites'	1 pkg	170	24.0	8.0
variety pack 'Granola Bites'	1 pkg	170	24.0	8.0
(Nature's Choice)				
chocolate chip 'Grrr-Nola Treats'	.75 oz	80	15.0	2.0
cinnamon toast 'Grrr-Nola Treats'	.75 oz	80	15.0	2.0
peanut butter and jelly 'Grrr-Nola Treats'	.75 oz	80	14.0	3.0
tutti-frutti 'Grrr-Nola Treats'	.75 oz	75	15.0	2.0

GRAPE

AMERICAN (Concord, Delaware, Niagara)

Food Name	Serv. Size	Total Cal.	Carbs GMS	Fat GMS
(Dole)	1.5 cup	85	24.0	0.0
Slipskin				
peeled and seeded	1 oz	18	4.9	0.1
trimmed	10 fruits	15	4.1	0.1
untrimmed	1 lb	165	45.1	0.9
untrimmed	1 cup	58	15.8	0.3

EUROPEAN (Muskat, Tokay, Thompson)

Food Name	Serv. Size	Total Cal.	Carbs GMS	Fat GMS
Adherent skin				
trimmed	10 fruits	35	8.9	0.3
untrimmed	1 lb	287	72.0	2.3
untrimmed	1 cup	114	28.4	0.9

Food Name	Serv. Size	Total Cal.	Carbs GMS	Fat GMS
untrimmed w/o seeds	1 lb	309	77.4	2.5
w/seeds	1/2 cup	57	14.2	0.5
w/seeds	1 oz	20	5.0	0.2
w/o seeds	1/2 cup	57	14.2	0.5
w/o seeds	1 oz	20	5.0	0.2
w/o seeds, approx 1.75 oz	10 grapes	36	8.9	0.3
GRAPE, CANNED				
THOMPSON, seedless				
in heavy syrup	1 cup	187	50.3	0.3
in heavy syrup	4 oz	83	22.3	0.1
in heavy syrup (S&W)	1/2 cup	100	25.0	0.0
in water	1 cup	98	25.2	0.3
in water	4 oz	45	11.7	0.1
GRAPE APPLE DRINK, bottle (Mott's)	10 oz	167	42.0	0.0
GRAPE DRINK				
Can, bottle, or box				
(A&P)	6 oz	100	25.0	<1.0
(All Sport) thirst quencher, caffeine-free	8 oz	70	20.0	0.0
(Bama)	8.45 oz	120	29.0	0.0
(Bright & Early) frozen, diluted	6 oz	100	24.0	0.0
(Crowley)	8 oz	130	32.0	0.0
(Fruitopia) 'The Grape Beyond' real fruit	8 oz	130	32.0	0.0
(Gatorade) low sodium, no caffeine	8 oz	50	14.0	0.0
(Hi-C) aseptic box	6 oz	90	23.0	0.0
(J. Hungerford)	9.03 oz	41	10.9	0.0
(Kool-Aid) 'Koolers'	8.45 oz	140	35.0	0.0
(Pathmark)	6 oz	90	22.0	0.0
(Squeezit) 'Grumpy Grape'	6.75 oz	120	30.0	0.0
(10-K) 'Clear'	8 oz	60	15.0	0.0
(Tropicana)	6 oz	90	22.0	<1.0
(Veryfine)	8 oz	130	34.0	0.0
(Wyler's) 'Fruit Slush'	4 oz	157	39.3	0.0
Prepared from mix				
(Finast)	8 oz	80	21.0	0.0
(Gatorade) instant 'Thirst Quencher'	8 oz	60	15.0	0.0
(Kool-Aid) sugar-sweetened	8 oz	80	20.0	0.0
(Kool-Aid) unsweetened, prepared w/sugar	8 oz	100	25.0	0.0
(Kool-Aid) unsweetened, prepared w/o sugar	8 oz	2	0.0	0.0
(Kool-Aid) w/NutraSweet	8 oz	4	0.0	0.0
(Pathmark) 'No Frills'	8 oz	90	22.0	0.0
(Pathmark) 'No Frills Sodium Free'	6 oz	80	22.0	0.0

Food Name	Serv. Size	Total Cal.	Carbs GMS	Fat GMS
GRAPE JUICE				
Can, bottle, or box				
(IGA) 'Unsweetened'	6 oz	120	30.0	0.0
(J. Hungerford)	9.03 oz	160	40.2	0.0
(J. Hungerford) 100% juice	9.03 oz	155	39.2	0.0
(J. Hungerford) 50% juice	9.03 oz	135	33.7	0.0
(J. Hungerford) 20% juice	9.03 oz	41	10.9	0.0
(Juicy Juice) blend	6 oz	100	25.0	0.0
(Juicy Juice) bottled	6 oz	90	22.0	0.0
(Juicy Juice) boxed	8.45 oz	130	31.0	0.0
(Knudsen & Sons)	8 oz	130	32.0	0.0
(Knudsen & Sons) Concord	8 oz	130	32.0	0.0
(Kraft) 'Pure 100% Unsweetened'	6 oz	104	25.0	0.0
(Pathmark) 'No Frills'	6 oz	113	27.0	0.0
(Lucky Leaf)	6 oz	130	32.0	0.0
(Minute Maid) aseptic box	6 oz	100	24.0	1.0
(Pathmark) 'Unsweetened'	6 oz	120	30.0	0.0
(S&W) Concord 'Unsweetened'	6 oz	100	25.0	0.0
(Sippin' Pak)	8.45 oz	130	32.0	0.0
(Squeezit 100) 'Caped Grape' 100% natural fruit juice	6.75 oz	100	24.0	0.0
(Veryfine) '100%'	8 oz	153	37.0	0.0
(Welch's) purple	6 oz	120	30.0	0.0
(Welch's) red	8.45 oz	170	43.0	0.0
(Welch's) red	6 oz	120	30.0	0.0
(Welch's) sparkling red	6 oz	128	30.0	0.0
(Welch's) sparkling white	6 oz	120	30.0	0.0
(Welch's) 'USDA'	6 oz	120	30.0	0.0
(Welch's) white	8.45 oz	160	39.0	0.0
(Welch's) white	6 oz	120	30.0	0.0
Frozen, diluted as directed				
(Minute Maid)	6 oz	90	24.0	0.0
(Sunkist)	6 oz	69	17.1	0.1
(Welch's) 'No Sugar Added'	6 oz	40	10.0	0.0
(Welch's) 'Orchard'	10 oz	170	43.0	0.0
(Welch's) 'Orchard'	6 oz	110	27.0	0.0
(Welch's) 'Orchard Cocktails-In-A-Box'	8.45 oz	150	38.0	0.0
(Welch's) purple	6 oz	100	25.0	0.0
(Welch's) white	6 oz	100	25.0	0.0
GRAPE JUICE DRINK				
(Hi-C)	8.45 oz	136	33.4	0.1
(Hi-C)	6 oz	96	23.7	0.1
(Sunkist) frozen, diluted	6 oz	69	17.0	0.1
(Tang) 'Fruit Box'	8.45 oz	130	34.0	0.0

Food Name	Serv. Size	Total Cal.	Carbs GMS	Fat GMS
GRAPE PUNCH				
(Minute Maid) chilled	6 oz	90	23.0	0.0
(Minute Maid) frozen concentrate	6 oz	90	23.0	0.0
GRAPEFRUIT				
PINK AND RED				
Arizona/California				
fresh, 3.75-inch diam	1/2 fruit	46	11.9	0.1
sections w/juice	1 cup	85	22.3	0.2
trimmed	1 oz	11	2.7	<.1
untrimmed	1 lb	86	22.4	0.2
Florida				
fresh (Ocean Spray)	1/2 med	50	13.0	0.0
fresh, 3.75-inch diam	1/2 fruit	37	9.2	0.1
sections w/juice	1 cup	69	17.3	0.2
trimmed	1 oz	9	2.1	<.1
untrimmed	1 lb	69	17.4	0.2
WHITE				
California				
fresh, 3.75-inch diam	1/2 fruit	44	10.7	0.1
sections w/juice	1 cup	85	20.9	0.2
trimmed	1 oz	10	2.6	<.1
untrimmed	1 lb	81	20.2	0.2
Florida				
fresh (Ocean Spray)	1/2 med	45	12.0	0.0
fresh, 3.75-inch diam	1/2 fruit	38	9.7	0.1
sections w/juice	1 cup	74	18.8	0.2
trimmed	1 oz	9	2.3	<.1
GRAPEFRUIT, CANNED				
(Featherweight) in juice	1/2 cup	40	9.0	0.0
(Finast) in light syrup	1/2 cup	80	20.0	<.1
(Kraft) chilled 'Pure'	1/2 cup	50	12.0	0.0
(S&W) in light syrup	1/2 cup	80	24.0	0.0
(S&W) 'Unsweetened'	1/2 cup	40	9.0	0.0
(S&W Nutradiet)	1/2 cup	40	9.0	0.0
(Stokely) in light syrup	1/2 cup	90	23.0	1.0
GRAPEFRUIT JUICE				
Can, bottle, or box				
(Del Monte)	6 oz	70	17.0	0.0
(J. Hungerford) regular	9.03 oz	120	29.8	0.0
(J. Hungerford) 100% juice	9.03 oz	98	24.2	0.0
(J. Hungerford) 50% juice	9.03 oz	109	26.9	0.0
(Knudsen & Sons)	8 oz	70	17.0	0.0
(Knudsen & Sons) pink	8 oz	80	18.0	0.0

Food Name	Serv. Size	Total Cal.	Carbs GMS	Fat GMS
(Kraft) '100% pure'	6 oz	70	16.0	0.0
(Libby's)	6 oz	70	17.0	0.0
(Minute Maid)	6 oz	70	17.0	0.0
(Minute Maid) 'Juices to Go'	6 oz	70	17.0	0.0
(Mott's)	9.5 oz	118	29.0	0.0
(Mott's)	10 oz	124	30.0	0.0
(Ocean Spray)	6 oz	70	16.0	0.0
(Ocean Spray) 100%	6 oz	60	18.0	0.0
(Ocean Spray) pink 'Pink Premium'	6 oz	60	15.0	0.0
(Ocean Spray) 'Ruby Red'	6 oz	100	24.0	0.0
(S&W)	6 oz	80	18.0	0.0
(Snapple)	8 oz	110	25.0	0.0
(Stokely)	6 oz	76	18.0	1.0
(Sunkist) 'Fresh Squeezed'	8 oz	96	22.7	0.2
(Tree Top)	6 oz	80	19.0	0.0
(TreeSweet) pink	6 oz	72	17.0	0.0
(TreeSweet) regular	6 oz	72	17.0	0.0
(Tropicana) 100% pure	6 oz	70	14.0	<1.0
(Tropicana) 'Ruby Red' 100% pure	6 oz	70	14.0	<1.0
(Veryfine) '100%'	8 oz	101	23.0	0.0
Fresh				
juice from one 3.75-inch diam fruit	6 oz	76	18.0	0.2
pink	1 cup	96	22.7	0.3
white	1 cup	96	22.7	0.3
Frozen, diluted as directed				
(A&P)	6 oz	80	18.0	<1.0
(Minute Maid)	6 oz	80	18.0	0.0
(Minute Maid) pink	6 oz	80	20.0	0.0
(Sunkist)	6 oz	56	13.3	0.2
(TreeSweet)	6 oz	78	18.0	0.0
GRAPEFRUIT JUICE COCKTAIL				
(IGA)	6 oz	80	20.0	0.0
(Minute Maid) 'Juices To Go'	6 oz	80	20.0	0.0
(Ocean Spray)	6 oz	80	20.0	0.0
(Pathmark)	6 oz	80	20.0	0.0
(TreeSweet) 'Lite'	6 oz	40	10.0	0.0
(Tropicana) 'Twister'	8 oz	110	28.0	0.0
(Tropicana) 'Twister Light' w/NutraSweet	6 oz	30	6.0	<1.0
(Veryfine)	8 oz	120	29.0	0.0
GRAPEFRUIT JUICE DRINK				
(Citrus Hill) 'Plus Calcium'	6 oz	70	19.0	<1.0
(Tropicana) 'Juice Sparkler'	8 oz	110	26.0	0.0
(Wyler's) 'Fruit Slush'	4 oz	157	39.3	0.0

Food Name	Serv. Size	Total Cal.	Carbs GMS	Fat GMS
GRAPESEED OIL				
....	1 cup	1927	0.0	218.0
....	1 oz	251	0.0	28.4
....	1 tbsp	120	0.0	13.6
GRAVY. See also SAUCE.				
AU JUS				
Canned or in jars				
(Franco-American)	2 oz	10	2.0	0.0
(Heinz) 'HomeStyle'	1/4 cup	18	2.0	1.0
Prepared from mix				
(French's)	1/4 cup	10	2.0	0.0
(Lawry's)	1 cup	84	11.1	1.8
(McCormick/Schilling)	1/4 cup	20	3.5	0.3
BEEF				
Canned				
(Franco-American)	2 oz	25	4.0	1.0
(Hormel) w/chunky beef 'Great Beginnings'	5 oz	136	7.0	7.0
BROWN				
Canned or in jars				
(Heinz) 'HomeStyle'	1/4 cup	25	3.0	1.0
(Heinz) 'HomeStyle' w/onions	1/4 cup	25	3.0	1.0
(LaChoy)	1/2 tsp	15	4.0	<1.0
Prepared from mix				
(French's)	1/4 cup	20	4.0	1.0
(Lawry's)	1 cup	94	16.5	1.4
(McCormick/Schilling)	1/3 cup	30	4.7	1.0
(McCormick/Schilling)	1/4 cup	23	3.5	0.8
(McCormick/Schilling) 'Lite'	1/4 cup	10	2.0	1.0
(Pillsbury)	1/4 cup	15	3.0	0.0
(Weight Watchers)	1/4 cup	10	2.0	0.0
(Weight Watchers) w/mushrooms	1/4 cup	10	2.0	0.0
(Weight Watchers) w/onions	1/4 cup	10	2.0	0.0
CHICKEN				
Canned or in jars				
(Franco-American)	2 oz	45	3.0	4.0
(Franco-American) giblet	2 oz	30	3.0	2.0
(Heinz) 'HomeStyle' w/mushrooms	1/4 cup	35	3.0	2.0
(Heinz) 'Homestyle' w/mushrooms and onions	1/4 cup	35	3.0	2.0
(Hormel) 'Great Beginnings' w/chunky chicken	5 oz	147	5.0	8.0
(Weight Watchers)	1/4 cup	10	2.0	0.0
Prepared from mix				
(French's)	1/4 cup	25	4.0	1.0
(Lawry's)	1 cup	99	15.5	2.8

Food Name	Serv. Size	Total Cal.	Carbs GMS	Fat GMS
(McCormick/Schilling)	1/4 cup	22	3.7	0.4
(Pillsbury)	1/4 cup	25	4.0	1.0
COUNTRY				
(Heinz) 'Homestyle' jar	2 oz	25	4.0	1.0
CREAM *(Franco-American)* canned	2 oz	35	4.0	2.0
HERB *(McCormick/Schilling)* mix, prepared	1/4 cup	20	3.0	0.5
MUSHROOM				
Canned or in jars				
(Franco-American)	2 oz	25	3.0	1.0
(Heinz) 'HomeStyle'	1/4 cup	25	3.0	1.0
Prepared from mix				
(French's)	1/4 cup	20	3.0	1.0
(McCormick/Schilling)	1/4 cup	19	3.0	0.5
ONION				
(French's) mix, prepared	1/4 cup	25	4.0	1.0
(McCormick/Schilling) mix, prepared	1/4 cup	22	3.6	0.6
PORK				
Canned or in jars				
(Franco-American)	1/4 cup	40	3.0	3.0
(Heinz) 'HomeStyle'	1/4 cup	25	3.0	1.0
(Hormel) 'Great Beginnings' w/chunky pork	5 oz	140	5.0	8.0
Prepared from mix				
(French's)	1/4 cup	20	4.0	1.0
(McCormick/Schilling)	1/4 cup	20	4.0	0.6
TURKEY				
Canned or in jars				
(Franco-American)	2 oz	30	3.0	2.0
(Heinz) 'HomeStyle'	1/4 cup	25	3.0	1.0
(Hormel) 'Great Beginnings' w/chunky turkey	5 oz	138	7.0	8.0
Prepared from mix				
(Lawry's)	1 cup	102	13.4	4.1
(McCormick/Schilling)	1/4 cup	22	4.0	0.5
GREAT NORTHERN BEAN				
boiled	4 oz	134	23.9	0.5
boiled, mature seeds	1/2 cup	104	18.6	0.4
raw	1/2 cup	308	56.8	1.0
raw	1 oz	96	17.7	0.3
Canned				
(A&P)	1 cup	210	38.0	1.0
(Allens)	1/2 cup	105	17.0	<1.0
(Allens) w/pork	1/2 cup	100	19.0	1.0
(Bush's Best)	1/2 cup	70	16.0	0.0
(Eden Foods) organically grown, w/liquid	1/2 cup	110	20.0	<1.0

Food Name	Serv. Size	Total Cal.	Carbs GMS	Fat GMS
(Green Giant)	1/2 cup	80	18.0	1.0
(Joan of Arc)	1/2 cup	80	18.0	1.0
(Luck's) w/pork	7.25 oz	220	32.0	5.0
GREEK SALAD, w/feta cheese and pitted Kalamata olives, refrigerated *(Trader Joe's)*	1 salad	310	10.0	28.0
GREEN BEAN/string bean				
boiled, drained	4 oz	40	8.9	0.3
boiled, drained	1/2 cup	22	4.9	0.2
raw, trimmed	1/2 cup	17	3.9	0.1
raw, trimmed	1 oz	9	2.0	<.1
raw, untrimmed	1 lb	123	28.5	0.5
GREEN BEAN, CANNED				
Cut				
(A&P)	1/2 cup	20	4.0	<1.0
(A&P) 'No Salt Added'	1/2 cup	20	4.0	<1.0
(Allens)	1/2 cup	20	4.0	<1.0
(Bush's Best)	1/2 cup	20	5.0	0.0
(Del Monte) w/liquid	1/2 cup	20	4.0	0.0
(Del Monte) w/liquid 'No Salt Added'	1/2 cup	20	4.0	0.0
(Bush's Best) 'Blue Lake'	1/2 cup	20	5.0	0.0
(Bush's Best) w/Shelly beans	1/2 cup	35	8.0	0.0
(Featherweight)	1/2 cup	25	5.0	0.0
(Finast)	1/2 cup	20	4.0	0.0
(Finast) 'No Salt Added'	1/2 cup	20	4.0	0.0
(Finast) 'Veri-Green'	1/2 cup	20	4.0	0.0
(Freshlike)	1/2 cup	20	4.0	0.0
(Freshlike) no salt added	1/2 cup	20	4.0	0.0
(Freshlike) no sugar or salt, in water	1/2 cup	20	4.0	0.0
(Freshlike) wax, water packed, w/o salt	1/2 cup	18	4.0	0.0
(Freshlike) wax, water packed, w/o sugar or salt	1/2 cup	18	4.0	0.0
(Green Giant)	1/2 cup	16	4.0	0.0
(Green Giant) 50% less salt	1/2 cup	16	4.0	0.0
(Green Giant) kitchen sliced	1/2 cup	16	4.0	0.0
(Green Giant) 'Pantry Express'	1/2 cup	12	3.0	0.0
(IGA)	1/2 cup	20	5.0	0.0
(Pathmark)	1/2 cup	20	4.0	0.0
(Pathmark) 'Blue Lake'	1/2 cup	20	4.0	0.0
(Pathmark) 'No Frills'	1 cup	35	8.0	0.0
(Pathmark) 'No Salt Added'	1/2 cup	20	5.0	0.0
(Quincy's)	4.3 oz	40	7.0	1.0
(S&W) 'Premium Blue Lake'	1/2 cup	20	4.0	0.0
(S&W) 'Premium Gold'	1/2 cup	20	5.0	0.0
(S&W) stringless, w/liquid	1/2 cup	20	4.0	0.0

Food Name	Serv. Size	Total Cal.	Carbs GMS	Fat GMS
(S&W Nutradiet)	1/2 cup	20	4.0	0.0
(Stokely)	1/2 cup	20	4.0	0.0
(Stokely) 'No Salt or Sugar'	1/2 cup	20	4.0	0.0
(Veg•All)	1/2 cup	20	4.0	0.0
French style				
(A&P)	1/2 cup	20	4.0	<1.0
(A&P) 'No Salt Added'	1/2 cup	20	4.0	<1.0
(Allens)	1/2 cup	20	4.0	<1.0
(Bush's Best)	1/2 cup	20	5.0	0.0
(Del Monte) seasoned, w/liquid	1/2 cup	20	4.0	0.0
(Finast)	1/2 cup	20	4.0	0.0
(Freshlike)	1/2 cup	20	4.0	0.0
(Freshlike) in water, w/o salt	1/2 cup	20	4.0	0.0
(Green Giant)	1/2 cup	16	4.0	0.0
(Pathmark) 'Blue Lake'	1/2 cup	20	4.0	0.0
(Pathmark) 'No Frills'	1 cup	35	8.0	0.0
(Pathmark) 'No Salt Added'	1/2 cup	20	5.0	0.0
(S&W) 'Premium Blue Lake'	1/2 cup	20	4.0	0.0
(S&W) stringless; w/liquid	1/2 cup	20	4.0	0.0
(Veg•All)	1/2 cup	20	4.0	0.0
Italian				
(Allens)	1/2 cup	18	3.0	<1.0
(Del Monte) cut	1/2 cup	25	6.0	0.0
Whole				
(A&P)	1/2 cup	20	4.0	<1.0
(Allens) Shelly beans	1/2 cup	35	6.0	<1.0
(Bush's Best)	1/2 cup	20	5.0	0.0
(Del Monte) w/liquid	1/2 cup	20	4.0	0.0
(Finast)	1/2 cup	25	4.0	0.0
(Freshlike)	1/2 cup	20	4.0	0.0
(Green Giant) amandine	1/2 cup	45	5.0	3.0
(IGA)	1 cup	45	8.0	0.0
(Pathmark)	1/2 cup	20	4.0	0.0
(S&W) dilled	1/2 cup	60	15.0	0.0
(S&W) stringless, w/liquid	1/2 cup	20	4.0	0.0
(S&W) 'Vertical Pak'	1/2 cup	20	4.0	0.0
GREEN BEAN, FREEZE-DRIED				
(Mountain House) diluted as directed	1/2 cup	35	6.0	0.0
GREEN BEAN, FROZEN				
Cut				
(A&P)	3 oz	25	6.0	<1.0
(Birds Eye)	3 oz	25	6.0	0.0
(Birds Eye) 'Portion Pack'	3 oz	25	6.0	0.0

Food Name	Serv. Size	Total Cal.	Carbs GMS	Fat GMS
(Finast)	3 oz	25	6.0	0.0
(Freshlike)	3 oz	25	6.0	0.0
(Frosty Acres)	3 oz	25	6.0	0.0
(Green Giant) 'Harvest Fresh'	1/2 cup	16	4.0	0.0
(Green Giant) in butter sauce	1/2 cup	30	4.0	1.0
(Seabrook)	3 oz	25	6.0	0.0
(Stokely) 'Singles'	3 oz	30	6.0	1.0
French style				
(A&P)	3 oz	25	6.0	<1.0
(Birds Eye)	3 oz	25	6.0	0.0
(Bird's Eye) w/almonds 'Combination Vegetables'	3 oz	50	8.0	2.0
(Finast)	3 oz	25	6.0	0.0
(Freshlike)	3 oz	25	6.0	0.0
(Frosty Acres)	3 oz	25	6.0	0.0
(Seabrook)	3 oz	25	6.0	0.0
(Southern)	3.5 oz	34	6.9	0.1
(Veg•All)	3 oz	25	6.0	0.0
Italian				
(Birds Eye)	3 oz	30	7.0	0.0
(Finast) cut	3 oz	30	7.0	0.0
(Freshlike)	3 oz	30	7.0	0.0
(Frosty Acres)	3 oz	30	7.0	0.0
(Seabrook)	3 oz	30	7.0	0.0
(Veg•All)	3 oz	30	7.0	0.0
Whole				
(Bird's Eye) Bavarian style, w/spaetzle	3.3 oz	100	11.0	5.0
(Birds Eye) 'Deluxe'	3 oz	25	5.0	0.0
(Bird's Eye) 'Farm Fresh Whole Vegetables'	4 oz	30	7.0	0.0
(Bird's Eye) petite 'Deluxe'	2.6 oz	20	5.0	0.0
(Freshlike)	3 oz	25	5.0	0.0
(Green Giant)	1/2 cup	14	4.0	0.0
(Green Giant) and creamy mushroom 'Garden Gourmet'	1 pkg	220	29.0	11.0
(Green Giant) in butter sauce 'One Serving'	5.5 oz	60	8.0	2.0
(Green Giant) 'Plain Polybag'	1/2 cup	14	4.0	0.0
(Seabrook)	3 oz	25	5.0	0.0
(Southern)	3.5 oz	33	6.8	0.1
(Stouffer's) mushroom casserole	4.75 oz	160	13.0	11.0
(Veg•All)	3 oz	25	5.0	0.0

GREEN ONION. See ONION, GREEN.

GRENADINE. See ALCOHOLIC BEVERAGES.

GRITS

Dry

| white *(Arrowhead Mills)* | 2 oz | 200 | 43.0 | 1.0 |

Food Name	Serv. Size	Total Cal.	Carbs GMS	Fat GMS
white, enriched	1 cup	579	124.2	1.9
white, enriched	1 tbsp	36	7.7	0.1
white, enriched 'Regular/Quick' (Aunt Jemima)	3 tbsp	101	22.4	0.2
white, unenriched	1 cup	579	124.2	1.9
white, unenriched	1 tbsp	36	7.7	0.1
yellow (Arrowhead Mills)	2 oz	200	44.0	1.0
yelllow, enriched	1 cup	579	124.2	1.9
yellow, enriched	1 tbsp	36	7.7	0.1
yellow, enriched (Quick)	3 tbsp	101	22.4	0.2
yellow, unenriched	1 cup	579	124.2	1.9
yellow, unenriched	1 tbsp	36	7.7	0.1
Prepared				
white, enriched, cooked w/water	1 cup	145	31.5	0.5
white, unenriched, cooked w/water	1 cup	145	31.5	0.5
yellow, enriched, cooked w/water	1 cup	145	31.5	0.5
yellow, unenriched, cooked w/water	1 cup	145	31.5	0.5
GRITS, CANNED				
golden (Allens)	1/2 cup	80	16.0	<1.0
golden (Bush's Best)	1/2 cup	45	11.0	0.0
golden (Van Camp's)	1 cup	128	27.9	0.6
golden, w/red and green peppers (Van Camp's)	1 cup	129	28.5	0.5
Mexican (Allens)	1/2 cup	80	16.0	<1.0
white	1 cup	115	22.8	1.4
white	4 oz	82	16.2	1.0
white (Allens)	1/2 cup	70	16.0	<1.0
white (Bush's Best)	1/2 cup	45	11.0	0.0
white (Van Camp's)	1 cup	138	30.0	0.7
yellow	1 cup	115	22.8	1.4
yellow	4 oz	82	16.2	1.0
GRITS, INSTANT				
white, hominy product, dry, one packet (Quaker)	.8 oz	79	17.7	0.1
w/imitation bacon bits, dry, one packet (Quaker)	1 oz	101	21.6	0.4
w/imitation ham bits, dry, one packet (Quaker)	1 oz	99	21.3	0.3
w/real cheddar cheese flavor, dry, one packet (Quaker)	1 oz	104	21.6	1.0
GRITS, QUICK-COOKING				
Dry				
white, enriched	1 cup	579	124.2	1.9
white, enriched	1 tbsp	36	7.7	0.1
white, unenriched	1 cup	579	124.2	1.9
white, unenriched	1 tbsp	36	7.7	0.1
yellow, enriched	1 cup	579	124.2	1.9
yellow, enriched	1 tbsp	36	7.7	0.1
yellow, enriched 'Quick' (Quaker)	3 tbsp	101	22.4	0.2

Food Name	Serv. Size	Total Cal.	Carbs GMS	Fat GMS
yellow, unenriched	1 cup	579	124.2	1.9
yellow, unenriched	1 tbsp	36	7.7	0.1
Prepared				
white, enriched, cooked w/water	1 cup	145	31.5	0.5
white, unenriched, cooked w/water	1 cup	145	31.5	0.5
yellow, enriched, cooked w/water	1 cup	145	31.5	0.5
yellow, unenriched, cooked w/water	1 cup	145	31.5	0.5
GROUND CHERRY. See CAPE GOOSEBERRY.				
GROUND HUSK TOMATO. See TOMATILLO.				
GROUPER, MIXED SPECIES				
broiled	4 oz	134	0.0	1.5
dry-heat cooked	4 oz	134	0.0	1.5
dry-heat cooked	3 oz	100	0.0	1.1
microwaved	4 oz	134	0.0	1.5
raw	1 lb	417	0.0	4.6
raw	3 oz	78	0.0	0.9
raw	1 oz	26	0.0	0.3
GUACAMOLE. See DIP, AVOCADO.				
GUACAMOLE SEASONING				
(Lawry's) 'Seasoning Blend' dry mix	1 pkg	60	12.6	0.4
(Old El Paso) dry mix	1/7 pkg	7	2.0	0.0
GUANABANA/soursop				
raw, approx 2.1 lb	1 med	416	105.3	1.9
trimmed	1 oz	19	4.8	0.1
trimmed	1/2 cup	75	18.9	0.3
untrimmed	1 lb	202	51.2	0.9
GUANABANA NECTAR (Libby's)	6 oz	110	26.0	0.0
GUANABANA PUNCH, 'Rain Forest' (Knudsen & Sons)	8 oz	125	29.0	0.0
GUAVA				
trimmed	1 cup	84	19.6	1.0
trimmed	1 fruit	46	10.7	0.5
trimmed	1 oz	15	3.4	0.2
untrimmed	1 lb	183	43.1	2.2
w/edible seeds (Sunfresh)	3.5 oz	70	18.0	0.0
GUAVA, STRAWBERRY				
trimmed	1 cup	168	42.4	1.5
trimmed	1 oz	20	4.9	0.2
trimmed	1 fruit	4	1.0	0.0
untrimmed	1 lb	268	66.9	2.3
GUAVA CRANBERRY JUICE				
organic 'Cruz' (Santa Cruz Natural)	8 oz	130	30.0	<1.0
GUAVA FRUIT DRINK				
Hawaiian 'Mauna La'i' (Ocean Spray)	6 oz	100	24.0	0.0

Food Name	Serv. Size	Total Cal.	Carbs GMS	Fat GMS
GUAVA JUICE				
'Orchard Tropicals' bottled, diluted *(Welch's)*	6 oz	100	25.0	0.0
'Orchard Tropicals' frozen, diluted *(Welch's)*	6 oz	100	25.0	0.0
GUAVA NECTAR				
(Kern's)	6 oz	110	28.0	0.0
(Libby's)	6 oz	110	26.0	0.0
GUAVA PASSION DRINK				
Hawaiian 'Hawaii' *(Pathmark)*	6 oz	100	25.0	0.0
Hawaiian 'Mauna La'i *(Ocean Spray)*	6 oz	100	25.0	0.0
GUAVA STRAWBERRY DRINK 'Refresher' *(Veryfine)*	8 oz	120	30.0	0.0
GUINEA HEN				
giblets, raw	100 gm	157	1.2	7.0
meat and skin, raw	1 lb	567	0.0	23.2
meat only, raw	1 oz	31	0.0	0.7
GUMBO. See OKRA.				
GUMBO FILE POWDER *(Tone's)*	1 tsp	8	1.7	0.2

H

Food Name	Serv. Size	Total Cal.	Carbs GMS	Fat GMS
HADDOCK				
baked	4 oz	127	0.0	1.1
broiled	4 oz	127	0.0	1.1
dry-heat cooked	3 oz	95	0.0	0.8
microwaved	4 oz	127	0.0	1.1
raw	1 lb	396	0.0	3.3
raw	3 oz	74	0.0	0.6
smoked	3 oz	99	0.0	0.8
HADDOCK FILLET, FROZEN				
(SeaPak)	4 oz	90	0.0	1.0
battered *(Van de Kamp's)*	2 pieces	250	19.0	15.0
battered, 'Crunchy' *(Mrs. Paul's)*	2 pieces	190	22.0	5.0
breaded *(Van de Kamp's)*	2 pieces	270	19.0	16.0
breaded, in lemon butter, 'Microwave' *(Gorton's)*	1 pkg	360	19.0	21.0
breaded, 'Light' *(Mrs. Paul's)*	1 piece	220	15.0	9.0
breaded, 'Light' *(Van de Kamp's)*	1 piece	240	21.0	11.0
'Fishmarket Fresh' *(Gorton's)*	5 oz	110	0.0	1.0
natural *(Van de Kamp's)*	4 oz	90	0.0	1.0
HALIBUT				
ATLANTIC				
broiled	4 oz	159	0.0	3.3
dry-heat cooked	4 oz	159	0.0	3.3

Food Name	Serv. Size	Total Cal.	Carbs GMS	Fat GMS
dry-heat cooked	3 oz	119	0.0	2.5
microwaved	4 oz	159	0.0	3.3
raw	1 lb	497	0.0	10.4
raw	3 oz	94	0.0	2.0
raw	1 oz	31	0.0	0.6
GREENLAND				
dry-heat cooked	3 oz	203	0.0	15.1
raw	1 lb	845	0.0	62.8
raw	3 oz	158	0.0	11.8
raw	1 oz	53	0.0	3.9
PACIFIC				
broiled	4 oz	159	0.0	3.3
dry-heat cooked	4 oz	159	0.0	3.3
dry-heat cooked	3 oz	119	0.0	2.5
microwaved	4 oz	159	0.0	3.3
raw	1 lb	497	0.0	10.4
raw	3 oz	94	0.0	2.0
raw	1 oz	31	0.0	0.6
raw, fillet portions, skinless *(Peter Pan Seafoods)*	3.5 oz	110	na	2.3
HALIBUT, FROZEN				
fillet, battered *(Van de Kamp's)*	2 pieces	150	16.0	6.0
steaks, w/o seasoning mix *(SeaPak)*	6-oz pkg	160	0.0	1.0
HAM. See HAM, ALTERNATIVE; HAM, CANNED; HAM, CURED; HAM, FRESH; HAM, MINCE HAM PATTY.				
HAM, ALTERNATIVE				
(Worthington) frozen, roll 'Wham' approx .9-oz slices	3 slices	120	3.0	7.0
HAM, CANNED				
chopped	1 oz	68	0.1	5.3
chopped	.75-oz slice	50	0.1	4.0
cured, extra lean, approx 4% fat, baked	3 oz	116	0.4	4.2
cured, extra lean, approx 4% fat, unheated	1 oz	34	0.0	1.3
cured, extra lean and regular, baked	3 oz	142	0.4	7.2
cured, extra lean and regular, unheated	1 oz	41	0.0	2.1
cured, regular, approx 13% fat, baked	3 oz	192	0.4	12.9
cured, regular, approx 13% fat, unheated	1 oz	54	0.0	3.7
(Armour) chopped	3 oz	190	1.0	14.0
(Black Label)				
'5-lb can'	4 oz	140	0.0	7.0
'3-lb can'	4 oz	140	0.0	7.0
'1 1/2-lb can'	4 oz	150	0.0	7.0
(Chi-Chi's) 'Black Label'	1 oz	37	2.0	1.0
(EXL) 'Deli Ham' 10-lb can	4 oz	130	0.0	6.0
(Holiday Glaze) '3-lb can'	4 oz	130	2.0	4.0

Food Name	Serv. Size	Total Cal.	Carbs GMS	Fat GMS
(Hormel)				
'Bone-In'	4 oz	210	1.0	15.0
chopped, '8-lb can'	3 oz	240	1.0	21.0
chopped, '12-oz can'	2 oz	120	0.0	9.0
chunk	6.75 oz	310	0.0	20.0
chunk	2.5 oz	110	1.0	7.0
'Cure/81'	4 oz	160	0.0	8.0
'Cure/81'	1 oz	31	2.0	1.0
'Curemaster'	4 oz	140	1.0	5.0
'Curemaster'	2 oz	60	1.0	2.0
'Light and Lean 97'	2 oz	60	1.0	2.0
roll	4 oz	170	0.0	10.0
spiced	3 oz	240	1.0	21.0
(JM) '95% Fat-free'	2 oz	60	1.0	2.0
(Light & Lean) 'Boneless'	2 oz	60	0.0	2.0
(Oscar Mayer) 'Jubilee'	1 oz	29	0.1	0.9
(Rath) hickory smoked, 'Black Hawk'	2 oz	60	1.0	2.0
HAM, CURED				
(NOTE: TRIMMED = Lean; separable fat removed. UNTRIMMED = Separable fat not removed.)				
BONELESS				
center slice, country-style, trimmed, unheated	1 oz	55	0.1	2.4
center slice, untrimmed, unheated	1 oz	58	0.0	3.7
extra lean, approx 5% fat, baked	3 oz	123	1.3	4.7
extra lean, approx 5% fat, unheated	1 oz	37	0.3	1.4
extra lean and regular, baked	3 oz	140	0.4	6.5
extra lean and regular, unheated	1 oz	46	0.7	2.4
extra lean and regular, unheated, 4 x 6 1/4 inch slice	1 slice	46	0.7	2.4
mini *(JM)*	3 oz	90	0.0	3.0
regular, approx 11% fat, baked	3 oz	151	0.0	7.7
regular, approx 11% fat, unheated	1 oz	52	0.9	3.0
steak, 'Jubilee' *(Oscar Mayer)*	2 oz	57	0.2	1.9
steak, unheated	2 oz	69	0.0	2.4
w/natural juices, 'EZ Cut' *(JM)*	2 oz	70	1.0	3.0
WHOLE				
trimmed, fully cooked, baked	3 oz	133	0.0	4.7
trimmed, fully cooked, unheated	1 oz	42	0.0	1.6
trimmed *(JM)*	3 oz	140	0.0	8.0
untrimmed, fully cooked, baked	3 oz	207	0.0	14.2
untrimmed, fully cooked, unheated	1 oz	70	0.0	5.3

Food Name	Serv. Size	Total Cal.	Carbs GMS	Fat GMS
HAM, FRESH. See also PORK.				
(NOTE: TRIMMED = Lean; separable fat removed. UNTRIMMED = Separable fat not removed.)				
LEG, RUMP HALF				
Trimmed				
raw	1 lb	621	0.0	23.5
raw	1 oz	39	0.0	1.5
roasted	3 oz	175	0.0	6.9
roasted, diced	1 cup	278	0.0	11.0
Untrimmed				
raw	1 lb	1007	0.0	71.2
raw	1 oz	63	0.0	4.4
roasted	3 oz	214	0.0	12.1
roasted	1.5 oz	117	0.0	7.6
roasted, diced	1 cup	340	0.0	19.3
LEG, SHANK HALF				
Trimmed				
raw	1 lb	631	0.0	25.5
raw	1 oz	39	0.0	1.6
roasted	3 oz	183	0.0	8.9
roasted, diced	1 cup	290	0.0	14.2
Untrimmed				
raw	1 lb	1193	0.0	95.4
raw	1 oz	75	0.0	6.0
roasted	3 oz	246	0.0	17.0
roasted	1.5 oz	129	0.0	9.4
roasted, diced	1 cup	390	0.0	27.1
LEG, WHOLE				
Trimmed				
raw	1 lb	617	0.0	24.5
raw	1 oz	39	0.0	1.5
roasted	3 oz	179	0.0	8.0
roasted	1.5 oz	94	0.0	4.7
roasted	1 cup	285	0.0	12.7
Untrimmed				
raw	1 lb	1111	0.0	85.6
raw	1 oz	69	0.0	5.3
roasted	3 oz	232	0.0	15.0
roasted	1.5 oz	125	0.0	8.8
roasted, diced	1 cup	369	0.0	23.8
HAM, MINCED	1 oz	75	0.5	5.9
HAM ENTRÉE, FROZEN				
and asparagus bake *(Stouffer's)*	9.5 oz	520	32.0	35.0
and cheese casserole, 'Microwave Classic' *(Pillsbury)*	1 pkg	470	34.0	29.0

Food Name	Serv. Size	Total Cal.	Carbs GMS	Fat GMS
dinner *(Morton)*	10 oz	290	49.0	4.0
'Platters' *(Banquet)*	10 oz	400	43.0	17.0
steak *(Le Menu)*	10 oz	300	31.0	11.0
steak 'Classics' *(Armour)*	10.75 oz	270	36.0	7.0
w/scalloped potatoes 'Homestyle Recipe' *(Swanson)*	9 oz	300	26.0	13.0
HAM LUNCHEON MEAT. See LUNCHEON MEAT.				
HAM PATTY				
canned *(Hormel)*	1 patty	180	0.0	16.0
canned, w/cheese *(Hormel)*	1 patty	190	0.0	18.0
cured, boneless steak, extra lean, unheated	2-oz slice	69	0.0	2.4
cured, unheated	1 oz	89	0.5	8.0
grilled	4 oz	388	1.9	35.0
'Premium Brown 'N Serve' *(Swift)*	1 patty	130	1.0	13.0
HAM SPREAD				
deviled	1 cup	790	0.0	72.7
deviled	4.5-oz can	449	0.0	41.3
deviled *(Hormel)*	1 oz	76	1.0	6.0
deviled *(Hormel)*	1 tbsp	35	0.0	3.0
deviled *(Underwood)*	2 1/8 oz	220	<1.0	19.0
deviled *(Underwood)* 'Light'	2 1/8 oz	120	1.0	8.0
deviled *(Underwood)* 'Smoked'	2 1/8 oz	190	<1.0	18.0
ham and cheese	1 oz	69	0.6	5.3
ham and cheese	1 tbsp	37	0.3	2.8
ham salad	1 oz	61	3.0	4.4
ham salad	1 tbsp	32	1.6	2.3
ham salad 'Spreadables' *(Libby's)*	1.9 oz	70	6.0	3.0
HAM TACO, refrigerated, 'Border Breakfasts' *(Owens)*	2.17 oz	90	13.0	6.0
HAMBURG PARSLEY. See PARSLEY ROOT.				
HAMBURGER. See BEEF, GROUND.				
HAMBURGER BUN. See BUN, HAMBURGER.				
HAMBURGER ENTRÉE MIX				
(Betty Crocker) 'Hamburger Helper'				
beef noodle, dry	1/5 pkg	140	26.0	2.0
beef noodle, prepared	1 cup	320	26.0	15.0
beef Romanoff, dry	1/5 pkg	180	31.0	3.0
beef Romanoff, prepared	1 cup	350	31.0	16.0
beef taco, dry	1/5 pkg	160	33.0	1.0
beef taco, prepared	1 cup	330	33.0	14.0
beef teriyaki, dry	1/5 pkg	180	38.0	1.0
beef teriyaki, prepared	1 cup	360	38.0	14.0
cheddar and bacon, dry	1/5 pkg	190	28.0	6.0
cheddar and bacon, prepared	1 cup	400	30.0	20.0
cheeseburger macaroni, dry	1/5 pkg	190	26.0	6.0

Food Name	Serv. Size	Total Cal.	Carbs GMS	Fat GMS
cheeseburger macaroni, prepared	1 cup	370	28.0	19.0
cheesy Italian, dry	1/5 pkg	160	27.0	3.0
cheesy Italian, prepared w/2% milk	1 cup	360	30.0	17.0
chili macaroni, dry	1/5 pkg	150	32.0	1.0
chili macaroni, prepared	1 cup	330	32.0	14.0
chili tomato, dry	1/5 pkg	150	31.0	1.0
chili tomato, prepared	1 cup	330	31.0	14.0
chili w/beans, dry	1/4 pkg	130	25.0	1.0
chili w/beans, prepared	1 1/4 cup	350	25.0	17.0
creamy Stroganoff, dry	1/5 pkg	190	30.0	5.0
creamy Stroganoff, prepared w/whole milk	1 cup	390	30.0	20.0
hamburger hash, dry	1/5 pkg	140	27.0	2.0
hamburger hash, prepared	1 cup	320	27.0	15.0
hamburger stew, dry	1/5 pkg	120	25.0	1.0
hamburger stew, prepared	1 cup	300	25.0	14.0
lasagna, dry	1/5 pkg	160	33.0	1.0
lasagna, prepared	1 cup	340	33.0	14.0
meat loaf, dry	1/5 pkg	70	13.0	1.0
meat loaf, prepared	1 cup	360	14.0	22.0
mushroom and wild rice, dry	1/5 pkg	180	34.0	3.0
mushroom and wild rice, prepared	1 cup	380	37.0	16.0
nacho cheese, dry	1/5 pkg	160	32.0	2.0
nacho cheese, prepared	1 cup	360	35.0	15.0
pizza dish, dry	1/5 pkg	180	37.0	1.0
pizza dish, prepared	1 cup	360	37.0	14.0
'Pizzabake' dry	1/6 pkg	150	29.0	2.0
'Pizzabake' prepared	4.5 oz	320	29.0	14.0
potato au gratin, dry	1/5 pkg	150	28.0	2.0
potato au gratin, prepared	1 cup	320	28.0	15.0
potato Stroganoff, dry	1/5 pkg	140	28.0	2.0
potato Stroganoff, prepared	1 cup	320	28.0	15.0
rice Oriental, dry	1/5 pkg	180	38.0	1.0
rice Oriental, prepared	1 cup	340	38.0	14.0
'Sloppy Joe Bake' dry	1/6 pkg	180	33.0	2.0
'Sloppy Joe Bake' prepared	5 oz	340	33.0	15.0
spaghetti, dry	1/5 pkg	170	32.0	2.0
spaghetti, prepared	1 cup	340	32.0	15.0
'Tacobake' dry	1/6 pkg	170	31.0	4.0
'Tacobake' prepared	5.75 oz	320	31.0	15.0
tamale pie, dry	1/5 pkg	200	39.0	3.0
tamale pie, prepared	1 cup	380	39.0	16.0
three cheese, dry	1/5 pkg	210	30.0	7.0
three cheese, prepared	1/5 pkg	400	32.0	20.0

Food Name	Serv. Size	Total Cal.	Carbs GMS	Fat GMS
zesty Italian, dry	1/5 pkg	170	35.0	1.0
zesty Italian, prepared	1 cup	340	35.0	13.0
HAWAIIAN YAM. See YAM, MOUNTAIN.				
HAWS/hawthorn tree fruit				
scarlet, flesh and skin, raw	100 gm	87	20.8	0.7
HAZELNUT, SHELLED/cobnut/filbert				
blanched	1 oz	191	4.5	19.1
dry-roasted, unblanched	1 oz	188	5.1	18.8
dry-roasted, unblanched, w/salt	1 oz	188	5.1	18.8
oil-roasted, unblanched	1 oz	187	5.4	18.1
oil-roasted, unblanched, w/salt	1 oz	187	5.4	18.1
unblanched	1 oz	179	4.4	17.8
unblanched, chopped	1 cup	727	17.6	72.0
HAZELNUT BUTTER, gourmet *(Roaster Fresh)*	1 oz	188	5.0	18.9
HAZELNUT OIL				
	1 cup	1927	0.0	218.0
	1 oz	251	0.0	28.4
	1 tbsp	120	0.0	13.6
HAZELNUT SPREAD, Nutella, with milk and cocoa *(Ferrero)*	1 tbsp	80	9.0	5.0
HEART NUT. See CASHEW.				
HERB AND GARLIC MARINADE, w/lemon *(Lawry's)*	2 tbsp	36	3.8	<1.0
HERB SEASONING MIX				
Italian, 'Bag 'n Season' *(Schilling)*	1 pkg	94	21.0	0.2
mixed, 'Pinch of Herbs' *(Lawry's)*	1 tsp	9	0.9	0.5
HERBAL TEA. See TEA.				
HERRING				
ATLANTIC				
broiled	4 oz	230	0.0	13.1
dry-heat cooked	4 oz	230	0.0	13.1
dry-heat cooked	3 oz	173	0.0	9.9
kippered	4 oz	246	0.0	14.0
kippered snacks, w/smoke flavoring, drained *(Beach Cliff)*	3.3 oz	220	1.0	17.0
microwaved	4 oz	230	0.0	13.1
pickled	4 oz	297	10.9	20.4
raw	1 lb	718	0.0	41.0
raw	3 oz	134	0.0	7.7
raw	1 oz	45	0.0	2.6
steaks, in soybean oil, drained *(Beach Cliff)*	3 oz	240	0.0	20.0
steaks, in water, drained *(Beach Cliff)*	3 oz	230	1.0	18.0
steaks, w/mustard, drained *(Beach Cliff)*	3 oz	227	4.0	18.0
steaks, w/tomato, drained *(Beach Cliff)*	3 oz	210	0.0	17.0
LAKE				
raw	1 lb	446	0.0	8.7

Food Name	Serv. Size	Total Cal.	Carbs GMS	Fa GM
raw	2.8-oz fillet	78	0.0	1.5
raw	1 oz	28	0.0	0.5
smoked	4 oz	201	0.0	13.5
PACIFIC				
dry-heat cooked	3 oz	213	0.0	15.1
raw	1 lb	885	0.0	63.0
raw	3 oz	166	0.0	11.8
raw	1 oz	55	0.0	3.9
HIBISCUS COOLER (Knudsen & Sons)	8 oz	95	24.0	0.0
HIBISCUS CRANBERRY JUICE (Knudsen & Sons)	8 oz	110	28.0	0.0
HICKORY NUT				
in shell	1 lb	954	26.5	93.4
shelled	1 oz	187	5.2	18.3
HOG PLUM. See JOBO.				
HOMINY GRITS. See GRITS.				
HONEY				
extracted	1 cup	1031	279.0	0.0
extracted	1 tbsp	64	17.3	0.0
strained	1 cup	1031	279.0	0.0
strained	1 tbsp	64	17.3	0.0
(Golden Blossom)	1 tbsp	60	16.0	0.0
(Knott's Berry Farm)	1 oz	90	23.0	0.0
(Knott's Berry Farm)	1 tbsp	60	17.0	0.0
(Knott's Berry Farm)	.5 oz	30	17.0	0.0
(Sioux)	1 tbsp	60	16.0	0.0
HONEY BUTTER	1 tbsp	50	11.0	1.0
HONEY ROLL SAUSAGE				
	1 oz	52	0.6	3.0
4-inch diam	1/8-inch slice	42	0.5	2.4
HONEYDEW MELON				
pulp	1 oz	10	2.6	<.1
raw, cubed	1 cup	59	15.6	0.2
raw, wedge	7 x 2 inches	45	11.8	0.1
untrimmed	1 lb	74	19.2	0.2
untrimmed (Dole)	7 x 2 inches	50	12.0	0.0
HORSE				
roasted	3 oz	149	0.0	5.1
roasted, diced	1 cup	245	0.0	8.5
raw	1 lb	603	0.0	20.9
raw	1 oz	37	0.0	1.3
HORSE BEAN. See FAVA BEAN.				

Food Name	Serv. Size	Total Cal.	Carbs GMS	Fat GMS
HORSERADISH				
Prepared				
. . . .	1 tbsp	6	1.4	0.0
. . . .	1 tsp	2	0.5	0.0
(Crowley)	1 oz	10	2.0	<1.0
(Kraft)	1 tbsp	10	1.0	0.0
(Kraft) cream style	1 tbsp	12	1.0	0.0
(Gold's) hot	1 tsp	4	<1.0	<1.0
(Gold's) red	1 tsp	4	<1.0	0.0
(Gold's) white	1 tsp	4	<1.0	<1.0
(Silver Spring) cream style	1 tsp	0	0.0	0.0
Raw	1 lb	288	65.3	1.0
HORSERADISH, JAPANESE. See WASABI.				
HORSERADISH TREE				
Leafy tips				
boiled, drained	4 oz	68	12.6	1.1
boiled, drained, chopped	1 cup	25	4.7	0.4
raw, chopped	1 cup	13	1.7	0.3
raw, trimmed	1 oz	18	2.3	0.4
raw, untrimmed	1 lb	181	23.3	3.9
Pods				
boiled, drained	4 oz	41	9.3	0.2
boiled, drained, sliced	1 cup	42	9.6	0.2
boiled, drained, sliced	1/2 cup	21	4.8	0.1
raw, sliced	1 cup	37	8.5	0.2
raw, trimmed	1 oz	10	2.4	0.1
raw, untrimmed	1 lb	88	20.1	0.5
raw, whole, approx 15 1/3 inches long	1 pod	4	0.9	0.0
HOT CHOCOLATE. See COCOA MIX.				
HOT DOG. See FRANKFURTER.				
HOT DOG BUN. See BUN, FRANKFURTER.				
HUBBARD SQUASH. See SQUASH, HUBBARD.				
HUMMUS				
mix, dry *(Casbah)*	1 oz	110	10.0	5.0
prepared	1/2 cup	210	24.8	10.4
prepared	1 oz	48	5.7	2.4
HUSHPUPPY, FROZEN, 'Regular' *(SeaPak)*	4 oz	330	56.0	9.0
HUSHPUPPY MIX				
deluxe, dry *(Golden Dipt)*	1.25 oz	120	26.0	0.0
jalapeño, dry *(Golden Dipt)*	1.25 oz	120	27.0	0.0
w/onion, dry *(Golden Dipt)*	1.25 oz	120	27.0	0.0
HYACINTH BEAN				
boiled, drained	4 oz	57	10.4	0.3

Food Name	Serv. Size	Total Cal.	Carbs GMS	Fat GMS
immature, boiled, drained	1/2 cup	22	4.1	0.1
immature, raw	1/2 cup	18	3.7	0.1
mature, boiled	1/2 cup	113	20.1	0.6
mature, raw	1/2 cup	361	63.8	1.8
raw, trimmed	1 oz	13	2.6	0.1
raw, untrimmed	1 lb	196	38.8	0.8
HYACINTH BEAN, DRIED				
mature, boiled	1/2 cup	114	20.1	0.6
mature, boiled	4 oz	133	23.5	0.7
mature, raw	1/2 cup	362	63.8	1.8
mature, raw	1 oz	98	17.2	0.5

I

Food Name	Serv. Size	Total Cal.	Carbs GMS	Fat GMS
ICE BARS AND DESSERTS. See also FRUIT BAR, FROZEN; SHERBET; SORBET.				
BAR				
'All Natural' all flavors (Popsicle)	1 bar	60	14.0	0.0
'Ice Stripes' 1.5 oz, all flavors (Good Humor)	1 bar	35	8.6	0.0
'Twin Pop' all flavors (Gold Bond)	1 bar	60	14.0	0.0
'Water Ice' all flavors except cherry and wildberry (Popsicle)	1 bar	50	12.0	0.0
Cherry				
'Calippo' 4.5 oz (Good Humor)	1 bar	138	34.9	0.1
'Jumbo Jet Star' 4.5 oz (Good Humor)	1 bar	85	19.5	0.7
'Water Ice' (Popsicle)	1 bar	70	17.0	0.0
Fruit				
and juice, 3 oz	1 bar	75	18.6	0.1
and water, aspartame-sweetened	1 bar	12	3.2	0.1
Lemon				
'Calippo' 4.5 oz (Good Humor)	1 bar	112	27.6	0.1
'Great White Shark' 3 oz (Good Humor)	1 bar	68	17.0	0.1
Orange				
'Calippo' 4.5 oz (Good Humor)	1 bar	111	27.2	0.2
Wildberry, 'Water Ice' (Popsicle)	1 bar	40	10.0	0.0
DESSERT				
cherry, Italian (Good Humor)	6 oz	138	34.2	0.1
daiquiri (Baskin-Robbins)	1 scoop	140	35.0	0.0
lime	4 oz	75	31.3	0.0
pineapple-coconut	4 oz	108	22.9	2.5

Food Name	Serv. Size	Total Cal.	Carbs GMS	Fat GMS
ICE CREAM. See also ICE CREAM, ALTERNATIVE; ICE CREAM BAR; ICE CREAM BAR, ALTERNATIVE; ICE CREAM CAKE; ICE CREAM CONE; ICE CREAM MIX; ICE CREAM SNACKS AND SANDWICHES; ICE MILK; ICE MILK BAR.				
ALMOND FUDGE *(Baskin-Robbins)* 'Jamoca'	1 scoop	270	30.0	14.0
BANANA				
(Baskin-Robbins) sugar-free 'Chunky Banana'	4 oz	100	20.0	1.0
(Ben & Jerry's) 'Chunky Monkey'	1/2 cup	280	29.0	19.0
BORDEAUX CHERRY *(Healthy Choice)* 'Dairy Dessert'	4 oz	120	23.0	2.0
BORDEAUX CHERRY CHOCOLATE CHIP				
(Healthy Choice) 'Dairy Dessert'	4 oz	120	23.0	2.0
BOYSENBERRY *(Good Humor)* 'King Cone'	5 oz	340	51.6	13.1
BROWNIES 'N CREME *(Weight Watchers)* 'ONE-ders'	4 oz	130	20.0	4.0
BUTTER ALMOND *(Breyers)*	4 oz	170	15.0	10.0
BUTTER CRUNCH *(Sealtest)*	4 oz	150	18.0	7.0
BUTTER PECAN				
(Ben & Jerry's)	1/2 cup	310	20.0	26.0
(Breyers)	4 oz	180	15.0	12.0
(Frusen Glädjé)	4 oz	280	16.0	21.0
(Häagen-Dazs)	4 oz	390	29.0	24.0
(Lady Borden)	4 oz	180	16.0	12.0
(Sealtest)	4 oz	160	16.0	9.0
BUTTER PECAN CRUNCH *(Healthy Choice)* 'Dairy Dessert'	4 oz	140	26.0	2.0
CHERRY				
(Ben & Jerry's) 'Cherry Garcia'	1/2 cup	240	25.0	16.0
(Breyers) vanilla	4 oz	150	17.0	7.0
CHOCOLATE				
(Baskin-Robbins)	1 scoop	270	32.0	14.0
(Baskin-Robbins) 'World Class'	1 scoop	280	35.0	14.0
(Ben & Jerry's) deep dark chocolate	1/2 cup	260	32.0	15.0
(Breyers)	4 oz	160	20.0	8.0
(Darigold)	4 oz	140	17.0	7.0
(Darigold) 'Alpine'	4 oz	140	17.0	7.0
(Darigold) 'Classic'	4 oz	180	16.0	13.0
(Frusen Glädjé)	4 oz	240	17.0	17.0
(Häagen-Dazs)	4 oz	270	24.0	17.0
(Häagen-Dazs) deep	4 oz	290	26.0	14.0
(Healthy Choice) 'Dairy Dessert'	4 oz	130	24.0	2.0
(Sealtest)	4 oz	140	18.0	6.0
CHOCOLATE, DUTCH *(Borden)* 'Olde Fashioned Recipe'	4 oz	130	16.0	6.0
CHOCOLATE CARAMEL NUT *(Baskin-Robbins)* light	4 oz	130	19.0	5.0
CHOCOLATE CHIP				
(Baskin-Robbins)	1 scoop	260	27.0	15.0
(Breyers)	4 oz	170	18.0	10.0

Food Name	Serv. Size	Total Cal.	Carbs GMS	Fat GMS
(Dreyer's)	4 oz	150	16.0	9.0
(Eskimo Pie) cone 'Cookie Dough'	1 cone	280	33.0	14.0
(Healthy Choice) 'Dairy Dessert'	4 oz	130	24.0	2.0
(Sealtest)	4 oz	150	17.0	8.0
(Weight Watchers) 'ONE-ders'	4 oz	120	19.0	4.0
CHOCOLATE CHIP CHOCOLATE (Häagen-Dazs)	4 oz	290	28.0	20.0
CHOCOLATE CHIP COOKIE DOUGH (Ben & Jerry's)	1/2 cup	270	30.0	17.0
CHOCOLATE CHOCOLATE CHIP (Frusen Glädjé)	4 oz	270	21.0	18.0
CHOCOLATE CHUNK				
(Ben & Jerry's) 'New York Super Fudge Chunk'	1/2 cup	290	28.0	20.0
CHOCOLATE FUDGE				
(Ben & Jerry's) 'Chocolate Fudge Brownie'	1/2 cup	250	31.0	14.0
(Ben & Jerry's) double chocolate fudge	1/2 cup	280	35.0	16.0
(Häagen-Dazs) deep	4 oz	290	26.0	14.0
CHOCOLATE MINT (Häagen-Dazs)	4 oz	300	26.0	20.0
CHOCOLATE PEANUT BUTTER COOKIE DOUGH				
(Ben & Jerry's)	1/2 cup	300	32.0	20.0
CHOCOLATE RASPBERRY TRUFFLE				
(Baskin-Robbins) 'International Creams'	1 scoop	310	35.0	17.0
CHOCOLATE SWIRL (Borden)	4 oz	130	18.0	6.0
CHOCOLATE TRIPLE STRIPES (Sealtest)	4 oz	140	17.0	7.0
CHOCOLATE-PEANUT BUTTER, DEEP (Häagen-Dazs)	4 oz	330	25.0	19.0
COCONUT ALMOND FUDGE CHIP (Ben & Jerry's)	1/2 cup	320	24.0	28.0
COFFEE				
(Baskin-Robbins) light 'Espresso and Cream'	4 oz	120	15.0	5.0
(Ben & Jerry's) Aztec harvest coffee	1/2 cup	230	22.0	16.0
(Breyers)	4 oz	150	16.0	8.0
(Häagen-Dazs)	4 oz	270	23.0	17.0
(Sealtest)	4 oz	140	16.0	7.0
COFFEE ALMOND FUDGE (Ben & Jerry's)	1/2 cup	290	24.0	20.0
COFFEE TOFFEE				
(Ben & Jerry's) 'Coffee Toffee Crunch'	1/2 cup	280	28.0	19.0
(Healthy Choice) 'Dairy Dessert'	4 oz	130	25.0	2.0
COOKIE DOUGH DYNAMO (Häagen-Dazs)	4 oz	300	31.0	18.0
COOKIES N' CREAM				
(Breyers)	4 oz	170	19.0	9.0
(Dreyer's)	4 oz	160	18.0	9.0
(Healthy Choice) 'Dairy Dessert'	4 oz	130	24.0	2.0
FUDGE, MARBLE (Dreyer's)	4 oz	150	18.0	8.0
FUDGE BROWNIE (Healthy Choice) 'Dairy Dessert'	4 oz	130	27.0	2.0
FUDGE ROYALE (Sealtest)	4 oz	140	19.0	7.0
FUDGE SWIRL, DOUBLE (Healthy Choice) 'Dairy Dessert'	4 oz	130	24.0	2.0

Food Name	Serv. Size	Total Cal.	Carbs GMS	Fat GMS
HEAVENLY HASH				
(Sealtest)	4 oz	150	19.0	7.0
(Weight Watchers) 'ONE-ders'	4 oz	130	22.0	3.0
MACADAMIA BRITTLE (Häagen-Dazs)	4 oz	280	25.0	18.0
MAPLE WALNUT (Sealtest)	4 oz	160	17.0	9.0
MINT CHOCOLATE (Breyers)	4 oz	170	18.0	10.0
MINT CHOCOLATE CHIP (Healthy Choice) 'Dairy Dessert'	4 oz	140	25.0	2.0
MINT WITH CHOCOLATE COOKIE (Ben & Jerry's)	1/2 cup	260	27.0	17.0
MOCHA ALMOND FUDGE (Breyers)	4 oz	190	20.0	10.0
MOCHA FUDGE (Ben & Jerry's)	1/2 cup	270	30.0	18.0
NEAPOLITAN (Healthy Choice) 'Dairy Dessert'	4 oz	120	22.0	2.0
PEACH				
(Baskin-Robbins) fat-free 'Just Peachy'	4 oz	100	22.0	0.0
(Breyers) natural	4 oz	130	18.0	6.0
PEANUT BUTTER CUP (Ben & Jerry's)	1/2 cup	370	30.0	26.0
PRALINE				
(Baskin-Robbins) light 'Praline Dream'	4 oz	130	17.0	6.0
(Baskin-Robbins) pralines 'n cream	1 scoop	280	35.0	14.0
(Healthy Choice) and caramel 'Dairy Dessert'	4 oz	130	26.0	2.0
(Weight Watchers) pralines 'n creme 'ONE-ders'	4 oz	120	19.0	4.0
RASPBERRY SWIRL (Healthy Choice) 'Dairy Dessert'	4 oz	120	23.0	2.0
ROCKY ROAD				
(Baskin-Robbins)	1 scoop	300	39.0	14.0
(Dreyer's)	4 oz	170	18.0	10.0
(Healthy Choice) 'Dairy Dessert'	4 oz	160	32.0	2.0
RUM RAISIN (Häagen-Dazs)	4 oz	250	21.0	17.0
STRAWBERRY				
(Baskin-Robbins) light 'Strawberry Royale'	4 oz	110	19.0	3.0
(Baskin-Robbins) 'Very Berry'	1 scoop	220	30.0	10.0
(Borden)	4 oz	130	18.0	6.0
(Borden) cream 'Olde Fashioned Recipe'	4 oz	130	19.0	5.0
(Breyers)	4 oz	130	16.0	6.0
(Frusen Glädjé)	4 oz	230	20.0	15.0
(Häagen-Dazs)	4 oz	250	23.0	15.0
(Healthy Choice) 'Dairy Dessert'	4 oz	120	23.0	2.0
(Sealtest)	4 oz	130	18.0	5.0
SUNDAE				
(Häagen-Dazs) caramel nut	4 oz	310	26.0	21.0
(Sealtest) chocolate-marshmallow	4 oz	150	21.0	6.0
(Sealtest) peanut fudge	4 oz	140	17.0	7.0
(Weight Watchers) hot caramel fudge	4.5 oz	160	27.0	4.0
(Weight Watchers) hot chocolate fudge	4.5 oz	160	26.0	4.0
(Weight Watchers) hot mocha fudge	4.5 oz	160	24.0	5.0

Food Name	Serv. Size	Total Cal.	Carbs GMS	Fat GMS
SWISS CHOCOLATE CANDY ALMOND *(Frusen Glädjé)*	4 oz	270	18.0	19.0
TOFFEE *(Ben & Jerry's)* 'English Toffee Crunch'	1/2 cup	310	30.0	21.0
VANILLA				
regular, 10% fat, hardened	1 oz	57	6.8	3.1
rich, 16% fat, hardened	1 oz	67	6.1	4.5
(Baskin-Robbins)	1 scoop	240	24.0	14.0
(Ben & Jerry's)	1/2 cup	230	21.0	17.0
(Ben & Jerry's) vanilla bean	1/2 cup	230	21.0	17.0
(Borden) 'Olde Fashioned Recipe'	4 oz	130	15.0	7.0
(Breyers)	4 oz	150	15.0	8.0
(Darigold)	4 oz	130	15.0	7.0
(Darigold) 'Alpine'	4 oz	130	15.0	7.0
(Darigold) 'Classic'	4 oz	180	16.0	12.0
(Dreyer's)	4 oz	160	14.0	10.0
(Eagle Brand) 'Homestyle'	4 oz	150	16.0	9.0
(Frusen Glädjé)	4 oz	230	16.0	17.0
(Good Humor) 'Cup'	3 oz	98	11.6	5.1
(Häagen-Dazs)	4 oz	260	23.0	17.0
(Healthy Choice) 'Dairy Dessert'	4 oz	120	21.0	2.0
(Sealtest)	4 oz	140	16.0	7.0
VANILLA, FRENCH				
(Baskin-Robbins)	1 scoop	280	25.0	18.0
(Sealtest)	4 oz	140	16.0	7.0
VANILLA CARAMEL FUDGE *(Ben & Jerry's)*	1/2 cup	280	33.0	17.0
VANILLA CRUNCH				
(Ben & Jerry's) 'Rainforest Crunch'	1/2 cup	300	24.0	23.0
(Ben & Jerry's) 'Wavy Gravy'	1/2 cup	330	29.0	24.0
VANILLA FUDGE *(Häagen-Dazs)*	4 oz	270	26.0	17.0
VANILLA FUDGE TWIRL *(Breyers)*	4 oz	160	19.0	8.0
VANILLA HONEY *(Häagen-Dazs)*	4 oz	250	22.0	16.0
VANILLA SWISS ALMOND				
(Frusen Glädjé)	4 oz	270	18.0	19.0
(Häagen-Dazs)	4 oz	290	24.0	19.0
VANILLA TOFFEE CHUNK *(Frusen Glädjé)*	4 oz	270	22.0	17.0
VANILLA-CHOCOLATE				
(Baskin-Robbins) fat-free 'Just Chocolate Vanilla'	4 oz	100	21.0	0.0
(Breyers)	4 oz	160	17.0	8.0
(Good Humor) cup 'Combo'	6 oz	201	25.6	9.2
VANILLA-CHOCOLATE-STRAWBERRY				
(Breyers)	4 oz	150	17.0	8.0
(Sealtest)	4 oz	140	18.0	6.0
(Sealtest) 'Cubic Scoops'	4 oz	130	17.0	6.0
VANILLA-PEANUT BUTTER SWIRL *(Häagen-Dazs)*	4 oz	280	19.0	21.0

Food Name	Serv. Size	Total Cal.	Carbs GMS	Fat GMS
WHITE RUSSIAN (Ben & Jerry's)	1/2 cup	240	23.0	16.0
ICE CREAM, ALTERNATIVE				
ALL FLAVORS (Lite Lite Tofutti)	4 oz	90	20.0	<1.0
BLACK CHERRY (Sealtest) 'Free'	4 oz	100	25.0	0.0
CAPPUCCINO				
(Rice Dream)	4 oz	130	17.0	5.0
(Tofutti) 'Love Drops'	4 oz	230	26.0	12.0
CAROB (Rice Dream)	4 oz	130	20.0	5.0
CAROB ALMOND (Rice Dream)	4 oz	140	20.0	6.0
CAROB CHIP (Rice Dream)	4 oz	140	20.0	6.0
CHOCOLATE				
(Lite Lite Tofutti) soft-serve	4 oz	90	20.0	<1.0
(Rice Dream) 'Dream Pie'	1 pie	380	47.0	19.0
(Sealtest) 'Free'	4 oz	100	23.0	0.0
(Simple Pleasures)	4 oz	140	25.0	<1.0
(Tofutti) 'Love Drops'	4 oz	230	26.0	13.0
(Tofutti) supreme	4 oz	210	20.0	13.0
(Weight Watchers)	4 oz	80	19.0	0.0
CHOCOLATE CHIP (Low, Lite 'n Luscious)	4 oz	100	19.0	2.0
CHOCOLATE SWIRL (Weight Watchers)	4 oz	90	22.0	0.0
COCOA MARBLE FUDGE (Rice Dream)	4 oz	140	19.0	6.0
COFFEE (Simple Pleasures)	4 oz	120	22.0	<1.0
COOKIES N' DREAM (Rice Dream)	4 oz	130	21.0	5.0
JAMOCA SWISS ALMOND (Low, Lite 'n Luscious)	4 oz	90	19.0	2.0
LEMON (Rice Dream)	4 oz	130	17.0	5.0
MINT (Rice Dream) 'Dream Pie'	1 pie	380	47.0	19.0
MINT CAROB CHIP (Rice Dream)	4 oz	140	20.0	6.0
MOCHA (Rice Dream) 'Dream Pie'	1 pie	380	47.0	19.0
NEAPOLITAN				
(Rice Dream)	4 oz	130	21.0	5.0
(Weight Watchers)	4 oz	80	19.0	0.0
PEACH				
(Sealtest) 'Free'	4 oz	100	23.0	0.0
(Simple Pleasures)	4 oz	135	24.0	<1.0
PEANUT BUTTER FUDGE (Rice Dream)	4 oz	160	19.0	7.0
PINEAPPLE COCONUT (Low, Lite 'n Luscious)	4 oz	90	19.0	1.0
RUM RAISIN (Simple Pleasures)	4 oz	130	25.0	<1.0
STRAWBERRY				
(Low, Lite 'n Luscious)	4 oz	80	17.0	1.0
(Rice Dream)	4 oz	130	17.0	5.0
(Sealtest) 'Free'	4 oz	100	23.0	0.0
(Simple Pleasures)	4 oz	120	22.0	<1.0

Food Name	Serv. Size	Total Cal.	Carbs GMS	Fat GMS
VANILLA				
(Lite Lite Tofutti) soft-serve	4 oz	90	20.0	<1.0
(Rice Dream)	4 oz	130	17.0	5.0
(Rice Dream) 'Dream Pie'	1 pie	380	47.0	19.0
(Sealtest) 'Free'	4 oz	100	24.0	0.0
(Tofutti)	4 oz	200	21.0	11.0
(Tofutti) 'Love Drops'	4 oz	220	26.0	12.0
(Weight Watchers)	4 oz	80	20.0	0.0
VANILLA ALMOND BARK (Tofutti)	4 oz	230	23.0	14.0
VANILLA CHOCOLATE (Tofutti) dipped 'O's'	1 piece	40	4.0	2.0
VANILLA SWISS ALMOND (Rice Dream)	4 oz	140	20.0	6.0
VANILLA-CHOCOLATE-STRAWBERRY (Sealtest) 'Free'	4 oz	100	23.0	0.0
VANILLA-FUDGE (Rice Dream)	4 oz	140	21.0	6.0
VANILLA-FUDGE ROYALE (Sealtest) 'Free'	4 oz	100	24.0	0.0
VANILLA-STRAWBERRY ROYALE (Sealtest) 'Free'	4 oz	100	25.0	0.0
WILDBERRY				
(Rice Dream)	4 oz	130	17.0	5.0
(Tofutti)	4 oz	210	22.0	12.0
ICE CREAM BAR				
ALMOND (Good Humor) toasted, 3 oz	1 bar	212	24.3	11.8
CARAMEL ALMOND (Häagen-Dazs) 'Crunch Bar'	1 bar	240	17.0	18.0
CHIP CANDY CRUNCH (Good Humor) 3 oz	1 bar	255	21.2	17.9
CHOCOLATE				
(Häagen-Dazs) w/dark chocolate coating	1 bar	390	32.0	27.0
(Klondike) 5 oz	1 bar	270	23.0	19.0
(Nestlé) w/milk chocolate coating 'Quik' 3 oz	1 bar	210	19.0	14.0
(Weight Watchers) 'Treat Bars' 2.75 oz	1 bar	100	18.0	1.0
CHOCOLATE DIP (Weight Watchers) 1.7 oz	1 bar	110	10.0	7.0
CHOCOLATE ECLAIR (Good Humor) 3 oz	1 bar	188	22.6	9.9
CHOCOLATE FUDGE				
(Baker's) sundae, crunchy 'Fudgetastic' 4 oz	1 bar	230	24.0	14.0
(Baker's) sundae 'Fudgetastic' 4 oz	1 bar	220	23.0	15.0
(Good Humor) cake, 6.3 oz	1 bar	214	18.1	15.0
(Weight Watchers) double, 1.75 oz	1.75 oz	60	12.0	1.0
CHOCOLATE MOUSSE				
(Weight Watchers) sugar-free, 1.75 oz	1 bar	35	9.0	<1.0
MILK CHOCOLATE				
(Nestlé) w/almonds, milk chocolate coating, 3.7 oz	1 bar	350	28.0	23.0
ORANGE-VANILLA (Weight Watchers) 'Sugar-free Treat Bars'	1 bar	30	8.0	<1.0
PEANUT BUTTER (Häagen-Dazs) 'Crunch Bar'	4 oz	270	16.0	21.0
STRAWBERRY SHORTCAKE (Good Humor) 3 oz	1 bar	176	23.8	8.2
VANILLA				
(Eskimo Pie) w/dark chocolate coating	1 bar	180	16.0	12.0

Food Name	Serv. Size	Total Cal.	Carbs GMS	Fat GMS
(Eskimo Pie) w/dark chocolate coating 'Sugar-freedom'	1 bar	140	13.0	11.0
(Eskimo Pie) w/milk chocolate coating	1 bar	190	18.0	12.0
(Eskimo Pie) w/milk chocolate coating and almonds 'Sugar-freedom'	1 bar	140	12.0	13.0
(Eskimo Pie) w/milk chocolate coating and crisp rice 'Sugar-freedom'	1 bar	150	12.0	11.0
(Good Humor) w/chocolate flavor coating, 3 oz	1 bar	198	16.8	13.7
(Häagen-Dazs) 'Crunch Bar' 4 oz	1 bar	220	16.0	16.0
(Häagen-Dazs) w/dark chocolate coating, 4 oz	1 bar	390	32.0	27.0
(Häagen-Dazs) w/milk chocolate coating, 4 oz	1 bar	360	26.0	27.0
(Häagen-Dazs) w/milk chocolate-almond coating, 4 oz	1 bar	370	27.0	27.0
(Häagen-Dazs) w/milk chocolate-brittle coating, 4 oz	1 bar	370	32.0	25.0
(Klondike) w/chocolate flavor coating 'Lite'	1 bar	110	14.0	6.0
(Nestlé) w/chocolate coating and crisp rice 'Crunch' 3 oz	1 bar	180	15.0	13.0
(Nestlé) w/chocolate coating and crisp rice 'Crunch Lite'	1 bar	120	16.0	5.0
(Nestlé) w/white chocolate coating 'Alpine Premium' 3.7 oz ..	1 bar	350	25.0	25.0
(Oh Henry!) w/caramel peanut, milk chocolate coating, 3 oz ..	1 bar	320	34.0	20.0
ICE CREAM BAR, ALTERNATIVE				
(Rice Dream) chocolate	1 bar	270	33.0	16.0
(Rice Dream) chocolate nutty bar	1 bar	330	29.0	23.0
(Rice Dream) strawberry	1 bar	260	31.0	14.8
(Rice Dream) vanilla	1 bar	275	33.0	15.8
(Rice Dream) vanilla nutty bar	1 bar	330	29.0	23.0
ICE CREAM CAKE (Breyers) 'Viennetta'	1 slice	190	18.0	12.0
ICE CREAM CONE				
Cup style, wafer				
(Bozo) cake	1 cone	16	3.0	0.0
(Keebler)	1 cone	15	4.0	1.0
(Keebler) assorted colors	1 cone	15	4.0	1.0
(Little Debbie)	1 cone	15	3.0	0.1
(Nabisco) 'Comet'	1 cone	18	4.0	<1.0
Sugar				
(Baskin-Robbins)	1 cone	60	11.0	1.0
(Bozo)	1 cone	53	11.0	1.0
(Keebler)	1 cone	45	11.0	1.0
(Nabisco)	1 cone	50	11.0	<1.0
(Nabisco) 'Comet'	1 cone	50	11.0	<1.0
Waffle, Baskin-Robbins	1 cone	140	28.0	2.0
ICE CREAM MIX				
Dutch chocolate, prepared (Salada)	8 oz	310	31.0	19.0
peach, prepared (Salada)	8 oz	310	32.0	18.0
vanilla, prepared (Salada)	8 oz	310	32.0	18.0
wild strawberry, prepared (Salada)	8 oz	310	32.0	18.0

Food Name	Serv. Size	Total Cal.	Carbs GMS	Fat GMS
ICE CREAM SNACKS AND SANDWICHES				
Nuggets				
vanilla, dark chocolate coated 'Bon Bons' *(Carnation)*	5 pieces	170	15.0	11.0
vanilla, milk chocolate coated 'Bon Bons' *(Carnation)*	5 pieces	165	14.0	11.0
Round novelties				
mocha, 4 oz *(Natural Nectar)*	1 bar	300	40.0	14.0
nectar, 4 oz *(Natural Nectar)*	1 bar	300	38.0	15.0
Sandwich				
chocolate chip cookie, 4 oz *(Good Humor)*	1 sandwich	246	35.1	10.5
chocolate chip cookie, 2.7 oz *(Good Humor)*	1 sandwich	204	30.1	8.3
vanilla *(Weight Watchers)*	1 sandwich	150	28.0	3.0
vanilla, 5 oz *(Klondike)*	1 sandwich	230	33.0	9.0
vanilla 'Lite' *(Klondike)*	1 sandwich	100	18.0	2.0
vanilla, 1.5-oz snacks *(Weight Watchers)*	1 sandwich	90	17.0	2.0
vanilla, 3 oz *(Good Humor)*	1 sandwich	191	31.1	5.7
vanilla, 2.5 oz *(Good Humor)*	1 sandwich	165	26.9	4.9
vanilla 'Sugar-freedom' *(Eskimo Pie)*	1 sandwich	170	26.0	6.0
Stick novelties				
banana cream *(Natural Nectar)*	1 bar	170	22.0	8.0
cocoa-fudge 'n cream *(Natural Nectar)*	1 bar	170	22.0	8.0
strawberries 'n cream *(Natural Nectar)*	1 bar	120	18.0	5.0
wildberry cream *(Natural Nectar)*	1 bar	120	22.0	3.0
ICE CREAM TOPPING. See individual toppings.				
ICE MILK				
CARAMEL NUT *(Light n' Lively)*	4 oz	120	18.0	4.0
CHOCOLATE				
(Breyers) 'Light'	4 oz	120	18.0	4.0
(Borden)	4 oz	100	18.0	2.0
(Darigold) 'Lite'	4 oz	110	19.0	3.0
(Weight Watchers) 'Grand Collection'	4 oz	110	18.0	3.0
CHOCOLATE CHIP				
(Light n' Lively)	4 oz	120	18.0	4.0
(Weight Watchers) 'Grand Collection'	4 oz	120	19.0	4.0
CHOCOLATE CHOCOLATE CHIP *(Breyers)* 'Light'	4 oz	140	20.0	5.0
CHOCOLATE FUDGE TWIRL *(Breyers)* 'Light'	4 oz	130	21.0	4.0
CHOCOLATE SWIRL *(Weight Watchers)* 'Grand Collection'	4 oz	120	19.0	3.0
COFFEE *(Light n' Lively)*	4 oz	100	16.0	3.0
COOKIES N' CREAM *(Light n' Lively)*	4 oz	110	18.0	3.0
HEAVENLY HASH				
(Breyers) 'Light'	4 oz	150	21.0	5.0
(Light n' Lively)	4 oz	120	20.0	4.0
NEAPOLITAN *(Weight Watchers)* 'Grand Collection'	4 oz	110	18.0	3.0

Food Name	Serv. Size	Total Cal.	Carbs GMS	Fat GMS
PECAN PRALINES 'N CREME				
(Weight Watchers) 'Grand Collection'	4 oz	120	20.0	4.0
PRALINE ALMOND *(Breyers)* 'Light'	4 oz	130	19.0	5.0
STRAWBERRY				
(Borden)	4 oz	90	17.0	2.0
(Breyers) 'Light'	4 oz	110	18.0	3.0
SWISS ALMOND FUDGE TWIRL *(Breyers)*	4 oz	150	21.0	6.0
TOFFEE FUDGE PARFAIT *(Breyers)* 'Light'	4 oz	140	22.0	5.0
VANILLA				
(Borden)	4 oz	90	17.0	2.0
(Breyers) 'Light'	4 oz	120	18.0	4.0
(Darigold)	4 oz	110	18.0	3.0
(Light n' Lively)	4 oz	100	16.0	3.0
(Light n' Lively) w/chocolate covered almonds	4 oz	120	17.0	4.0
(Weight Watchers) 'Grand Collection'	4 oz	100	16.0	3.0
VANILLA-CHOCOLATE-STRAWBERRY				
(Breyers) 'Light'	4 oz	120	18.0	4.0
(Light n' Lively)	4 oz	100	17.0	3.0
VANILLA-FUDGE TWIRL *(Light n' Lively)*	4 oz	110	18.0	3.0
VANILLA-RASPBERRY				
(Breyers) parfait 'Light'	4 oz	130	23.0	3.0
(Light n' Lively) swirl	4 oz	110	19.0	3.0
ICE MILK BAR				
CHOCOLATE ALMOND CRUNCH *(Weight Watchers)*	1 bar	120	12.0	7.0
CHOCOLATE FUDGE, DOUBLE *(Light n' Lively)* nonfat	1 bar	50	11.0	0.0
CHOCOLATE MOUSSE *(Light n' Lively)* nonfat	1 bar	50	12.0	0.0
CHOCOLATE W/FUDGE SWIRL *(Sealtest)* nonfat 'Free'	1 bar	80	19.0	0.0
ORANGE VANILLA *(Light n' Lively)* nonfat	1 bar	40	10.0	0.0
PRALINE *(Weight Watchers)* 'Crispy Praline 'N Creme'	1 bar	120	13.0	6.0
STRAWBERRY *(Light n' Lively)* nonfat	1 bar	80	12.0	0.0
TOFFEE *(Weight Watchers)* 'English Toffee Crunch'	1 bar	120	11.0	8.0
VANILLA				
(Light n' Lively) chocolate dipped	1 bar	110	14.0	6.0
(Sealtest) w/fudge swirl, nonfat 'Free'	1 bar	80	18.0	0.0
(Sealtest) w/strawberry swirl, nonfat 'Free'	1 bar	70	17.0	0.0
ICED TEA. See TEA, ICED.				
IMBU. See JOBO.				
INDIAN DATE. See TAMARIND.				
INDIAN FRY BREAD. See BREAD.				
INFANT FORMULA. See BABY FOOD.				
IRISH MOSS. See SEAWEED.				
ITALIAN SEASONING *(Schilling)* 'Spice Blends'	1/4 tsp	1	0.1	na
ITALIAN STONE PINE NUT. See PINE NUT.				

J

Food Name	Serv. Size	Total Cal.	Carbs GMS	Fat GMS
JACK BEAN. See FAVA BEAN.				
JACKFRUIT				
trimmed	1 oz	27	6.8	0.1
untrimmed	1 lb	119	30.5	0.4
JALAPEÑO. See PEPPER, JALAPEÑO.				
JAM. See also FRUIT SPREAD; JELLY; PRESERVES.				
(Bama) all flavors	2 tsp	30	8.0	0.0
(Estee) all flavors	1 tsp	2	0.0	0.0
(Featherweight) all flavors	1 tsp	4	1.0	0.0
(Kraft) all flavors	1 tsp	17	4.0	0.0
(S&W Nutradiet) all flavors	1 tsp	4	1.0	0.0
APRICOT				
(Finast)	2 tsp	35	9.0	0.0
(Smucker's) natural ingredients	1 tsp	18	4.0	0.0
APRICOT-PINEAPPLE *(Smucker's)* natural ingredients	1 tsp	18	4.0	0.0
BLACK RASPBERRY *(Smucker's)* natural ingredients	1 tsp	18	4.0	0.0
BLACKBERRY				
(Finast)	2 tsp	16	4.0	0.0
(Smucker's) natural ingredients	1 tsp	18	4.0	0.0
BLUEBERRY				
(Finast)	2 tsp	16	4.0	0.0
(Smucker's) natural ingredients	1 tsp	18	4.0	0.0
BOYSENBERRY *(Smucker's)* natural ingredients	1 tsp	18	4.0	0.0
CHERRY				
(Finast)	2 tsp	25	9.0	0.0
(Smucker's) natural ingredients	1 tsp	18	4.0	0.0
GRAPE				
(Finast) Concord or regular	2 tsp	35	9.0	0.0
(Polaner)	2 tsp	35	9.0	0.0
(Smucker's) Concord, natural ingredients	1 tsp	18	4.0	0.0
(Welch's)	2 tsp	35	9.0	0.0
ORANGE MARMALADE *(Polaner)*	2 tsp	35	9.0	0.0
PEACH				
(Finast)	2 tsp	35	9.0	0.0
(Smucker's) natural ingredients	1 tsp	18	4.0	0.0
PINEAPPLE				
(Finast)	2 tsp	35	9.0	0.0
(Smucker's) natural ingredients	1 tsp	18	4.0	0.0
PLUM *(Smucker's)* natural ingredients	1 tsp	18	4.0	0.0
RASPBERRY				
(Finast)	2 tsp	35	9.0	0.0

Food Name	Serv. Size	Total Cal.	Carbs GMS	Fat GMS
(Smucker's) natural ingredients, seedless	1 tsp	18	4.0	0.0
RASPBERRY-APPLE *(Welch's)*	2 tsp	35	9.0	0.0
STRAWBERRY				
(Finast)	2 tsp	35	9.0	0.0
(Kraft) 'Reduced Calorie'	1 tsp	6	2.0	0.0
(Piedmont)	2 tsp	35	9.0	0.0
(Smucker's) natural ingredients, seedless	1 tsp	18	4.0	0.0
(Welch's)	2 tsp	35	9.0	0.0
TOMATO *(Smucker's)* natural ingredients	1 tsp	18	4.0	0.0
JAMAICAN BREADNUT. See BREADNUT TREE SEEDS.				
JAMBERRY, fresh *(Frieda's)*	3.5 oz	25	4.2	0.5
JAMBOLAN. See JAVA PLUM.				
JAPANESE MEDLAR. See LOQUAT.				
JAPANESE WHITE RADISH. See RADISH, ORIENTAL.				
JAVA PLUM/jambolan				
raw	1 cup	81	21.0	0.3
raw	3 fruits	5	1.4	0.0
w/seeds	1 lb	222	57.2	0.9
w/o seeds	1 oz	17	4.4	0.1
JELLY. See also JAM; FRUIT SPREAD; PRESERVES.				
(Bama) and peanut butter, spread, all flavors	2 tbsp	150	20.0	7.0
(Estee) all flavors	1 tsp	2	0.0	0.0
(Featherweight) all flavors, except grape	1 tsp	4	1.0	0.0
(Kraft) all flavors	1 tsp	17	4.0	0.0
(Smucker's) 'Slenderella' all flavors	1 tsp	7	2.0	0.0
APPLE				
(Bama)	2 tsp	30	8.0	0.0
(Finast)	2 tsp	35	9.0	0.0
(Lucky Leaf)	1 oz	80	20.0	0.0
(Musselman's)	1 oz	80	20.0	0.0
(Polaner)	2 tsp	35	9.0	0.0
(Smucker's) cinnamon-flavored, natural ingredients	1 tsp	18	4.0	0.0
(Smucker's) mint-flavored, natural ingredients	1 tsp	18	4.0	0.0
(Smucker's) natural ingredients	1 tsp	18	4.0	0.0
APPLE-BLACKBERRY *(Musselman's)*	1 oz	80	19.0	0.0
APPLE-CHERRY *(Musselman's)*	1 oz	80	19.0	0.0
APPLE-GRAPE				
(Musselman's)	1 oz	80	20.0	0.0
(Welch's)	2 tsp	35	9.0	0.0
APPLE-RASPBERRY *(Musselman's)*	1 oz	80	19.0	0.0
APPLE-STRAWBERRY *(Musselman's)*	1 oz	80	20.0	0.0
APRICOT-PINEAPPLE				
(Knott's Berry Farm) 'Light' w/NutraSweet	1 tsp	8	2.0	0.0

Food Name	Serv. Size	Total Cal.	Carbs GMS	Fat GMS
BLACK RASPBERRY *(Smucker's)* natural ingredients	1 tsp	18	4.0	0.0
BLACKBERRY				
(Bama)	2 tsp	30	8.0	0.0
(Knott's Berry Farm) 'Light' w/NutraSweet	1 tsp	8	2.0	0.0
(Smucker's) natural ingredients	1 tsp	18	4.0	0.0
BOYSENBERRY *(Knott's Berry Farm)* 'Light' w/NutraSweet	1 tsp	8	2.0	0.0
CHERRY *(Smucker's)* natural ingredients	1 tsp	18	4.0	0.0
CRABAPPLE *(Smucker's)* natural ingredients	1 tsp	18	4.0	0.0
CURRANT				
(Finast)	2 tsp	35	9.0	0.0
(Polaner)	2 tsp	35	9.0	0.0
(Smucker's) natural ingredients	1 tsp	18	4.0	0.0
ELDERBERRY *(Smucker's)* natural ingredients	1 tsp	18	4.0	0.0
GRAPE				
(Bama)	2 tsp	30	8.0	0.0
(Featherweight)	1 tsp	4	1.0	0.0
(Finast)	2 tsp	35	9.0	0.0
(Kraft) 'Reduced Calorie'	1 tsp	6	2.0	0.0
(Musselman's)	1 oz	80	20.0	0.0
(Polaner)	2 tsp	35	9.0	0.0
(Smucker's) Concord, natural ingredients	1 tsp	18	4.0	0.0
(Welch's)	2 tsp	35	9.0	0.0
GREEN PEPPER *(Great Impressions)*	1 tbsp	50	12.6	0.0
GUAVA *(Smucker's)* natural ingredients	1 tsp	18	4.0	0.0
JALAPEÑO				
(Great Impressions)	1 tbsp	58	14.6	0.0
(Knott's Berry Farm)	1 oz	70	18.0	0.0
(Knott's Berry Farm)	1 tsp	18	4.0	0.0
MINT				
(Finast)	2 tsp	35	9.0	0.0
(Polaner)	2 tsp	35	9.0	0.0
MIXED FRUIT *(Smucker's)* natural ingredients	1 tsp	18	4.0	0.0
PLUM *(Smucker's)* natural ingredients	1 tsp	18	4.0	0.0
QUINCE *(Smucker's)* natural ingredients	1 tsp	18	4.0	0.0
RASPBERRY				
(Knott's Berry Farm) 'Light' w/NutraSweet	1 tsp	8	2.0	0.0
(Polaner)	2 tsp	35	9.0	0.0
(Smucker's) natural ingredients	1 tsp	18	4.0	0.0
RED PEPPER *(Great Impressions)*	1 tbsp	50	12.6	0.0
STRAWBERRY				
(Finast)	2 tsp	35	9.0	0.0
(Knott's Berry Farm) 'Light' w/NutraSweet	1 tsp	8	2.0	0.0
(Polaner)	2 tsp	35	9.0	0.0

Food Name	Serv. Size	Total Cal.	Carbs GMS	Fat GMS
(Smucker's) natural ingredients	1 tsp	18	4.0	0.0
STRAWBERRY-APPLE (Polaner)	2 tsp	35	9.0	0.0

JERKY. See BEEF JERKY.

JERUSALEM ARTICHOKE. See ARTICHOKES, JERUSALEM.

JEW'S EAR. See CHINESE FUNGUS.

JICAMA/Chinese yam/fon goot yam/Mexican potato/sicama/yambean tuber

boiled, drained	4 oz	52	11.8	0.1
raw, trimmed	1 oz	12	2.5	0.1
raw, trimmed, sliced	1/2 cup	25	5.3	0.1
raw, untrimmed	1 lb	170	36.5	0.3

JOBO/hog plum/imbu/yellow mombin

seeded	1 oz	20	3.9	0.6

JUICE. See individual listings.

JUJUBE, CHINESE

dried	100 gm	287	73.6	1.1
dried	1 oz	81	20.1	0.3
raw	100 gm	79	20.2	0.2
raw	1 oz	22	5.7	0.1
raw, w/seeds	1 lb	331	85.3	0.8

JUNKET MIX

CHOCOLATE

mix only, dry	2-oz pkg	207	52.2	1.9
mix only, dry	1 tbsp	33	8.2	0.3
prepared (Junket)	1/2 cup	120	15.0	4.0
prepared w/2% milk	1/2 cup	110	18.4	2.9
prepared w/whole milk	1/2 cup	125	18.1	4.5

STRAWBERRY OR RASPBERRY

mix only, dry	1.5-oz pkg	165	42.6	0.0
mix only, dry	1 tbsp	38	9.9	0.0
prepared (Junket)	1/2 cup	120	16.0	4.0
prepared w/whole milk	1 cup	238	32.0	9.0

VANILLA

mix only, dry	1.5-oz pkg	165	42.6	0.0
mix only, dry	1 tbsp	41	10.7	0.0
prepared (Junket)	1/2 cup	120	16.0	4.0
prepared w/2% milk	1/2 cup	101	16.4	2.4
prepared w/whole milk	1/2 cup	116	16.2	4.1

JUTE POTHERB

boiled, drained	4 oz	42	8.3	0.2
raw, trimmed	1 oz	10	1.6	0.1
raw, untrimmed	1 lb	96	16.3	0.7

K

Food Name	Serv. Size	Total Cal.	Carbs GMS	Fat GMS
KALE/borecole/cole/colewort				
boiled, drained	4 oz	36	6.4	0.5
boiled, drained, chopped	1 cup	42	7.3	0.5
chopped (Dole)	1/2 cup	17	3.0	0.5
raw, chopped	1 cup	33	6.7	0.5
raw, trimmed	1 oz	14	2.8	0.2
raw, untrimmed	1 lb	137	27.7	1.9
Canned, chopped (Allen's)	1/2 cup	25	3.0	<1.0
Frozen				
boiled, drained	4 oz	34	5.9	0.6
boiled, drained, chopped	1 cup	39	6.8	0.6
chopped (Frosty Acres)	3.3 oz	25	5.0	0.0
chopped (Seabrook)	3.3 oz	25	5.0	0.0
chopped (Southern)	3.5 oz	30	4.8	0.5
unprepared, 10-oz pkg	3.3 oz	26	4.6	0.4
KALE, SCOTCH				
boiled, drained	4 oz	32	6.4	0.5
boiled, drained, chopped	1 cup	36	7.3	0.5
raw, chopped	1 cup	28	5.6	0.4
raw, trimmed	1 oz	12	2.4	0.2
raw, untrimmed	1 lb	115	23.0	1.7
KANPYO/dried gourd strips				
	1 lb	1169	295.0	2.5
	1 oz	73	18.4	0.2
	1/2 cup	70	17.6	0.2
KANTEN				
raw	1 lb	116	30.6	0.1
raw	1 oz	7	1.9	tr
KASHA. See BUCKWHEAT GROATS.				
KATSUO. See TUNA, SKIPJACK.				
KATURAY/sesbania flower				
raw, approx .1 oz	1 flower	1	0.2	tr
raw, trimmed	1 cup	5	1.4	<.1
raw, trimmed	1 oz	8	1.9	<.1
raw, untrimmed	1 lb	106	25.9	0.2
steamed	4 oz	25	5.9	0.1
KAUAI PUNCH, organic (Santa Cruz Natural)	8 oz	120	28.0	1.0
KEFIR, CULTURED				
black cherry (Alta•Dena)	1 cup	200	24.0	9.0
boysenberry (Alta•Dena)	1 cup	200	24.0	9.0
peach (Alta•Dena)	1 cup	200	24.0	9.0

Food Name	Serv. Size	Total Cal.	Carbs GMS	Fat GMS
red raspberry *(Alta•Dena)*	1 cup	200	24.0	9.0

KELP. See SEAWEED.

KETCHUP. See CATSUP.

KIDNEY BEAN

California red, mature

boiled	4 oz	141	25.4	0.1
boiled	1/2 cup	109	19.7	0.1
raw	1/2 cup	304	55.0	0.2
raw	1 oz	94	17.0	0.1

Red, mature

boiled	1/2 cup	112	20.1	0.4
boiled	4 oz	144	25.9	0.6
boiled *(A&P)*	1 cup	230	41.0	1.0
raw	1/2 cup	310	56.4	1.0
raw	1 oz	96	17.4	0.1
raw *(Arrowhead Mills)*	2 oz	190	35.0	1.0

Royal red, mature

boiled	4 oz	139	24.8	0.2
boiled	1/2 cup	108	19.2	0.2
raw	1/2 cup	303	53.7	0.4
raw	1 oz	93	16.5	0.1

Sprouted, mature

boiled, drained	4 oz	37	5.4	0.7
raw	1 lb	132	18.6	2.3
raw	1 cup	53	7.5	0.9
raw	1 oz	8	1.2	0.1

KIDNEY BEAN, CANNED

Dark red

(Allens)	1/2 cup	105	20.0	<1.0
(Bush's Best)	1/2 cup	70	17.0	0.0
(Finast)	1/2 cup	110	20.0	2.0
(Green Giant)	1/2 cup	90	20.0	<1.0
(Green Giant) 50% less salt	1/2 cup	90	20.0	<1.0
(Joan of Arc)	1/2 cup	90	20.0	<1.0
(Joan of Arc) 50% less salt	1/2 cup	90	20.0	<1.0
(Pathmark)	1/2 cup	110	18.0	0.0
(S&W) 50% less salt 'Lite'	1/2 cup	120	22.0	1.0
(S&W) 'Premium'	1/2 cup	120	22.0	1.0
(Stokely)	1/2 cup	110	20.0	1.0
(Van Camp's)	1 cup	182	35.0	0.5

Light red

(Allens)	1/2 cup	105	2.0	<1.0
(Bush's Best)	1/2 cup	70	17.0	0.0

Food Name	Serv. Size	Total Cal.	Carbs GMS	Fat GMS
(Finast)	1/2 cup	110	20.0	2.0
(Green Giant)	1/2 cup	90	20.0	<1.0
(Green Giant) 50% less salt	1/2 cup	90	20.0	<1.0
(Joan of Arc)	1/2 cup	90	20.0	<1.0
(Joan of Arc) 50% less salt	1/2 cup	90	20.0	<1.0
(Stokely)	1/2 cup	110	20.0	1.0
(Van Camp's)	1 cup	184	36.0	0.5
Red				
(A&P)	1/2 cup	110	20.0	<1.0
(B&M) baked	8 oz	250	42.0	7.0
(Eden Foods) organic, very low sodium, no salt added	1/2 cup	60	18.0	<1.0
(Friends) baked	8 oz	340	57.0	4.0
(Friends) baked, w/pork	8 oz	270	55.0	4.0
(Green Giant)	1/2 cup	90	20.0	0.0
(Hunt's)	4 oz	120	21.0	0.0
(Joan of Arc)	1/2 cup	90	20.0	0.0
(Pathmark)	1/2 cup	110	18.0	0.0
(Progresso)	1/2 cup	100	21.0	<1.0
(S&W) 50% less salt 'Lite'	1/2 cup	120	22.0	1.0
(S&W) 'Premium'	1/2 cup	120	22.0	1.0
(S&W Nutradiet)	1/2 cup	90	16.0	1.0
(Stokely)	1/2 cup	110	20.0	1.0
(Van Camp's)	1 cup	184	36.0	0.5
(Van Camp's) 'New Orleans Style'	1 cup	178	34.0	0.6
KIELBASA/kolbassy				
'Bun Size' *(Hillshire Farm)*	2 oz	180	2.0	16.0
'Kolbase' *(Hormel)*	3 oz	220	1.0	19.0
'Lean Supreme Polska' *(Eckrich)*	1 oz	72	1.0	6.0
'Polska Flavorseal' *(Hillshire Farm)*	2 oz	190	2.0	17.0
'Polska Flavorseal' beef *(Hillshire Farm)*	2 oz	190	1.0	17.0
'Polska Flavorseal Lite' *(Hillshire Farm)*	2 oz	160	2.0	13.0
'Polska Flavorseal' mild *(Hillshire Farm)*	2 oz	190	2.0	17.0
'Polska Links' *(Hillshire Farm)*	2 oz	190	2.0	17.0
'Polska' skinless *(Eckrich)*	1 link	180	2.0	16.0
skinless *(Hormel)*	1/2 link	180	1.0	14.0
KIWI FRUIT/Chinese gooseberry				
fresh, raw, w/o skin	1 large	56	13.5	0.4
fresh, raw, w/o skin	1 med	46	11.3	0.3
trimmed	1 oz	17	4.2	0.1
untrimmed *(Dole)*	2 fruit	90	18.0	1.0
w/skin	1 lb	237	58.1	1.7
KIWI NECTAR *(Knudsen & Sons)*	8 oz	60	14.0	0.0

Food Name	Serv. Size	Total Cal.	Carbs GMS	Fat GMS
KNACKWURST				
.... 4-inch link	209	1.2	18.9
.... 1 oz	87	0.5	7.9
beef *(Hebrew National)* .... 3-oz link	263	<1.0	25.0
'Links' *(Hillshire Farm)* .... 2 oz	180	1.0	16.0
KOHLRABI/cabbage turnip				
boiled, drained .... 4 oz	33	7.6	0.1
boiled, drained, sliced .... 1/2 cup	24	5.5	0.1
raw, sliced .... 1/2 cup	19	4.3	0.1
raw, trimmed .... 1 oz	8	1.8	<.1
raw, untrimmed .... 1 lb	57	12.9	0.2
KOLBASSY. See KIELBASA				
KOOL-AID. See individual flavors.				
KOYADOFU. See TOFU.				
KUMQUAT				
raw, trimmed .... 1 fruit	12	3.1	0.0
w/seeds .... 1 lb	266	69.3	0.4

L

Food Name	Serv. Size	Total Cal.	Carbs GMS	Fat GMS
LAMB, DOMESTIC				
(NOTE: All USDA choice grade. TRIMMED = Lean; separable fat removed. UNTRIMMED = Separable fat not removed.)				
BRAINS				
braised .... 3 oz	123	0.0	8.6
braised, yield from 1 lb raw .... 12.25 oz	503	0.0	35.3
pan-fried .... 3 oz	232	0.0	18.9
raw .... 4 oz	138	0.0	9.7
COMPOSITE CUTS/LEG AND SHOULDER				
Trimmed				
braised, cubes .... 3 oz	190	0.0	7.5
broiled, cubes .... 3 oz	158	0.0	6.2
broiled, ground .... 3 oz	241	0.0	16.7
raw, cubes .... 1 lb	608	0.0	24.0
raw, cubes .... 1 oz	38	0.0	1.5
raw, ground .... 1 lb	1279	0.0	106.2
raw, ground .... 1 oz	79	0.0	6.6
stewed, cubes .... 4 oz	253	0.0	10.0
HEART				
braised .... 3 oz	157	1.6	6.7
raw .... 4 oz	138	0.2	6.4

Food Name	Serv. Size	Total Cal.	Carbs GMS	Fat GMS
simmered	4 oz	210	2.2	9.0
KIDNEYS				
braised	3 oz	116	0.8	3.1
raw	4 oz	110	0.9	3.3
LEG/FORESHANK				
Trimmed				
braised	3 oz	159	0.0	5.1
braised	1 oz	53	0.0	1.7
braised, diced	1 cup	262	0.0	8.4
broiled, ground	1 cup	328	0.0	23.1
broiled, ground	4 oz	321	0.0	22.3
raw	1 lb	544	0.0	14.9
raw	1 oz	34	0.0	0.9
raw, ground	1 cup	637	0.0	52.9
stewed	4 oz	212	0.0	6.8
stewed	1 oz	53	0.0	1.7
stewed, diced	1 cup	262	0.0	8.4
Untrimmed				
braised	3 oz	207	0.0	11.4
braised	1 oz	69	0.0	3.8
braised, diced	1 cup	340	0.0	18.8
raw	1 lb	912	0.0	60.7
raw	1 oz	56	0.0	3.8
stewed	1 oz	69	0.0	3.8
stewed, diced	1 cup	340	0.0	18.8
LEG/SHANK				
Trimmed				
raw	1 lb	567	0.0	19.0
raw	1 oz	35	0.0	1.2
roasted	3 oz	153	0.0	5.7
roasted	1 oz	51	0.0	1.9
roasted, diced	1 cup	252	0.0	9.3
Untrimmed				
raw	1 lb	912	0.0	61.2
raw	1 oz	56	0.0	3.8
roasted	3 oz	191	0.0	10.6
roasted	1 oz	64	0.0	3.5
roasted, diced	1 cup	315	0.0	17.4
LEG/SIRLOIN				
Trimmed				
raw	1 lb	608	0.0	23.0
raw	1 oz	38	0.0	1.4
roasted	3 oz	173	0.0	7.8

Food Name	Serv. Size	Total Cal.	Carbs GMS	Fat GMS
roasted	1 oz	58	0.0	2.6
roasted, diced	1 cup	286	0.0	12.8
Untrimmed				
raw	1 lb	1234	0.0	100.3
raw	1 oz	76	0.0	6.2
roasted	3 oz	248	0.0	17.6
roasted	1 oz	83	0.0	5.9
roasted, diced	1 cup	409	0.0	28.9
LEG/WHOLE				
Trimmed				
raw	1 lb	581	0.0	20.5
raw	1 oz	36	0.0	1.3
roasted	3 oz	162	0.0	6.6
roasted	1 oz	54	0.0	2.2
roasted, diced	1 cup	267	0.0	10.8
Untrimmed				
raw	1 lb	1043	0.0	77.4
raw	1 oz	64	0.0	4.8
roasted	3 oz	219	0.0	14.0
roasted	1 oz	73	0.0	4.7
roasted, diced	1 cup	361	0.0	23.0
LIVER				
braised	3 oz	187	2.2	7.5
pan-fried	3 oz	202	3.2	10.8
raw	4 oz	158	2.0	5.7
LOIN				
Trimmed				
broiled	3 oz	184	0.0	8.3
raw	1 oz	40	0.0	1.7
roasted	3 oz	172	0.0	8.3
Untrimmed				
broiled	3 oz	269	0.0	19.6
roasted	3 oz	263	0.0	20.0
LUNGS				
braised	3 oz	96	0.0	2.6
raw	4 oz	108	0.0	3.0
PANCREAS				
braised	3 oz	199	0.0	12.8
raw	4 oz	172	0.0	11.1
RIB				
Trimmed				
broiled	3 oz	200	0.0	11.0
raw	1 lb	767	0.0	41.9

Food Name	Serv. Size	Total Cal.	Carbs GMS	Fe GM
raw	1 oz	47	0.0	2
roasted	3 oz	197	0.0	11
Untrimmed				
broiled	3 oz	307	0.0	25
raw	1 lb	1687	0.0	156
raw	1 oz	104	0.0	9
roasted	3 oz	305	0.0	25
SHOULDER/ARM				
Trimmed				
braised	3 oz	237	0.0	12
broiled	3 oz	170	0.0	7.
raw	1 oz	37	0.0	1
roasted	3 oz	163	0.0	7
Untrimmed				
braised	3 oz	294	0.0	20
broiled	3 oz	239	0.0	16.
raw	1 oz	73	0.0	5.
roasted	3 oz	237	0.0	17.
SHOULDER/BLADE				
Trimmed				
braised	1 oz	81	0.0	4.
broiled	3 oz	179	0.0	9.
raw	3 oz	128	0.0	6.
roasted	3 oz	178	0.0	9
Untrimmed				
braised	3 oz	293	0.0	21.
broiled	3 oz	236	0.0	17.
raw	1 lb	1175	0.0	94.
raw	1 oz	73	0.0	5.
roasted	3 oz	239	0.0	17.
SHOULDER/WHOLE				
Trimmed				
braised	4 oz	321	0.0	10.
braised, diced	1 cup	396	0.0	22.
broiled	4 oz	238	0.0	11.
roasted	4 oz	231	0.0	12.
roasted, diced	1 cup	286	0.0	15.
stewed	4 oz	321	0.0	10.
stewed, diced	1 cup	396	0.0	22.
Untrimmed				
braised, diced	1 cup	482	0.0	34.
broiled	4 oz	315	0.0	21.
broiled, diced	1 cup	389	0.0	27.

Food Name	Serv. Size	Total Cal.	Carbs GMS	Fat GMS
roasted	4 oz	313	0.0	22.6
roasted, diced	1 cup	386	0.0	28.0
stewed	4 oz	390	0.0	27.8
stewed, diced	1 cup	482	0.0	34.4
SPLEEN				
braised	3 oz	133	0.0	4.1
raw	4 oz	115	0.0	3.5
TONGUE				
braised	3 oz	234	0.0	17.2
raw	4 oz	252	0.0	19.5
LAMB, NEW ZEALAND, FROZEN				
COMPOSITE CUTS				
Trimmed				
cooked	4 oz	234	0.0	10.0
raw	1 oz	36	0.0	1.3
Untrimmed				
raw	1 oz	182	0.0	19.2
LEG/FORESHANK				
Trimmed				
braised	3 oz	158	0.0	5.1
braised, diced	1 cup	260	0.0	8.5
raw	1 lb	535	0.0	14.9
raw	1 oz	33	0.0	0.9
stewed	4 oz	211	0.0	6.8
stewed, diced	1 cup	260	0.0	8.5
Untrimmed				
braised	3 oz	219	0.0	13.5
braised, diced	1 cup	361	0.0	22.2
raw	1 lb	1012	0.0	73.3
raw	1 oz	62	0.0	4.5
stewed	4 oz	293	0.0	18.0
stewed, diced	1 cup	361	0.0	22.2
LEG/WHOLE				
Trimmed				
raw	1 lb	558	0.0	17.2
raw	1 oz	34	0.0	1.1
roasted	3 oz	154	0.0	6.0
roasted, diced	1 cup	253	0.0	9.8
Untrimmed				
raw	1 lb	980	0.0	69.4
raw	1 oz	60	0.0	4.3
roasted	3 oz	209	0.0	13.2
roasted, diced	1 cup	344	0.0	21.8

Food Name	Serv. Size	Total Cal.	Carbs GMS	Fa GM
LOIN				
Trimmed				
broiled	4 oz	226	0.0	9.
raw	1 oz	36	0.0	1.2
roasted	3 oz	169	0.0	7.0
Untrimmed				
broiled	3 oz	268	0.0	20.
raw	1 oz	85	0.0	7.3
RIB				
Trimmed				
raw	1 lb	644	0.0	27.5
raw	1 oz	40	0.0	1.7
roasted	3 oz	167	0.0	8.6
Untrimmed				
raw	1 lb	1569	0.0	142.
raw	1 oz	97	0.0	8.1
roasted	3 oz	289	0.0	24.4
SHOULDER/WHOLE				
Trimmed				
braised	3 oz	242	0.0	13.2
braised, diced	1 cup	399	0.0	21.7
raw	1 lb	612	0.0	24.6
raw	1 oz	38	0.0	1.5
stewed	6.5 oz	522	0.0	28.3
stewed, diced	1 cup	399	0.0	21.7
Untrimmed				
braised	3 oz	303	0.0	22.3
braised, diced	1 cup	491	0.0	35.5
raw	1 lb	1234	0.0	100.8
stewed	4 oz	398	0.0	28.8
stewed, diced	1 cup	491	0.0	35.5
LAMB'S-QUARTER				
boiled, drained	4 oz	36	5.7	0.8
boiled, drained, chopped	1 cup	58	9.0	1.3
raw	100 gm	43	7.3	0.8
raw, trimmed	1 lb	195	33.1	3.6
raw, trimmed	1 oz	12	2.1	0.2
LARD				
pork, fresh	1 cup	1849	0.0	205.0
pork, fresh	1 tbsp	115	0.0	12.8
pork leaf, fresh	1 oz	243	0.0	26.7
LASAGNA ENTRÉE, FROZEN				
(Banquet) 'Extra Helping'	16.5 oz	645	88.0	23.0

Food Name	Serv. Size	Total Cal.	Carbs GMS	Fat GMS
(Celentano)	10 oz	460	40.0	24.0
(Celentano)	8 oz	370	32.0	19.0
(Celentano)	6.25 oz	230	22.0	14.0
(Chef Boyardee)	5.97 oz	280	42.0	8.0
(Green Giant) 'Entrées'	12 oz	490	44.0	20.0
(Stouffer's) 96-oz tray	9.75 oz	400	37.0	14.0
(Stouffer's) 21-oz pkg	10.5 oz	360	33.0	13.0
(Stouffer's) 10-oz pkg	10 oz	340	40.0	12.0
(Tyson) 'Gourmet Selection'	11.5 oz	380	47.0	14.0
(Weight Watchers)	10.25 oz	270	29.0	6.0
CHEESE				
(Budget Gourmet) three cheese	10 oz	400	38.0	17.0
(Dining Lite)	9 oz	260	36.0	6.0
(Lean Cuisine) casserole 'Lunch Express'	9.5 oz	290	42.0	6.0
(Weight Watchers) Italian	11 oz	290	29.0	7.0
FLORENTINE *(Smart Ones)* w/spinach cheese	11 oz	220	34.0	1.0
IN SAUCE *(Buitoni)* 'Family Style'	7.3 oz	370	30.0	13.0
LOW FAT *(Celentano)* 'Great Choice'	10 oz	260	42.0	2.0
MEAT *(Buitoni)* 'Single Serving'	9 oz	580	57.0	19.0
PRIMAVERA *(Celentano)*	11 oz	330	34.0	14.0
SAUSAGE *(Budget Gourmet)* Italian	10 oz	420	38.0	20.0
SEAFOOD *(Mrs. Paul's)* seafood 'Light'	9.5 oz	290	39.0	8.0
TOFU				
(Amy's Kitchen) vegetable, organic	9.5 oz	310	36.0	10.0
(Legume) and sauce 'Classic'	8 oz	210	20.0	8.0
TUNA *(Lean Cuisine)* w/spinach noodles	9.75 oz	240	29.0	7.0
VEGETABLE				
(Amy's Kitchen) organic	9.5 oz	310	36.0	8.5
(Le Menu) garden 'Light Style'	10.5 oz	260	35.0	8.0
(Legume) w/tofu and sauce	12 oz	240	26.0	8.0
(Stouffer's)	10.5 oz	430	35.0	23.0
(Stouffer's) 96-oz tray	9.5 oz	400	33.0	20.0
(Weight Watchers) garden 'Lowfat'	11 oz	260	30.0	7.0
W/MEAT SAUCE				
(Banquet) 'Family Entrees'	7 oz	270	30.0	10.0
(Dining Lite)	9 oz	240	36.0	5.0
(Freezer Queen) 'Deluxe Family Suppers'	7 oz	200	28.0	6.0
(Healthy Choice)	10 oz	260	37.0	5.0
(Le Menu) 'LightStyle'	10 oz	290	36.0	8.0
(Lean Cuisine)	10.25 oz	280	36.0	6.0
(Swanson) 'Homestyle Recipe'	10.5 oz	400	39.0	15.0
ZUCCHINI				
(Healthy Choice)	11.5 oz	250	41.0	3.0

Food Name	Serv. Size	Total Cal.	Carbs GMS	Fat GMS
(Lean Cuisine)	11 oz	260	34.0	6.0
LASAGNA ENTRÉE, MICROWAVE				
(Chef Boyardee)	7.5 oz	230	31.0	9.0
(Chef Boyardee) hearty 'Main Meals'	10.5 oz	290	41.0	8.0
(Chef Boyardee) in garden vegetable sauce	7.5 oz	170	14.0	1.0
(Hormel)	7.5 oz	250	25.0	13.0
(Libby's) w/meat sauce 'Diner'	7.75 oz	200	29.0	5.0
(Lunch Bucket) w/meat sauce	7.5 oz	220	38.0	4.0
LASAGNA ENTRÉE, PACKAGED				
(Dinty Moore) w/meat sauce 'American Classics'	10 oz	320	33.0	14.0
(Top Shelf) Italian	10 oz	350	30.0	16.0
(Top Shelf) vegetable	10.6 oz	275	34.0	8.0
(Ultra Slim Fast) vegetable	12 oz	240	39.0	4.0
(Ultra Slim Fast) w/meat sauce	12 oz	330	38.0	9.0
LASAGNA NOODLE. See PASTA.				
LAVER. See SEAWEED.				
LEEK				
boiled, drained	4 oz	35	8.6	0.2
boiled, drained, chopped	1/4 cup	8	2.0	0.1
raw, chopped	1/2 cup	32	7.4	0.2
raw, trimmed	1 oz	17	4.0	0.1
raw, untrimmed	1 lb	122	28.2	0.6
LEEK, FREEZE-DRIED				
bulb-lower leaf portion	1 oz	91	21.2	0.6
bulb-lower leaf portion	1/4 cup	3	0.6	0.0
bulb-lower leaf portion	1 tbsp	1	0.2	0.0
LEMON				
w/peel, approx 3.9 oz	1 med	22	11.6	0.3
w/peel, whole	1 lb	89	47.6	1.3
w/o peel, approx 3.9 oz	1 med	17	5.4	0.2
w/o peel, approx 5.6 oz	1 large	24	7.8	0.3
w/o peel, trimmed	1-oz wedge	5	2.9	0.1
LEMON AND HERB SEASONING				
(Schilling) 'Spice Blends'	1/4 tsp	1	0.2	0.1
LEMON DILL SEASONING MIX				
(Schilling) 'Bag 'n Season'	1 pkg	161	15.0	11.0
LEMON DRINK. See also LEMONADE.				
(Crowley) chilled	8 oz	130	32.0	0.0
(Gatorade) 'Thirst Quencher'	8 oz	50	14.0	0.0
(Pathmark) 'No Frills' mix, prepared	8 oz	90	20.0	0.0
LEMON GINGER JUICE				
(Santa Cruz Natural) organic 'Cruz'	8 oz	125	29.0	<1.0
LEMON HERB MARINADE *(Golden Dipt)*	1 oz	130	2.0	14.0

Food Name	Serv. Size	Total Cal.	Carbs GMS	Fat GMS
LEMON JUICE				
	1 cup	61	21.1	0.0
	1 oz	8	2.6	0.0
	1 tbsp	4	1.3	0.0
Canned or bottled				
(A&P) reconstituted, natural strength	1 oz	6	2.0	<1.0
(Lucky Leaf)	6 oz	30	6.0	0.0
(ReaLemon) reconstituted, natural strength, refrigerated	1 oz	6	2.0	0.0
(ReaLemon) reconstituted, '100%'	1 oz	6	2.0	0.0
Frozen				
single strength	1/2 cup	27	7.9	0.4
single strength	1 tbsp	3	1.0	0.1
(Minute Maid) concentrate	6 oz	8	2.0	0.0
(Sunkist)	1 oz	7	2.0	0.1
LEMON PEEL				
candied	1 oz	88	22.6	0.1
raw	1 tbsp	na	1.0	0.0
raw	1 tsp	na	0.3	0.0
LEMON PEPPER				
Dry seasoning				
(Lawry's)	1 tsp	6	1.2	0.1
(Schilling) 'Parsley Patch'	1 tsp	13	1.0	0.6
(Schilling) 'Spice Blends'	1 tsp	7	0.8	0.0
Marinade *(Lawry's)*	1 oz	20	2.1	1.1
LEMONADE				
Can, bottle, or box				
(Fruitopia) 'Lemonade, Love & Hope' real fruit	8 oz	110	28.0	0.0
(Fruitopia) 'Pink Lemonade Euphoria' real fruit	8 oz	120	29.0	0.0
(Hi-C)	8.45 oz	109	27.2	0.1
(J. Hungerford) pink, 20% plus juice	9.03 oz	41	10.7	0.0
(Knudsen & Sons) 'Natural'	8 oz	100	26.0	0.0
(Minute Maid)	6 oz	80	21.0	0.0
(Minute Maid) country style	6 oz	80	21.0	0.0
(Minute Maid) cranberry	6 oz	90	23.0	0.0
(Minute Maid) pink	6 oz	80	21.0	0.0
(Minute Maid) raspberry	6 oz	90	23.0	0.0
(Santa Cruz Natural) organic	8 oz	60	21.0	<1.0
(Santa Cruz Natural) organic 'Sparkling'	8 oz	85	20.0	<1.0
(Shasta)	12 oz	146	39.0	0.0
(Sunkist)	8 oz	141	36.0	0.0
(10-K) pink	8 oz	60	15.0	0.0
(Tropicana)	6 oz	100	22.0	<1.0
(Tropicana) 'Single Serve'	8 oz	120	30.0	0.0

Food Name	Serv. Size	Total Cal.	Carbs GMS	Fat GMS
(Veryfine)	8 oz	120	30.0	0.0
(Wyler's)	6 oz	64	16.5	0.0
(Wyler's) pink 'Fruit Slush'	4 oz	157	39.3	0.0
LEMONADE DRINK MIX				
Prepared from dry mix				
(Country Time)	8 oz	80	20.0	0.0
(Country Time) pink	8 oz	80	20.0	0.0
(Country Time) pink, 'Sugar Free'	8 oz	4	0.0	0.0
(Country Time) pink, sugar sweetened	8 oz	80	20.0	0.0
(Country Time) pink, sugar-free, w/NutraSweet	8 oz	4	0.0	0.0
(Country Time) 'Sugar-free'	8 oz	4	0.0	0.0
(Crystal Light) 'Sugar-free'	8 oz	4	0.0	0.0
(Crystal Light) sugar-free, w/NutraSweet	8 oz	4	0.0	0.0
(Finast)	8 oz	80	20.0	0.0
(Gatorade) instant 'Thirst Quencher'	8 oz	60	15.0	0.0
(Kool-Aid) pink, unsweetened, prepared w/sugar	8 oz	100	25.0	0.0
(Kool-Aid) pink, unsweetened, prepared w/o sugar	8 oz	2	0.0	0.0
(Kool-Aid) sugar free, w/NutraSweet	8 oz	4	0.0	0.0
(Kool-Aid) sugar sweetened	8 oz	80	20.0	0.0
(Wyler's) 'Crystals' 32-serving pkg	8 oz	78	19.4	0.0
Prepared from frozen concentrate				
(A&P)	8 oz	110	28.0	<1.0
(A&P) pink	8 oz	110	28.0	<1.0
(Minute Maid)	6 oz	90	22.0	0.0
(Minute Maid) country style	6 oz	90	22.0	0.0
(Minute Maid) cranberry	6 oz	90	22.0	0.0
(Minute Maid) pink	6 oz	90	22.0	0.0
(Minute Maid) raspberry	6 oz	90	22.0	0.0
(Sunkist)	8 oz	92	24.2	0.0
LEMONADE PUNCH MIX *(Country Time)* sugar sweetened	8 oz	80	20.0	0.0
LEMON-LIME DRINK				
Can, bottle, or box				
(All-Sports) thirst quencher, caffeine-free	8 oz	70	19.0	0.0
(Gatorade) 'Thirst Quencher'	8 oz	50	14.0	0.0
(Gatorade) 'Thirst Quencher Light'	8 oz	25	7.0	0.0
(PowerAde) thirst quencher, high energy	8 oz	70	19.0	0.0
(10-K)	8 oz	60	15.0	0.0
(Veryfine)	8 oz	120	30.0	0.0
Prepared from dry mix				
(Crystal Light) w/NutraSweet	8 oz	4	0.0	0.0
(GatorAde) instant 'Thirst Quencher'	8 oz	60	15.0	0.0
(Kool-Aid) unsweetened, prepared w/sugar	8 oz	100	25.0	0.0
(Kool-Aid) unsweetened, prepared w/o sugar	8 oz	2	0.0	0.0

Food Name	Serv. Size	Total Cal.	Carbs GMS	Fat GMS
LENTIL				
boiled	1/2 cup	115	19.9	0.4
boiled	4 oz	132	22.8	0.4
boiled *(A&P)*	1 cup	210	39.0	1.0
raw	1/2 cup	324	54.8	0.9
raw	1 oz	96	16.2	0.3
raw, green *(Arrowhead Mills)*	2 oz	190	35.0	1.0
raw, red *(Arrowhead Mills)*	2 oz	195	34.0	1.0
raw, sprouted	1 oz	30	6.3	0.2
LENTIL DINNER, CANNED				
hearty, w/garden vegetables 'Fast Menu' fat-free *(Health Valley)*	7.5 oz	160	18.0	4.0
hearty, w/garden vegetables 'Fast Menu' fat-free *(Health Valley)*	5 oz	80	12.0	0.0
LETTUCE				
BIBB, BOSTON, OR BUTTERHEAD				
raw, approx 7.75 oz, 5-inch diam	1 head	21	3.8	0.4
trimmed	1 oz	4	0.7	0.1
untrimmed	1 lb	45	7.8	0.7
COS				
raw, shredded	1/2 cup	4	0.7	0.1
trimmed	1 oz	5	0.7	0.1
untrimmed	1 lb	68	10.1	0.9
ICEBERG				
raw, 6-inch diam	1 head	70	11.3	1.0
trimmed	1 oz	4	0.6	0.1
untrimmed	1 lb	55	9.0	0.8
LEAF, shredded *(Dole)*	1.5 cups	12	1.0	0.0
LOOSELEAF				
raw, shredded	1/2 cup	5	1.0	0.1
trimmed	1 oz	5	1.0	0.1
untrimmed	1 lb	52	10.2	0.9
ROMAINE				
raw, shredded	1/2 cup	4	0.7	0.1
trimmed	1 oz	5	0.7	0.1
untrimmed	1 lb	68	10.1	0.9
LIMA BEAN /butterbean				
boiled, drained	4 oz	139	26.8	0.4
raw, trimmed	1 oz	32	5.7	0.2
raw, untrimmed	1 lb	226	40.2	1.7
MATURE, DRY				
Baby				
boiled	4 oz	143	26.4	0.4

Food Name	Serv. Size	Total Cal.	Carbs GMS	Fat GMS
boiled (A&P)	1 cup	230	40.0	1.0
boiled, thin-seeded	1/2 cup	115	21.2	0.4
raw	1 oz	95	17.8	0.3
raw, thin-seeded	1/2 cup	338	63.5	0.9
Large				
boiled	4 oz	130	23.7	0.4
boiled	1/2 cup	108	19.6	0.4
boiled (A&P)	1 cup	230	35.0	1.0
raw	1/2 cup	301	56.4	0.6
raw	1 oz	96	18.0	0.2
LIMA BEAN, CANNED				
(A&P)	1/2 cup	110	20.0	<1.0
(Allens) large	1/2 cup	110	18.0	<1.0
(Featherweight)	1/2 cup	80	16.0	0.0
(Freshlike)	1/2 cup	80	16.0	0.0
(Freshlike) water packed, w/o salt	1/2 cup	80	16.0	0.0
(Green Giant)	1/2 cup	80	16.0	0.0
(Joan of Arc)	1/2 cup	80	16.0	0.0
(S&W)	1/2 cup	100	19.0	1.0
(Stokely)	1/2 cup	80	16.0	0.0
(Stokely) 'No Salt or Sugar Added'	1/2 cup	80	16.0	0.0
(Van Camp's)	1 cup	162	30.0	0.5
(Veg•All)	1/2 cup	80	16.0	0.0
FORDHOOK (Stokely)	1/2 cup	80	14.0	0.0
GREEN				
(A&P)	1/2 cup	80	15.0	<1.0
(Allens) medium	1/2 cup	90	15.0	<1.0
(Allens) tiny, small	1/2 cup	90	15.0	<1.0
(Bush's Best)	1/2 cup	90	17.0	0.0
(Del Monte) w/liquid	1/2 cup	70	14.0	0.0
(Luck's) small, w/pork	7.5 oz	220	33.0	7.0
(S&W) small 'Fancy'	1/2 cup	80	16.0	0.0
GREEN AND WHITE				
(Allens)	1/2 cup	90	15.0	<1.0
(Bush's Best) gem	1/2 cup	80	17.0	0.0
W/HAM (Dennison's)	7.5 oz	250	33.0	7.0
W/PORK (Luck's)	7.5 oz	230	34.0	7.0
LIMA BEAN, FROZEN				
(Green Giant)	1/2 cup	100	19.0	0.0
(Green Giant) 'Harvest Fresh'	1/2 cup	80	18.0	0.0
(Green Giant) in butter sauce	1/2 cup	100	17.0	2.0
(Health Valley)	1/2 cup	94	18.0	0.0

Food Name	Serv. Size	Total Cal.	Carbs GMS	Fat GMS
BABY				
boiled, drained	10-oz pkg	376	71.4	1.3
boiled, drained	4 oz	119	22.1	0.3
boiled, drained, immature seeds	10-oz pkg	327	60.5	0.9
boiled, drained, immature seeds	1/2 cup	94	17.5	0.3
unprepared, immature seeds	10-oz pkg	375	71.4	1.3
unprepared, immature seeds	1/2 cup	108	20.6	0.4
(A&P) green	3.3 oz	130	24.0	<1.0
(Birds Eye)	3.3 oz	130	24.0	0.0
(Freshlike)	3.3 oz	130	24.0	1.0
(Frosty Acres)	3.3 oz	130	24.0	0.0
(Seabrook)	3.3 oz	130	24.0	0.0
(Seabrook) butter	3.3 oz	140	26.0	1.0
(Southern)	3.5 oz	135	25.2	0.5
(Stokely) in butter sauce 'Singles'	4 oz	140	25.0	2.0
(Veg•All)	3.3 oz	130	24.0	1.0
FORDHOOK				
boiled, drained	10-oz pkg	301	56.3	1.0
boiled, drained	4 oz	113	21.3	0.4
boiled, drained, immature seeds	10-oz pkg	311	58.5	1.1
boiled, drained, immature seeds	1/2 cup	85	16.0	0.3
unprepared, immature seeds	1/2 cup	85	15.9	0.3
(A&P)	3.3 oz	100	19.0	<1.0
(Birds Eye)	3.3 oz	100	19.0	0.0
(Frosty Acres)	3.3 oz	100	19.0	0.0
(Seabrook)	3.3 oz	100	19.0	0.0
(Southern)	3.5 oz	105	19.1	0.3
SPECKLED				
(Seabrook)	3.3 oz	120	23.0	0.0
(Southern)	3.5 oz	135	25.0	0.4
TINY *(Seabrook)*	3.3 oz	110	21.0	1.0
LIME				
peeled and seeded	1 oz	9	3.0	0.1
raw, 2-inch diam	1 med	20	7.1	0.1
untrimmed	1 lb	115	40.2	0.8
LIME JUICE				
fresh	1 cup	66	22.2	0.3
fresh	1 oz	8	2.8	<.1
fresh	1 tbsp	4	1.4	0.0
Canned or bottled				
	1/2 cup	26	8.2	0.3
	1 tbsp	3	1.0	<.1
unsweetened	1 cup	52	16.5	0.6

Food Name	Serv. Size	Total Cal.	Carbs GMS	Fat GMS
unsweetened	1 tbsp	3	1.0	0.0
(ReaLime) reconstituted, natural strength	1 oz	6	2.0	0.0
(Roses)	1 oz	48	12.0	0.0
(Santa Cruz Natural) organic, 'Cruz'	8 oz	120	27.0	<1.0
LIMEADE				
(Minute Maid) frozen concentrate, diluted	6 oz	70	19.0	0.0
(Santa Cruz Natural) organic, 'Sparkling'	8 oz	60	23.0	<1.0
LING				
dry-heat cooked	3 oz	94	0.0	0.7
raw	1 lb	394	0.0	2.9
raw	3 oz	74	0.0	0.5
raw	1 oz	25	0.0	0.2
LINGCOD				
dry-heat cooked	3 oz	93	0.0	1.2
raw	1 lb	385	0.0	4.8
raw	3 oz	72	0.0	0.9
raw	1 oz	24	0.0	0.3
LINGUINE ENTRÉE				
Frozen				
(Banquet) w/meat sauce 'Healthy Balance'	11.5 oz	290	49.0	6.0
(Budget Gourmet) w/shrimp	10 oz	330	33.0	15.0
(Healthy Choice) w/shrimp	9.5 oz	230	40.0	2.0
(Lean Cuisine) w/clam sauce	9 5/8 oz	280	36.0	8.0
Packaged (Top Shelf) w/clam sauce	1 serving	330	30.0	18.0
Refrigerated				
(Contadina) egg, angel hair 'Fresh'	3 oz	260	45.0	3.0
(DiGiorno) herb, approx 1 1/3 cups cooked	3 oz	250	46.0	3.0
LINGUINE NOODLE. See PASTA.				
LINSEED OIL				
edible	1/2 cup	964	0.0	109.0
edible	1 oz	251	0.0	28.4
edible	1 tbsp	120	0.0	13.6
LIQUEUR. See ALCOHOLIC BEVERAGES.				
LIQUOR. See ALCOHOLIC BEVERAGES.				
LITCHI/lychee				
Dried				
	100 gm	277	70.7	1.2
	1 oz	79	20.0	0.3
Raw				
approx .6 oz	1 med	6	1.6	<.1
shelled and seeded	1/2 cup	63	15.7	0.4
shelled and seeded	1 oz	19	4.7	0.1
untrimmed	1 lb	179	45.0	1.2

Food Name	Serv. Size	Total Cal.	Carbs GMS	Fat GMS
LIVER. See individual animal listings.				
LIVERWURST. See LUNCHEON MEATS.				
LIVERWURST SPREAD				
(Hormel) canned	.5 oz	35	0.0	3.0
(Underwood) canned	2 1/8 oz	180	4.0	15.0
LOBSTER, NORTHERN				
boiled	1 cup	142	1.9	0.9
boiled	4 oz	111	1.5	0.7
moist-heat cooked	1 cup	142	1.9	0.9
moist-heat cooked	3 oz	83	1.1	0.5
poached	1 cup	142	1.9	0.9
poached	4 oz	111	1.5	0.7
raw	1 lb	410	2.3	4.1
raw	3 oz	77	0.4	0.8
raw	1 oz	26	0.1	0.3
steamed	1 cup	142	1.9	0.9
steamed	4 oz	111	1.5	0.7
LOBSTER, SPINY, MIXED SPECIES				
moist-heat cooked	3 oz	122	2.7	1.6
raw	1 lb	506	11.0	6.9
raw	3 oz	95	2.1	1.3
raw	1 oz	32	0.7	0.4
LOBSTER PASTE, canned	1 tsp	13	0.1	0.7
LOGANBERRY				
fresh, trimmed	1 lb	281	67.6	2.7
fresh, trimmed	1 cup	89	21.5	0.9
fresh, untrimmed	1 lb	267	64.2	2.6
frozen	1 cup	81	19.1	0.5
frozen	4 oz	62	14.8	0.4
LONGAN				
raw, approx .2 oz	1 med	2	0.5	tr
raw, shelled and seeded	1 oz	17	4.3	<.1
raw, untrimmed	1 lb	144	36.4	0.2
LONGAN, DRIED				
	100 gm	286	74.0	0.4
	1 oz	81	21.0	0.1
LONGBEAN				
boiled, drained	4 oz	53	10.4	0.1
boiled, drained, sliced	1/2 cup	25	4.8	0.1
boiled, drained, 13 1/4 inches long x 1/4 inch diam	1 pod	7	1.3	<.1
raw, sliced	1/2 cup	22	3.8	0.2
raw, 13 1/4 inches long x 1/4 inch diam	1 pod	6	1.0	0.1
raw, trimmed	1 oz	13	2.4	0.1

Food Name	Serv. Size	Total Cal.	Carbs GMS	Fat GMS
raw, untrimmed	1 lb	203	36.0	1.7
LONGBEAN, DRIED				
boiled	1/2 cup	102	18.1	0.4
boiled	4 oz	134	23.9	0.5
raw	1/2 cup	292	52.0	1.1
raw	1 oz	98	17.6	0.4
LOOFAH GOURD. See GOURD, DISHCLOTH.				
LOQUAT/Japanese medlar				
peeled and seeded	1 oz	13	3.4	0.1
trimmed, .6 oz	1 med	5	1.2	0.0
untrimmed	1 lb	132	34.1	0.6
LOTTE. See MONKFISH.				
LOTUS ROOT				
boiled, drained	4 oz	75	18.2	0.1
boiled, drained, 2.5-inch diam	10 slices	59	14.3	0.1
raw, 2.5-inch diam	10 slices	45	14.0	0.1
raw, 9.5 inches long	1 root	64	19.8	0.1
raw, trimmed	1 oz	16	4.9	<.1
raw, untrimmed	1 lb	201	61.8	0.4
LOTUS SEED				
dried	1 cup	106	20.6	0.6
dried, approx 42 medium seeds	1 oz	94	18.3	0.6
raw	1 oz	25	4.9	0.2
raw, in shell	1 lb	214	41.5	1.3
LOX. See SALMON, CHINOOK.				
LUNCHEON MEAT				
BARBECUE LOAF *(Oscar Mayer)*	1 oz	46	1.7	2.3
BOLOGNA				
(Eckrich)	1 oz	100	1.0	9.0
(Eckrich) 'German Brand'	1 oz	80	1.0	7.0
(Eckrich) 'Lean Supreme'	1 oz	70	1.0	6.0
(Eckrich) 'Sandwich'	1 oz	100	1.0	9.0
(Eckrich) 'Smorgas Pac'	1 oz	100	1.0	9.0
(Eckrich) 'Thick Sliced, 1-lb pkg'	1.8 oz	170	2.0	15.0
(Hillshire Farm) 'Large'	1 oz	90	<1.0	8.0
(Hillshire Farm) 'Ring'	1 oz	89	<1.0	8.0
(Hormel) 'Fine Ground, 1-lb'	2 oz	170	1.0	16.0
(Hormel) 'Perma-Fresh'	2 slices	180	0.0	16.0
(JM)	1 oz	90	1.0	8.0
(JM) 'German Brand'	1 oz	70	1.0	6.0
(Kahn's)	1 slice	90	1.0	8.0
(Kahn's) 'Deluxe Club'	1 slice	90	1.0	8.0
(Kahn's) 'Deluxe Club Family Pack'	1 slice	70	1.0	6.0

Food Name	Serv. Size	Total Cal.	Carbs GMS	Fat GMS
(Kahn's) 'Giant Deluxe'	1 slice	90	1.0	8.0
(Kahn's) 'Giant Thick Deluxe'	1 slice	110	1.0	10.0
(Kahn's) 'Thick Deluxe'	1 slice	140	1.0	13.0
(Kahn's) 'Thin Sliced Deluxe'	1 slice	60	1.0	5.0
(Light & Lean)	2 slices	140	2.0	12.0
(Light & Lean) 'Thin Sliced'	2 slices	70	1.0	6.0
(OHSE)	1 oz	75	3.0	6.0
(Oscar Mayer)	1.6 oz	144	1.1	13.3
(Oscar Mayer)	1 oz	90	0.7	8.3
(Oscar Mayer)	.53 oz	48	0.4	4.4
(Oscar Mayer) 'Light'	1 oz	64	0.7	5.4
(Oscar Mayer) Wisconsin made, ring	1 oz	90	<1.0	8.0
(Oscar Mayer) w/cheese	.8 oz	74	0.6	6.8
(Pilgrim's Pride)	1 oz	59	0.6	4.4
Beef				
(Boar's Head)	1 oz	74	<1.0	7.0
(Boar's Head) 'Premium' low cholesterol	1 oz	70	1.0	7.0
(Eckrich)	1 oz	90	1.0	8.0
(Eckrich) 'Thick Sliced'	1.5 oz	130	2.0	12.0
(Hebrew National) 'Original Deli Style'	1 oz	90	<1.0	3.0
(Hormel) 'Coarse Ground, 1 lb'	2 oz	160	1.0	14.0
(Hormel) 'Perma-Fresh'	2 slices	170	1.0	16.0
(JM)	1 oz	90	1.0	8.0
(Kahn's)	1 slice	90	1.0	8.0
(Kahn's) 'Family Pack'	1 slice	70	1.0	6.0
(Kahn's) 'Giant'	1 slice	90	1.0	8.0
(Kahn's) 'Pounder'	1 slice	90	1.0	8.0
(OHSE)	1 oz	85	1.0	8.0
(Oscar Mayer)	1.6 oz	143	1.0	13.3
(Oscar Mayer)	1 oz	89	0.6	8.2
(Oscar Mayer)	.53 oz	48	0.3	4.4
(Oscar Mayer) 'Light'	1 oz	64	0.9	5.3
Beef and cheddar *(Kahn's)*	1 slice	90	1.0	8.0
Beef and pork				
(Boar's Head)	1 oz	80	<1.0	7.0
(Boar's Head) 'Premium' low cholesterol	1 oz	80	1.0	7.0
(Healthy Deli)	1 oz	41	1.1	2.0
Chicken				
(Health Valley)	1 slice	85	1.0	8.0
(OHSE) '15% Chicken'	1 oz	90	1.0	8.0
(Tyson)	1 slice	44	3.7	0.5
Garlic				
(Eckrich)	1 oz	90	1.0	9.0

Food Name	Serv. Size	Total Cal.	Carbs GMS	Fat GMS
(Eckrich) w/cheese	1 oz	90	1.0	9.0
(JM)	1 oz	90	1.0	8.0
(Kahn's)	1 slice	90	1.0	8.0
Ham				
(Boar's Head)	1 oz	40	1.0	2.0
(Oscar Mayer)	1 oz	90	0.7	8.3
Lebanon (Oscar Mayer)	.8 oz	46	0.4	2.9
Turkey				
(Butterball) 'Cold Cuts'	1 oz	70	2.0	6.0
(Butterball) 'Deli/Slice 'n Serve'	1 oz	70	2.0	6.0
(Butterball) 'Turkey Variety Pak'	.75 oz	50	1.0	4.0
(Healthy Choice) beef and pork	.75-oz slice	25	1.0	1.0
(Longacre) sliced	1 oz	61	0.0	5.0
(Louis Rich)	1 oz	61	0.6	5.0
(Louis Rich) mild	1 oz	59	0.7	4.5
(Norbest) 'Blue Label' 2-2.5 lb	1 oz	68	0.5	5.6
(Norbest) 'Blue Label' 5-lb	1 oz	57	0.3	4.4
(OHSE)	1 oz	70	2.0	6.0
CHICKEN				
Breast				
(Healthy Choice) deli-thin, 97% fat-free	1 slice	10	<1.0	<1.0
(Healthy Choice) oven roasted, 97% fat-free	1 slice	30	1.0	<1.0
(Healthy Favorites) oven roasted	.4-oz slice	12	<1.0	<1.0
(Hillshire Farm) smoked 'Deli Select'	1 oz	31	<1.0	0.2
(Longacre) 'Premium'	1 oz	45	1.0	3.0
(Louis Rich) hickory smoked	1 oz	30	0.6	0.8
(Louis Rich) oven roasted 'Deluxe'	1 oz	30	0.6	0.8
(Louis Rich) oven roasted 'Thin Sliced'	.4-oz slice	12	0.2	0.3
(Louis Rich) oven roasted, white meat	1-oz slice	35	0.1	1.7
(Mr. Turkey)	1 oz	32	0.6	1.1
(Oscar Mayer) oven roasted	1 oz	29	0.6	0.7
(Oscar Mayer) smoked	1 oz	25	0.2	0.4
(Oscar Mayer) 'Thin Sliced'	.4-oz slice	13	0.3	0.4
(Tyson) hickory smoked	1 slice	25	0.8	1.0
(Tyson) honey flavored	1 slice	25	0.8	1.0
(Tyson) mesquite, oven roasted	1 slice	25	0.8	1.0
(Tyson) oven roasted	1 slice	25	0.8	0.5
Roll				
(Longacre)	1 oz	60	1.0	5.0
(Pilgrim's Pride)	1-oz slice	35	0.4	1.2
(Tyson)	1 slice	26	1.4	0.5
CHICKEN HAM				
(Healthy Favorites) smoked, w/natural juices	.4-oz slice	13	0.2	0.4

Food Name	Serv. Size	Total Cal.	Carbs GMS	Fat GMS
(Pilgrim's Pride)	1-oz slice	35	0.8	1.8
CORNED BEEF LOAF, jellied	1 oz	43	0.0	1.7
DUTCH BRAND LOAF				
	1-oz slice	68	1.6	5.1
(Eckrich)	1-oz slice	70	2.0	6.0
(Eckrich) 'Lean Supreme'	1-oz slice	60	2.0	4.0
(Eckrich) 'Smorgas Pac'	1-oz slice	70	2.0	6.0
(Kahn's)	1 slice	80	1.0	7.0
HAM				
(Boar's Head) boiled 'Deluxe'	1 oz	28	1.0	<1.0
(Boar's Head) deluxe 'Deli-trition' low cholesterol	1 oz	30	1.0	1.0
(Boar's Head) 'Lower Salt'	1 oz	28	<1.0	<1.0
(Healthy Deli)	1 oz	33	0.2	0.8
(Healthy Deli) 'Deluxe'	1 oz	31	1.1	0.9
(Healthy Deli) 'Lessalt'	1 oz	32	1.4	0.9
(Healthy Deli) 'Light AM'	1 oz	27	1.4	0.6
(Healthy Deli) 'Taverne'	1 oz	31	0.3	0.8
(Healthy Favorites) boiled	.4-oz slice	12	<1.0	<1.0
(Hormel)	1 oz	29	1.0	1.0
(JM)	1 oz	30	1.0	1.0
(JM) 'Slice 'n Eat' 93% fat-free	2 oz	70	1.0	3.0
(JM) 'Slice 'n Eat' 95% fat-free, presliced	2 slices	60	1.0	2.0
(Jones Dairy Farm) 'Farm'	1 slice	50	tr	1.1
(Jones Dairy Farm) 'Four Family Ham'	1 oz	35	tr	1.2
(Kahn's)	1 slice	30	1.0	1.0
(Kahn's) 'Low Salt'	1 slice	30	1.0	1.0
(Light & Lean)	2 slices	50	0.0	2.0
(OHSE)	1 oz	30	1.0	1.0
(Oscar Mayer) boiled	.75-oz slice	23	0.3	0.7
(Oscar Mayer) boiled 'Thin Sliced'	.4 oz	13	0.2	0.4
(Oscar Mayer) 'Breakfast Ham'	1.5-oz slice	47	1.2	1.5
(Oscar Mayer) 'Jubilee'	1 oz	43	0.1	2.4
(Oscar Mayer) 'Lower Salt'	.7 oz	23	0.6	0.7
(Swift) 'Premium Hostess'	1 oz	30	0.0	1.0
(Swift) 'Premium Sugar Plum'	1 oz	30	1.0	1.0
Baked				
(Healthy Deli) Virginia	1 oz	34	1.6	0.9
(Healthy Deli) Virginia 'Lessalt'	1 oz	32	1.4	0.9
(Louis Rich) 'Carving Board' cooked w/natural juices	22 grams	22	0.5	0.4
(Oscar Mayer)	.75-oz slice	21	0.4	0.5
Barbecue (Light & Lean)	2 slices	50	0.0	2.0
Black Forest (Healthy Deli)	1 oz	32	0.4	0.6
Cajun (Hillshire Farm) 'Deli Select'	1 oz	31	<1.0	0.9

Food Name	Serv. Size	Total Cal.	Carbs GMS	Fat GMS
Capocollo *(Hormel)*	1 oz	80	0.0	6.0
Chopped				
(Eckrich)	1-oz slice	45	<1.0	2.0
(Eckrich) 'Lean Supreme'	1-oz slice	35	<1.0	2.0
(Hormel) 'Black Label'	1 oz	70	1.0	6.0
(Hormel) 'Perma-Fresh'	2 slices	88	0.0	5.0
(JM)	1-oz slice	80	1.0	7.0
(Kahn's)	1 slice	50	1.0	3.0
(Light & Lean)	2 slices	70	0.0	4.0
(OHSE)	1 oz	65	1.0	5.0
(Oscar Mayer)	1-oz slice	41	0.7	2.3
Glazed *(Light & Lean)*	2 slices	50	0.0	2.0
Honey				
(Boar's Head) 'Premium' low cholesterol	1 oz	35	2.0	1.0
(Carl Buddig) 'Lean' smoked, chopped	1 oz	50	1.0	3.0
(Healthy Choice) 'Deli-Thin'	1 slice	10	<1.0	<1.0
(Healthy Deli) 'Honey Valley'	1 oz	31	1.2	0.8
(Healthy Favorites)	1 slice	14	<1.0	<1.0
(Healthy Favorites) 'Breakfast' water added	1 oz	30	0.7	0.9
(Hillshire Farm) 'Deli Select'	1 oz	31	<1.0	0.9
(Louis Rich) 'Carving Board' w/natural juices	2.1 oz	68	1.8	1.9
(Oscar Mayer)	.75-oz slice	23	0.5	0.6
(Oscar Mayer) 'Thin Sliced'	.4-oz slice	13	0.3	0.4
Jalapeño *(Healthy Deli)*	1 oz	25	0.8	0.6
Peppered				
(Light & Lean) black pepper	2 slices	50	0.0	2.0
(Light & Lean) red pepper	2 slices	50	0.0	2.0
(Oscar Mayer) cracked black pepper	.75-oz slice	22	0.2	0.8
Prosciutto *(Hormel)*	1 oz	90	0.0	7.0
Smoked				
(Carl Buddig) 'Lean' chopped	1 oz	50	1.0	3.0
(Eckrich) 'Slender Sliced'	1 oz	40	1.0	2.0
(Healthy Favorites)	.4-oz slice	14	<1.0	<1.0
(Hillshire Farm) 'Deli Select'	1 oz	31	<1.0	0.9
(JM) golden	2 oz	80	1.0	5.0
(JM) golden, water added	2 oz	70	4.0	2.0
(Light & Lean)	2 slices	50	0.0	2.0
(Louis Rich) 'Carving Board' w/natural juices	10 grams	11	0.0	0.4
(OHSE) '95% Fat-Free'	1 oz	30	1.0	1.0
(Oscar Mayer)	.75-oz slice	22	0.1	0.7
HAM AND CHEESE LOAF				
(Eckrich)	1-oz slice	50	1.0	4.0
(Hormel) '8 lb' canned	3 oz	260	1.0	22.0

Food Name	Serv. Size	Total Cal.	Carbs GMS	Fat GMS
(Hormel) 'Perma-Fresh'	2 slices	110	0.0	7.0
(Kahn's)	1 slice	70	1.0	6.0
(Light & Lean)	2 slices	90	0.0	6.0
(OHSE)	1 oz	65	2.0	5.0
(Oscar Mayer)	1-oz slice	66	1.0	5.0
HEAD CHEESE (Oscar Mayer)	1-oz slice	55	0.1	4.0
HONEY LOAF				
(Eckrich)	1-oz slice	35	2.0	1.0
(Eckrich) 'Smorgas Pac'	1-oz slice	35	2.0	1.0
(Hormel) 'Perma-Fresh'	2 slices	90	0.0	5.0
(Kahn's)	1 slice	40	1.0	2.0
(Oscar Mayer)	1-oz slice	34	1.0	1.0
IOWA BRAND LOAF (Hormel) 'Perma-Fresh'	2 slices	90	0.0	6.0
JALAPEÑO LOAF (Kahn's)	1 slice	70	2.0	6.0
LIVER CHEESE				
(JM)	1-oz slice	70	1.0	6.0
(Oscar Mayer)	1.34-oz slice	116	0.5	10.0
LIVER LOAF				
(Hormel) 'Perma-Fresh'	2 slices	160	1.0	13.0
(Kahn's)	1 slice	170	3.0	15.0
LIVERWURST/liver sausage				
(Hickory Farms)	1 oz	97	1.0	9.0
(Jones Dairy Farm) 'Farm Club'	1 oz	80	tr	6.3
(Jones Dairy Farm) 'Farm Slices'	1 slice	75	tr	6.6
LOAF				
(Hormel) spiced, canned	3 oz	280	2.0	26.0
(JM) 'P&B'	1-oz slice	70	2.0	5.0
(Kahn's) 'P&B'	1 slice	40	1.0	2.0
(OHSE)	1 oz	75	1.0	6.0
MACARONI AND CHEESE LOAF				
(Eckrich)	1-oz slice	75	3.0	6.0
(OHSE)	1 oz	60	4.0	3.0
OLD-FASHIONED LOAF (Oscar Mayer)	1-oz slice	62	2.4	4.0
OLIVE LOAF				
(Eckrich)	1-oz slice	80	2.0	6.0
(Hormel) 'Perma-Fresh'	2 slices	110	5.0	7.0
(Oscar Mayer)	1-oz slice	63	3.2	4.3
PASTRAMI. See also TURKEY PASTRAMI.				
(Boar's Head) 'Round'	1 oz	40	<1.0	1.5
(Carl Buddig) 'Lean' smoked, chopped, sliced	1 oz	40	1.0	2.0
(Healthy Deli) 'Deli Round'	1 oz	34	0.8	1.1
(Hillshire Farm) 'Deli Select'	1 oz	31	<1.0	0.4
(Oscar Mayer)	.6-oz slice	16	0.1	0.3

Food Name	Serv. Size	Total Cal.	Carbs GMS	Fat GMS
PEPPERED BEEF				
(Carl Buddig) 'Lean' smoked, chopped, sliced	1 oz	40	1.0	2.0
(Eckrich)	1-oz slice	35	2.0	1.0
(Kahn's)	1 slice	40	1.0	2.0
(Oscar Mayer)	1-oz slice	39	1.2	1.5
PICKLE LOAF				
(Eckrich)	1-oz slice	80	2.0	6.0
(Eckrich) 'Smorgas-Pac'	1-oz slice	80	2.0	6.0
(Hormel) 'Perma-Fresh'	2 slices	102	3.0	7.0
(Kahn's)	1 slice	80	2.0	7.0
(Kahn's) 'Family-Pack'	1 slice	70	2.0	6.0
(Light & Lean)	2 slices	100	3.0	6.0
(OHSE)	1 oz	60	2.0	4.0
PICKLE-PIMIENTO LOAF (Oscar Mayer)	1-oz slice	66	4.1	4.1
PORK LOAF (Eckrich) 'Slender Sliced'	1 oz	45	1.0	2.0
ROAST BEEF				
(Healthy Deli)	1 oz	30	0.2	0.4
(Healthy Deli) Italian	1 oz	31	0.1	0.6
(Hillshire Farm) 'Deli Select' oven roasted, cured, w/o added ingredients	1 oz	31	<1.0	0.5
(Oscar Mayer) 'Thin Sliced'	.4-oz slice	14	0.2	0.4
SALAMI. See also TURKEY SALAMI.				
Beef				
(Boar's Head)	1 oz	60	<1.0	4.0
(Hebrew National) 'Original Deli-Style'	1 oz	80	<1.0	7.0
(Hormel) 'Party'	1 oz	90	0.0	8.0
(Hormel) 'Perma-Fresh'	2 slices	50	0.0	5.0
(Kahn's)	1 slice	70	1.0	6.0
(Kahn's) 'Family-Pack'	1 slice	60	1.0	5.0
(Oscar Mayer) 'Machiaeh Brand'	.8-oz slice	60	0.0	5.0
Beer				
(Eckrich)	1-oz slice	70	1.0	6.0
(Oscar Mayer) 'Salami for Beer'	.8-oz slice	50	0.4	4.0
(Oscar Mayer) 'Salami for Beer' beef	.8-oz slice	63	0.4	5.6
Cooked				
(Kahn's)	1 slice	60	1.0	4.0
(OHSE)	1 oz	65	1.0	5.0
Cotto				
(Eckrich)	1-oz slice	70	1.0	6.0
(Eckrich) beef	1.3 oz	100	2.0	8.0
(Hormel) 'Club'	1 oz	100	0.0	5.0
(Hormel) 'Perma-Fresh'	2 slices	105	1.0	7.0
(JM)	1-oz slice	80	2.0	6.0

Food Name	Serv. Size	Total Cal.	Carbs GMS	Fat GMS
(Kahn's) 'Family Pack'	1 slice	45	1.0	3.0
(Light & Lean)	2 slices	80	0.0	6.0
(Oscar Mayer) beef	.8-oz slice	45	0.4	3.4
(Oscar Mayer) beef	.5-oz slice	29	0.3	2.2
Dry or hard				
(Hickory Farms)	1 oz	120	0.0	10.0
(Hormel)	1 oz	110	0.0	10.0
(Hormel) 'Homeland'	1 oz	117	2.0	10.0
(Hormel) 'National Brand'	1 oz	120	0.0	11.0
(Hormel) 'Perma-Fresh'	2 slices	80	0.0	7.0
(Hormel) 'Sliced'	1 oz	110	0.0	10.0
(JM)	1-oz slice	110	1.0	9.0
(Oscar Mayer)	.8-oz slice	52	0.4	4.2
(Oscar Mayer) 'Hard'	.3-oz slice	33	0.1	2.8
Genoa				
(Hickory Farms)	1 oz	110	0.0	10.0
(Hormel)	1 oz	110	0.0	10.0
(Hormel) 'DiLusso'	1 oz	100	0.0	8.0
(Hormel) 'Gran Valore'	1 oz	110	0.0	10.0
(Hormel) 'San Remo Brand'	1 oz	118	0.0	10.0
(JM)	1-oz slice	100	1.0	8.0
(Oscar Mayer)	.3-oz slice	34	0.1	2.8
Piccolo (Hormel) 'Stick'	1 oz	120	0.0	11.0
SOUSE LOAF (Kahn's)	1 slice	90	1.0	7.0
SPICE LOAF				
(Hormel) canned	3 oz	280	2.0	26.0
(Hormel) 'Perma-Fresh'	2 slices	118	1.0	9.0
(JM)	1-oz slice	70	1.0	6.0
(Kahn's) 'Family Pack'	1 slice	70	1.0	6.0
(Kahn's) 'Family Pack' beef	1 slice	60	1.0	5.0
(Kahn's) 'Luncheon Loaf'	1 slice	80	1.0	7.0
TURKEY. See also TURKEY LOAF/ROLL.				
(Boar's Head) 'Premium' skin on, low cholesterol	1 oz	35	1.0	1.0
(Butterball) 'Cold Cuts'	1 oz	30	1.0	1.0
(Butterball) 'Deli No Salt Added'	1 oz	45	0.0	2.0
(Healthy Choice) 97% fat-free	1 slice	30	<1.0	1.0
(Healthy Deli) 'Gourmet'	1 oz	28	0.5	0.6
(Healthy Deli) 'Lessalt'	1 oz	25	0.4	0.5
(Hormel) 'Perma-Fresh'	2 slices	60	0.0	2.0
(Light & Lean)	2 slices	60	0.0	2.0
(Longacre) 'Catering'	1 oz	35	<1.0	1.0
(Norbest) white meat, diced	1 oz	31	1.0	0.9
(Tyson)	1 slice	20	0.3	0.4

Food Name	Serv. Size	Total Cal.	Carbs GMS	Fat GMS
Honey roasted *(Healthy Deli)*	1 oz	28	0.5	0.5
Honey roasted and smoked				
(Healthy Choice)	1-oz slice	35	1.0	1.0
(Healthy Choice) deli thin	1 slice	10	<1.0	<1.0
Oven roasted				
(Healthy Choice) deli thin	1 slice	10	<1.0	<1.0
(Healthy Choice) 97% fat-free	1-oz slice	30	<1.0	1.0
(Healthy Deli)	1 oz	26	0.4	0.2
(Healthy Favorites)	.4-oz slice	12	<1.0	<1.0
(Hillshire Farm) 'Deli Select'	1 oz	31	<1.0	0.2
(Longacre)	1 oz	30	1.0	1.0
(Louis Rich)	1 oz	31	1.1	0.8
(Louis Rich) 'Thin Sliced'	.4-oz slice	12	0.4	0.3
(Oscar Mayer)	.75-oz slice	23	0.5	0.5
(Oscar Mayer) 'Thin Sliced'	.4-oz slice	12	0.3	0.2
Smoked				
(Butterball) 'Cold Cuts'	1 oz	35	0.0	1.0
(Butterball) 'Turkey Variety Pak'	.75 oz	25	1.0	1.0
(Carl Buttig) 'Lean' chopped, sliced	1 oz	50	1.0	3.0
(Healthy Choice) deli thin	1 slice	10	<1.0	<1.0
(Healthy Deli) '3 lb'	1 oz	29	0.5	0.5
(Healthy Favorites)	1 slice	12	<1.0	<1.0
(Hillshire Farm) 'Deli Select'	1 oz	31	<1.0	0.2
(Longacre)	1 oz	26	1.0	<1.0
(Louis Rich)	.74-oz slice	21	0.2	0.3
(Louis Rich) 'Thin Sliced'	.4-oz slice	11	0.1	0.1
(Mr. Turkey)	1 oz	31	0.3	0.7
(Oscar Mayer)	.75-oz slice	20	0.2	0.2
TURKEY HAM				
(Butterball) 'Cold Cuts'	1 oz	35	1.0	1.0
(Butterball) 'Deli Thin'	1 oz	35	1.0	1.0
(Butterball) 'Slice 'n Serve'	1 oz	35	1.0	2.0
(Longacre)	1 oz	33	0.0	1.0
(Longacre) lean lite 'Deli'	1 oz	37	0.0	2.0
(Louis Rich) cured	1 oz	25	0.6	0.7
Chopped				
(Louis Rich)	1 oz	46	0.2	2.8
(Louis Rich) 92% fat-free, water added	1 oz	45	<1.0	2.0
(Mr. Turkey)	1 oz	37	0.3	1.6
Chunk *(Longacre)*	1 oz	37	0.0	2.0
Honey cured				
(Butterball) 'Cold Cuts'	1 oz	35	1.0	1.0
(Butterball) 'Cold Cuts' chopped	1 oz	35	2.0	1.0

Food Name	Serv. Size	Total Cal.	Carbs GMS	Fat GMS
(Butterball) 'Slice 'n Serve'	1 oz	40	1.0	2.0
(Louis Rich) 96% fat-free	1 oz	25	<1.0	<1.0
(Mr. Turkey)	1 oz	32	0.3	1.0
(Mr. Turkey) breakfast	1 oz	33	0.4	1.3
(Mr. Turkey) buffet style	1 oz	32	0.4	1.3
(Mr. Turkey) 'Chub'	1 oz	32	0.4	1.3
Smoked				
(Louis Rich) 'Deli Thin' 96% fat-free	1 slice	15	<1.0	<1.0
(Louis Rich) 94% fat-free, water added	1 oz	35	<1.0	2.0
(Louis Rich) 'Round'	1 oz	34	0.4	1.2
(Louis Rich) 'Round' 95% fat-free, water added	1-oz slice	30	<1.0	1.0
(Louis Rich) 'Square'	.75-oz slice	24	0.3	0.7
(Louis Rich) 'Square' 96% fat-free	1-oz slice	25	<1.0	<1.0
(Louis Rich) 'Thin Sliced'	.4-oz slice	12	0.1	0.4
(Louis Rich) 'Water Added'	1 oz	33	0.4	1.4
(Norbest) roll	1 oz	31	0.5	1.1
(Norbest) thigh meat, Canadian style	1 oz	35	0.3	1.4
(Norbest) thigh meat 'Gold Label'	1 oz	27	0.3	0.7
(Norbest) thigh meat 'Tavern' 5-6 lb, whole	1 oz	27	0.3	0.8
(Norbest) thigh meat 'Tavern' 2-2.5 lb, half	1 oz	29	0.6	0.8
(OHSE)	1 oz	30	2.0	1.0
TURKEY LOAF/ROLL				
(Louis Rich)	1 oz	45	0.4	2.8
(Louis Rich) 89% fat-free	1 oz	45	<1.0	3.0
(Mr. Turkey) spiced	1 oz	51	0.5	3.6
TURKEY PASTRAMI				
(Butterball) 'Cold Cuts'	1 oz	30	0.0	1.0
(Butterball) 'Slice 'n Serve'	1 oz	35	1.0	1.0
(Longacre)	1 oz	32	0.0	1.0
(Louis Rich) 'Deli Thin' 96% fat-free	1 oz	10	<1.0	<1.0
(Louis Rich) 'Round'	1 oz	32	0.3	1.1
(Louis Rich) 'Round' 96% fat-free	1 oz	35	<1.0	1.0
(Louis Rich) 'Square'	1 oz	24	0.1	0.7
(Louis Rich) 'Square' 96% fat-free	1 oz	25	<1.0	<1.0
(Louis Rich) Thin Sliced	1 oz	11	0.1	0.4
(Mr. Turkey)	1 oz	28	0.1	0.9
(Norbest) '5-6 lb Slab'	1 oz	29	0.5	0.6
(Norbest) '3 lb'	1 oz	29	0.3	0.8
TURKEY SALAMI				
(Butterball) 'Cold Cuts'	1 oz	50	1.0	4.0
(Butterball) 'Deli/Slice 'n Serve'	1 oz	50	1.0	4.0
(Butterball) 'Turkey Variety Pak'	.75 oz	40	1.0	3.0
(Longacre)	1 oz	52	1.0	4.0

Food Name	Serv. Size	Total Cal.	Carbs GMS	Fat GMS
(Louis Rich)	1 oz	54	0.2	4.0
(Louis Rich) cotto	1 oz	53	0.3	3.8
(Louis Rich) cotto, 85% fat-free	1-oz slice	55	<1.0	4.0
(Louis Rich) 85% fat-free	1-oz slice	55	<1.0	4.0
(Mr. Turkey) cotto	1 oz	45	0.4	2.9
(Norbest) 'Blue Label' 5 lb	1 oz	46	0.5	2.9
(Norbest) 'Blue Label' 2-2.5 lb	1 oz	45	0.9	2.6
(OHSE)	1 oz	50	1.0	3.0

LUNCHEON MEAT, ALTERNATIVE

Food Name	Serv. Size	Total Cal.	Carbs GMS	Fat GMS
(Worthington) canned 'Numete' 1/2-inch slice	2.4 oz	160	6.0	11.0
(Worthington) canned 'Protose' 1/2-inch slice	2.7 oz	180	9.0	8.0

BOLOGNA TYPE

Food Name	Serv. Size	Total Cal.	Carbs GMS	Fat GMS
(Worthington) frozen 'Bolono' approx .65-oz slices	2 slices	60	2.0	2.0

SALAMI TYPE

Food Name	Serv. Size	Total Cal.	Carbs GMS	Fat GMS
(Worthington) frozen, roll, approx 1.5-oz slices	2 slices	90	3.0	5.0
(Worthington) frozen, sliced, approx 1.3-oz slices	2 slices	80	3.0	4.0

LUNCHEON MEAT, CANNED. See also POTTED MEAT SPREAD; SANDWICH SPREAD.

Food Name	Serv. Size	Total Cal.	Carbs GMS	Fat GMS
(Armour) 'Treet'	2 oz	200	3.0	17.0
(Armour) 'Treet' low salt	2 oz	190	3.0	16.0
(Spam)	1 oz	86	<2.0	8.0
(Spam) less salt	2 oz	176	1.0	15.0
(Spam) lite	2 oz	140	1.0	12.0
(Spam) smoke flavored	2 oz	170	0.0	15.0
(Spam) w/cheese chunks	2 oz	170	0.0	16.0

LUNCHEON MEAT COMBINATIONS, PACKAGED

(Eckrich) 'Lunch Makers'

Food Name	Serv. Size	Total Cal.	Carbs GMS	Fat GMS
ham/Swiss cheese/crackers	1 pc each	40	2.0	2.0
turkey/cheddar cheese/crackers	1 pc each	40	2.0	2.0

(Hillshire Farms) 'Lunch 'n Munch'

Food Name	Serv. Size	Total Cal.	Carbs GMS	Fat GMS
bologna/American cheese/crackers/Snickers	4.25 oz	490	31.0	34.0
bologna/American cheese/crackers/Snickers/6-oz drink	4.25 oz	590	55.0	34.0
chicken/Monterey jack cheese/crackers/Snickers	4.25 oz	400	31.0	23.0
ham/cheddar cheese/crackers/Snickers	4.25 oz	400	32.0	23.0
ham/cheddar cheese/crackers/Snickers/6-oz drink	4.25 oz	500	56.0	23.0
ham/Swiss cheese/crackers/Oreo	4.1 oz	370	30.0	21.0
turkey/cheddar cheese/crackers/brownie	4.5 oz	400	34.0	22.0

(Louis Rich) 'Lunch Breaks'

Food Name	Serv. Size	Total Cal.	Carbs GMS	Fat GMS
turkey/cheddar cheese	1 pkg	410	23.0	26.0
turkey/Monterey jack cheese	1 pkg	400	27.0	25.0
turkey ham/Swiss cheese	1 pkg	380	25.0	22.0
turkey salami/cheddar cheese	1 pkg	430	25.0	29.0

(Oscar Mayer) 'Lunchables'

Food Name	Serv. Size	Total Cal.	Carbs GMS	Fat GMS
bologna/American cheese/crackers	4.5 oz	480	20.0	38.0

Food Name	Serv. Size	Total Cal.	Carbs GMS	Fat GMS
chicken/Monterey jack cheese/crackers/pudding	6.2 oz	380	32.0	21.0
ham/American cheese/crackers/pudding	6.2 oz	410	33.0	23.0
ham/cheddar cheese/crackers	4.5 oz	370	18.0	25.0
ham/Swiss cheese/crackers	4.5 oz	340	18.0	21.0
ham/Swiss cheese/crackers/cookie	4.2 oz	380	29.0	23.0
turkey/cheddar cheese/crackers	4.5 oz	360	19.0	22.0
turkey/cheddar cheese/crackers/trail mix	5 oz	460	41.0	26.0
turkey/ham, deluxe variety pak	5.1 oz	370	23.0	20.0
turkey/Monterey jack cheese/wheat crackers	4.5 oz	360	18.0	22.0
LUPIN, mature seeds				
boiled	4 oz	135	11.2	3.3
boiled	1/2 cup	99	8.2	2.4
raw	1/2 cup	334	36.3	8.8
raw	1 oz	105	11.4	2.8

LYCHEE. See LITCHI.

M

Food Name	Serv. Size	Total Cal.	Carbs GMS	Fat GMS
MACADAMIA NUT/bushnut				
in shell	1 lb	987	19.3	103.7
shelled	1 cup	941	18.4	98.8
shelled	1 oz	199	3.9	20.9
shelled, oil roasted, chopped	1 cup	790	14.2	84.2
shelled, oil roasted, kernels, 10-12	1 oz	204	3.7	21.7
shelled, oil roasted, whole or halves	1 cup	962	17.3	102.5
shelled, w/salt *(Maunu Loa)*	1 oz	210	4.0	21.0
MACADAMIA NUT BUTTER, roasted *(Maranatha Natural)*	2 tbsp	200	6.0	19.0
MACARONI. See PASTA.				
MACARONI ENTRÉE, CANNED				
(Chef Boyardee) shells	7.5 oz	150	31.0	1.0
(Heinz)	7.5 oz	190	26.0	8.0
W/BEEF, IN TOMATO SAUCE				
(Heinz)	7.5 oz	200	23.0	8.0
(Pathmark) 'No Frills'	7.5 oz	200	22.0	8.0
W/CHEESE				
(Chef Boyardee)	7.5 oz	170	33.0	2.0
(Franco-American)	7 3/8 oz	170	24.0	6.0
Shells w/cheddar *(Lipton)* 'Hearty Ones'	11 oz	367	60.0	7.4
MACARONI ENTRÉE, FROZEN				
W/BEEF				
(Swanson)	12 oz	370	48.0	15.0

Food Name	Serv. Size	Total Cal.	Carbs GMS	Fat GMS
(Weight Watchers)	9 oz	220	31.0	4.0
In tomato sauce (Lean Cuisine)	10 oz	250	35.0	6.0
W/tomatoes (Stouffer's)	11.5-oz pkg	340	38.0	12.0
W/CHEESE				
(Banquet)	10 oz	420	46.0	20.0
(Banquet) 'Casserole'	8 oz	350	36.0	17.0
(Banquet) 'Family Entrees'	8 oz	290	32.0	13.0
(Budget Gourmet) 'Side Dish'	5.3 oz	210	23.0	8.0
(Freezer Queen) 'Family Side Dish'	4 oz	110	19.0	2.0
(Green Giant)	5.7 oz	220	27.0	8.0
(Green Giant) 'One Serving'	5.7 oz	230	28.0	9.0
(Healthy Choice)	9 oz	280	45.0	6.0
(Healthy Choice)	8.5 oz	260	42.0	5.0
(Kid Cuisine) 'Mega Meal'	12.45 oz	470	75.0	13.0
(Lean Cuisine)	9 oz	290	37.0	9.0
(Myers)	3.5 oz	168	16.0	9.0
(Stouffer's) 76-oz pkg	9.5 oz	440	39.0	24.0
(Stouffer's) 12-oz pkg	6 oz	250	23.0	13.0
(Swanson)	12.25 oz	370	43.0	15.0
(Swanson) 'Homestyle Recipe'	10 oz	390	37.0	19.0
Casserole (Morton)	6.5 oz	290	30.0	14.0
Organic (Amy's Kitchen)	9 oz	452	58.0	18.0
Pot pie (Swanson)	7 oz	200	24.0	8.0
W/broccoli (Lean Cuisine) 'Lunch Express'	9.75 oz	240	32.0	7.0
W/cheddar and parmesan cheese (Budget Gourmet) 'Light & Healthy'	10.5 oz	330	49.0	8.0
W/mini franks (Kid Cuisine)	9 oz	380	55.0	14.0
W/soy cheese, organic (Amy's Kitchen)	9 oz	380	42.0	14.0
W/three cheeses (Weight Watchers)	9 oz	280	43.0	6.0
MACARONI ENTRÉE, MICROWAVE				
W/BEEF				
(Chef Boyardee) 'Beefaroni'	7.5 oz	220	31.0	7.0
(Chef Boyardee) elbows in sauce	7.5 oz	210	29.0	7.0
(Kid's Kitchen) microwave cup	7.5 oz	200	25.0	6.0
(Nalley's)	7.5 oz	180	29.0	3.0
W/CHEESE				
(Chef Boyardee)	7.5 oz	180	27.0	5.0
(Hormel) micro cup	7.5 oz	189	26.0	6.0
(Kid's Kitchen) microwave cup	7.5 oz	260	28.0	11.0
(Libby's) 'Diner' microwave cup	7.5 oz	360	27.0	22.0
(Lunch Bucket) microwave cup	7.5 oz	210	24.0	9.0
MACARONI ENTRÉE, PACKAGED				
(Ultra Slim Fast) w/cheese sauce, prepared	1 cup	230	46.0	3.0

Food Name	Serv. Size	Total Cal.	Carbs GMS	Fat GMS
MACARONI ENTRÉE MIX				
(Kraft) 'Dinner' spirals, prepared	3/4 cup	340	36.0	18.0
MEXICAN STYLE				
(Velveeta) 'Touch of Mexico' shells, prepared	1/2 cup	210	27.0	8.0
W/CHEDDAR				
(Fantastic Foods) 'Traditional' prepared	1/2 cup	112	19.0	2.0
(Golden Grain) dry mix	1.81 oz	190	35.6	2.1
(Golden Grain) prepared	1 serving	310	36.0	15.0
W/CHEESE				
(Kraft) 'Deluxe Dinner' prepared	3/4 cup	260	36.0	8.0
(Kraft) 'Dinner' prepared	3/4 cup	290	34.0	13.0
(Kraft) 'Dinomac Dinner' prepared	3/4 cup	310	36.0	14.0
(Kraft) 'Family Size Dinner' prepared	3/4 cup	290	34.0	13.0
(Kraft) 'Teddy Bears Dinner' prepared	3/4 cup	310	36.0	14.0
(Kraft) 'Wild Wheels Dinner' prepared	3/4 cup	310	36.0	14.0
(Velveeta) 'Bits of Bacon' shells, w/bacon, prepared	1/2 cup	240	27.0	10.0
(Velveeta) shells, prepared	1/2 cup	210	25.0	8.0
W/CURRY				
(Tofu Classics) 'Shells 'n Curry' prepared w/tofu	1/2 cup	103	15.0	3.0
(Tofu Classics) 'Shells 'n Curry' prepared w/tofu and salted butter	1/2 cup	143	15.0	7.0
W/PARMESAN AND HERBS				
(Fantastic Foods) prepared w/whole milk	1/2 cup	109	19.0	2.0
MACE				
ground	1 oz	135	14.3	9.2
ground	1 tbsp	25	2.7	1.7
ground	1 tsp	8	0.9	0.6
ground *(Durkee)*	1 tsp	10	0.0	<0.1
ground *(Laurel Leaf)*	1 tsp	10	0.0	<0.1
ground *(Spice Islands)*	1 tsp	10	0.8	0.7
MACKEREL				
ATLANTIC				
baked	4 oz	297	0.0	20.2
broiled	4 oz	297	0.0	20.2
dry-heat cooked	3 oz	223	0.0	15.1
microwaved	4 oz	297	0.0	20.2
raw	1 lb	929	0.0	63.0
raw	3 oz	174	0.0	11.8
raw	1 oz	58	0.0	3.9
JACK, mixed species				
canned, drained	1 cup	296	0.0	12.0
canned, drained	4 oz	177	0.0	7.1
dry-heat cooked	3 oz	171	0.0	8.6

Food Name	Serv. Size	Total Cal.	Carbs GMS	Fa GM
raw	1 lb	712	0.0	35.
raw	3 oz	134	0.0	6.
raw	1 oz	45	0.0	2.
KING				
dry-heat cooked	3 oz	114	0.0	2.
raw	1 lb	475	0.0	9.
raw	3 oz	89	0.0	1.
raw	1 oz	30	0.0	0.
PACIFIC, mixed species				
dry-heat cooked	3 oz	171	0.0	8.
raw	1 lb	712	0.0	35.
raw	3 oz	134	0.0	6.
raw	1 oz	45	0.0	2.
SPANISH				
baked	5.1-oz fillet	230	0.0	9.
baked	4 oz	179	0.0	7.
broiled	5.1-oz fillet	230	0.0	9.
broiled	4 oz	179	0.0	7.
dry-heat cooked	3 oz	134	0.0	5.
microwaved	5.1-oz fillet	230	0.0	9.
microwaved	4 oz	179	0.0	7.
raw	1 lb	631	0.0	28.
raw	3 oz	118	0.0	5.
raw	1 oz	39	0.0	1.
MAHI MAHI/dolphin fish				
dry-heat cooked	3 oz	93	0.0	0.
raw	1 lb	387	0.0	3.
raw	3 oz	72	0.0	0.
raw	1 oz	24	0.0	0.
Fillet portions *(Peter Pan Seafoods)* raw	3.5 oz	85	na	0.
MALACCA APPLE, w/o seeds	1 oz	9	2.3	<
MALT, DRY	1 oz	103	21.7	0.
MALT EXTRACT, DRIED	1 oz	103	25.0	0.
MALT LIQUOR. See ALCOHOLIC BEVERAGES.				
MALT SYRUP				
	1 cup	1221	273.8	0.
	1 tbsp	76	17.1	0.
MALTED MILK DRINK MIX. See also BREAKFAST DRINK MIX, INSTANT.				
CHOCOLATE FLAVOR				
	1 oz	106	24.9	1.
w/added nutrients	1 oz	101	23.9	1.
w/added nutrients	4-5 heap tsp	75	17.7	0.
(Carnation)	3 heap tsp	80	18.0	0.

Food Name	Serv. Size	Total Cal.	Carbs GMS	Fat GMS
(Kraft) 'Instant'	3 tsp	90	18.0	1.0
NATURAL FLAVOR				
	1 oz	117	21.5	2.2
w/added nutrients	1 oz	109	23.0	0.8
w/added nutrients	4-5 heap tsp	80	17.0	0.6
w/o added nutrients	3/4 oz	87	15.9	1.7
(Carnation) 'Original'	3 heap tsp	90	15.0	1.8
(Kraft) 'Instant'	3 tsp	90	16.0	2.0
MAMMY APPLE				
peeled, w/o seeds	1 oz	14	3.5	0.1
raw	3 1/2 oz	51	12.5	0.5
raw, trimmed, approx 3.1 lb	1 med	431	105.8	4.2
raw, untrimmed	1 lb	139	34.0	1.4
MANDARIN ORANGE				
fresh, whole, approx 2 3/8-inch diam, 4.1 oz	1 med	37	9.4	0.2
peeled, w/o seeds	1 oz	12	3.2	0.1
sections, w/o membrane	1/2 cup	43	10.9	0.2
untrimmed	1 lb	144	36.6	0.6
MANDARIN ORANGE, CANNED *(Dole)* sections	1/2 cup	70	19.0	<1.0
MANDARIN ORANGE DRINK				
w/papaya *(Tropicana)* 'Twister'	6 oz	90	21.0	<1.0
MANGO				
peeled, w/o seed	1 oz	18	4.8	0.1
raw, sliced	1 cup	107	28.1	0.5
raw, trimmed, approx 10.6 oz	1 med	135	35.2	0.6
raw, untrimmed	1 lb	204	53.2	0.9
sliced, chilled, in jar *(Sun Fresh)*	3.5 oz	89	21.0	0.3
MANGO DRINK				
(Arizona) 'Mucho Mango Cowboy Cocktail'	8 oz	100	27.0	0.0
(Kern's) nectar, canned or bottled	6 oz	100	28.0	0.0
(Libby's) nectar, canned or bottled	6 oz	110	26.0	0.0
MANGO FLAVOR DRINK MIX *(Tang)* prepared	6 oz	80	20.0	0.0
MANGO-PEACH JUICE *(Knudsen & Sons)*	8 oz	110	29.0	0.0
MANHATTAN. See ALCOHOLIC BEVERAGES.				
MANICOTTI ENTRÉE, FROZEN				
(Budget Gourmet) cheese, w/meat sauce	10 oz	450	33.0	26.0
(Buitoni) 'Single Serving'	9 oz	470	45.0	14.0
(Celentano)	8 oz	300	36.0	11.0
(Celentano) cheese, w/sauce	10 oz	380	45.0	14.0
(Celentano) cheese, w/sauce	7 oz	360	35.0	16.0
(Celentano) low-fat, 'Great Choice'	10 oz	250	41.0	3.0
(Healthy Choice) cheese	9.25 oz	220	34.0	3.0
(Le Menu) three cheese	11.75 oz	390	44.0	15.0

Food Name	Serv. Size	Total Cal.	Carbs GMS	Fat GMS
(Legume) cheese, w/spinach, tofu, and sauce	11 oz	260	30.0	7.0
(Legume) cheese, w/tofu and sauce, 'Classic'	8 oz	220	24.0	11.0
(Weight Watchers) cheese	9.25 oz	260	31.0	8.0
MANICOTTI NOODLE. See PASTA.				
MANIOC. See CASSAVA.				
MAPLE SYRUP. See also PANCAKE SYRUP.				
	1 cup	825	211.7	0.6
	1 tbsp	52	13.4	0.0
(Knudsen & Sons) 'Fruit 'N Maple'	1 oz	105	26.0	<1.0
(Maple House) 100% pure	1 oz	100	61.0	0.0
MARGARINE				
hydrogenated and regular corn oil	1 stick	815	1.0	91.3
hydrogenated and regular corn oil	1 tsp	34	0.0	3.8
hydrogenated and regular soybean oil	1 stick	815	1.0	91.3
hydrogenated and regular soybean oil	1 tsp	34	0.0	3.8
hydrogenated safflower and soybean oil	1 stick	815	1.0	91.3
hydrogenated safflower and soybean oil	1 tsp	34	0.0	3.8
hydrogenated soybean and cottonseed oil	1 stick	815	1.0	91.3
hydrogenated soybean and cottonseed oil	1 tsp	34	0.0	3.8
(A&P)				
'Corn Oil Quarters'	1 tbsp	100	<1.0	11.0
'Premium'	1 tbsp	100	<1.0	11.0
(Ann Page) 'Quarters'	1 tbsp	100	<1.0	11.0
(Blue Bonnet) stick	1 tbsp	100	0.0	11.0
(Canoleo) 100% canola oil, all natural, dairy-free	1 tbsp	100	0.0	11.0
(Fleischmann's)				
reduced calorie, 'Diet'	1 tbsp	50	0.0	6.0
stick	1 tbsp	100	0.0	11.0
unsalted, stick	1 tbsp	100	0.0	11.0
(Hain)				
safflower oil	1 tbsp	100	0.0	11.0
safflower oil, unsalted	1 tbsp	100	0.0	11.0
(Hollywood)				
safflower oil	1 tbsp	100	0.0	11.0
safflower oil, unsalted	1 tbsp	100	0.0	11.0
(Imperial) reduced calorie, 'Diet'	1 tbsp	50	0.0	6.0
(Land O'Lakes)				
premium, corn oil, stick	1 tsp	35	0.0	4.0
regular, soy oil, stick	1 tsp	35	0.0	4.0
tub	1 tsp	35	0.0	4.0
(Mazola)				
reduced calorie, 'Diet'	1 tbsp	50	0.0	6.0
regular	1 tbsp	100	0.0	11.0

Food Name	Serv. Size	Total Cal.	Carbs GMS	Fat GMS
unsalted	1 tbsp	100	0.0	11.0
(Nucoa)	1 tbsp	100	0.0	11.0
(Parkay)	1 tbsp	100	0.0	11.0
(Quincy's)	1 oz	204	<1.0	22.0
(Spectrum Naturals) non-hydrogenated canola oil, 100% dairy-free	1 tbsp	94	0.0	11.0
MARGARINE, ALTERNATIVE				
hydrogenated and regular corn oil	1 cup	801	0.9	90.0
hydrogenated and regular corn oil	1 tsp	17	0.0	1.9
hydrogenated soybean and cottonseed oil	1 cup	801	0.9	90.0
hydrogenated soybean and cottonseed oil	1 tsp	17	0.0	1.9
hydrogenated soybean oil	1 cup	801	0.9	90.0
hydrogenated soybean oil	1 tsp	17	0.0	1.9
MARGARINE, SOFT				
(A&P) bowl	1 tbsp	100	<1.0	11.0
(Blue Bonnet)	1 tbsp	100	0.0	11.0
(Chiffon)				
cup	1 tbsp	90	0.0	10.0
stick	1 tbsp	100	0.0	11.0
unsalted	1 tbsp	90	0.0	10.0
(Fleischmann's)				
lightly salted	1 tbsp	100	0.0	11.0
unsalted	1 tbsp	100	0.0	11.0
(Imperial)	1 tbsp	100	0.0	11.0
(Nucoa)	1 tbsp	90	0.0	10.0
(Parkay)				
reduced calorie, 'Diet'	1 tbsp	50	0.0	6.0
regular	1 tbsp	100	0.0	11.0
'Squeezable'	1 tbsp	90	0.0	10.0
MARGARINE, WHIPPED				
(Blue Bonnet) stick	1 tbsp	70	0.0	7.0
(Chiffon)	1 tbsp	70	0.0	8.0
(Fleischmann's)				
lightly salted	1 tbsp	70	0.0	7.0
unsalted	1 tbsp	70	0.0	7.0
(Miracle Brand)				
cup	1 tbsp	60	0.0	7.0
stick	1 tbsp	70	0.0	7.0
(Parkay)				
cup	1 tbsp	70	0.0	7.0
stick	1 tbsp	70	0.0	7.0
MARGARINE SPREAD				
hydrogenated soybean and cottonseed oil, tub	1 cup	1236	0.0	139.2

Food Name	Serv. Size	Total Cal.	Carbs GMS	Fat GMs
hydrogenated soybean and cottonseed oil, tub	1 tsp	26	0.0	2.9
hydrogenated soybean and hydrogenated and regular palm oils	1 tsp	26	0.0	2.9
hydrogenated soybean and hydrogenated and regular palm oils, tub	1 cup	1236	0.0	139.2
hydrogenated soybean and palm oil, stick	1 cup	1236	0.0	139.2
hydrogenated soybean and palm oil, stick	1 tsp	26	0.0	2.9
60% corn oil margarine, 40% butter	1 stick	811	0.7	91.2
60% corn oil margarine, 40% butter	1 tsp	36	0.0	4.0
(Blue Bonnet)				
48% vegetable oil	1 tbsp	60	<1.0	6.0
75% vegetable oil	1 tbsp	90	0.0	11.0
whipped, 60% vegetable oil	1 tbsp	80	0.0	8.0
(Blue Bonnet) 'Better Blend'				
soft	1 tbsp	90	0.0	11.0
stick	1 tbsp	90	0.0	11.0
unsalted	1 tbsp	90	0.0	11.0
(Country Crock)				
'Churn Style' stick	1 tbsp	80	0.0	9.0
regular	1 tbsp	60	0.0	7.0
(Fleischmann's) 'Move Over Butter'	1 tbsp	90	0.0	10.0
(Hollywood) soft	1 tbsp	90	1.0	10.0
(Imperial) 'Light'	1 tbsp	60	0.0	6.0
(Kraft) 'Touch of Butter'				
bowl	1 tbsp	50	0.0	6.0
stick	1 tbsp	90	0.0	10.0
(Land O'Lakes) 'Country Morning Blend'				
stick	1 tsp	35	0.0	4.0
tub	1 tsp	30	0.0	3.0
unsalted, stick	1 tsp	35	0.0	4.0
unsalted, tub	1 tsp	30	0.0	3.0
(Land O'Lakes) 'Country Morning Light'				
stick	1 tsp	20	0.0	2.0
tub	1 tsp	20	0.0	2.0
(Land O'Lakes) w/sweet cream				
stick	1 tsp	30	0.0	4.0
tub	1 tsp	25	0.0	3.0
unsalted	1 tsp	30	0.0	4.0
(Mazola) 'Corn Oil Light'	1 tbsp	50	0.0	6.0
(Nucoa) 'Heart Beat'				
regular	1 tbsp	25	0.0	3.0
unsalted	1 tbsp	24	0.0	3.0
(P&Q) 60% vegetable oil, stick	1 tbsp	80	<1.0	8.0

Food Name	Serv. Size	Total Cal.	Carbs GMS	Fat GMS
(Parkay) 50% vegetable oil	1 tbsp	60	0.0	7.0
(Promise)				
'Extra Light'	1 tbsp	50	0.0	6.0
regular	1 tbsp	90	0.0	10.0
'Ultra' fat-free	1 tbsp	5	0.0	0.0
'Ultra' w/canola oil	1 tbsp	35	0.0	4.0
(Shedd's Spread) 52% vegetable oil	1 tbsp	60	0.0	7.0
(Van Den Bergh Foods) 'I Can't Believe It's Not Butter'				
light	1 tbsp	60	0.0	7.0
regular	1 tbsp	90	0.0	10.0
(Weight Watchers)				
'Country Cottage Farms' extra light, sweet, unsalted	1 tbsp	50	0.0	6.0
'Country Cottage Farms' extra light, tub	1 tbsp	45	2.0	4.0
'Country Cottage Farms' light	1 tbsp	50	0.0	6.0
light, stick	1 tbsp	60	0.0	7.0

MARGARITA. See ALCOHOLIC BEVERAGES.

MARINADE. See individual listings.

MARJORAM

dried	1 oz	77	17.2	2.0
dried	1 tbsp	5	1.0	0.1
dried	1 tsp	2	0.4	0.0
dried *(Durkee)*	1 tsp	2	0.0	tr
dried *(Laurel Leaf)*	1 tsp	2	0.0	tr
dried *(Spice Islands)*	1 tsp	4	0.7	0.1

MARMALADE, ORANGE

(Finast)	2 tsp	35	9.0	0.0
(Knott's Berry Farm) light, w/NutraSweet	1 tsp	8	2.0	0.0
(Knudsen & Sons)	2 tsp	35	8.0	<1.0
(Smucker's)	1 tsp	18	4.0	0.0
(Smucker's) low-sugar	1 tsp	8	2.0	0.0
(Smucker's) 'Simply Fruit'	1 tsp	16	4.0	0.0
(Smucker's) sweet, natural ingredients	1 tsp	18	4.0	0.0

MARMALADE PLUM. See SAPOTE.

MARROW BEAN

boiled	4 oz	158	28.5	0.4
boiled	1/2 cup	125	22.5	0.3
raw	1/2 cup	337	60.9	0.9
raw	1 oz	94	17.1	0.2
small, boiled	4 oz	161	29.3	0.7
small, boiled	1/2 cup	127	23.2	0.6
small, raw	1/2 cup	363	67.2	1.3
small, raw	1 oz	95	17.6	0.3

MARROW SQUASH. See SQUASH, MARROW.

Food Name	Serv. Size	Total Cal.	Carbs GMS	Fc GM
MARSHMALLOW				
(Campfire) large	2 pieces	40	10.0	0.
(FunMallows)	1 piece	30	7.0	0.
(FunMallows) miniature	10 pieces	18	5.0	0.
(Kraft) 'Jet Puffed'	1 piece	25	6.0	0.
(Kraft) miniature	10 pieces	18	5.0	0.
MARSHMALLOW CREME TOPPING				
(Finast)	1 oz	95	23.0	0.
(Kraft)	1 oz	90	23.0	0.
(Marshmallow Fluff)	1 tsp	59	15.0	0.
(Smucker's)	2 tbsp	120	29.0	0.
MARTINI. See ALCOHOLIC BEVERAGES.				
MASA HARINA. See CORN FLOUR.				
MATAI. See WATER CHESTNUT, CHINESE.				
MATZO. See cracker.				
MAYONNAISE				
(Bama)	1 tbsp	100	0.0	11.
(Bennett's) 'Real'	1 tbsp	110	1.0	12.
(Best Foods)	1 tbsp	100	0.0	11.
(Cains)	1 tbsp	100	0.0	11.0
(Finast)	1 tbsp	100	0.0	11.
(Hain) cold processed	1 tbsp	110	0.0	12.
(Hellmann's)	1 tbsp	100	0.0	11.
(Hollywood)	1 tbsp	110	0.0	12.0
(Kraft) 'Real'	1 tbsp	100	0.0	12.
(Pathmark)	1 tbsp	100	0.0	11.
(Pathmark) 'No Frills'	1 tbsp	100	0.0	11.0
(Rokeach)	1 tbsp	100	0.0	11.0
(Westbrae)	1 tbsp	100	0.0	11.0
CANOLA				
(Hain)	1 tbsp	100	<1.0	11.0
(Hollywood)	1 tbsp	100	<1.0	11.0
(Spectrum Naturals)	1 tbsp	100	0.0	12.0
(Spectrum Naturals) 'Lite Mayo'	1 tbsp	35	1.0	3.0
(Westbrae)	1 tbsp	100	0.0	11.0
LOW-SODIUM				
(Hain) 'Real No Salt Added'	1 tbsp	110	0.0	12.0
(Weight Watchers) 'Low Sodium'	1 tbsp	50	1.0	5.0
REDUCED CALORIE				
(Best Foods) 'Light'	1 tbsp	50	1.0	5.0
(Estee)	1 tbsp	50	1.0	5.0
(Featherweight)	1 tbsp	30	3.0	2.0
(Finast) 'Lite'	1 tbsp	40	1.0	4.0

Food Name	Serv. Size	Total Cal.	Carbs GMS	Fat GMS
(Hain) 'Light Low Sodium'	1 tbsp	60	2.0	6.0
(Hellmann's) 'Light'	1 tbsp	50	1.0	5.0
(Janet Lee) 'Light'	1 tbsp	50	1.0	5.0
(Kraft) 'Light'	1 tbsp	50	1.0	5.0
(Pathmark)	1 tbsp	40	1.0	4.0
(Smart Beat) 'Golden Corn Light'	1 tbsp	40	1.0	4.0
(Weight Watchers) 'Light'	1 tbsp	50	1.0	5.0
SAFFLOWER				
(Hain)	1 tbsp	110	0.0	12.0
(Hollywood)	1 tbsp	100	0.0	12.0
SAFFLOWER AND SOYBEAN	1 tbsp	99	0.4	11.0
SOYBEAN				
	1 tbsp	99	0.4	11.0
(Featherweight) 'Soyamaise'	1 tbsp	100	0.0	11.0
MAYONNAISE, ALTERNATIVE				
(Best Foods) 'Cholesterol Free'	1 tbsp	50	1.0	5.0
(Hain) 'Eggless No Salt Added'	1 tbsp	110	0.0	12.0
(Hellman's) 'Cholesterol Free'	1 tbsp	50	1.0	5.0
(Kraft) 'Free'	1 tbsp	8	3.0	0.0
(Nucoa) 'Heart Beat'	1 tbsp	40	1.0	4.0
(Weight Watchers) 'Cholesterol Free'	1 tbsp	50	1.0	5.0
CANOLA *(Hain)* reduced calorie	1 tbsp	60	2.0	5.0
MILK CREAM	1 tbsp	15	1.7	0.8
SOYBEAN	1 tbsp	35	2.4	2.9
SUNFLOWER *(Life)* 'All Natural'	1 tbsp	71	1.0	8.0
TOFU *(Nasoya)* 'Nayonaise'	1 tbsp	40	1.0	4.0
MEAT. See individual listings.				
MEAT, ALTERNATIVE. See also individual listings.				
chops *(Worthington)* 'Choplets' canned	2 slices	100	5.0	2.0
cutlet *(Worthington)* 'Multigrain' canned	2 slices	90	6.0	1.0
unflavored *(Heartline)* lite	.5 oz	22	1.0	0.0
MEAT EXTENDER				
soybean	1 cup	275	33.7	2.6
soybean	1 oz	88	10.7	0.8
MEAT LOAF ENTRÉE, FROZEN				
(Armour) 'Classics'	11.25 oz	360	32.0	17.0
(Banquet)	11 oz	440	27.0	27.0
(Banquet) 'Cookin' Bags'	4 oz	200	8.0	14.0
(Freezer Queen)	10 oz	350	26.0	19.0
(Freezer Queen) 'Family Suppers' w/tomato sauce	7 oz	230	15.0	13.0
(Healthy Choice) low-fat, low-cholesterol	12 oz	340	48.0	8.0
(Lean Cuisine) w/macaroni and cheese	9 3/8 oz	280	26.0	8.0
(Morton)	10 oz	310	26.0	17.0

Food Name	Serv. Size	Total Cal.	Carbs GMS	Fat GMS
(Stouffer's) homestyle, in gravy, w/whipped potatoes	9 7/8 oz	370	25.0	20.0
(Swanson)	10.75 oz	360	41.0	15.0
MEAT LOAF ENTRÉE, PACKAGED				
(Dinty Moore) 'American Classics' w/mashed potatoes				
and gravy	10 oz	262	26.0	9.0
(Ultra Slim Fast) w/tomato sauce	10.5 oz	340	52.0	9.0
MEAT LOAF MIX				
(Hunt's) 'Meatloaf Fixins'	2.222 oz	23	3.9	0.4
(Lipton) 'Microeasy' homestyle	1/4 pkg	90	15.0	1.0
MEAT LOAF MIX, ALTERNATIVE				
(Natural) 'Touch Loaf Mix' vegetarian	4 oz	180	7.0	7.0
MEAT LOAF SEASONING				
(French's)	1/8 pkg	20	5.0	0.0
(Lawry's) 'Seasoning Blends'	1 pkg	355	64.5	1.2
(Schilling) 'Bag 'n Season'	1 pkg	111	26.0	0.7
MEAT MARINADE MIX *(French's)*	1/8 pkg	10	2.0	0.0
MEAT STICKS				
smoked	1 oz	156	1.5	14.1
smoked	1 stick	109	1.1	9.8
MEAT TENDERIZER				
(Tone's) seasoned	1 tsp	7	1.2	0.2
(Tone's) unseasoned	1 tsp	7	1.2	0.2
MEATBALL, ALTERNATIVE				
vegetarian *(Worthington)* 'Non-Meat Balls'	3 pieces	100	4.0	6.0
MEATBALL ENTRÉE				
Canned, stew				
(Chef Boyardee)	8 oz	350	24.0	24.0
(Dinty Moore)	8 oz	240	14.0	16.0
Frozen, BBQ homestyle *(Banquet)* 'Healthy Balance'	10.25 oz	270	43.0	5.0
Microwave *(Dinty Moore)* microwave cup	7.5 oz	240	14.0	16.0
MEATBALL SEASONING *(French's)* dry mix	1/4 pkg	35	7.0	0.0
MELBA TOAST. See CRACKER.				
MELON. See individual listings.				
MELON, BITTER. See BALSAM PEAR.				
MELON BALLS, FROZEN				
cantaloupe and honeydew	1 lb	144	36.0	1.1
cantaloupe and honeydew	1 cup	57	13.7	0.4
cantaloupe and honeydew	1 oz	9	2.3	0.1
MENUDO MIX				
(Gebhardt)	1 tsp	5	1.0	<1.0
(Gebhardt) spice	.0141 oz	1	0.1	0.0
MESQUITE MARINADE *(Lawry's)*	2 tbsp	24	3.0	0.4
MESQUITE SEASONING *(Tone's)*	1 tsp	13	3.2	<.1

Food Name	Serv. Size	Total Cal.	Carbs GMS	Fat GMS
MEXICAN FOODS. See individual listings.				
MEXICAN POTATO. See JICAMA.				
MEXICAN SEASONING (Tone's)	1 tsp	6	1.3	0.1
MEXICAN STYLE DINNER, FROZEN. See also individual listings.				
(Banquet)	12 oz	490	62.0	18.0
(Banquet) combination	12 oz	520	72.0	17.0
(Morton)	10 oz	300	44.0	10.0
(Patio)	13.25 oz	540	64.0	25.0
(Patio) 'Fiesta'	12.25 oz	470	55.0	20.0
(Swanson) combination	14.25 oz	490	62.0	18.0
(Swanson) 'Hungry Man'	20.25 oz	820	88.0	41.0
(Van de Kamp's)	1/2 pkg	220	25.0	10.0
MILK, ALTERNATIVE. See RICE BEVERAGE; SOY BEVERAGE.				
MILK, COW'S, CANNED				
CONDENSED, SWEETENED				
	1 cup	982	166.5	26.6
(Borden)	1/3 cup	320	54.0	8.0
(Carnation)	1/3 cup	320	56.0	8.0
(Diehl) 'Jerzee'	1/3 cup	320	52.0	9.0
(Eagle)	1/2 cup	320	52.0	9.0
EVAPORATED				
	1/2 cup	169	12.6	9.5
(Carnation)	1/2 cup	170	12.0	10.0
(Diehl)	1/2 cup	170	12.0	10.0
(Finast)	1/2 cup	170	12.0	10.0
(IGA)	1/2 cup	170	12.0	10.0
(Pathmark)	1/2 cup	170	12.0	10.9
(Pet)	1/2 cup	170	12.0	10.0
Filled (Pet)	1/2 cup	150	12.0	8.0
Low-fat (Carnation)	1/2 cup	110	12.0	3.0
Skim				
	1/2 cup	100	14.5	0.3
(Carnation) 'Lite'	1/2 cup	100	14.0	<1.0
(Diehl)	1/2 cup	100	14.0	<1.0
(Finast)	1/2 cup	100	14.0	<1.0
(Pathmark)	1/2 cup	100	14.0	0.0
(Pet) 'Lite'	1/2 cup	100	14.0	<1.0
MILK, COW'S, DRY				
LOW-FAT				
(Milkman)	1/4 pkg	90	12.0	1.0
(Milkman) reconstituted	1 quart	380	48.0	5.0
SKIM				
(Alba) reconstituted	8 oz	80	13.0	0.0

Food Name	Serv. Size	Total Cal.	Carbs GMS	Fat GMS
(Carnation)	1/3 cup	80	12.0	0.0
(Lucerne)	1/3 cup	80	12.0	0.0
(Saco Foods)	5 tbsp	80	12.0	<1.0
(Sanalac) 'Dairy Fresh' reconstituted	8 oz	80	12.0	0.1
(Sanalac) reconstituted	9.03 oz	80	12.3	0.1
(Weight Watchers) 'Dairy Creamer'	1 pkt	10	1.0	0.0

MILK, COW'S, FLUID

WHOLE

Food Name	Serv. Size	Total Cal.	Carbs GMS	Fat GMS
(A&P)	1 cup	150	11.0	8.0
(Borden)	1 cup	150	11.0	8.0
(Borden) 'Hi-Calcium'	1 cup	150	11.0	8.0
(Carnation)	1 cup	150	12.0	8.0
(Crowley)	1 cup	150	11.0	8.0
(Darigold)	1 cup	150	11.0	8.0
(Knudsen)	1 cup	160	12.0	8.0
Low-sodium	1 cup	149	10.9	8.4
3.7% fat	1 cup	157	11.4	8.9
3.3% fat	1 cup	150	11.4	8.1

2% FAT

Food Name	Serv. Size	Total Cal.	Carbs GMS	Fat GMS
	1 cup	121	11.7	4.7
Protein-fortified				
	1 cup	137	13.5	4.9
(A&P)	1 cup	120	12.0	5.0
(Borden) 'Hi-Protein'	1 cup	140	13.0	5.0
(Crowley) 'Tone Acidophilus'	1 cup	120	11.0	5.0
(Darigold) 'Nutrish Acidophilus'	1 cup	120	11.0	5.0
(Finast)	1 cup	130	12.0	5.0
(Knudsen) 'Sweet Acidophilus'	1 cup	140	13.0	5.0
(Viva)	1 cup	120	11.0	5.0
W/non-fat milk solids added	1 cup	125	12.2	4.7

1% FAT

Food Name	Serv. Size	Total Cal.	Carbs GMS	Fat GMS
	1 cup	102	11.7	2.6
(Crowley)	1 cup	100	11.0	2.0
Protein-fortified				
	1 cup	119	13.6	2.9
(A&P)	1 cup	100	12.0	3.0
(Borden)	1 cup	100	11.0	2.0
(Crowley)	1 cup	120	14.0	2.0
(Crowley) 'Lactaid'	1 cup	100	11.0	2.0
(Darigold)	1 cup	100	13.0	2.0
(Knudsen) 'Nice n' Light'	1 cup	130	15.0	3.0
W/calcium added *(Darigold)*	1 cup	100	11.0	2.0
W/non-fat milk solids added	1 cup	104	12.2	2.4

Food Name	Serv. Size	Total Cal.	Carbs GMS	Fat GMS
SKIM				
....	1 cup	86	11.9	0.4
Protein-fortified				
(A&P)	1 cup	90	12.0	<1.0
(Borden)	1 cup	90	12.0	1.0
(Borden) 'Skim-Line'	1 cup	100	13.0	1.0
(Crowley)	1 cup	90	12.0	<1.0
(Darigold) 'Trim'	1 cup	80	11.0	1.0
(Knudsen)	1 cup	80	12.0	(mq)
(Weight Watchers)	1 cup	90	13.0	<1.0
W/non-fat milk solids added	1 cup	90	12.3	0.6
W/vitamin A added	1 cup	86	11.9	0.4
MILK, GOAT'S				
evaporated *(Meyenberg)* canned, undiluted	4 oz	143	10.0	7.9
fluid, whole	1 cup	168	10.9	10.1
fluid, whole	1 oz	20	1.3	1.2
MILK, HUMAN				
fluid, whole	1 cup	171	17.0	10.8
fluid, whole	1 oz	21	2.1	1.4
fluid, whole	1 tbsp	11	1.1	0.7
MILK, INDIA BUFFALO				
fluid, whole	1 cup	236	12.6	16.8
fluid, whole	1 oz	27	1.5	2.0
MILK, LACTOSE-REDUCED				
2% FAT				
(Lactaid) 70% lactose reduced, w/vitamins A and D	1 cup	130	12.0	5.0
(Lucerne) 70% lactose reduced, w/vitamins A and D	1 cup	120	12.0	5.0
1% FAT				
(First Alternative) lactose free	1 cup	80	6.0	2.0
SKIM				
(Lactaid) 70% lactose reduced, w/calcium and vitamins A and D	1 cup	80	13.0	0.0
(Lactaid) 70% lactose reduced, w/vitamins A and D	1 cup	80	13.0	0.0
(Lactaid 100) lactose free, w/vitamins A and D	1 cup	80	13.0	0.0
(Lucerne) 70% lactose reduced, w/vitamins A and D	1 cup	80	12.0	0.0
MILK, REINDEER	1 cup	580	10.2	48.6
MILK, SHEEP'S				
fluid, whole	1 cup	264	13.1	17.2
fluid, whole	1 oz	31	1.5	2.0
MILKFISH. See AWA.				
MILKSHAKE				
chocolate, thick	10.6 oz	356	63.5	8.1
vanilla, thick	11 oz	350	55.6	9.5

Food Name	Serv. Size	Total Cal.	Carbs GMS	Fat GMS
(MicroMagic) chocolate, frozen	11.5 oz	340	55.0	8.0
(MicroMagic) chocolate, frozen	7 oz	200	32.0	4.0
(MicroMagic) strawberry, frozen	11.5 oz	340	54.0	9.0
(MicroMagic) vanilla, frozen	11.5 oz	380	60.0	13.0
MILKSHAKE MIX				
(Alba '77) chocolate 'Fit'N' prepared	6 oz	346	56.0	2.5
(Alba '77) chocolate marshmallow 'Fit'N' prepared	6 oz	346	51.5	3.6
(Alba '77) double fudge, frosty 'Fit'N' prepared	6 oz	346	52.2	3.3
(Alba '77) strawberry 'Fit'N' prepared	6 oz	333	55.0	1.7
(Alba '77) vanilla 'Fit'N' prepared	6 oz	333	54.5	1.4
(Weight Watchers) chocolate fudge	1 pkt	70	11.0	1.0
(Weight Watchers) orange sherbet	1 pkt	70	11.0	0.0
MILLET				
pearl, cooked	1/2 cup	143	28.4	1.2
pearl, cooked	4 oz	135	26.8	1.1
pearl, raw	1/2 cup	378	72.9	4.2
pearl, raw	1 oz	107	20.7	1.2
pearl, raw, hulled *(Arrowhead Mills)*	1 oz	90	21.0	1.0
Proso/hog millet, whole grain	3 1/2 oz	327	72.9	2.9
MILLET FLOUR, whole grain *(Arrowhead Mills)*	2 oz	185	41.0	2.0
MINCEMEAT. See PIE FILLING.				
MISO				
	1/2 cup	284	38.6	8.4
	1 oz	58	7.9	1.7
w/barley malt/mugi-koji	1 oz	56	8.0	1.2
w/rice malt, dark yellow/kome-koji	1 oz	53	5.4	1.6
w/rice malt, sweet/kome-koji	1 oz	62	10.4	0.9
w/soybean malt/mame-koji	1 oz	62	3.2	3.9
(Eden Foods) barley/mugi, organic	1 tbsp	25	3.0	<1.0
(Eden Foods) brown rice/genmai, organic	1 tbsp	25	3.0	1.0
(Eden Foods) rice/shiro, organic	1 tbsp	35	5.0	1.0
(Eden Foods) soybean and rice/kome, organic	1 tbsp	25	3.0	1.0
(Eden Foods) soybean/hacho, organic	1 tbsp	35	2.0	2.0
(Westbrae) barley, pasteurized	1 tsp	12	2.0	0.0
(Westbrae) brown rice, pasteurized	1 tsp	10	2.0	0.0
(Westbrae) red, instant	.35 oz	35	3.0	1.0
(Westbrae) red, pasteurized	1 tsp	10	1.0	0.0
(Westbrae) soybean, pasteurized	1 tsp	12	1.0	0.0
(Westbrae) soybean/hacho	1 tsp	14	1.0	0.0
(Westbrae) white, instant	.35 oz	35	4.0	1.0
MOLASSES				
	1 cup	872	225.7	0.3
	1 tbsp	53	13.8	0.0

Food Name	Serv. Size	Total Cal.	Carbs GMS	Fat GMS
Barbados	1 cup	889	229.6	0.0
Barbados	1 oz	111	28.7	0.0
1st extraction/light	1 cup	827	213.2	0.0
1st extraction/light	1 oz	103	26.7	0.0
2nd extraction/medium	1 cup	761	196.8	0.0
2nd extraction/medium	1 oz	95	24.6	0.0
3rd extraction/blackstrap	1 cup	771	199.4	0.0
3rd extraction/blackstrap	1 tbsp	47	12.2	0.0
(Br'er Rabbit) dark	1 oz	110	28.0	0.0
(Br'er Rabbit) light	1 oz	110	29.0	0.0
(Grandma's) mild flavor, gold	1 tbsp	70	17.0	0.0
(Grandma's) robust flavor, green	1 tbsp	70	16.0	0.0
(LaChoy) bead	.7055 oz	52	12.5	0.0
(LaChoy) bead	1/2 tsp	7	2.0	0.0
MONKFISH/angler fish/bellyfish/frogfish/goosefish/lotte/sea devil				
dry-heat cooked	3 oz	82	0.0	1.7
raw	1 lb	343	0.0	6.9
raw	3 oz	65	0.0	1.3
raw	1 oz	22	0.0	0.4
MONOSODIUM GLUTAMATE/MSG				
flavor enhancer (Tone's) 'MSG'	1 tsp	0	0.0	0.0
MOOSE				
raw	1 lb	463	0.0	3.4
raw	1 oz	29	0.0	0.2
roasted	3 oz	114	0.0	0.8
roasted, diced	1 cup	188	0.0	1.4
MOSTACCIOLI. See PASTA.				
MOSTACCIOLI ENTRÉE				
(Banquet) frozen, w/meat sauce 'Family Entrees'	7 oz	170	28.0	3.0
MOTH BEAN				
boiled	4 oz	133	23.8	0.6
boiled	1/2 cup	103	18.4	0.5
raw	1/2 cup	336	60.3	1.6
raw	1 oz	97	17.4	0.5
MOUNTAIN YAM. See YAM.				
MOUSSE (Estee) orange chocolate	1/2 cup	70	9.0	3.0
MOUSSE, FROZEN				
(Weight Watchers) 'Sweet Celebrations' chocolate	2.5 oz	170	24.0	6.0
(Weight Watchers) 'Sweet Celebrations' praline pecan	2.75 oz	190	27.0	7.0
(Weight Watchers) 'Sweet Celebrations' triple chocolate caramel	2.75 oz	170	31.0	4.0
MOUSSE MIX				
(Jell-O) 'Rich & Luscious' chocolate, dry mix	1 pkg	110	18.0	3.0

Food Name	Serv. Size	Total Cal.	Carbs GMS	Fat GMS
(Jell-O) 'Rich & Luscious' chocolate, prepared	1/2 cup	150	21.0	6.0
(Jell-O) 'Rich & Luscious' chocolate fudge, dry mix	1 pkg	110	18.0	4.0
(Jell-O) 'Rich & Luscious' chocolate fudge, prepared	1/2 cup	140	20.0	6.0
(Weight Watchers) chocolate, prepared w/skim milk	1/2 cup	60	9.0	3.0
(Weight Watchers) chocolate cheesecake, prepared w/skim milk	1/2 cup	60	12.0	2.0
(Weight Watchers) chocolate raspberry, prepared w/skim milk	1/2 cup	60	12.0	3.0
(Weight Watchers) white chocolate almond, prepared w/skim milk	1/2 cup	60	6.0	3.0
MSG. See MONOSODIUM GLUTAMATE.				
MUFFIN. See also ENGLISH MUFFIN.				
APPLE				
(Awrey's) 1.5-oz muffin	1 muffin	130	17.0	6.0
(Awrey's) 2.5-oz muffin	1 muffin	220	30.0	10.0
(Awrey's) w/banana nut 'Grande' 4.2-oz muffin	1 muffin	260	27.0	16.0
(Hostess) w/banana walnut, mini muffin	5 muffins	160	17.0	9.0
APPLE SPICE				
(Dunkin' Donuts) 3.5-oz muffin	1 muffin	300	52.0	8.0
(Health Valley) fat-free	1 muffin	130	30.0	0.0
APPLE STREUSEL *(Awrey's)* 'Grande' 4.2-oz muffin	1 muffin	340	50.0	13.0
BANANA *(Health Valley)* fat-free	1 muffin	130	29.0	0.0
BANANA NUT				
(Break Cake) .5-oz muffin	1 muffin	60	7.0	3.0
(Dunkin' Donuts) 3.6-oz muffin	1 muffin	310	49.0	10.0
BLUEBERRY				
(Awrey's) 1.5-oz muffin	1 muffin	130	18.0	5.0
(Awrey's) 2.5-oz muffin	1 muffin	210	31.0	8.0
(Awrey's) 'Grande' 4.2-oz muffin	1 muffin	360	52.0	14.0
(Break Cake)	1 muffin	60	8.0	3.0
(Dunkin' Donuts) 3.6-oz muffin	1 muffin	280	46.0	8.0
(Entenmann's)	1 muffin	200	29.0	8.0
(Hostess) mini muffin	5 muffins	240	29.0	13.0
BLUEBERRY-APPLE *(Health Valley)* fat-free, twin pack	1 muffin	140	32.0	0.0
BRAN *(Dunkin' Donuts)* w/raisins, 3.7-oz muffin	1 muffin	310	51.0	9.0
CARROT *(Health Valley)* fat-free, twin pack	1 muffin	130	30.0	0.0
CINNAMON APPLE *(Hostess)* mini muffin	5 muffins	260	27.0	16.0
CORN				
(Awrey's) 1.5-oz muffin	1 muffin	130	20.0	5.0
(Awrey's) 2.5-oz muffin	1 muffin	220	33.0	8.0
(Dunkin' Donuts) 3.4-oz muffin	1 muffin	340	51.0	12.0
CRANBERRY *(Awrey's)* 1.5-oz muffin	1 muffin	120	20.0	4.0
CRANBERRY NUT *(Dunkin' Donuts)* 3.5-oz muffin	1 muffin	290	44.0	9.0

Food Name	Serv. Size	Total Cal.	Carbs GMS	Fat GMS
OAT BRAN				
(Awrey's) 2.75-oz muffin	1 muffin	180	27.0	7.0
(Awrey's) pineapple raisin, 2.75-oz muffin	1 muffin	180	26.0	6.0
(Dunkin' Donuts) 3.4-oz muffin	1 muffin	330	50.0	11.0
(Hostess)	1 muffin	160	21.0	7.0
(Hostess) banana nut	1 muffin	140	20.0	5.0
(Health Valley) almond and date	1 muffin	180	31.0	4.0
(Health Valley) blueberry	1 muffin	180	32.0	4.0
(Health Valley) 'Fancy Fruit Muffins' raisin	1 muffin	180	31.0	5.0
RAISIN				
(Dunkin' Donuts)	1 muffin	310	51.0	9.0
(Wonder) 'Raisin Rounds'	1 muffin	140	27.0	2.0
RAISIN BRAN				
(Awrey's) 1.5-oz muffin	1 muffin	110	18.0	4.0
(Awrey's) 2.5-oz muffin	1 muffin	190	30.0	7.0
(Awrey's) 'Grande' 4.2-oz muffin	1 muffin	320	50.0	12.0
RAISIN SPICE (Health Valley) fat-free	1 muffin	140	32.0	0.0
RASPBERRY (Health Valley) fat-free, twin pack	1 muffin	130	30.0	0.0
RICE BRAN-RAISIN (Health Valley)	1 muffin	215	35.0	7.0
SOURDOUGH (Wonder)	1 muffin	130	27.0	1.0
MUFFIN, FROZEN				
APPLE SPICE				
(Healthy Choice) 2.5-oz muffin	1 muffin	190	40.0	4.0
(Sara Lee) 2.5-oz muffin	1 muffin	220	36.0	8.0
(Weight Watchers) 'Microwave' 2.5-oz muffin	1 muffin	160	29.0	5.0
BANANA NUT				
(Healthy Choice) 2.5-oz muffin	1 muffin	180	32.0	6.0
(Weight Watchers) 'Microwave' 2.5-oz muffin	1 muffin	170	32.0	5.0
BLUEBERRY				
(Healthy Choice) 2.5-oz muffin	1 muffin	190	39.0	4.0
(Pepperidge Farm) 'Old Fashioned'	1 muffin	170	27.0	7.0
(Sara Lee) 2.5-oz muffin	1 muffin	200	34.0	8.0
(Sara Lee) 'Free & Light'	1 muffin	120	28.0	0.0
(Weight Watchers) 'Microwave' 2.5-oz muffin	1 muffin	170	32.0	5.0
CHEESE STREUSEL (Sara Lee) 2.1-oz muffin	1 muffin	220	27.0	11.0
CHOCOLATE CHUNK (Sara Lee) 2.1-oz muffin	1 muffin	220	33.0	8.0
CINNAMON SWIRL (Pepperidge Farm) 'Old Fashioned'	1 muffin	190	30.0	6.0
CORN (Pepperidge Farm) 'Old Fashioned'	1 muffin	180	27.0	7.0
HONEY BRAN				
(Sara Lee) golden, 2.5-oz muffin	1 muffin	250	31.0	13.0
(Weight Watchers) 2.5-oz muffin	1 muffin	160	32.0	4.0
OAT BRAN				
(Pepperidge Farm) apple 'Old Fashioned Cholesterol Free'	1 muffin	190	29.0	7.0

Food Name	Serv. Size	Total Cal.	Carbs GMS	Fat GMS
(Sara Lee) 2.5-oz muffin	1 muffin	210	35.0	8.0
(Sara Lee) apple, 2.5-oz muffin	1 muffin	210	35.0	8.0
RAISIN BRAN				
(Pepperidge Farm) 'Old Fashioned Cholesterol Free'	1 muffin	170	30.0	6.0
(Sara Lee) 2.5-oz muffin	1 muffin	220	37.0	7.0
MUFFIN MIX				
ALMOND *(Krusteaz)* w/poppy seed, prepared	1 muffin	160	29.0	4.0
APPLE CINNAMON				
(Betty Crocker) prepared w/egg, 2% milk	1/12 recipe	120	18.0	4.0
(Betty Crocker) prepared w/egg white, skim milk	1/12 recipe	110	18.0	3.0
(General Mills) prepared	1 muffin	100	17.0	3.0
(General Mills) prepared w/egg, 1/2 cup 2% milk	1 muffin	120	18.0	4.0
(General Mills) prepared w/egg white, skim milk	1 muffin	110	18.0	3.0
(Krusteaz) prepared	1 muffin	180	36.0	3.0
(Martha White) prepared	1/16 recipe	140	25.0	3.0
(Martha White) prepared w/2% milk	1 muffin	140	25.0	3.0
APPLE STREUSEL				
(Betty Crocker) Dutch, prepared w/egg, whole milk	1/12 recipe	200	32.0	7.0
APPLESAUCE				
(Gold Medal) 'Pouch Mix' prepared w/egg, whole milk	1/6 recipe	160	26.0	5.0
(Robin Hood) 'Pouch Mix' prepared w/egg, whole milk	1/6 recipe	160	26.0	5.0
BANANA				
(Gold Medal) 'Pouch Mix' prepared w/egg, whole milk	1/12 recipe	150	24.0	5.0
(Robin Hood) 'Pouch Mix' prepared w/egg, whole milk	1/12 recipe	150	24.0	5.0
BANANA NUT				
(Betty Crocker) prepared w/egg, 2% milk	1/12 recipe	120	17.0	5.0
(Betty Crocker) prepared w/egg white, skim milk	1/12 recipe	110	17.0	4.0
(General Mills) prepared	1 muffin	110	17.0	4.0
(General Mills) prepared w/egg, 1/3 cup 2% milk	1 muffin	120	18.0	4.0
(General Mills) prepared w/egg white, skim milk	1 muffin	120	18.0	4.0
(Martha White) prepared w/2% milk	1 muffin	180	23.0	8.0
BLACKBERRY				
(Martha White) prepared	1/6 recipe	140	25.0	3.0
(Martha White) prepared w/2% milk	1 muffin	140	25.0	3.0
BLUEBERRY				
(Betty Crocker) streusel 'Bake Shop' prepared	1/12 recipe	210	31.0	8.0
(Betty Crocker) wild blueberries, prepared w/egg, 2% milk	1/12 recipe	120	18.0	4.0
(Betty Crocker) wild blueberries, prepared w/egg white, skim milk	1/12 recipe	110	18.0	3.0
(Duncan Hines) 'Bakery Style' prepared	1 muffin	190	32.0	6.0
(Duncan Hines) prepared	1 muffin	120	21.0	3.0
(General Mills) 'Twice the Blueberries' prepared	1 muffin	100	17.0	3.0

Food Name	Serv. Size	Total Cal.	Carbs GMS	Fat GMS
(General Mills) 'Twice the Blueberries' prepared, no cholesterol recipe	1 muffin	110	18.0	3.0
(General Mills) 'Twice the Blueberries' prepared w/egg, 1/2 cup 2% milk	1 muffin	120	18.0	4.0
(Gold Medal) 'Pouch Mix' prepared w/egg, whole milk	1/6 recipe	170	26.0	6.0
(Krusteaz) prepared	1 muffin	150	27.0	4.0
(Lovin' Lites) dry mix	1/12 pkg	100	21.0	1.0
(Lovin' Lites) prepared w/egg, water	1/12 recipe	100	21.0	1.0
(Lovin' Lites) prepared w/2 egg whites, water	1/12 recipe	100	21.0	1.0
(Martha White) prepared	1/6 recipe	140	25.0	3.0
(Martha White) prepared w/2% milk	1 muffin	140	25.0	3.0
(Robin Hood) 'Pouch Mix' prepared w/egg, whole milk	1/6 recipe	170	26.0	6.0
BRAN				
(Duncan Hines) w/honey 'Bakery Style' prepared	1 muffin	200	32.0	7.0
(Martha White) prepared	1/6 recipe	150	24.0	5.0
(Martha White) prepared w/2% milk	1 muffin	150	24.0	5.0
CARAMEL				
(Gold Medal) 'Pouch Mix' prepared w/egg, whole milk	1/6 recipe	150	23.0	5.0
(Robin Hood) 'Pouch Mix' prepared w/egg, whole milk	1/6 recipe	150	23.0	5.0
CARROT NUT				
(Betty Crocker) prepared w/egg, 2% milk	1/12 recipe	150	22.0	5.0
(Betty Crocker) prepared w/egg white, skim milk	1/12 recipe	150	22.0	5.0
CHOCOLATE CHIP				
(Betty Crocker) prepared	1/12 recipe	140	22.0	5.0
(Betty Crocker) prepared w/egg, 2% milk	1/12 recipe	150	22.0	6.0
(Krusteaz) prepared	1 muffin	200	35.0	5.0
CINNAMON				
(Betty Crocker) streusel, prepared w/egg, 2% milk	1/12 recipe	200	27.0	9.0
(Duncan Hines) swirl 'Bakery Style' prepared	1 muffin	200	32.0	7.0
(General Mills) streusel, prepared	1 muffin	190	27.0	8.0
CORN				
(Arrowhead Mills) blue, prepared	1 muffin	110	15.0	4.0
(Dromedary) dry mix	3 1/2 tbsp	110	20.0	3.0
(Dromedary) prepared	1 muffin	120	20.0	4.0
(Flako) prepared	1 muffin	116	19.8	3.3
(Gold Medal) prepared w/egg, whole milk	1/6 pkg	130	24.0	2.0
(Krusteaz) prepared	1 muffin	220	36.0	7.0
(Martha White) yellow, prepared w/water	1 muffin	160	30.0	3.0
(Robin Hood) prepared w/egg, whole milk	1/6 pkg	130	24.0	2.0
CRANBERRY-ORANGE NUT				
(Duncan Hines) 'Bakery Style' prepared	1 muffin	200	30.0	8.0
HONEY BRAN				
(Gold Medal) 'Pouch Mix' prepared w/egg, whole milk	1/6 recipe	170	25.0	6.0

Food Name	Serv. Size	Total Cal.	Carbs GMS	Fat GMS
(Krusteaz) prepared	1 muffin	140	23.0	4.0
(Martha White) w/poppy seed, prepared w/2% milk	1 muffin	200	30.0	9.0
(Robin Hood) 'Pouch Mix' prepared w/egg, whole milk	1/6 recipe	170	25.0	6.0
OAT				
(Gold Medal) 'Pouch Mix' prepared w/egg, 2% milk	1/6 recipe	150	23.0	5.0
(Robin Hood) 'Pouch Mix' prepared w/egg, 2% milk	1/6 recipe	150	23.0	5.0
OAT BRAN				
(Arrowhead Mills) apple spice, prepared	1 muffin	120	15.0	4.0
(General Mills) prepared	1 muffin	170	26.0	6.0
(Krusteaz) prepared	1 muffin	190	33.0	5.0
(Hain) apple cinnamon, prepared	1 muffin	140	28.0	3.0
(Hain) banana nut, prepared	1 muffin	140	26.0	4.0
(Hain) raspberry spice, prepared	1 muffin	140	27.0	3.0
OATMEAL RAISIN				
(Arrowhead Mills) wheat-free, prepared	1 muffin	100	11.0	5.0
(Betty Crocker) prepared w/egg, 2% milk	1/8 recipe	190	25.0	8.0
(Betty Crocker) prepared w/egg white, skim milk	1/8 recipe	180	25.0	7.0
(General Mills) prepared w/egg, 1/2 cup 2% milk	1 muffin	180	26.0	7.0
(General Mills) prepared w/egg white, skim milk	1 muffin	170	26.0	6.0
ORANGEBERRY				
(Martha White) prepared	1/6 recipe	140	25.0	3.0
(Martha White) prepared w/2% milk	1 muffin	140	25.0	3.0
PECAN CRUNCH *(Duncan Hines)* 'Bakery Style' prepared	1 muffin	220	27.0	11.0
RASPBERRY				
(Martha White) prepared	1/6 recipe	140	25.0	3.0
(Martha White) prepared w/2% milk	1 muffin	140	25.0	3.0
STRAWBERRY				
(Arrowhead Mills) wheat bran, prepared	2 muffins	270	43.0	7.0
(Betty Crocker) prepared w/egg, 2% milk	1/10 recipe	150	24.0	5.0
(Betty Crocker) prepared w/egg white, skim milk	1/10 recipe	140	24.0	4.0
(Martha White) prepared	1/6 recipe	140	25.0	3.0
(Martha White) prepared w/2% milk	1 muffin	140	25.0	3.0
WILD BERRY				
(General Mills) 'Light' prepared	1 muffin	90	20.0	<1.0
(General Mills) 'Light' prepared w/egg	1 muffin	90	20.0	1.0
(General Mills) prepared	1 muffin	100	18.0	3.0
(General Mills) prepared w/egg, 1/2 cup 2% milk	1 muffin	120	19.0	4.0
(General Mills) prepared w/egg white, skim milk	1 muffin	110	19.0	3.0
MUFFIN/PASTRY, TOASTER				
APPLE				
(Kellogg's) Dutch, 'Frosted Pop-Tarts' 1.8 oz each	1 pastry	210	37.0	6.0
(Pastry Poppers) fruit juice sweetened, low-sodium, 2 oz each	1 pastry	212	38.0	5.4

Food Name	Serv. Size	Total Cal.	Carbs GMS	Fat GMS
(Pillsbury) 'Toaster Strudel'	1/6 pkg	200	26.0	9.0
(Toastettes) 'Frosted Tarts' 1.5 oz each	1 pastry	190	35.0	5.0
(Toastettes) 'Tarts' 1.5 oz each	1 pastry	190	36.0	5.0
APPLE SPICE *(Toaster)* 'Muffins'	1 muffin	130	21.0	5.0
APPLE-CINNAMON				
(Pepperidge Farm) 'Croissant Toaster Tarts'	1 pastry	170	25.0	7.0
BANANA NUT				
(Pastry Poppers) fruit juice sweetened, low-sodium,				
2 oz each	1 pastry	212	38.0	4.5
(Thomas') 'Toast-r-Cakes'	1 muffin	111	16.7	4.4
(Toaster) 'Muffins'	1 muffin	130	19.0	6.0
(Toaster) 'Strudel Breakfast Pastries'	1 pastry	190	28.0	8.0
BLUEBERRY				
(Kellogg's) 'Frosted Pop-Tarts' 1.8 oz each	1 pastry	210	37.0	6.0
(Kellogg's) 'Pop-Tarts' 1.8 oz each	1 pastry	210	37.0	6.0
(Pillsbury) 'Toaster Strudel'	1/6 pkg	190	26.0	9.0
(Thomas') 'Toast-r-Cakes'	1 muffin	108	18.0	3.3
(Toaster) 'Strudel Breakfast Pastries'	1 pastry	190	28.0	8.0
(Toaster) wild, Maine	1 muffin	120	23.0	3.0
(Toastettes) 'Frosted Tarts' 1.5 oz each	1 pastry	190	35.0	5.0
(Toastettes) 'Tarts' 1.5 oz each	1 pastry	190	35.0	5.0
BRAN *(Thomas')* 'Toast-r-Cakes'	1 muffin	103	17.6	2.9
BROWN SUGAR-CINNAMON				
(Kellogg's) 'Frosted Pop-Tarts'	1 pastry	210	34.0	7.0
(Toastettes) 'Frosted Tarts' 1.5 oz each	1 pastry	190	35.0	5.0
(Kellogg's) 'Pop-Tarts' 1.8 oz each	1 pastry	210	33.0	8.0
CHEESE *(Pepperidge Farm)* 'Croissant Toaster Tarts'	1 pastry	190	22.0	10.0
CHERRY				
(Kellogg's) 'Frosted Pop-Tarts' 1.8 oz each	1 pastry	200	37.0	5.0
(Kellogg's) 'Pop-Tarts' 1.8 oz each	1 pastry	210	37.0	6.0
(Pastry Poppers) fruit juice sweetened, low-sodium,				
2 oz each	1 pastry	212	38.0	4.5
(Toaster) 'Strudel Breakfast Pastries'	1 pastry	190	26.0	9.0
(Toastettes) 'Frosted Tarts' 1.5 oz each	1 pastry	190	35.0	5.0
(Toastettes) 'Tarts' 1.5 oz each	1 pastry	190	35.0	5.0
CHOCOLATE FUDGE				
(Kellogg's) 'Frosted Pop-Tarts' 1.8 oz each	1 pastry	200	37.0	5.0
CHOCOLATE-VANILLA CREME				
(Kellogg's) 'Frosted Pop-Tarts' 1.8 oz each	1 pastry	200	37.0	5.0
CINNAMON				
(Pillsbury) 'Toaster Strudel'	1/6 pkg	200	23.0	10.0
(Toaster) 'Strudel Breakfast Pastries'	1 pastry	190	26.0	8.0

Food Name	Serv. Size	Total Cal.	Carbs GMS	Fat GMS
CORN				
(Thomas') 'Toast-r-Cakes'	1 muffin	120	19.2	4.0
(Toaster) 'Old Fashioned Muffins'	1 muffin	120	17.0	5.0
FRUIT PUNCH (Toastettes) 'Frosted Tarts' 1.5 oz each	1 pastry	190	35.0	5.0
FUDGE (Toastettes) 'Frosted Tarts' 1.5 oz each	1 pastry	200	34.0	5.0
GRAPE (Kellogg's) 'Frosted Pop-Tarts' 1.8 oz each	1 pastry	200	37.0	5.0
OAT BRAN (Awrey's) 'Toastums' w/raisins	1 muffin	130	17.0	5.0
PEACH-APRICOT (Pastry Poppers) fruit juice sweetened, low-sodium, 2 oz each	1 pastry	212	38.0	4.5
RAISIN BRAN (Toaster) 'Muffins'	1 muffin	120	16.0	5.0
RASPBERRY				
(Kellogg's) 'Frosted Pop-Tarts' 1.8 oz each	1 pastry	200	37.0	5.0
(Pastry Poppers) fruit juice sweetened, low-sodium, 2 oz each	1 pastry	212	38.0	4.5
(Toaster) 'Strudel Breakfast Pastries'	1 pastry	190	27.0	8.0
STRAWBERRY				
(Kellogg's) 'Frosted Pop-Tarts' 1.8 oz each	1 pastry	200	37.0	5.0
(Kellogg's) 'Pop-Tarts' 1.8 oz each	1 pastry	210	37.0	6.0
(Pastry Poppers) fruit juice sweetened, low-sodium, 2 oz each	1 pastry	212	38.0	4.5
(Pepperidge Farm) 'Croissant Toaster Tarts'	1 pastry	190	28.0	7.0
(Pillsbury) 'Toaster Strudel'	1/6 pkg	190	26.0	9.0
(Toaster) 'Strudel Breakfast Pastries'	1 pastry	190	27.0	8.0
(Toastettes) 'Frosted Tarts' 1.5 oz each	1 pastry	190	35.0	5.0
(Toastettes) 'Tarts' 1.5 oz each	1 pastry	190	35.0	5.0
MULBERRY				
raw	1 lb	197	44.5	1.8
raw	1 cup	60	13.7	0.6
raw	1/2 cup	31	6.9	0.3
raw	1 oz	12	2.8	0.1
MULLANGI. See DAIKON.				
MULLET, STRIPED				
baked	4 oz	170	0.0	5.5
broiled	4 oz	170	0.0	5.5
dry-heat cooked	3 oz	127	0.0	4.1
microwaved	4 oz	170	0.0	5.5
raw	1 lb	530	0.0	17.2
raw	3 oz	99	0.0	3.2
raw	1 oz	33	0.0	1.1
MUNG BEAN				
boiled	4 oz	119	21.7	0.4
boiled	1/2 cup	106	19.3	0.4
raw	1/2 cup	361	65.1	1.2

Food Name	Serv. Size	Total Cal.	Carbs GMS	Fat GMS
raw	1 oz	98	17.8	0.3
sprouted, boiled, drained	4 oz	24	4.8	0.1
sprouted, boiled, drained	1/2 cup	13	2.6	0.1
sprouted, raw	1 lb	136	26.9	0.8
sprouted, raw	1/2 cup	16	3.1	0.1
sprouted, raw	1 oz	9	1.7	0.1
sprouted, stir-fried	4 oz	57	12.0	0.2
sprouted, stir-fried	1/2 cup	31	6.6	0.1
MUNG BEAN, CANNED				
drained	4 oz	14	2.4	0.1
sprouted *(LaChoy)*	2 oz	8	1.0	0.1
sprouted, drained	1/2 cup	7	1.3	0.0
MUNG BEAN LONG RICE				
dehydrated	1/2 cup	246	60.3	0.0
dehydrated	1 oz	99	24.4	tr
MUNGO BEAN				
boiled	1/2 cup	94	16.5	0.5
raw	1/2 cup	365	63.5	1.9
MUSHROOM, ENOKI				
raw	1 large	2	0.4	0.0
raw	1 med	1	0.2	0.0
MUSHROOM, JAPANESE HONEY/hon shimeji				
trimmed	1 lb	136	20.0	1.4
trimmed	1 oz	9	1.2	<.1
MUSHROOM, OYSTER/abalone/hiritake/shimeji/tree mushroom				
(Frieda's)	1 lb	113	20.9	1.8
(Frieda's)	1 oz	7	1.3	0.1
MUSHROOM, SHIITAKE				
cooked	4 oz	62	16.2	0.2
cooked, pieces	1 cup	80	20.7	0.3
dried	1 lb	1343	341.9	4.5
dried	1 oz	84	21.4	0.3
MUSHROOM, STRAW				
(Green Giant) canned	2 oz	12	2.0	0.0
(Green Giant) canned, whole	1/4 cup	12	2.0	0.0
MUSHROOM, WHITE				
boiled, drained	4 oz	31	5.8	0.5
boiled, drained, pieces	1/2 cup	21	4.0	0.4
raw, pieces	1/2 cup	9	1.6	0.2
raw, trimmed	1 oz	7	1.3	0.1
raw, untrimmed	1 lb	111	20.5	1.9
Canned				
drained	4 oz	27	5.6	0.3

Food Name	Serv. Size	Total Cal.	Carbs GMS	Fat GMS
pieces, drained	1/2 cup	19	3.9	0.2
(Allens) pieces and stems	1/2 cup	20	3.0	<1.0
(B In B)	1/4 cup	12	2.0	0.0
(B In B) w/garlic	1/4 cup	12	2.0	0.0
(Empress) pieces and stems	2 oz	14	2.0	na
(Green Giant) in butter sauce	1/2 cup	30	4.0	1.0
(Green Giant) whole, pieces and stems	1/4 cup	12	2.0	0.0
Frozen				
(Birds Eye) whole 'Deluxe'	2.6 oz	20	4.0	0.0
(Freshlike)	3.5 oz	30	4.0	0.0
(Green Giant) creamy 'Right for Lunch'	9.5-oz pkg	220	29.0	11.0
(Stilwell) battered 'Quick Krisp'	2 oz	140	15.0	8.0
(Veg•All)	3.5 oz	30	4.0	0.0
MUSKMELON. See CANTALOUPE.				
MUSKRAT				
raw	1 lb	735	0.0	36.7
raw	1 oz	45	0.0	2.3
roasted	3 oz	199	0.0	10.0
roasted, diced	1 cup	258	0.0	12.9
MUSSEL, BLUE				
moist-heat cooked	4 oz	195	8.4	5.1
moist-heat cooked	3 oz	146	6.3	3.8
raw	1 lb	391	16.8	10.2
raw	1 cup	129	5.5	3.4
raw	3 oz	73	3.1	1.9
MUSTARD, DRY. See MUSTARD POWDER.				
MUSTARD, PREPARED				
(Featherweight)	1 tsp	5	0.0	0.0
(French's) 'Medford'	1 tbsp	16	1.0	1.0
(Grey Poupon) 'Parisian'	1 tsp	6	0.0	0.0
(Kraft) 'Pure'	1 tbsp	11	1.0	1.0
(Life) 'English All Natural'	1 tbsp	22	<1.0	2.0
(Westbrae) 'Mt. Fuji'	1 tbsp	16	1.0	1.0
DIJON				
(French's)	1 tsp	8	0.0	1.0
(Grey Poupon)	1 tbsp	18	0.0	1.0
(Grey Poupon) 'Country Style'	1 tsp	6	0.0	0.0
(Westbrae)	1 tbsp	16	1.0	1.0
HORSERADISH				
(French's)	1 tbsp	16	1.0	1.0
(Kraft)	1 tbsp	14	1.0	1.0
JALAPEÑO (Great Impressions)	2 tsp	7	0.7	0.3
ONION (French's)	1 tsp	8	2.0	

Food Name	Serv. Size	Total Cal.	Carbs GMS	Fat GMS
SPICY				
(French's) 'Bold 'n Spicy'	1 tsp	6	0.0	0.0
(Gulden's) hot, 'Diablo'	.25 oz	8	0.0	0.0
(Gulden's) 'Spicy Brown'	.25 oz	8	0.0	0.0
(Heinz) 'Brown'	1 tbsp	14	1.0	1.0
STONE GROUND				
(Hain)	1 tbsp	14	1.0	1.0
(Hain) no salt added	1 tbsp	14	1.0	1.0
(Westbrae)	1 tbsp	16	1.0	1.0
(Westbrae) no salt added	1 tbsp	16	1.0	1.0
YELLOW				
(French's)	1 tbsp	10	1.0	1.0
(Gulden's) 'Creamy Mild'	.25 oz	6	0.0	0.0
(Heinz)	1 tsp	3	0.2	0.2
(Heinz) 'Mild'	1 tbsp	8	1.0	1.0
(Westbrae)	1 tbsp	16	1.0	1.0
MUSTARD BLEND (Best Foods) 'Dijonnaise'	1 tsp	12	1.0	1.0
MUSTARD GREENS				
boiled, drained	4 oz	17	2.4	0.3
boiled, drained, chopped	1/2 cup	10	1.5	0.2
raw, chopped	1/2 cup	7	1.4	0.1
raw, untrimmed	1 lb	109	20.7	0.8
Canned (Allens) chopped	1/2 cup	20	2.0	<1.0
Frozen				
boiled, drained	10-oz pkg	40	6.6	0.5
boiled, drained	4 oz	22	3.5	0.3
boiled, drained, chopped	1/2 cup	14	2.3	0.2
chopped	1/2 cup	15	2.5	0.2
unprepared	10-oz pkg	57	9.7	0.8
(Frosty Acres)	3.3 oz	20	3.0	0.0
(Seabrook) chopped	3.3 oz	20	3.0	0.0
(Southern) chopped	3.5 oz	25	3.6	0.3
MUSTARD OIL				
	1 cup	1927	0.0	218.0
	1 oz	251	0.0	28.4
	1 tbsp	124	0.0	14.0
MUSTARD POWDER				
ground (Durkee)	1 tsp	19	0.0	<0.1
ground (Laurel Leaf)	1 tsp	19	0.0	<0.1
ground (Spice Islands)	1 tsp	9	0.3	0.6
MUSTARD SEED, YELLOW				
whole	1 oz	133	9.9	8.2
whole	1 tbsp	53	3.9	3.2

Food Name	Serv. Size	Total Cal.	Carbs GMS	Fat GMS
whole	1 tsp	15	1.1	1.0
MUSTARD SPINACH/tendergreen				
boiled, drained	4 oz	18	3.2	0.2
boiled, drained, chopped	1/2 cup	14	2.5	0.2
raw, chopped	1/2 cup	16	2.9	0.2
raw, trimmed	1 oz	6	1.1	0.1
raw, untrimmed	1 lb	93	16.5	1.3
MUSTARD TALLOW	1 oz	256	0.0	28.4
MUTTON TALLOW				
	1 cup	1849	0.0	205.0
	1 tbsp	115	0.0	12.8

MUTTONFISH. See OCEAN POUT.

N

Food Name	Serv. Size	Total Cal.	Carbs GMS	Fat GMS
NACHO CHIPS. See CORN CHIPS AND SNACKS.				
NACHO SEASONING (Lawry's) 'Seasoning Blends'	1 pkg	141	15.0	6.8
NAPA CABBAGE. See CABBAGE, NAPA.				
NATAL PLUM. See CARISSA.				
NATTO. See SOYBEAN, FERMENTED.				
NAVY BEAN				
boiled	4 oz	161	29.8	0.6
boiled	1/2 cup	129	23.9	0.5
cooked 'Michigan #1' (A&P)	1 cup	220	40.0	1.0
raw	1/2 cup	348	63.1	1.3
raw	1 oz	95	17.2	0.4
NAVY BEAN, CANNED				
(Allens)	1/2 cup	160	24.0	<1.0
(Bush's Best)	1/2 cup	60	17.0	0.0
(Eden Foods) organic, very low sodium	1/2 cup	70	18.0	<1.0
(Hunt's) w/ham 'Homestyle'	9.03 oz	239	37.6	2.7
NAVY BEAN, SPROUTED				
boiled, drained	4 oz	88	17.0	0.9
raw	1 lb	306	59.2	3.2
raw	1/2 cup	35	6.8	0.4
raw	1 oz	19	3.7	0.2
NECTAR. See individual flavors.				
NECTARINE				
pitted	1 oz	14	3.3	0.1
sliced	1 cup	68	16.3	0.6
trimmed, approx 2.5-inch diam	1 med	67	16.0	0.6

Food Name	Serv. Size	Total Cal.	Carbs GMS	Fat GMS
untrimmed *(Dole)*	1 med	70	16.0	1.0
whole	1 lb	204	48.6	1.9

NEW ZEALAND SPINACH. See SPINACH, NEW ZEALAND.

NOODLE. See NOODLE, CHINESE; NOODLE, EGG; NOODLE, JAPANESE; PASTA.

NOODLE, CHINESE

Food Name	Serv. Size	Total Cal.	Carbs GMS	Fat GMS
cellophane, dehydrated	1 lb	1594	390.6	0.3
cellophane, dehydrated	2 oz	199	48.8	<.1
chow mein	1 cup	237	25.9	13.8
chow mein	1.5 oz	227	24.7	13.2
long rice, dehydrated	1 lb	1594	390.6	0.3
long rice, dehydrated	2 oz	199	48.8	<.1

NOODLE, EGG

(NOTE: All of the following egg noodles are dry unless otherwise noted.)

Food Name	Serv. Size	Total Cal.	Carbs GMS	Fat GMS
DUMPLING *(Creamette)* w/pasteurized eggs	2 oz	220	40.0	3.0
ENRICHED				
	2 oz	217	40.5	2.4
cooked	1 cup	213	39.7	2.3
EXTRA WIDE *(American Beauty)* enriched	2 oz	220	42.0	3.0
FINE				
(American Beauty) enriched	2 oz	220	42.0	3.0
(Herb's)	2 oz	230	40.0	2.0
JERUSALEM ARTICHOKE				
(De Boles)	2 oz	210	41.0	1.0
(De Boles) w/garlic and parsley	2 oz	210	41.0	1.0
MEDIUM *(American Beauty)* enriched	2 oz	220	42.0	3.0
PLAIN				
cooked	4 oz	151	28.2	1.7
(Creamette) enriched	2 oz	221	40.0	2.5
(Gioia)	2 oz	220	40.0	3.0
(Golden Grain)	2 oz	210	39.3	2.2
(Goodman's) 'Country Style'	2 oz	220	40.0	3.0
(Mrs. Grass)	2 oz	220	40.0	3.0
(Mueller's)	2 oz	220	40.0	3.0
(P&R)	2 oz	220	42.0	3.0
(Prince)	2 oz	210	40.0	2.0
(San Giorgio)	2 oz	220	42.0	3.0
SPINACH				
cooked	4 oz	150	27.5	1.8
enriched	1 cup	145	26.7	1.7
enriched	2 oz	218	40.1	2.6
enriched, cooked	1 cup	211	38.8	2.5
SUBSTITUTE *(No Yolks)* broad	2 oz	200	40.0	1.0

Food Name	Serv. Size	Total Cal.	Carbs GMS	Fat GMS
UNENRICHED				
....	2 oz	74	16.1	0.2
cooked	1 cup	213	39.7	2.3
VERY LOW SODIUM (Ronzoni) 'Egg Pastina'	2 oz	220	42.0	3.0
WIDE				
(American Beauty) enriched	2 oz	220	42.0	3.0
(Creamette) w/pasteurized eggs 'Fancy'	2 oz	220	40.0	3.0
(Hospitality) enriched 'Valu Pack'	1 1/4 cup	235	43.0	2.5
(Ronzoni) enriched 'Country Kitchen Style'	2 oz	220	42.0	3.0
NOODLE, JAPANESE				
GENMAI, dry (Westbrae)	2 oz	200	41.0	1.0
SOBA/BUCKWHEAT				
cooked	1 cup	113	24.4	0.1
dry	1 lb	1526	338.5	3.2
dry	2 oz	192	42.5	0.4
dry (Westbrae)	2 oz	190	40.0	2.0
SOMEN/WHEAT				
cooked	1 cup	231	48.5	0.3
cooked	4 oz	149	31.2	0.2
dry	2 oz	203	42.2	0.5
whole wheat, dry (Westbrae)	2 oz	200	41.0	1.0
TRADITIONAL, dry (Westbrae)	2 oz	190	41.0	2.0
UDON/WHEAT				
cooked	4 oz	115	23.0	0.6
dry	2 oz	159	32.3	0.7
whole wheat, organic, dry (Westbrae)	2 oz	200	41.0	1.0
NOODLE ENTRÉE/DISH				
(Dinty Moore)				
and chicken 'American Classics'	10 oz	230	24.0	7.0
tuna casserole 'American Classics'	10 oz	240	28.0	7.0
(LaChoy)				
and beef	9.03 oz	156	26.8	3.5
and chicken	8.995 oz	163	24.4	3.3
and vegetables	9.383 oz	131	26.6	1.3
chow mein	2 tbsp	140	17.0	6.1
chow mein, narrow	1/2 cup	150	16.0	8.0
chow mein, wide	1/2 cup	150	16.0	8.0
crispy, wide	2 tbsp	148	17.1	7.8
rice	1/2 cup	130	21.0	5.0
rice	2 tbsp	122	21.9	3.1
(Westbrae)				
brown rice, steamed 'Ramen'	1 oz	100	21.0	1.0
buckwheat, steamed 'Ramen'	1 oz	100	20.0	0.0

Food Name	Serv. Size	Total Cal.	Carbs GMS	Fat GMS
carrot, steamed 'Ramen'	1 oz	100	20.0	1.0
curry, steamed 'Ramen'	1 oz	100	20.0	1.0
five-spice, steamed 'Ramen'	1 oz	100	20.0	1.0
miso, steamed 'Ramen'	1 oz	100	20.0	1.0
mushroom, steamed 'Ramen'	1 oz	100	20.0	1.0
onion, steamed 'Ramen'	1 oz	100	20.0	1.0
seaweed, steamed 'Ramen'	1 oz	100	20.0	1.0
spinach, steamed 'Ramen'	1 oz	100	20.0	1.0
tofu, steamed 'Ramen'	1 oz	100	20.0	1.0
whole wheat, steamed 'Ramen'	1 oz	110	22.0	1.0
NOODLE ENTRÉE/DISH, CANNED				
(Heinz)				
and chicken	7.5 oz	160	19.0	7.0
w/beef, in sauce	7.5 oz	170	17.0	8.0
w/tuna	7.5 oz	170	20.0	5.0
(Nalley's)				
and chicken	7 3/8 oz	150	17.0	5.0
and chicken w/vegetables	7 3/8 oz	160	18.0	5.0
(Van Camp's) w/franks 'Noodle Weenee'	1 cup	245	32.9	8.5
NOODLE ENTRÉE/DISH, FREEZE-DRIED				
(Mountain House) w/chicken, prepared	1 cup	270	34.0	10.0
NOODLE ENTRÉE/DISH, FROZEN				
(Banquet)				
and beef w/gravy 'Family Entrées'	8 oz	200	22.0	7.0
and julienne beef w/sauce 'Family Entrées'	7 oz	170	22.0	3.0
w/chicken	10 oz	350	42.0	15.0
w/chicken 'Family Favorites'	10 oz	340	42.0	15.0
(Stouffer's) Romanoff	6 oz	260	23.0	14.0
(Swanson) w/chicken	10.5 oz	280	45.0	8.0
NOODLE ENTRÉE/DISH, MICROWAVE				
(Hormel) and chicken 'Micro-Cup'	7.5 oz	180	18.0	8.0
(Kid's Kitchen) rings and chicken	7.5 oz	150	17.0	4.0
(Minute)				
Alfredo, family size, prepared w/salted butter	1/2 cup	170	23.0	6.0
Alfredo, single size, prepared w/salted butter	1/2 cup	160	23.0	5.0
chicken or chicken flavor, family size, prepared	1/2 cup	160	23.0	5.0
chicken or chicken flavor, single size, prepared	1/2 cup	160	25.0	4.0
Parmesan, family size, prepared w/salted butter	1/2 cup	170	23.0	6.0
Parmesan, single size, prepared w/salted butter	1/2 cup	160	23.0	5.0
w/cheddar cheese, family size, prepared w/salted butter	1/2 cup	160	20.0	7.0
w/cheddar cheese, single size, prepared w/salted butter	1/2 cup	160	20.0	6.0

Food Name	Serv. Size	Total Cal.	Carbs GMS	Fat GMS
NOODLE ENTRÉE/DISH, MIX				
(Kraft)				
cheese 'Dinner' prepared	3/4 cup	340	37.0	17.0
chicken flavor 'Dinner' prepared	3/4 cup	240	32.0	9.0
(LaChoy)				
beef flavor 'Ramen' prepared	1 cup	225	33.0	8.0
chicken flavor 'Ramen' prepared	1 cup	200	29.0	7.0
(Lipton)				
Alfredo 'Noodles and Sauce' dry mix	1/4 pkg	150	22.0	4.0
beef 'Noodles and Sauce' dry mix	1/4 pkg	120	23.0	2.0
broccoli 'Noodles and Sauce' dry mix	1/4 pkg	130	22.0	2.0
butter 'Noodles and Sauce' dry mix	1/4 pkg	150	23.0	4.0
butter and herb 'Noodles and Sauce' dry mix	1/4 pkg	140	23.0	3.0
carbonara Alfredo 'Noodles and Sauce' dry mix	1/4 pkg	140	20.0	4.0
cheese 'Noodles and Sauce' dry mix	1/4 pkg	140	25.0	2.0
chicken flavor 'Noodles and Sauce' dry mix	1/4 pkg	130	23.0	2.0
Parmesan 'Noodles and Sauce' dry mix	1/4 pkg	140	21.0	4.0
sour cream and chives 'Noodles and Sauce' dry mix	1/4 pkg	150	24.0	3.0
Stroganoff 'Noodles and Sauce' dry mix	1/4 pkg	130	22.0	3.0
(Mueller's)				
Alfredo 'Chef's Series' prepared	1/2 cup	190	23.0	9.0
chicken flavor 'Chef's Series' prepared	1/2 cup	160	21.0	8.0
garlic and butter 'Chef's Series' prepared	1/2 cup	170	21.0	7.0
sour cream and chives 'Chef's Series' prepared	1/2 cup	190	22.0	8.0
Stroganoff 'Chef's Series' prepared	1/2 cup	190	22.0	9.0
(Noodle Roni)				
angel hair pasta, w/Parmesan cheese, prepared	1/2 cup	210	26.0	9.0
fettuccini, prepared	1/2 cup	300	29.0	18.0
garlic, creamy, prepared	1/2 cup	300	29.0	17.0
herb and butter, prepared	1/2 cup	160	19.0	7.0
mushroom, prepared	1/2 cup	160	25.0	4.0
Parmesan, prepared	1/2 cup	240	23.0	13.0
Parmesano 'Less Fat' prepared	1/2 cup	190	24.0	8.0
Romanoff, prepared	1/2 cup	240	28.0	11.0
Stroganoff, prepared	1/2 cup	350	37.0	17.0
(Ultra Slim Fast) w/Alfredo sauce, prepared	8 oz	240	47.0	4.0
NORI. See SEAWEED.				
NORWAY HADDOCK. See OCEAN PERCH, ATLANTIC.				
NUT TOPPING				
(Fisher) fancy	1 oz	170	7.0	15.0
(Fisher) oil-roasted, w/peanuts	1 oz	160	7.0	14.0
(Planters)	1 oz	180	6.0	16.0
(Smucker's) pecan, in syrup	2 tbsp	130	28.0	1.0

Food Name	Serv. Size	Total Cal.	Carbs GMS	Fat GMS
(Smucker's) walnut, in syrup	2 tbsp	130	27.0	1.0
NUTMEG				
ground	1 oz	149	14.0	10.3
ground	1 tbsp	37	3.5	2.5
ground	1 tsp	12	1.1	0.8
ground *(Durkee)*	1 tsp	12	0.0	<0.1
ground *(Laurel Leaf)*	1 tsp	12	0.0	<0.1
ground *(Spice Islands)*	1 tsp	11	0.9	0.7
NUTMEG BUTTER OIL				
	1 cup	1927	0.0	218.0
	1 oz	251	0.0	28.4
	1 tbsp	120	0.0	13.6
NUTRASWEET. See SUGAR, ALTERNATIVE.				
NUTS, MIXED				
(Guy's) w/peanuts	1 oz	170	3.0	14.0
(Planters) 'Select Mix' cashews, almonds, and peanuts	1 oz	170	7.0	14.0
(Planters) 'Select Mix' cashews, almonds, and pecans	1 oz	180	6.0	16.0
(Planters) 'Select Mix' cashews, pecans, and peanuts	1 oz	180	6.0	16.0
Dry-roasted				
(Finast) 'No Frills' w/peanuts, salted	1 oz	180	7.0	14.0
(Fisher) lightly salted	1 oz	170	7.0	15.0
(Fisher) salted	1 oz	170	7.0	15.0
(Pathmark) 'No Frills' w/peanuts, salted	1 oz	180	7.0	14.0
(Planters)	1 oz	160	7.0	14.0
(Planters) sesame nut mix	1 oz	160	8.0	12.0
(Planters) 'Unsalted'	1 oz	170	7.0	15.0
w/peanuts	1 cup	814	34.7	70.5
w/peanuts	1 oz	169	7.2	14.6
w/peanuts, salted	1 cup	814	34.7	70.5
w/peanuts, salted	1 oz	169	7.2	14.6
Honey-roasted				
(Fisher) peanuts and cashews	1 oz	150	6.0	13.0
(Planters)	1 oz	170	9.0	13.0
(Planters) cashews and peanuts	1 oz	170	9.0	12.0
Oil-roasted				
(Fisher) lightly salted	1 oz	170	6.0	16.0
(Fisher) salted	1 oz	170	6.0	16.0
(Flavor House)	1 oz	180	6.0	18.0
(Pathmark) 'No Frills' salted	1 oz	180	7.0	15.0
(Pathmark) 'No Frills' w/peanuts, salted	1 oz	180	5.0	15.0
(Pathmark) 'No Frills Fancy' salted	1 oz	180	7.0	15.0
(Planters)	1 oz	180	6.0	16.0
(Planters) 'Deluxe'	1 oz	180	6.0	17.0

Food Name	Serv. Size	Total Cal.	Carbs GMS	Fat GMS
(Planters) lightly salted	1 oz	180	6.0	16.0
(Planters) sesame nut mix	1 oz	160	8.0	13.0
salted	1 cup	886	32.1	80.9
salted	1 oz	175	6.3	15.9
w/peanuts	1 cup	876	30.4	80.0
w/peanuts	1 oz	175	6.1	16.0
w/peanuts, salted	1 cup	876	30.4	80.0
w/peanuts, salted	1 oz	175	6.1	16.0

O

Food Name	Serv. Size	Total Cal.	Carbs GMS	Fat GMS
OAT. See also CEREAL, HOT.				
cooked	1 cup	87	25.1	1.9
cooked	4 oz	45	13.0	1.0
raw	1 cup	231	62.2	6.6
raw	1 oz	70	18.8	2.0
steel-cut (Arrowhead Mills)	2 oz	220	37.0	4.0
whole grain	1 cup	607	103.4	10.8
whole grain	1 oz	110	18.8	2.0
OAT BRAN. See CEREAL, HOT.				
OAT FLOUR				
(Arrowhead Mills) whole grain	2 oz	200	43.0	1.0
(Gold Medal) blend	1 cup	390	81.0	3.0
OAT GROATS (Arrowhead Mills)	2 oz	220	38.0	4.0
OAT VEGETABLE OIL				
	1 cup	1927	0.0	218.0
	1 tbsp	120	0.0	13.6
OATMEAL. See CEREAL, HOT.				
OCEAN CATFISH. See WOLF FISH.				
OCEAN PERCH, ATLANTIC/Norway haddock/red perch/redfish/rosefish/sea perch				
baked	4 oz	137	0.0	2.4
broiled	4 oz	137	0.0	2.4
dry-heat cooked	3 oz	103	0.0	1.8
microwaved	4 oz	137	0.0	2.4
raw	1 lb	427	0.0	7.4
raw	1 oz	27	0.0	0.5
OCEAN PERCH, FROZEN				
(Booth)	4 oz	100	0.0	1.0
(Gorton's) 'Fishmarket Fresh'	5 oz	140	2.0	3.0
(Van de Kamp's) breaded 'Light'	1 piece	280	21.0	14.0
(Van de Kamp's) 'Natural'	4 oz	130	0.0	5.0

Food Name	Serv. Size	Total Cal.	Carbs GMS	Fat GMS
OCEAN POUT/muttonfish				
dry-heat cooked	3 oz	87	0.0	1.0
raw	1 lb	360	0.0	4.1
raw	1 oz	22	0.0	0.3
OCEANIC BONITO. See TUNA, SKIPJACK.				
OCTOBER BEAN, CANNED, w/pork *(Luck's)*	7.25 oz	230	32.0	6.0
OCTOPUS				
moist-heat cooked	3 oz	139	3.7	1.8
raw	1 lb	372	10.0	4.7
raw	1 oz	23	0.6	0.3
OHELOBERRY				
raw	1 lb	126	31.0	1.0
raw	1 cup	39	9.6	0.3
raw	1 oz	8	1.9	0.1
raw, approx .4 oz	10 fruits	3	0.8	0.0
OIL. See individual listings.				
OKRA/gumbo				
boiled, drained	4 oz	36	8.2	0.2
boiled, drained, approx 3 inches long	8 pods	27	6.1	0.1
boiled, drained, sliced	1/2 cup	26	5.8	0.1
raw, approx 3 inches long	8 pods	36	7.3	0.1
raw, sliced	1/2 cup	19	3.8	0.1
raw, trimmed	1 oz	11	2.2	<.1
raw, untrimmed	1 lb	148	29.8	0.4
OKRA, FROZEN				
boiled, drained	10 oz	94	20.8	0.8
boiled, drained, sliced	1/2 cup	34	7.5	0.3
cut *(Freshlike)*	3.3 oz	25	6.0	0.0
cut *(Seabrook)*	3.3 oz	25	6.0	0.0
cut *(Southern)*	3.5 oz	31	6.5	0.2
cut *(Veg•All)*	3.3 oz	25	6.0	0.0
whole *(Freshlike)*	3.3 oz	30	7.0	0.0
whole *(Seabrook)*	3.3 oz	30	7.0	0.0
whole *(Southern)*	3.5 oz	35	7.4	0.2
whole *(Veg•All)*	3.3 oz	30	7.0	0.0
whole, baby *(Frosty Acres)*	3.3 oz	30	7.0	0.0
OLD FASHIONED. See ALCOHOLIC BEVERAGES.				
OLIVE				
all varieties, all sizes, pickled *(S&W)*	1 oz	46	0.0	5.1
black, jumbo, canned	1 olive	7	0.5	0.6
black, large, canned	1 olive	5	0.3	0.5
black, small, canned	1 olive	4	0.2	0.3
black, super colossal, canned	1 olive	12	0.9	1.0

Food Name	Serv. Size	Total Cal.	Carbs GMS	Fat GMS
mixed varieties, chopped, pickled *(Lindsay)*	1 oz	29	1.7	2.7
mixed varieties, pitted, pickled *(Vlasic)*	1 oz	37	0.7	3.9
mixed varieties, sliced, pickled *(Lindsay)*	1/2 cup	70	4.1	6.5
mixed varieties, sliced, pickled *(Lindsay)*	1 oz	29	1.7	2.7
salad, pickled *(Progresso)*	1/2 cup	120	1.0	15.0
OLIVE, ASCOLANO				
all sizes, pitted, pickled	1 oz	23	1.6	1.9
all sizes, pitted, pickled *(Lindsay)*	1 oz	23	1.6	1.9
colossal, pitted, pickled *(Lindsay)*	10 olives	90	6.3	7.7
jumbo, pitted, pickled	10 olives	67	4.7	5.7
jumbo, pitted, pickled *(Lindsay)*	10 olives	66	4.7	5.7
super colossal, pitted, pickled	10 olives	123	8.5	10.4
super colossal, pitted, pickled *(Lindsay)*	10 olives	122	8.5	10.4
OLIVE, GREEK				
all sizes, pitted, salt-cured, oil-coated, pickled	1 oz	96	2.5	10.2
extra large, w/pits, salt-cured, oil-coated, pickled	10 olives	89	2.3	9.5
extra large, w/pits, salt-cured, pickled	10 olives	89	2.3	9.5
medium, w/pits, salt-cured, oil-coated, pickled	10 olives	65	1.7	6.9
medium, w/pits, salt-cured, pickled	10 olives	65	1.7	6.9
OLIVE, GREEN				
all sizes, pitted, pickled	1 oz	33	0.4	3.6
giant, w/pits, pickled	10 olives	76	0.9	8.3
large, w/pits, pickled	10 olives	45	0.5	4.9
small, select, w/pits, pickled	10 olives	33	0.4	3.6
small, standard, w/pits, pickled	10 olives	33	0.4	3.6
OLIVE, MANZANILLA				
all sizes, pitted, pickled	1 oz	33	1.8	3.0
all sizes, pitted, pickled *(Lindsay)*	1 oz	32	1.8	3.0
extra large, pitted, pickled *(Lindsay)*	10 olives	63	3.5	5.9
large, pitted, pickled	10 olives	51	2.8	4.7
large, pitted, pickled *(Lindsay)*	10 olives	50	2.8	4.8
medium, pitted, pickled *(Lindsay)*	10 olives	44	2.4	4.1
small, pitted, pickled	10 olives	37	2.0	3.4
small, pitted, pickled *(Lindsay)*	10 olives	37	2.0	3.5
OLIVE, MISSION				
all sizes, pitted, pickled	1 oz	33	1.8	3.0
all sizes, pitted, pickled *(Lindsay)*	1 oz	32	1.8	3.0
extra large, pitted, pickled *(Lindsay)*	10 olives	63	3.5	5.9
large, pitted, pickled	10 olives	51	2.8	4.7
large, pitted, pickled *(Lindsay)*	10 olives	50	2.8	4.8
medium, pitted, pickled *(Lindsay)*	10 olives	44	2.4	4.1
small, pitted, pickled	10 olives	37	2.0	3.4
small, pitted, pickled *(Lindsay)*	10 olives	37	2.0	3.5

Food Name	Serv. Size	Total Cal.	Carbs GMS	Fat GMS
OLIVE, SEVILLANO				
all sizes, pitted, pickled	1 oz	23	1.6	1.9
all sizes, pitted, pickled *(Lindsay)*	1 oz	23	1.6	1.9
colossal, pitted, pickled *(Lindsay)*	10 olives	90	6.3	7.7
jumbo, pitted, pickled	10 olives	67	4.7	5.7
jumbo, pitted, pickled *(Lindsay)*	10 olives	66	4.7	5.7
super colossal, pitted, pickled	10 olives	123	8.5	10.4
super colossal, pitted, pickled *(Lindsay)*	10 olives	122	8.5	10.4
OLIVE APPETIZER				
(Progresso)	1/2 cup	180	6.0	21.0
(Progresso) 'Condite'	1/2 cup	130	5.0	14.0
OLIVE OIL				
	1/2 cup	955	0.0	108.0
	1 oz	251	0.0	28.4
(Amore) 'Extra Virgin'	1 tbsp	130	0.0	14.0
(Amore) 'Pure'	1 tbsp	130	0.0	14.0
(Bertolli)	1 tbsp	120	0.0	14.0
(Filippo Berio)	1 tbsp	120	0.0	14.0
(Hain)	1 tbsp	120	0.0	14.0
(Pope) 100% Italian cold press, no salt	1 tbsp	120	0.0	14.0
(Progresso) all varieties	1 tbsp	119	0.0	14.0
(Spectrum Naturals)	1 tbsp	120	0.0	14.0
(Spectrum Naturals) organic	1 tbsp	120	0.0	14.0
(Wesson)	1 tbsp	120	0.0	14.0
OMELET, FROZEN				
(Healthy Choice) turkey sausage, on English muffin	1 serving	210	30.0	4.0
(Healthy Choice) western style, on English muffin	1 serving	200	29.0	3.0
(Weight Watchers) ham and cheese 'Handy'	4 oz	180	18.0	5.0
ONION				
Mature				
boiled, drained	4 oz	50	11.5	0.2
chopped, boiled, drained	1/2 cup	46	10.7	0.2
chopped, boiled, drained	1 tbsp	7	1.5	0.0
raw *(Dole)*	1 med	60	14.0	0.0
raw, chopped	1/2 cup	30	6.9	0.1
raw, chopped	1 tbsp	4	0.9	<.1
raw, trimmed	1 oz	11	2.4	<.1
raw, untrimmed	1 lb	154	35.2	0.7
ONION, CANNED				
sweet *(Heinz)*	1 oz	40	9.0	0.0
whole, small *(Pathmark)*	1/2 cup	35	7.0	0.0
whole, small *(S&W)*	1/2 cup	35	9.0	0.0
w/liquid	4 oz	22	4.5	0.1

Food Name	Serv. Size	Total Cal.	Carbs GMS	Fat GMS
w/liquid, chopped	1/2 cup	21	4.5	0.1
ONION, COCKTAIL, lightly spiced *(Vlasic)*	1 oz	4	1.0	0.0
ONION, DRIED				
flakes	1 oz	92	23.6	0.1
flakes	1/4 cup	45	11.7	0.1
flakes	1 tbsp	16	4.2	0.0
w/green onion, minced *(Lawry's)*	1 tsp	7	1.6	0.2
ONION, FROZEN				
Chopped				
boiled, drained	1/2 cup	29	6.9	0.1
boiled, drained	4 oz	32	7.5	0.1
boiled, drained	1 tbsp	4	1.0	0.0
unprepared	10 oz	82	19.3	0.3
(Ore-Ida)	2 oz	20	4.0	<1.0
(Seabrook)	1 oz	8	2.0	0.0
Diced				
(Freshlike)	3.3 oz	8	2.0	0.0
(Veg•All)	3.3 oz	8	2.0	0.0
Whole				
boiled, drained	4 oz	32	7.6	0.1
(Birds Eye) small	4 oz	40	10.0	0.0
(Birds Eye) small, w/cream sauce 'Combination Vegetables'	5 oz	140	12.0	10.0
(Freshlike)	3.3 oz	35	8.0	0.0
(Seabrook) small	3.3 oz	35	8.0	0.0
(Veg•All)	3.3 oz	35	8.0	0.0
ONION, GREEN/scallion/spring onion				
chopped *(Dole)*	1 tbsp	2	0.3	0.1
trimmed, w/top	1 oz	19	2.1	<.1
trimmed, w/top, chopped	1/2 cup	16	3.7	0.1
trimmed, w/top, chopped	1 tbsp	2	0.4	<.1
untrimmed	1 lb	140	32.0	0.8
ONION, SPRING. See ONION, GREEN.				
ONION, WELSH				
trimmed	1 lb	160	28.8	1.6
trimmed	1 oz	10	1.8	0.1
ONION POWDER				
ground	1 tbsp	23	5.2	0.1
ground	1 tsp	7	1.7	0.0
ground *(Durkee)*	1 tsp	8	0.0	tr
ground *(Laurel Leaf)*	1 tsp	8	0.0	tr
ground *(Spice Islands)*	1 tsp	8	1.7	<.1
ONION RINGS, FROZEN				
breaded, partially fried in vegetable oil, prepared in oven	4 oz	462	43.3	30.3

Food Name	Serv. Size	Total Cal.	Carbs GMS	Fat GMS
breaded, partially fried in vegetable oil, prepared in oven ...	2 rings	81	7.6	5.3
breaded, partially fried in vegetable oil, unprepared	16 oz	1171	138.6	64.0
breaded, partially fried in vegetable oil, unprepared	9 oz	658	77.8	36.0
(Farm Rich) battered, precooked 'Batter Dipt'	4 oz	260	32.0	13.0
(Farm Rich) crispy 'Onion O's'	5 rings	190	26.0	9.0
(Mrs. Paul's) crispy	2.5 oz	190	19.0	12.0
(Ore-Ida) 'Onion Ringers'	2 oz	140	18.0	7.0
(Stilwell) battered	3 oz	250	22.0	16.0
ONION SALT (Tone's)	1 tsp	1	0.4	tr
OPOSSUM				
roasted	4 oz	251	0.0	11.6
roasted	3 oz	188	0.0	8.7
roasted, diced	1 cup	309	0.0	14.3
ORANGE				
All commercial varieties				
approx 2 5/8-inch diam	1 med	62	15.4	0.2
peeled and seeded	1 oz	13	3.3	<.1
sections, w/o membrane	1 cup	85	21.1	0.2
untrimmed	1 lb	156	38.9	0.4
California navel				
approx 2 7/8-inch diam	1 med	64	16.3	0.1
peeled and seeded	1 oz	13	3.3	<.1
sections, w/o membrane	1 cup	76	19.2	0.2
untrimmed	1 lb	142	35.9	0.3
California Valencia				
approx 2 5/8-inch diam	1 med	59	14.4	0.4
peeled and seeded	1 oz	14	3.4	0.1
sections, w/o membrane	1 cup	88	21.4	0.5
untrimmed	1 lb	167	40.5	1.0
Florida				
approx 2 5/8-inch diam	1 med	69	17.4	0.3
peeled and seeded	1 oz	13	3.3	0.1
sections, w/o membrane	1 cup	85	21.4	0.4
untrimmed	1 lb	153	38.7	0.7
ORANGE APRICOT DRINK (Tropicana) 'Twister'	8 oz	115	30.0	0.0
ORANGE APRICOT JUICE (Musselman's) 'Breakfast Cocktail'	6 oz	90	21.0	0.0
ORANGE APRICOT JUICE DRINK	1 oz	16	4.0	0.0
ORANGE BANANA NECTAR (Kern's)	6 oz	110	25.0	0.0
ORANGE CRANBERRY JUICE (Santa Cruz Natural) organic				
'Cruz'	8 oz	125	29.0	<1.0
ORANGE CRANBERRY JUICE DRINK				
(Ocean Spray) 'Refreshers'	6 oz	100	26.0	0.0
(Tropicana) 'Single Serve'	10 oz	175	43.0	0.0

Food Name	Serv. Size	Total Cal.	Carbs GMS	Fat GMS
(Tropicana) 'Twister'	8 oz	115	30.0	0.0
(Tropicana) 'Twister'	6 oz	100	23.0	<1.0
(Tropicana) 'Twister Light' w/NutraSweet	6 oz	18	5.0	<1.0
ORANGE DRINK				
Can, bottle, or box				
	8 oz	128	32.0	tr
(Bama)	8.45 oz	120	29.0	0.0
(Crowley)	8 oz	130	32.0	0.0
(Hawaiian Punch)	6 oz	100	24.0	0.0
(Hi-C)	8.45 oz	134	32.9	<.1
(Hi-C)	6 oz	95	23.3	<.1
(Hi-C) aseptic box	6 oz	90	23.0	0.0
(J. Hungerford) 20% plus juice	9.03 oz	41	10.8	0.0
(Pathmark) 'No Frills Sodium Free'	6 oz	80	22.0	0.0
(Squeezit) 'Smarty Arty Orange'	6.75 oz	100	26.0	0.0
(Sunny Delight) California style	8 oz	130	31.0	0.0
(Tropicana)	6 oz	90	22.0	<1.0
(Tropicana) 'Single Serve'	10 oz	132	33.0	0.0
(Veryfine)	8 oz	130	33.0	0.0
(Wyler's) 'Fruit Slush'	4 oz	157	39.3	0.0
Chilled *(Hi-C)*	6 oz	90	23.0	0.0
Frozen, w/juice and pulp, diluted	6 oz	85	21.2	0.0
Mix				
(Finast) breakfast, prepared	8 oz	80	20.0	0.0
(Kool-Aid) sugar-free, w/NutraSweet, prepared	8 oz	4	0.0	0.0
(Kool-Aid) sugar-sweetened, prepared	8 oz	80	20.0	0.0
(Kool-Aid) unsweetened, prepared w/sugar	8 oz	100	25.0	0.0
(Kool-Aid) unsweetened, prepared w/o sugar	8 oz	2	0.0	0.0
(Pathmark) breakfast 'No Frills' prepared	4 oz	60	15.0	0.0
ORANGE FLAVOR DRINK				
Can, bottle, or box	12 oz	729	182.0	2.2
Chilled *(Bright & Early)* diluted	6 oz	90	20.8	0.2
Frozen				
(Bright & Early) diluted	6 oz	90	20.8	0.2
w/orange pulp, diluted	1 oz	15	3.8	tr
Mix				
powder, unprepared	1 oz	109	28.0	<.1
powder, unprepared	.3 rounded tsp	93	23.7	tr
(Tang) crystals, prepared	6 oz	90	22.0	0.0
(Tang) crystals 'Sugar-free' prepared	6 oz	6	1.0	0.0
ORANGE FRUIT JUICE BLEND				
(Mott's)	10 oz	144	35.0	0.0
(Mott's)	9.5 oz	139	34.0	0.0

Food Name	Serv. Size	Total Cal.	Carbs GMS	Fat GMS
ORANGE GRAPEFRUIT JUICE				
canned	8 oz	106	25.4	0.3
canned	1 oz	13	3.2	0.0
(Kraft) chilled 'Pure 100%'	6 oz	80	19.0	0.0
ORANGE JUICE				
fresh squeezed	8 oz	112	25.8	0.5
Can, bottle, or box				
	6 oz	78	18.4	0.3
(Del Monte) 'Unsweetened'	6 oz	80	19.0	0.0
(J. Hungerford)	9.03 oz	112	27.8	0.0
(Minute Maid) blend 'Juices to Go'	6 oz	90	22.0	0.0
(Minute Maid) 'Juices to Go'	6 oz	80	20.0	0.0
(Ocean Spray)	6 oz	80	19.0	0.0
(S&W)	6 oz	83	18.0	0.0
(Sippin' Pak)	8.45 oz	110	26.0	0.0
(Snapple)	8 oz	130	29.0	0.0
(Stokely) 'Unsweetened'	6 oz	89	21.0	1.0
(Sunkist)	6 oz	84	20.0	0.1
(Tree Top)	6 oz	90	22.0	0.0
(TreeSweet)	6 oz	78	18.0	0.0
(Tropicana) '100% Pure'	8 oz	109	24.9	0.0
(Tropicana) 'Pure Premium' 100% pure	6 oz	80	19.0	<1.0
(Tropicana) reconstituted, 100% pure	6 oz	80	16.0	<1.0
(Veryfine) blend '100%'	8 oz	120	30.0	0.0
(Veryfine) '100%'	8 oz	121	24.0	0.0
Chilled				
	8 oz	110	25.0	0.7
(Citrus Hill) 'Plus Calcium'	6 oz	90	20.0	<1.0
(Citrus Hill) 'Select'	6 oz	90	20.0	<1.0
(Crowley)	8 oz	110	26.0	0.0
(Kraft) 'Pure 100% Unsweetened'	6 oz	80	19.0	0.0
(Minute Maid) calcium fortified	6 oz	80	20.0	0.0
(Minute Maid) country style	6 oz	80	20.0	0.0
(Minute Maid) country style, premium choice	6 oz	90	21.0	0.0
(Minute Maid) premium choice	6 oz	90	21.0	0.0
(Minute Maid) regular	6 oz	80	20.0	0.0
(Sunkist)	6 oz	84	20.0	0.1
(Sunkist) 'Fresh Squeezed'	6 oz	77	17.7	0.3
Frozen				
(A&P) diluted	6 oz	80	19.0	<1.0
(Minute Maid) calcium fortified	6 oz	80	20.0	0.0
(Minute Maid) country style	6 oz	80	20.0	0.0
(Minute Maid) reduced acid	6 oz	80	20.0	0.0

Food Name	Serv. Size	Total Cal.	Carbs GMS	Fat GMS
(Minute Maid) regular	6 oz	80	20.0	0.0
(Sunkist) '8-16 servings per pkg' diluted	6 oz	112	26.8	0.1
(TreeSweet) diluted	6 oz	84	20.0	0.0
ORANGE JUICE COCKTAIL				
(Musselman's) w/grapefruit juice 'Breakfast Cocktail'	6 oz	90	22.0	0.0
(Ocean Spray)	6 oz	100	25.0	0.0
(Welch's) 'Orchard'	10 oz	150	37.0	0.0
ORANGE JUICE DRINK				
(Citrus Hill) 'Lite Premium'	6 oz	60	14.0	<1.0
(Kool-Aid) 'Koolers'	8.45 oz	110	30.0	0.0
(Tang) 'Fruit Box'	8.45 oz	130	32.0	0.0
(Tropicana) tropical 'Juice Sparkler'	8 oz	110	26.0	0.0
ORANGE JUICE FLOAT *(Knudsen & Sons)*	8 oz	120	27.0	0.0
ORANGE KIWI PASSION JUICE *(Tropicana)* 100% pure	6 oz	80	17.0	<1.0
ORANGE MANGO DRINK *(Tropicana)* 'Twister'	6 oz	90	21.0	<1.0
ORANGE MANGO JUICE *(Knudsen & Sons)*	8 oz	110	24.0	0.0
ORANGE PASSION DRINK				
(Tropicana) 'Twister'	8 oz	90	22.0	0.0
(Tropicana) 'Twister'	6 oz	80	19.0	<1.0
ORANGE PEACH DRINK				
(Tropicana) 'Twister'	8 oz	115	30.0	0.0
(Tropicana) 'Twister'	6 oz	90	21.0	<1.0
ORANGE PEACH MANGO JUICE *(Tropicana)* 100% pure	6 oz	80	19.0	<1.0
ORANGE PEEL				
candied	1 oz	88	22.6	0.1
fresh	1 oz	na	7.1	0.1
fresh	1 tbsp	na	1.5	<.1
fresh	1 tsp	na	0.5	tr
ORANGE PINEAPPLE JUICE				
(Kraft) 'Pure 100%'	6 oz	80	19.0	0.0
(Musselman's) 'Breakfast Cocktail'	6 oz	90	23.0	0.0
(Tropicana) 100% pure	6 oz	80	19.0	<1.0
ORANGE PUNCH *(Minute Maid)* aseptic box	6 oz	80	20.0	0.0
ORANGE RASPBERRY DRINK				
(Tropicana) 'Twister'	6 oz	80	20.0	<1.0
(Tropicana) 'Twister Light'	6 oz	30	6.0	<1.0
ORANGE ROUGHY/slimehead				
dry-heat cooked	3 oz	76	0.0	0.8
raw	1 lb	571	0.0	31.8
raw	1 oz	36	0.0	2.0
ORANGE STRAWBERRY BANANA JUICE				
(Tropicana) 100% pure	6 oz	80	18.0	<1.0

Food Name	Serv. Size	Total Cal.	Carbs GMS	Fat GMS
ORANGE STRAWBERRY DRINK				
(Tropicana) w/banana 'Twister'	6 oz	80	20.0	<1.0
(Tropicana) w/banana 'Twister Light'	6 oz	25	6.0	<1.0
(Tropicana) w/guava 'Twister'	6 oz	80	20.0	<1.0
ORANGEADE				
(Santa Cruz Natural) organic	8 oz	90	22.0	<1.0
(Santa Cruz Natural) organic 'Sparkling'	8 oz	90	24.0	<1.0
OREGANO				
dried (Golden Dipt)	2 grams	6	1.0	0.0
dried (Spice Islands)	1 tsp	6	1.0	0.1
ground	1 tbsp	14	2.9	0.5
ground	1 tsp	5	1.0	0.2
ground (Durkee)	1 tsp	5	0.0	tr
ground (Laurel Leaf)	1 tsp	5	0.0	tr
ORIENTAL SEASONING MIX (Schilling) 'Bag 'n Season'	1 pkg	152	31.0	8.0
OYSTER, CANNED				
Eastern	1 cup	171	9.7	6.1
Eastern	3 oz	59	3.3	2.1
Eastern, w/liquid	4 oz	78	4.4	2.8
(Bumble Bee)	1 cup	218	15.4	5.3
(S&W) mole 'Fancy'	2 oz	95	4.0	3.0
OYSTER, EASTERN				
Farmed				
dry-heat cooked	3 oz	67	6.2	1.8
dry-heat cooked	6 med	47	4.3	1.3
raw, approx 3 oz	6 med	50	4.7	1.3
Wild				
dry-heat cooked	3 oz	61	4.1	1.6
dry-heat cooked	6 med	42	2.8	1.1
moist-heat cooked	4 oz	155	8.9	5.6
moist-heat cooked	3 oz	116	6.7	4.2
moist-heat cooked, approx 1.5 oz	6 med	58	3.3	2.1
raw	1 cup	169	9.7	6.1
raw	1 oz	20	1.1	0.7
raw, approx 3 oz	6 med	57	3.3	2.1
OYSTER, PACIFIC				
moist-heat cooked	3 oz	139	8.4	3.9
moist-heat cooked	1 med	41	2.5	1.1
raw	1 lb	370	22.5	10.4
raw	3 oz	69	4.2	2.0
raw	1 oz	23	1.4	0.7
raw, approx 1.75 oz	1 med	41	2.5	1.1
OYSTER PLANT. See SALSIFY.				

Food Name	Serv. Size	Total Cal.	Carbs GMS	Fat GMS

OYSTER STEW. See SOUP.

P

Food Name	Serv. Size	Total Cal.	Carbs GMS	Fat GMS
PALM KERNEL OIL/babassu oil				
....	1 cup	1927	0.0	218.0
....	1/2 cup	964	0.0	109.0
....	1 oz	251	0.0	28.4
....	1 tbsp	120	0.0	13.6
PALM OIL				
....	1 oz	251	0.0	28.4
....	1 tbsp	120	0.0	13.6
PAM COOKING SPRAY. See COOKING SPRAY.				
PANANG CURRY BASE (A Taste of Thai)	1 tbsp	25	2.0	2.0
PANCAKE, FROZEN				
(Aunt Jemima) blueberry ....:	3.5 oz	220	42.3	3.7
(Aunt Jemima) buttermilk 'Lite Microwave'	3.5 oz	140	28.0	3.0
(Aunt Jemima) buttermilk 'Microwave'	3.5 oz	210	41.3	3.0
(Aunt Jemima) 'Original Microwave'	3.5 oz	211	40.3	3.6
(Downyflake)	3 pancakes	280	45.0	9.0
(Downyflake) blueberry	3 pancakes	290	48.0	9.0
(Downyflake) buttermilk	3 pancakes	280	45.0	9.0
(Krusteaz) blueberry, 4.5 oz	3 pancakes	280	49.0	5.0
(Krusteaz) buttermilk, 4.75 oz	3 pancakes	290	53.0	5.0
(Krusteaz) mini, microwave	6 pancakes	120	21.0	2.0
(Krusteaz) whole wheat honey, 4.75 oz	3 pancakes	250	45.0	4.0
(Pillsbury) blueberry 'Microwave'	3 pancakes	250	49.0	4.0
(Pillsbury) buttermilk 'Microwave'	3 pancakes	260	51.0	4.0
(Pillsbury) harvest wheat 'Microwave'	3 pancakes	240	48.0	4.0
(Pillsbury) 'Original Microwave'	3 pancakes	240	47.0	4.0
(Weight Watchers) buttermilk 'Microwave' approx 2.5 oz ...	1/2 pkg	140	22.0	3.0
PANCAKE BATTER, FROZEN				
(Aunt Jemima) blueberry	3.6 oz	204	38.7	4.0
(Aunt Jemima) buttermilk	3.6 oz	180	36.0	2.3
(Aunt Jemima) 'Original'	3.6 oz	183	36.5	2.4
PANCAKE ENTRÉE, FROZEN				
(Aunt Jemima) and sausages 'Homestyle'	6 oz	420	57.0	16.0
(Aunt Jemima) lite, w/lite links 'Homestyle'	6 oz	310	43.0	10.0
(Aunt Jemima) lite, w/lite syrup 'Homestyle'	6 oz	260	53.0	3.0
(Downyflake) and sausages	5.5 oz	430	47.0	23.0
(Swanson) and sausages 'Great Starts'	6 oz	460	52.0	22.0

Food Name	Serv. Size	Total Cal.	Carbs GMS	Fat GMS
(Swanson) silver dollar, and sausage 'Great Starts'	3.75 oz	310	37.0	14.0
(Swanson) whole wheat, w/lite links 'Great Starts'	5.5 oz	350	39.0	16.0
(Swanson) w/bacon 'Great Starts'	4.5 oz	400	47.0	20.0
PANCAKE MIX. See also PANCAKE/WAFFLE MIX.				
(NOTE: Unless otherwise stated, all pancakes are 4 inches in diameter.)				
(Hungry Jack) dry	1/14 pkg	180	33.0	3.0
(Hungry Jack) prepared w/water	3 pancakes	180	33.0	3.0
BLUEBERRY *(Krusteaz)* imitation, prepared	3 pancakes	205	39.0	4.0
BLUEBERRY, WILD				
(Hungry Jack) dry	1/5 pkg	170	38.0	1.0
(Hungry Jack) prepared w/milk/oil/egg	3 pancakes	320	41.0	14.0
BUCKWHEAT *(Krusteaz)* prepared	3 pancakes	215	40.0	3.0
BUTTERMILK				
(Health Valley) 'Biscuit & Pancake'	1 oz	100	20.0	1.0
(Hungry Jack) 'Complete' dry	1/17 pkg	180	38.0	1.0
(Hungry Jack) 'Complete' prepared w/water	3 pancakes	180	38.0	1.0
(Hungry Jack) dry	1/25 pkg	120	26.0	0.0
(Hungry Jack) prepared w/skim milk/oil/egg whites	3 pancakes	200	28.0	7.0
(Hungry Jack) prepared w/2% milk/oil/egg	3 pancakes	210	28.0	9.0
(Krusteaz) prepared	3 pancakes	200	39.0	3.0
EXTRA LIGHT				
(Hungry Jack) 'Complete' dry	1/17 pkg	180	38.0	3.0
(Hungry Jack) dry	1/17 pkg	180	38.0	3.0
(Hungry Jack) dry	1/26 pkg	120	26.0	0.1
(Hungry Jack) prepared w/skim milk/oil/egg whites	3 pancakes	170	28.0	4.0
(Hungry Jack) prepared w/2% milk/oil/egg	3 pancakes	190	28.0	6.0
OAT BRAN *(Krusteaz)* 'Lite'	3 pancakes	130	36.0	1.0
WHOLE WHEAT *(Krusteaz)* honey	3 pancakes	215	42.0	1.0
PANCAKE MIX, MICROWAVE				
(Hungry Jack) blueberry, dry	3/4 pkg	230	47.0	4.0
(Hungry Jack) buttermilk, dry	3/4 pkg	260	51.0	4.0
(Hungry Jack) harvest wheat, dry	3/4 pkg	230	46.0	4.0
(Hungry Jack) oat bran, dry	3/4 pkg	230	45.0	4.0
(Hungry Jack) original, dry	3/4 pkg	240	49.0	4.0
PANCAKE SYRUP. See also MAPLE SYRUP.				
15% maple	1 cup	879	236.9	0.3
15% maple	1 tbsp	56	15.0	0.0
2% maple	1 cup	762	202.9	0.6
2% maple	1 tbsp	48	12.9	0.0
reduced calorie	100 gm	164	44.3	0.0
(Aunt Jemima)				
'ButterLite'	1 oz	50	13.0	0.0
'Lite'	1 oz	54	13.1	0.1

Food Name	Serv. Size	Total Cal.	Carbs GMS	Fat GMS
'Original' rich maple taste	1 oz	100	26.0	0.0
(Br'er Rabbit)				
dark	1 oz	120	31.0	0.0
light	1 oz	120	31.0	0.0
(Estee)				
	1 tbsp	4	1.0	0.0
'Breakfast'	1 tbsp	12	3.0	0.0
(Featherweight)	1 tbsp	16	4.0	0.0
(Hungry Jack)				
'Lite'	2 tbsp	50	14.0	0.0
regular	2 tbsp	100	26.0	0.0
(Knott's Berry Farm)				
	1 oz	110	28.0	0.0
'Country'	1 oz	110	27.0	0.0
'Light' microwavable	1 oz	45	11.0	0.0
w/30% real maple syrup, microwavable	1 oz	110	28.0	0.0
(Log Cabin)				
'Country Kitchen'	1 oz	100	26.0	0.0
'Country Kitchen' butter flavor	1 oz	100	27.0	0.0
'Country Kitchen Lite'	1 oz	50	13.0	0.0
'Lite' reduced calorie	1 oz	50	13.0	0.0
'Pancake and Waffle'	1 oz	100	26.0	0.0
(Maple Valley)				
maple syrup substitute	2 tbsp	110	27.0	0.0
maple syrup substitute 'Lite'	2 tbsp	60	16.0	0.0
(Mrs. Butterworth's) thick 'n rich 'Lite'	2 tbsp	60	15.0	0.0
(Mrs. Richardson's)				
'Lite'	1 oz	50	13.0	0.0
original recipe	1 oz	100	25.0	0.0
(S&W) maple flavor, saccharin sweetened	1 tsp	4	1.0	0.0
(Vermont Maid)	1 tbsp	50	13.0	0.0
(Weight Watchers) 'Reduced Calorie'	1 tbsp	25	7.0	0.0
PANCAKE/WAFFLE MIX. See also PANCAKE MIX.				
(NOTE: Unless otherwise stated, all pancakes are 4 inches in diameter.)				
(Arrowhead Mills) 'Griddle Lite' prepared	1/2 cup	260	50.0	3.0
(Aunt Jemima) 'Original' prepared	3 pancakes	116	25.4	0.8
(Aunt Jemima) 'Original Complete' prepared	3 pancakes	253	50.2	3.6
(Bisquick) 'Shake 'n Pour' prepared	3 pancakes	260	48.0	5.0
(Estee) prepared, 3 inches each	3 pancakes	100	21.0	0.0
(Featherweight) prepared	3 pancakes	140	24.0	2.0
(Gold Medal) 'Pouch Mix' prepared w/egg	1/8 pouch	100	17.0	2.0
(Hungry Jack) 'Panshakes' prepared	3 pancakes	250	43.0	6.0
(Krusteaz) Belgian waffle, prepared, 4-inch square	1 waffle	170	22.0	7.0

Food Name	Serv. Size	Total Cal.	Carbs GMS	Fat GMS
(Martha White) 'FlapStax' 1/4-cup batter per pancake ...	1 pancake	80	17.0	1.0
(Martha White) 'Light Crust' dry	2 oz	120	20.0	3.0
(Robin Hood) 'Pouch Mix' prepared w/egg	1/8 pouch	100	17.0	2.0
APPLE CINNAMON *(Bisquick)* 'Shake 'n Pour' prepared	3 pancakes	270	49.0	5.0
BLUE CORN *(Arrowhead Mills)* prepared	1/2 cup	330	36.0	5.0
BLUEBERRY				
(Bisquick) 'Shake 'n Pour' prepared	3 pancakes	280	53.0	5.0
(Hungry Jack) prepared	3 pancakes	320	41.0	15.0
BUCKWHEAT				
(Arrowhead Mills) prepared	1/2 cup	270	53.0	2.0
(Aunt Jemima) prepared	3 pancakes	143	31.7	1.6
BUTTERMILK				
(Aunt Jemima) 'Complete' prepared	3 pancakes	231	46.4	2.8
(Aunt Jemima) 'Lite Complete' prepared	3 pancakes	130	25.0	2.0
(Aunt Jemima) prepared	3 pancakes	122	26.1	0.7
(Betty Crocker) complete, dry	1/2 cup	210	41.0	3.0
(Betty Crocker) complete, prepared	3 pancakes	210	41.0	3.0
(Betty Crocker) dry	1/2 cup	170	36.0	1.0
(Betty Crocker) prepared w/milk/oil/egg	3 pancakes	280	39.0	10.0
(Bisquick) 'Shake 'n Pour' prepared	3 pancakes	260	47.0	5.0
(Hungry Jack) 'Complete' prepared	3 pancakes	180	39.0	1.0
(Hungry Jack) 'Complete Packets' prepared	3 pancakes	180	35.0	3.0
(Hungry Jack) prepared	3 pancakes	240	29.0	11.0
EXTRA LIGHT *(Hungry Jack)* 'Complete' prepared w/water	3 pancakes	180	38.0	3.0
MULTIGRAIN *(Arrowhead Mills)* prepared	1/2 cup	350	70.0	2.0
OAT BRAN				
(Arrowhead Mills) prepared	1/2 cup	200	64.0	2.0
(Bisquick) 'Shake 'n Pour' prepared	3 pancakes	240	45.0	4.0
WHOLE WHEAT *(Aunt Jemima)* prepared	3 pancakes	161	34.5	1.0
PAPAYA				
peeled and seeded	1 oz	11	2.8	<.1
raw *(Calavo Growers)*	1/2 med	80	19.0	0.0
raw *(Del Monte)*	1/3 med	60	15.0	0.0
raw, approx 3 1/2-inch diam	1 med	119	29.8	0.4
raw, cubed	1 cup	55	13.7	0.2
raw, slices in light syrup *(Sunfresh)*	2/3 cup	80	19.0	0.0
PAPAYA DRINK *(Knudsen & Sons)* concentrate	1.5 oz	90	22.0	0.0
PAPAYA JUICE *(Knudsen & Sons)* cream	2 oz	25	6.0	0.0
PAPAYA LIME JUICE *(Knudsen & Sons)*	8 oz	115	29.0	0.0
PAPAYA NECTAR				
canned	1 cup	142	36.3	0.4
canned	1 oz	18	4.5	0.1
(Kern's)	6 oz	110	27.0	0.0

Food Name	Serv. Size	Total Cal.	Carbs GMS	Fat GMS
(Knudsen & Sons)	8 oz	100	26.0	0.0
(Knudsen & Sons) concentrate	1.5 oz	90	22.0	0.0
(Libby's)	6 oz	110	28.0	0.0
PAPAYA PUNCH (Veryfine)	8 oz	120	30.0	0.0
PAPRIKA				
ground	1 oz	82	15.8	3.7
ground	1 tbsp	20	3.8	0.9
ground	1 tsp	6	1.2	0.3
ground (Durkee)	1 tsp	8	0.0	tr
ground (Laurel Leaf)	1 tsp	8	0.0	tr
ground (Spice Islands)	1 tsp	7	1.1	0.2
PARANUT. See BRAZIL NUT.				
PARFAIT				
chocolate (Pearson)	1 oz	120	23.0	3.0
chocolate (Swiss Miss)	4 oz	170	27.0	6.0
chocolate vanilla, fat-free (Swiss Miss)	4 oz	104	23.3	0.3
peanut butter (Pearson)	1 oz	120	23.0	3.0
vanilla (Swiss Miss)	4 oz	180	29.0	6.0
vanilla chocolate (Swiss Miss)	4 oz	164	24.5	6.0
vanilla chocolate 'Light' (Swiss Miss)	4 oz	100	20.0	1.0
PARROT FISH/pollyfish				
raw	1 lb	390	0.0	1.8
raw	1 oz	24	0.0	0.1
PARSLEY				
dried	1 oz	78	14.6	1.3
dried	1 tbsp	4	0.7	0.1
dried	1 tsp	1	0.2	tr
dried (Durkee)	1 tsp	1	0.0	tr
dried (Laurel Leaf)	1 tsp	1	0.0	tr
dried flakes (Spice Islands)	1 tsp	4	0.6	0.1
freeze-dried	1 oz	77	12.0	1.5
freeze-dried	1/4 cup	4	0.6	0.1
freeze-dried	1 tbsp	1	0.2	tr
raw	10 sprigs	4	0.6	0.1
raw, chopped	1/2 cup	11	1.9	0.2
raw, trimmed	1 oz	9	2.0	0.1
raw, untrimmed	1 lb	140	29.8	1.3
PARSLEY ROOT/hamburg parsley/turnip-rooted parsley				
fresh	1 lb	50	10.4	2.7
fresh	1 oz	3	0.7	0.2
PARSLEY SEASONING				
(Schilling) all-purpose 'Parsley Patch'	1 tsp	6	1.0	0.0

Food Name	Serv. Size	Total Cal.	Carbs GMS	Fat GMS
PARSNIP				
boiled, drained	4 oz	92	22.1	0.3
boiled, drained, 9 inches long	1 parsnip	130	31.3	0.5
boiled, drained, slices	1/2 cup	63	15.2	0.2
raw, slices	1/2 cup	50	12.0	0.2
raw, trimmed	1 oz	21	5.1	0.1
raw, untrimmed	1 lb	289	69.4	1.2
PASSION FRUIT/granadilla				
purple, trimmed	1 oz	27	6.6	0.2
purple, trimmed, approx 1.2 oz	1 med	17	4.2	0.1
purple, untrimmed	1 lb	230	55.1	1.7
PASSION FRUIT BEVERAGES				
COCKTAIL				
fresh, purple	1 cup	126	33.6	0.1
fresh, purple	1 oz	16	4.2	0.0
fresh, yellow	1 cup	148	35.7	0.4
(Welch's) bottled 'Orchard Tropicals' diluted	6 oz	100	25.0	0.0
(Welch's) frozen 'Orchard Tropicals' diluted	6 oz	100	25.0	0.0
(Welch's) 'Orchard Tropicals Cocktails-In-A-Box'	8.45 oz	140	34.0	0.0
JUICE				
fresh, yellow	1 oz	19	4.5	0.1
(Knudsen & Sons) raspberry	8 oz	130	32.0	0.0
(Snapple) passion juice 'Passion Supreme'	8 oz	160	39.0	0.0
(Veryfine) refresher, w/orange, tropical	8 oz	110	26.0	0.0
PASTA/macaroni. See also NOODLE, CHINESE; NOODLE, EGG; NOODLE, JAPANESE; TORTELLINI PASTA.				
(NOTE: 2 ounces uncooked pasta = approximately 1 cup cooked.)				
ACINI PEPE *(Ronzoni)* dry	2 oz	210	42.0	1.0
AGNOLOTTI, refrigerated, 'Fresh' *(Contadina)*	3 oz	270	38.0	7.0
ANGEL HAIR				
Dry				
corn *(Westbrae)*	2 oz	210	46.0	2.0
Jerusalem artichoke *(De Boles)*	2 oz	210	41.0	1.0
Jerusalem artichoke, garlic and parsley *(De Boles)*	2 oz	210	41.0	1.0
Jerusalem artichoke, tomato and basil *(De Boles)*	2 oz	210	41.0	1.0
100% durum wheat semolina *(American Beauty)*	2 oz	210	42.0	1.0
wheat *(Creamette)*	2 oz	210	42.0	1.0
wheat *(DiGiorno)*	3 oz	250	47.0	3.0
whole wheat *(De Boles)*	2 oz	210	40.0	2.0
Refrigerated, fresh				
'Fresh' *(Contadina)*	3 oz	260	45.0	3.0
BOW TIE. See FARFELLE.				

Food Name	Serv. Size	Total Cal.	Carbs GMS	Fat GMS
CAPELLINI				
100% durum wheat semolina *(American Beauty)* dry	2 oz	210	42.0	1.0
CURLY				
100% durum wheat semolina 'Curly-Roni'				
(American Beauty) dry	2 oz	210	42.0	1.0
ELBOW				
Dry				
corn *(Westbrae)*	2 oz	210	46.0	2.0
corn, wheat-free *(De Boles)*	2 oz	210	45.0	1.0
Jerusalem artichoke *(De Boles)*	2 oz	210	41.0	1.0
100% durum wheat semolina *(American Beauty)*	2 oz	210	42.0	1.0
'Primavera' *(De Boles)*	2 oz	210	41.0	<1.0
quinoa 'Supergrain Wheat Free' *(Ancient Harvest)*	2 oz	180	36.0	2.0
quinoa 'Supergrain Wheat Free' *(Quinoa)*	2 oz	180	36.0	2.0
'Valu Pack' *(Hospitality)*	1/2 cup	240	48.0	0.5
wheat *(Creamette)*	2 oz	210	42.0	1.0
whole wheat	1 cup	365	78.8	1.5
whole wheat *(De Boles)*	2 oz	210	40.0	2.0
FARFELLE/bow tie				
Dry				
wheat *(De Cecco)*	2 oz	210	41.0	1.0
wheat *(Ronzoni)*	2 oz	210	42.0	1.0
FETTUCCINE				
Dry				
basil *(Al Dente)*	2 oz	220	40.0	2.0
curry *(Al Dente)*	2 oz	220	40.0	2.0
dill *(Al Dente)*	2 oz	220	40.0	2.0
egg noodle *(Antoine's)*	2 oz	210	41.0	1.0
egg noodle, extra long *(Ronzoni)*	2 oz	220	42.0	3.0
egg noodle 'Home-Style' *(De Cecco)*	2 oz	210	40.0	3.0
Jerusalem artichoke *(De Boles)*	2 oz	210	41.0	1.0
spinach *(Al Dente)*	2 oz	220	40.0	2.0
spinach *(DiGiorno)*	3 oz	250	46.0	3.0
spinach, Jerusalem artichoke *(De Boles)*	2 oz	210	41.0	<1.0
spinach and egg 'Florentine' *(American Beauty)*	2 oz	220	42.0	3.0
tarragon *(Al Dente)*	2 oz	220	40.0	2.0
wheat *(DiGiorno)*	3 oz	250	47.0	3.0
wheat, bell pepper/basil, organic *(Herb's)*	2 oz	220	40.0	2.0
whole wheat *(Al Dente)*	2 oz	210	42.0	1.0
Refrigerated, fresh				
spinach 'Fresh' *(Contadina)*	3 oz	260	45.0	4.0

Food Name	Serv. Size	Total Cal.	Carbs GMS	Fat GMS
FUSILLI				
Dry				
rainbow *(Antoine's)*	2 oz	210	41.0	1.0
spinach *(De Cecco)*	2 oz	210	41.0	1.0
tricolor *(Antoine's)*	2 oz	210	41.0	1.0
tricolor, vegetable *(Antoine's)*	2 oz	210	41.0	1.0
vegetable *(Antoine's)*	2 oz	210	41.0	1.0
wheat *(De Cecco)*	2 oz	210	41.0	1.0
GEMELLI *(Antoine's)* dry	2 oz	210	41.0	1.0
LASAGNA				
Dry				
curly edge *(Ronzoni)*	2 oz	210	42.0	1.0
Jerusalem artichoke *(De Boles)*	2 oz	210	41.0	1.0
100% durum wheat semolina *(American Beauty)*	2 oz	210	42.0	1.0
100% semolina *(Creamette)*	2 oz	210	42.0	1.0
100% semolina *(De Cecco)*	2 oz	210	41.0	1.0
spinach, whole wheat, no egg *(Westbrae)*	2 oz	210	40.0	2.0
whole wheat *(De Boles)*	2 oz	210	40.0	2.0
whole wheat *(Health Valley)*	2 oz	170	40.0	1.0
whole wheat, no egg *(Westbrae)*	2 oz	210	40.0	2.0
whole wheat, spinach *(Health Valley)*	2 oz	170	40.0	1.0
LINGUINE				
Dry				
Jerusalem artichoke *(De Boles)*	2 oz	210	41.0	1.0
quinoa 'Supergrain Wheat Free' *(Ancient Harvest)*	2 oz	180	35.0	2.0
quinoa 'Supergrain Wheat Free' *(Quinoa)*	2 oz	180	35.0	2.0
wheat *(Creamette)*	2 oz	210	42.0	1.0
wheat *(De Cecco)*	2 oz	210	41.0	1.0
wheat *(DiGiorno)*	3 oz	250	46.0	3.0
wheat *(Ronzoni)*	2 oz	210	42.0	1.0
Refrigerated, fresh				
(DiGiorno)	3 oz	250	47.0	3.0
MANICOTTI, extra fancy *(Ronzoni)* dry	2 oz	210	42.0	1.0
MOSTACCIOLI				
Dry				
100% durum wheat semolina *(American Beauty)*	2 oz	210	42.0	1.0
wheat *(Creamette)*	2 oz	210	42.0	1.0
wheat *(Ronzoni)*	2 oz	210	40.0	1.0
ORZO *(Ronzoni)* dry	2 oz	210	42.0	3.0
PENNE RIGATI				
Dry				
(Antoine's)	2 oz	210	41.0	1.0
(De Cecco)	2 oz	210	41.0	1.0

Food Name	Serv. Size	Total Cal.	Carbs GMS	Fat GMS
PENNONI *(De Cecco)* dry	2 oz	210	41.0	1.0
QUINOA				
Dry				
garden pagodas 'Supergrain Wheat Free' *(Ancient Harvest)*	2 oz	180	35.0	2.0
veggie curls 'Supergrain Wheat Free' *(Ancient Harvest)*	2 oz	180	35.0	2.0
veggie curls 'Supergrain Wheat Free' *(Quinoa)*	2 oz	180	35.0	2.0
RADIATORE				
Dry				
tomato and spinach, tri-color *(Ronzoni)*	2 oz	210	42.0	1.0
wheat *(Antoine's)*	2 oz	210	41.0	1.0
RAINBOW				
100% durum wheat semolina 'Rainbo Twirl'				
(American Beauty) dry	2 oz	210	42.0	1.0
RIBBON				
Dry				
spinach *(Creamette)*	2 oz	210	42.0	1.0
wheat, mixed vegetable, organic *(Herb's)*	2 oz	220	40.0	2.0
wheat, paella, w/saffron, organic *(Eden Foods)*	2 oz	228	44.0	<1.0
wheat, parsley garlic, organic *(Eden Foods)*	2 oz	228	44.0	<1.0
whole wheat *(De Boles)*	2 oz	210	40.0	2.0
yolk-free 'Pennsylvania Dutch' *(Creamette)*	2 oz	210	42.0	1.0
RIGATONI				
Dry				
(Creamette)	2 oz	210	42.0	1.0
(De Cecco)	2 oz	210	41.0	1.0
(Ronzoni)	2 oz	210	42.0	1.0
Refrigerated, fresh				
'Fresh' *(Contadina)*	2.3 oz	200	34.0	3.0
Jerusalem artichoke *(De Boles)*	2 oz	210	41.0	1.0
ROTELLE				
Dry				
100% durum wheat semolina *(American Beauty)*	2 oz	210	42.0	1.0
quinoa 'Supergrain Wheat Free' *(Ancient Harvest)*	2 oz	180	35.0	2.0
quinoa 'Supergrain Wheat Free' *(Quinoa)*	2 oz	180	35.0	2.0
wheat *(Creamette)*	2 oz	210	42.0	1.0
wheat *(De Cecco)*	2 oz	210	41.0	1.0
wheat *(Ronzoni)*	2 oz	210	40.0	1.0
ROTINI				
Dry				
garlic and parsley *(De Boles)*	2 oz	210	41.0	1.0
Jerusalem artichoke *(De Boles)*	2 oz	210	41.0	1.0
100% durum wheat semolina *(American Beauty)*	2 oz	210	42.0	1.0
quinoa 'Supergrain' *(Ancient Harvest)*	2 oz	210	40.0	1.0

Food Name	Serv. Size	Total Cal.	Carbs GMS	Fat GMS
vegetable 'Primavera' (De Boles)	2 oz	210	41.0	<1.0
vegetable, tomato, and basil (De Boles)	2 oz	210	41.0	1.0
SALAD PASTA				
100% durum wheat semolina 'Salad-Roni'				
(American Beauty) dry	2 oz	210	42.0	1.0
SEASHELL				
durum wheat semolina (American Beauty) dry	2 oz	210	42.0	1.0
SHELL				
Dry				
corn (Westbrae)	2 oz	210	46.0	2.0
corn, wheat-free (De Boles)	2 oz	210	45.0	1.0
extra fancy (Ronzoni)	2 oz	210	42.0	1.0
jumbo (Ronzoni)	2 oz	210	42.0	1.0
medium (Creamette)	2 oz	210	42.0	1.0
medium, 100% durum wheat semolina (American Beauty)	2 oz	210	42.0	1.0
100% durum wheat semolina 'Shel-Roni'				
(American Beauty) dry	2 oz	210	42.0	1.0
quinoa 'Supergrain Wheat Free' (Ancient Harvest)	2 oz	180	35.0	2.0
quinoa 'Supergrain Wheat Free' (Quinoa)	2 oz	180	35.0	2.0
'Primavera' (De Boles)	2 oz	210	41.0	<1.0
wheat (Ronzoni)	2 oz	210	42.0	1.0
wheat, vegetable, no eggs, organic (Eden Foods)	2 oz	228	44.0	<1.0
whole wheat (De Boles)	2 oz	210	40.0	2.0
SPAGHETTI				
Dry				
amaranth (Health Valley)	2 oz	170	40.0	1.0
corn (Westbrae)	2 oz	210	46.0	2.0
corn, wheat-free (De Boles)	2 oz	210	45.0	1.0
Jerusalem artichoke (De Boles)	2 oz	210	41.0	1.0
oat bran (Health Valley)	2 oz	120	23.0	1.0
100% durum wheat semolina (American Beauty)	2 oz	210	42.0	1.0
100% semolina (Hospitality)	2 oz	210	42.0	0.5
pepper 'Three Pepper Pasta' (Al Dente)	2 oz	220	40.0	2.0
protein-fortified	2 oz	213	37.4	1.3
quinoa 'Supergrain' (Ancient Harvest)	2 oz	210	40.0	1.0
quinoa 'Supergrain' (Quinoa)	2 oz	210	40.0	1.0
quinoa 'Supergrain Wheat Free' (Ancient Harvest)	2 oz	180	35.0	2.0
quinoa 'Supergrain Wheat Free' (Quinoa)	2 oz	180	35.0	2.0
spinach	2 oz	212	42.6	0.9
spinach, Jerusalem artichoke (De Boles)	2 oz	210	41.0	<1.0
spinach, whole wheat, no egg (Westbrae)	2 oz	210	40.0	2.0
thin (Creamette)	2 oz	210	42.0	1.0
thin (Ronzoni)	2 oz	210	42.0	1.0

Food Name	Serv. Size	Total Cal.	Carbs GMS	Fat GMS
thin, 100% durum wheat semolina *(American Beauty)*	2 oz	210	42.0	1.0
unenriched	2 oz	211	42.6	0.9
wheat *(DiGiorno)*	3 oz	250	47.0	3.0
wheat *(Rummo)*	2 oz	210	41.0	1.0
whole wheat	2 oz	198	42.8	0.8
whole wheat *(De Boles)*	2 oz	210	40.0	2.0
whole wheat *(Health Valley)*	2 oz	170	40.0	1.0
whole wheat, no egg *(Westbrae)*	2 oz	210	40.0	2.0
whole wheat, spinach *(Health Valley)*	2 oz	170	40.0	1.0
SPAGHETTINI *(De Cecco)* dry	2 oz	210	41.0	1.0
SPIRAL				
Dry				
spicy *(Antoine's)*	2 oz	210	41.0	1.0
vegetable	1 cup	308	62.9	0.9
wheat, sesame rice, organic *(Eden Foods)*	2 oz	212	40.0	1.0
wheat, vegetable, no eggs, organic *(Eden Foods)*	2 oz	228	44.0	<1.0
TRICOLOR				
Dry				
'Primavera' *(De Boles)*	2 oz	200	41.0	1.0
spirals	1 cup	308	62.9	0.9
wheat *(Creamette)*	2 oz	210	42.0	1.0
TRIO ITALIANO				
rotini, mostaccioli, shells *(American Beauty)* dry	2 oz	210	42.0	1.0
VERMICELLI				
Dry				
extra thin *(Creamette)*	2 oz	210	42.0	1.0
100% durum wheat semolina *(American Beauty)*	2 oz	210	42.0	1.0
wheat *(Ronzoni)*	2 oz	210	42.0	1.0
ZITI Jerusalem artichoke *(De Boles)* dry	2 oz	210	41.0	1.0
ZITI RIGATI *(Ronzoni)* dry	2 oz	210	42.0	1.0
PASTA DINNER, FROZEN				
penne, w/tomato sauce, Italian sausage *(Budget Gourmet)*	10 oz	320	53.0	9.0
primavera *(Healthy Choice)*	11 oz	280	51.0	3.0
stuffed, shells, three-cheese 'LightStyle' *(Le Menu)*	10 oz	280	34.0	8.0
w/chicken and herb tomato sauce *(Lean Cuisine)*	9.5 oz	270	38.0	6.0
zesty tomato sauce over ziti 'Classics' *(Healthy Choice)*	12 oz	350	59.0	5.0
PASTA DINNER MIX				
artichoke elbow 'Mac & Cheese' dry *(De Boles)*	2 oz	210	40.0	2.0
artichoke elbow 'Mac & Cheese' prepared *(De Boles)*	3/4 cup	220	31.0	7.0
artichoke shells and cheddar, dry *(De Boles)*	2 oz	210	40.0	2.0
artichoke shells and cheddar, prepared *(De Boles)*	3/4 cup	220	31.0	7.0
wheat elbow 'Mac & Cheese' dry *(De Boles)*	2 oz	210	39.0	3.0
wheat elbow 'Mac & Cheese' prepared *(De Boles)*	3/4 cup	200	27.0	8.0

Food Name	Serv. Size	Total Cal.	Carbs GMS	Fat GMS
w/beef flavored sauce, prepared *(Ultra Slim Fast)*	8 oz	230	45.0	3.0
w/chicken flavored sauce, prepared *(Ultra Slim Fast)*	8 oz	220	45.0	3.0
w/tomato herb sauce, prepared *(Ultra Slim Fast)*	8 oz	220	46.0	3.0
w/zesty cheese sauce, prepared *(Ultra Slim Fast)*	8 oz	230	44.0	4.0

PASTA DISH MIX. See also NOODLE ENTRÉE/DISH MIX; ROTINI ENTRÉE MIX; SPAGHETTI ENTRÉE MIX.

Food Name	Serv. Size	Total Cal.	Carbs GMS	Fat GMS
Alfredo 'Pasta For One' *(Villa Lorenzo)*	2.3 oz	270	39.0	8.0
butter and herbs 'Pasta For One' *(Villa Lorenzo)*	2.3 oz	270	43.0	7.0
cream sauce and mushrooms 'Pasta For One' *(Villa Lorenzo)*	2.3 oz	260	42.0	6.0
cream sauce and spinach 'Pasta For One' *(Villa Lorenzo)*	2.3 oz	270	43.0	6.0
pesto and herbs 'Pasta For One' *(Villa Lorenzo)*	2.3 oz	260	41.0	6.0
three cheese and broccoli 'Pasta For One' *(Villa Lorenzo)*	2.3 oz	260	43.0	5.0
zesty tomato 'Pasta For One' *(Villa Lorenzo)*	2.3 oz	250	47.0	3.0

PASTA ENTRÉE, CANNED. See also NOODLE ENTRÉE/DISH, CANNED; RAVIOLI ENTRÉE; SPAGHETTI ENTRÉE, CANNED.

(Chef Boyardee)

Food Name	Serv. Size	Total Cal.	Carbs GMS	Fat GMS
and chicken	7.5 oz	180	30.0	2.0
in cheese sauce 'ABC's & 123's'	8.6 oz	200	42.0	1.0
in cheese sauce 'Dinosaurs'	8.6 oz	200	42.0	1.0
in cheese sauce 'Dinosaurs'	7.5 oz	160	33.0	1.0
in cheese sauce 'Sharks'	7.5 oz	170	34.0	1.0
in cheese sauce 'Smurfs'	7.5 oz	150	29.0	1.0
in cheese sauce 'Tic Tac Toes'	8.6 oz	190	41.0	1.0
in cheese sauce 'Tic Tac Toes'	7.5 oz	160	31.0	1.0
in chicken sauce 'Pac Man'	7.5 oz	170	22.0	7.0
in meat sauce, shells	7.5 oz	190	31.0	6.0
in pizza sauce, spirals	7.5 oz	180	35.0	3.0
in sauce 'ABC's & 123's'	7.5 oz	160	31.0	1.0
in sauce 'Turtles'	7.5 oz	150	31.0	1.0
in tomato sauce 'Pac Man'	7.5 oz	150	30.0	1.0
mini bites	7.5 oz	260	30.0	12.0
'Roller Coasters'	7.5 oz	230	28.0	10.0
w/meatballs 'ABC's & 123's'	8.6 oz	280	35.0	11.0
w/meatballs 'Dinosaurs'	8.6 oz	280	36.0	11.0
w/meatballs 'Pac Man'	7.5 oz	230	32.0	9.0
w/meatballs 'Sharks'	7.5 oz	230	31.0	8.0
w/meatballs 'Smurfs'	7.5 oz	240	31.0	9.0
w/meatballs 'Tic Tac Toes'	8.6 oz	290	39.0	11.0
w/meatballs 'Tic Tac Toes'	7.5 oz	240	31.0	9.0
w/meatballs 'Turtles'	7.5 oz	220	30.0	8.0
w/meatballs in sauce 'Zooroni'	7.5 oz	240	33.0	8.0
w/mini meatballs 'ABC's & 123's'	7.5 oz	240	33.0	9.0

Food Name	Serv. Size	Total Cal.	Carbs GMS	F... G...
w/mini meatballs 'Dinosaurs'	7.5 oz	230	32.0	8.

PASTA ENTRÉE, FROZEN. See also NOODLE ENTRÉE/DISH, FROZEN; RAVIOLI ENTRÉE; ROTINI ENTRÉE, FROZEN; SPAGHETTI ENTRÉE, FROZEN; TORTELLINI PASTA DISH/ ENTRÉE, FROZEN; ZITI ENTRÉE, FROZEN.

Food Name	Serv. Size	Total Cal.	Carbs GMS	F... G...
angel hair *(Smart Ones)*	8.55 oz	120	18.0	<1.
angel hair pasta *(Lean Cuisine)*	10 oz	240	38.0	5
baked, and cheese *(Celentano)*	6 oz	290	29.0	13
broccoli stuffed shells, low fat 'Great Choice' *(Celentano)*	10 oz	190	31.0	4.
creamy cheddar 'Pasta Accents' *(Green Giant)*	1/2 cup	90	14.0	3.
Dijon 'Microwave Garden Gourmet' *(Green Giant)*	1 pkg	300	24.0	20.
garden herb seasoning 'Pasta Accents' *(Green Giant)*	1/2 cup	80	12.0	3.
garlic seasoning 'Pasta Accents' *(Green Giant)*	1/2 cup	100	14.0	4.
Italiano *(Ultimate 200)*	8 oz	190	19.0	4.
'Looney Tunes Bugs Bunny & Tazmanian Devil' *(Tyson)*	8 oz	290	41.0	8.
'Looney Tunes Daffy Duck' spaghetti & meatballs *(Tyson)*	8.65 oz	340	49.0	10.
'Looney Tunes Daffy Duck & Elmer Fudd' *(Tyson)*	8 oz	270	40.0	7.
'Looney Tunes Foghorn Leghorn & Henry Hawk' *(Tyson)*	8 oz	230	39.0	4.
'Looney Tunes Sylvester & Tweety' *(Tyson)*	8 oz	250	41.0	4.
'Looney Tunes Tweety' macaroni and cheese *(Tyson)*	8 oz	340	49.0	10.
Parmesan, w/sweet peas 'One Serving' *(Green Giant)*	5.5 oz	160	21.0	5.
Portafino, in wine sauce *(Smart Ones)*	9.5 oz	160	30.0	1.
primavera 'Pasta Accents' *(Green Giant)*	1/2 cup	110	15.0	4.
Romanoff supreme *(Weight Watchers)*	9 oz	230	29.0	7.
shells, cheese, w/tomato sauce *(Stouffer's)*	9.25 oz	300	28.0	13.
shells, stuffed *(Celentano)*	8 oz	330	41.0	11.
shells, stuffed, in tomato sauce 'Classics' *(Healthy Choice)*	12 oz	330	53.0	3.
shells, stuffed, low fat 'Great Choice' *(Celentano)*	10 oz	250	41.0	2.
shells, stuffed 'Single Serving' *(Buitoni)*	9 oz	460	46.0	13.
shells, stuffed, w/sauce *(Celentano)*	10 oz	410	51.0	14.0
shells, stuffed, w/sauce *(Celentano)*	6.25 oz	340	31.0	16.
shells, stuffed, w/vegetables, tofu, sauce *(Legume)*	11 oz	240	26.0	12.
shells and beef *(Budget Gourmet)*	10 oz	340	34.0	14.
teriyaki pasta, w/chicken 'Classics' *(Healthy Choice)*	12.6 oz	350	58.0	3.0
trio 'Gourmet Selection' *(Tyson)*	11 oz	450	53.0	17.
w/shrimp 'Classics' *(Healthy Choice)*	12.5 oz	270	44.0	4.
w/turkey, Dijon sauce 'Lunch Express' *(Lean Cuisine)*	9 7/8 oz	290	39.0	7.

PASTA ENTRÉE, MICROWAVE. See also NOODLE ENTRÉE/DISH, MICROWAVE; RAVIOLI ENTRÉE; SPAGHETTI ENTRÉE, MICROWAVE.

(Chef Boyardee)

Food Name	Serv. Size	Total Cal.	Carbs GMS	F... G...
in cheese sauce 'ABC's & 123's'	7.5 oz	180	37.0	1.
in cheese sauce 'Dinosaurs'	7.5 oz	180	36.0	1.0
in cheese sauce 'Tic Tac Toes'	7.5 oz	170	36.0	1.0
in sauce 'Turtles'	7.5 oz	160	33.0	1.0

Food Name	Serv. Size	Total Cal.	Carbs GMS	Fat GMS
rings and franks	7.5 oz	190	31.0	5.0
rings and meatballs	7.5 oz	220	33.0	8.0
shells, in meat sauce	7.5 oz	210	32.0	6.0
shells, in mushroom sauce	7.5 oz	170	35.0	1.0
w/meatballs 'Dinosaurs'	7.5 oz	240	32.0	9.0
w/meatballs 'Tic Tac Toes'	7.5 oz	250	32.0	10.0
w/meatballs 'Turtles'	7.5 oz	210	30.0	8.0
w/mini meatballs 'ABC's & 123's'	7.5 oz	260	32.0	11.0
(Lunch Bucket)				
and garden vegetables 'Light 'n Healthy'	7.5 oz	150	30.0	1.0
elbows, in tomato sauce	7.5 oz	190	38.0	2.0
in wine sauce, beef 'Light 'n Healthy'	7.5 oz	130	21.0	3.0
Italian style chicken 'Light 'n Healthy'	7.5 oz	130	23.0	1.0
'Pasta 'n Chicken'	7.5 oz	180	22.0	6.0
PASTA SALAD MIX				
Caesar, dry *(Suddenly Salad)*	1/6 pkg	110	20.0	1.0
Caesar, prepared *(Suddenly Salad)*	1/2 cup	170	20.0	8.0
creamy macaroni, dry *(Suddenly Salad)*	1/6 pkg	100	20.0	1.0
creamy macaroni, prepared *(Suddenly Salad)*	1/2 cup	200	21.0	10.0
garden primavera, dry *(Kraft)*	1/6 box	170	21.0	7.0
Italian 'Light' dry *(Kraft)*	1/6 box	120	22.0	1.0
pasta, classic, dry *(Suddenly Salad)*	1/6 pkg	120	23.0	1.0
pasta, classic, prepared *(Suddenly Salad)*	1/2 cup	160	23.0	6.0
pasta primavera, dry *(Suddenly Salad)*	1/6 pkg	90	19.0	1.0
pasta primavera, prepared *(Suddenly Salad)*	1/2 cup	190	20.0	10.0
ranch and bacon, dry *(Suddenly Salad)*	1/6 pkg	110	21.0	1.0
ranch and bacon, prepared *(Suddenly Salad)*	1/2 cup	210	22.0	11.0
tortellini, Italiano, dry *(Suddenly Salad)*	1/5 pkg	120	21.0	2.0
tortellini, Italiano, prepared *(Suddenly Salad)*	1/2 cup	160	21.0	7.0
PASTA SAUCE. See SAUCE.				
PASTRAMI. See LUNCHEON MEAT.				
PASTRY. See also BREAD, SWEET; BUN, SWEET; CAKE; DANISH PASTRY; MUFFIN; PIE; ROLL, SWEET; TURNOVER.				
(Charlette Russe) w/lady fingers, whipped cream filling	1 serving	326	38.2	16.6
(Pillsbury) pocket, refrigerated	1 piece	240	25.0	13.0
PASTRY, BAVARIAN CREAM				
(Entenmann's)	1.3 oz	80	20.0	0.0
(Rich's) puff, frozen	1 piece	150	17.0	8.0
PASTRY, CINNAMON *(Entenmann's)* filbert ring	1.5 oz	190	19.0	12.0
PASTRY, DATE NUT *(Awrey's)* 1 piece	1.6 oz	230	35.0	10.0
PASTRY, ÉCLAIR				
(Rich's) frozen, chocolate, 2 oz	1 piece	210	27.0	10.0
(Weight Watchers) frozen, chocolate 'Sweet Celebrations'	2.1 oz	150	26.0	4.0

Food Name	Serv. Size	Total Cal.	Carbs GMS	Fat GMS
PATÉ, CANNED				
chicken liver	1 oz	57	1.9	3.7
chicken liver	1 tbsp	26	0.9	1.7
foie gras, goose liver, smoked	1 oz	131	1.3	12.4
foie gras, goose liver, smoked	1 tbsp	60	0.6	5.7
liver *(Sells)*	2 1/8 oz	190	4.0	16.0
PATTYPAN SQUASH. See SQUASH, SCALLOP.				
PEACH				
peeled, pitted	1 oz	12	3.1	<.1
peeled, sliced	1/2 cup	37	9.4	0.1
raw, approx 4 oz	1 med	37	9.7	0.1
raw, slices	1 cup	73	18.9	0.2
untrimmed	1 lb	148	38.2	0.3
untrimmed *(Dole)*	2 pieces	70	19.0	0.0
PEACH, CANNED				
'Fruit Pak' *(Mott's)*	3.75 oz	75	18.0	0.0
halves *(Hunt's)*	4 oz	90	23.0	<1.0
slices *(Hunt's)*	4 oz	90	23.0	<1.0
FREESTONE				
halves *(Del Monte)*	1/2 cup	90	23.0	0.0
halves *(S&W Nutradiet)*	1/2 cup	30	7.0	0.0
halves 'Lite' *(Del Monte)*	1/2 cup	60	13.0	0.0
in heavy syrup, halves *(S&W)*	1/2 cup	100	26.0	0.0
in heavy syrup, slices *(S&W)*	1/2 cup	100	26.0	0.0
slices *(Del Monte)*	1/2 cup	90	23.0	0.0
slices *(S&W Nutradiet)*	1/2 cup	30	7.0	0.0
slices 'Lite' *(Del Monte)*	1/2 cup	60	13.0	0.0
YELLOW CLING				
diced 'Fruit Cup' *(Del Monte)*	5 oz	110	28.0	0.0
halves *(Del Monte)*	1/2 cup	80	22.0	0.0
halves *(S&W Nutradiet)*	1/2 cup	30	8.0	0.0
halves 'Lite' *(Del Monte)*	1/2 cup	50	13.0	0.0
halves 'Lite' *(Finast)*	1/2 cup	50	14.0	0.0
in heavy syrup, halves *(A&P)*	1/2 cup	100	25.0	<1.0
in heavy syrup, halves *(S&W)*	1/2 cup	100	25.0	0.0
in heavy syrup, slices *(A&P)*	1/2 cup	100	25.0	<1.0
in heavy syrup, slices *(Finast)*	1/2 cup	100	25.0	0.0
in heavy syrup, slices *(Pathmark)*	1/2 cup	100	25.0	0.0
in heavy syrup, slices *(S&W)*	1/2 cup	100	25.0	0.0
in heavy syrup, whole, spiced *(S&W)*	1/2 cup	90	23.0	0.0
in juice *(A&P)*	1/2 cup	50	12.0	<1.0
in juice, halves *(A&P)*	1/2 cup	50	12.0	<1.0
in juice, halves *(Featherweight)*	1/2 cup	50	14.0	0.0

Food Name	Serv. Size	Total Cal.	Carbs GMS	Fat GMS
in juice, halves 'Lite' *(Libby's)*	1/2 cup	50	13.0	0.0
in juice, slices *(Featherweight)*	1/2 cup	50	14.0	0.0
in juice, slices *(IGA)*	1/2 cup	50	14.0	0.0
in juice, slices *(Pathmark)*	1/2 cup	50	14.0	0.0
in juice, slices 'Lite' *(Libby's)*	1/2 cup	50	13.0	0.0
in juice, slices, sweetened *(S&W)*	1/2 cup	90	20.0	0.0
in light syrup, slices 'No Frills' *(Pathmark)*	1/2 cup	140	36.0	0.0
slices *(Del Monte)*	1/2 cup	80	22.0	0.0
slices 'Lite' *(Del Monte)*	1/2 cup	50	13.0	0.0
slices 'Lite' *(Finast)*	1/2 cup	50	14.0	0.0
slices, unsweetened *(S&W Nutradiet)*	1/2 cup	30	8.0	0.0
spiced, w/pits *(Del Monte)*	3.5 oz	80	20.0	0.0
PEACH, DRIED				
sulfured, cooked, sweetened	4 oz	117	30.2	0.2
sulfured, cooked, sweetened, halves	1/2 cup	139	35.9	0.3
sulfured, cooked, unsweetened	4 oz	87	22.3	0.3
sulfured, cooked, unsweetened, halves	1/2 cup	91	25.4	0.3
sulfured, uncooked	4 oz	271	69.5	0.9
sulfured, uncooked, approx 4.6 oz	10 halves	311	79.7	1.0
sulfured, uncooked, halves	1/2 cup	192	49.1	0.6
(Del Monte) uncooked	2 oz	140	35.0	0.0
(Mountain House) freeze-dried, prepared	1/4 cup	50	12.0	0.0
(Sun•Maid)	2 oz	140	38.0	0.0
(SunSweet)	2 oz	140	38.0	0.0
PEACH, FROZEN				
slices, sweetened	10-oz pkg	267	68.1	0.4
slices, sweetened	1/2 cup	118	30.0	0.2
slices, sweetened	4 oz	107	27.2	0.1
PEACH BUTTER *(Smucker's)*	1 tsp	15	4.0	0.0
PEACH DRINK				
(Hi-C)	6 oz	101	24.8	<.1
(Ocean Spray) citrus 'Refreshers'	6 oz	90	23.0	0.0
PEACH JUICE				
(Dole) orchard blend 'Pure & Light'	6 oz	90	24.0	0.0
(Smucker's) 'Naturally 100%'	8 oz	120	30.0	0.0
(Snapple) 'Dixie Peach'	8 oz	160	39.0	0.0
PEACH NECTAR				
w/added ascorbic acid	1 cup	134	34.7	0.1
w/added ascorbic acid	1 oz	17	4.3	0.0
w/o added ascorbic acid	1 cup	134	34.7	0.1
w/o added ascorbic acid	1 oz	17	4.3	0.0
(Kern's)	6 oz	110	26.0	0.0
(Knudsen & Sons)	8 oz	107	32.0	0.0

Food Name	Serv. Size	Total Cal.	Carbs GMS	Fat GMS
(Libby's)	6 oz	100	24.0	0.0
PEANUT, SHELLED				
(Beer Nuts)	1 oz	180	7.0	14.0
(Frito Lay) salted	1 oz	170	6.0	15.0
(Little Debbie) salted	1.25 oz	230	5.0	18.0
(Pathmark) 'Sweet and Crunchy'	1 oz	140	15.0	8.0
(Planters)				
hot spicy 'Heat'	1 oz	170	5.0	14.0
mild spicy 'Heat'	1 oz	170	5.0	14.0
'Sweet-N-Crunchy'	1 oz	140	15.0	8.0
(Weight Watchers)	1 pouch	100	4.0	7.0
BOILED				
salted	1/2 cup	102	6.8	7.0
salted	1 oz	90	6.0	6.2
DRY-ROASTED				
(Finast)				
lightly salted	1 oz	160	5.0	14.0
salted	1 oz	160	6.0	14.0
(Flavor House)				
salted	1 oz	180	5.0	14.0
unsalted	1 oz	180	5.0	14.0
(Frito Lay) salted	1 1/8 oz	190	7.0	16.0
(Guy's) salted	1 oz	170	3.0	14.0
(Pathmark)				
'No Frills' salted	1 oz	170	5.0	14.0
'No Frills' unsalted	1 oz	180	5.0	14.0
(Planters)				
lightly salted	1 oz	170	5.0	15.0
salted	1 oz	160	6.0	14.0
unsalted	1 oz	170	5.0	15.0
HONEY-ROASTED				
(Eagle) 'Honey Roast'	1 oz	170	7.0	13.0
(Fisher)				
lightly salted	1 oz	150	5.0	13.0
salted	1 oz	150	5.0	13.0
(Flavor House)	1 oz	160	9.0	11.0
(Little Debbie)	1.13 oz	190	9.0	13.0
(Pathmark)	1 oz	170	8.0	13.0
(Planters)	1 oz	170	8.0	13.0
(Weight Watchers)	1 pouch	100	4.0	7.0
OIL-ROASTED				
(Fisher) salted	1 oz	160	6.0	14.0
(Flavor House) salted	1 oz	170	5.0	15.0

Food Name	Serv. Size	Total Cal.	Carbs GMS	Fat GMS
(Pathmark) salted	1 oz	180	5.0	14.0
(Planters)				
cocktail	1 oz	170	5.0	15.0
cocktail, unsalted	1 oz	170	5.0	15.0
lightly salted	1 oz	170	5.0	14.0
redskin	1 oz	170	5.0	15.0
salted	1 oz	170	5.0	15.0
unsalted	1 oz	170	5.0	14.0
PEANUT, SPANISH				
DRY-ROASTED *(Planters)*	1 oz	160	6.0	14.0
OIL-ROASTED				
salted	1/2 cup	426	12.8	36.0
salted	1 oz	162	4.9	13.7
salted *(Flavor House)*	1 oz	170	5.0	15.0
salted *(Planters)*	1 oz	170	5.0	15.0
shelled, salted *(Flavor House)*	1 oz	170	5.0	15.0
shelled, salted *(Guy's)*	1 oz	170	3.0	14.0
unsalted	1/2 cup	426	12.8	36.0
unsalted	1 oz	162	4.9	13.7
RAW				
	1 cup	832	23.1	72.4
	1 oz	160	4.4	13.9
(Planters)	1 oz	160	5.0	14.0
PEANUT, VALENCIA				
oil-roasted	1 cup	848	23.5	73.8
oil-roasted	1/2 cup	424	11.7	36.9
oil-roasted	1 oz	165	4.6	14.4
raw	1/2 cup	417	15.3	34.7
raw	1 oz	160	5.8	13.3
PEANUT, VIRGINIA				
oil-roasted, unsalted	1 cup	827	28.4	69.5
oil-roasted, unsalted	1 oz	162	5.6	13.6
raw	1 cup	822	24.2	71.2
raw	1 oz	158	4.6	13.6
PEANUT BUTTER				
(Hollywood) 'Unsalted'	1 tbsp	35	1.0	3.0
(Pathmark) 'Natural'	2 tbsp	200	5.0	17.0
(Roaster Fresh) gourmet	1 oz	166	5.0	14.0
(S&W Nutradiet)	1 tbsp	93	2.0	8.0
(Smucker's)				
honey sweetened	2 tbsp	200	7.0	16.0
no salt added 'Natural'	2 tbsp	200	6.0	16.0

Food Name	Serv. Size	Total Cal.	Carbs GMS	Fat GMS
CHUNKY				
(Arrowhead Mills)	2 tbsp	190	6.0	16.0
(Bama)	2 tbsp	200	6.0	17.0
(Estee)	2 tbsp	200	6.0	18.0
(Featherweight)	1 tbsp	90	2.0	7.0
(Finast) 'Crunchy'	2 tbsp	195	6.0	17.0
(Health Valley) 'No Salt Added'	2 tbsp	180	6.0	14.0
(Hollywood)	1 tbsp	35	1.0	3.0
(Jif)				
regular	2 tbsp	190	6.0	16.0
'Simply Jif'	2 tbsp	180	5.0	16.0
(Maranatha Natural) crunchy	2 tbsp	190	7.0	15.0
(Pathmark) 'Super Chunky'	2 tbsp	200	6.0	17.0
(Peter Pan)				
'Extra Crunchy'	2 tbsp	190	5.1	16.3
regular	2 tbsp	190	5.0	16.0
'Salt Free'	2 tbsp	190	5.0	17.0
(Skippy) 'Super Chunk'	2 tbsp	190	4.0	17.0
(Smucker's) 'Chunky Natural'	2 tbsp	200	6.0	16.0
(Westbrae)				
'Natural' w/salt	2 tbsp	190	7.0	16.0
'Natural' w/o salt	2 tbsp	190	7.0	16.0
SMOOTH				
(Arrowhead Mills)	2 tbsp	190	6.0	16.0
(Bama)	2 tbsp	200	6.0	17.0
(Estee)	1 tbsp	100	3.0	8.0
(Featherweight)	1 tbsp	90	2.0	7.0
(Finast)	2 tbsp	195	6.0	17.0
(Health Valley) 'No Salt Added'	2 tbsp	180	6.0	14.0
(Hollywood)	1 tbsp	35	1.0	3.0
(Jif)				
regular	2 tbsp	190	6.0	16.0
'Simply Jif'	2 tbsp	180	5.0	16.0
(Pathmark) 'No Frills Creamy'	2 tbsp	200	6.0	17.0
(Peter Pan)				
'Creamy'	2 tbsp	190	5.7	16.4
'Creamy Salt Free'	2 tbsp	195	5.3	17.1
(Skippy) 'Creamy'	2 tbsp	190	4.0	17.0
(Smucker's)				
'Natural'	2 tbsp	200	6.0	16.0
'No Salt Added Natural'	2 tbsp	200	6.0	17.0
(Westbrae) 'Natural' no salt	2 tbsp	190	7.0	16.0
(Woodstock) 'Old Fashioned Unsalted'	2 tbsp	200	6.0	16.0

Food Name	Serv. Size	Total Cal.	Carbs GMS	Fat GMS
W/JELLY				
(Bama)	2 tbsp	150	20.0	7.0
(Smucker's)				
'Goober Grape'	2 tbsp	180	18.0	10.0
'Goober Strawberry'	2 tbsp	180	18.0	10.0
PEANUT BUTTER CHIPS (Hershey's) 'Reese's'	1.5 oz	230	19.0	13.0
PEANUT BUTTER TOPPING (Smucker's) caramel	2 tbsp	150	29.0	2.0
PEANUT FLOUR				
defatted	1 cup	196	20.8	0.3
defatted	1 oz	92	9.7	0.2
low-fat	1 cup	257	18.8	13.1
low-fat	1 oz	120	8.8	6.1
PEANUT OIL				
	1/2 cup	955	0.0	108.0
	1 oz	251	0.0	28.4
(Hain)	1 tbsp	120	0.0	14.0
(Planters)	1 tbsp	120	0.0	14.0
(Spectrum Naturals)	1 tbsp	120	0.0	14.0
(Wesson)	1 tbsp	122	0.0	13.6
PEAR				
Asian, raw	1 fruit	51	13.0	0.3
raw, slices	1 cup	97	24.9	0.7
trimmed, w/skin	1 oz	17	4.3	0.1
untrimmed	1 lb	247	63.1	1.7
untrimmed (Dole)	1 fruit	100	25.0	1.0
w/skin, sliced	1/2 cup	49	12.5	0.3
PEAR, CANNED				
in extra heavy syrup	4 oz	110	28.6	0.1
in extra heavy syrup, halves	1/2 cup	127	33.0	0.2
in extra heavy syrup, solid and liquid, halves	1 cup	253	65.9	0.3
in extra light syrup	4 oz	53	13.8	0.1
in extra light syrup, halves	1/2 cup	58	15.1	0.1
in extra light syrup, solid and liquid, halves	1 cup	116	30.1	0.3
in heavy syrup	4 oz	84	21.7	0.1
in heavy syrup, halves	1/2 cup	94	24.4	0.2
in heavy syrup, solid and liquid, halves	1 cup	189	48.9	0.3
in juice	4 oz	57	14.7	0.1
in juice, halves	1/2 cup	62	16.0	0.1
in juice, solid and liquid, halves	1 cup	124	32.1	0.2
in light syrup	4 oz	65	17.2	<.1
in light syrup, halves	1/2 cup	72	19.0	<.1
in light syrup, solid and liquid, halves	1 cup	143	38.1	0.1
in water	4 oz	33	8.9	<.1

Food Name	Serv. Size	Total Cal.	Carbs GMS	Fat GMS
in water, halves	1/2 cup	36	9.5	<.1
in water, solid and liquid, halves	1 cup	71	19.1	0.1
(A&P)				
in heavy syrup, halves or slices	1/2 cup	95	25.0	<1.0
in juice, halves or slices	1/2 cup	60	15.0	<1.0
in light syrup, halves or slices	1/2 cup	70	20.0	<1.0
(Del Monte)				
Bartlett, halves 'Lite'	1/2 cup	50	14.0	0.0
Bartlett, halves or slices	1/2 cup	80	22.0	0.0
Bartlett, slices 'Lite'	1/2 cup	50	14.0	0.0
(Featherweight) in juice, halves	1/2 cup	60	15.0	0.0
(Finast)				
Bartlett, halves or slices, in heavy syrup	1/2 cup	100	25.0	0.0
Bartlett, halves or slices, 'Lite No Sugar Added'	1/2 cup	60	15.0	0.0
(Hunt's) halves	4 oz	90	23.0	1.0
(IGA) Bartlett, halves, unsweetened	1/2 cup	60	15.0	0.0
(Libby's) in juice, halves or slices, 'Lite'	1/2 cup	60	19.0	0.0
(Pathmark)				
Bartlett, halves, in heavy syrup	1/2 cup	90	23.0	0.0
Bartlett, halves, in juice	1/2 cup	60	15.0	0.0
Bartlett, in light syrup 'No Frills'	1 cup	140	38.0	0.0
Bartlett, slices, in heavy syrup	1 cup	180	46.0	0.0
(S&W Nutradiet)				
Bartlett, peeled, unsweetened	1/2 cup	35	10.0	0.0
in heavy syrup, halves	1/2 cup	100	25.0	0.0
in juice, slices, sweetened 'Natural Style'	1/2 cup	80	20.0	0.0
peeled, quarters	1/2 cup	35	10.0	0.0
PEAR, DRIED				
Sulfured				
cooked, sweetened	4 oz	159	42.1	0.3
cooked, unsweetened	4 oz	144	38.3	0.4
stewed, w/added sugar, halves	1/2 cup	196	52.0	0.4
stewed, w/o added sugar, halves	1/2 cup	163	43.3	0.4
uncooked	10 halves	458	122.0	1.1
uncooked	4 oz	297	79.0	0.7
PEAR JUICE				
(Knudsen & Sons)	8 oz	110	28.0	0.0
(Santa Cruz Natural) organic 'Cruz'	8 oz	135	32.0	<1.0
PEAR NECTAR				
(Kern's)	6 oz	120	28.0	0.0
(Libby's)	6 oz	110	28.0	0.0
PEAS, CROWDER				
(Allens) canned, 'Fresh'	1/2 cup	80	15.0	<1.0

Food Name	Serv. Size	Total Cal.	Carbs GMS	Fat GMS
(Seabrook) frozen	3 oz	130	23.0	1.0

PEAS, GREEN

(NOTE: All peas are shelled unless otherwise noted.)

boiled, drained	4 oz	95	17.7	0.2
boiled, drained	1/2 cup	67	12.5	0.2
boiled, drained, in pod	4 oz	48	8.0	0.3
boiled, drained, in pod	1/2 cup	34	5.6	0.2
raw	1/2 cup	58	10.4	0.3
raw	1 oz	23	4.1	0.1
raw, in pod	1 lb	140	24.9	0.7
raw, trimmed	1/2 cup	30	5.4	0.1
raw, trimmed	1 oz	12	2.1	0.1
raw, untrimmed	1 lb	180	32.2	0.9

CANNED

dietary pack, drained solids	1/2 cup	59	10.7	0.3
dietary pack, solids and liquid	1/2 cup	61	11.1	0.4
drained, low-sodium	4 oz	78	14.3	0.4
regular pack, drained solids	1/2 cup	59	10.7	0.3
regular pack, solids and liquid	1/2 cup	61	11.1	0.4

Early/June

(A&P)	1/2 cup	70	15.0	<1.0
(Allens) dry	1/2 cup	80	15.0	<1.0
(Del Monte) small, w/liquid	1/2 cup	50	9.0	0.0
(Green Giant)	1/2 cup	50	12.0	0.0
(Green Giant) very young, small	1/2 cup	50	12.0	0.0
(S&W) 'Petit Pois'	1/2 cup	70	12.0	0,0
(Stokely)	1/2 cup	60	12.0	0.0

Mixed sizes

(A&P)	1/2 cup	60	12.0	<1.0
(IGA) 'No Salt or Sugar Added'	1/2 cup	50	10.0	0.0

Sweet

wrinkled, dietary pack, drained, low-sodium	1 lb	82	15.4	0.0
wrinkled, dietary pack, drained, low-sodium	1 oz	5	1.0	0.0
wrinkled, regular pack, drained	1 lb	100	19.5	0.0
wrinkled, regular pack, drained	1 oz	6	1.2	0.0
(Featherweight)	1/2 cup	70	12.0	0.0
(Finast)	1/2 cup	70	13.0	1.0
(Finast) 'No Salt Added'	1/2 cup	60	12.0	0.0
(Green Giant)	1/2 cup	50	11.0	0.0
(Green Giant) 50% less salt	1/2 cup	50	11.0	0.0
(Green Giant) mini	1/2 cup	50	12.0	0.0
(Green Giant) mini, in brine	1/2 cup	60	12.0	<1.0
(Green Giant) very young, small	1/2 cup	50	12.0	0.0

Food Name	Serv. Size	Total Cal.	Carbs GMS	Fat GMS
(Green Giant) very young, tender	1/2 cup	50	11.0	0.0
(IGA) tiny, early/June	1/2 cup	70	12.0	0.0
(Pathmark) garden, fancy	1/2 cup	70	12.0	1.0
(Pathmark) large, tender	1/2 cup	70	12.0	1.0
(Pathmark) 'Little Gem'	1/2 cup	70	12.0	1.0
(Pathmark) mixed sizes 'No Salt Added'	1/2 cup	50	10.0	0.0
(Pathmark) 'No Frills'	1 cup	120	25.0	1.0
(Pathmark) small	1/2 cup	70	12.0	1.0
(S&W) 'Perfection'	1/2 cup	70	12.0	0.0
(S&W Nutradiet)	1/2 cup	40	8.0	0.0
(Stokely)	1/2 cup	60	10.0	0.0
W/liquid				
low-sodium	4 oz	56	10.2	0.3
(Del Monte)	1/2 cup	60	10.0	0.0
(Del Monte) 'No Salt Added'	1/2 cup	60	11.0	0.0
FREEZE-DRIED (Mountain House) prepared	1/2 cup	70	12.0	1.0
FROZEN				
boiled, drained	4 oz	88	16.2	0.3
boiled, drained	1/2 cup	62	11.4	0.2
unprepared	1/2 cup	55	9.9	0.3
(Birds Eye)	3.3 oz	80	13.0	0.0
(Birds Eye) 'Portion Pack'	3 oz	70	12.0	0.0
(Freshlike)	3.3 oz	80	13.0	0.0
(Frosty Acres)	3.3 oz	80	13.0	0.0
(Health Valley)	1/2 cup	65	11.0	0.0
(Seabrook)	3.3 oz	80	13.0	0.0
(Southern)	3.5 oz	79	14.0	0.5
(Stokely) 'Singles'	3 oz	65	12.0	1.0
(Veg•All)	3.3 oz	80	13.0	0.0
Chinese				
(Chun King)	1.5 oz	20	3.0	0.0
(Seabrook)	2 oz	20	4.0	0.0
Combinations				
(Bird's Eye) w/cream sauce 'Combination Vegetables'	5 oz	180	16.0	11.0
(Bird's Eye) w/pearl onions 'Combination Vegetables'	3.3 oz	70	13.0	0.0
(Bird's Eye) w/potatoes, cream sauce 'Combination Vegetables'	5 oz	190	17.0	12.0
(Budget Gourmet) and cauliflower, in cream sauce	5.75 oz	170	16.0	7.0
(Budget Gourmet) Oriental, and water chestnuts 'Side Dish'	5 oz	120	15.0	3.0
(Green Giant) 'LeSueur Valley'	1/2 cup	70	12.0	2.0
(Green Giant) mini, pea pods, water chestnut, butter 'LeSueur Valley'	1/2 cup	80	10.0	2.0

Food Name	Serv. Size	Total Cal.	Carbs GMS	Fat GMS
(Green Giant) w/onions and carrots in butter sauce				
'LeSueur Valley'	1/2 cup	80	11.0	3.0
Early/June				
(Finast) in butter sauce	1/2 cup	80	15.0	4.0
(Green Giant) 'Harvest Fresh'	1/2 cup	60	12.0	1.0
(Green Giant) in butter sauce 'One Serving'	4.5 oz	90	16.0	2.0
(Green Giant) in butter sauce 'Select LeSueur'	1/2 cup	80	14.0	2.0
(Southern) petite	3.5 oz	64	11.0	0.4
Sweet				
(Finast)	3.3 oz	80	13.0	0.0
(Green Giant)	1/2 cup	50	11.0	0.0
(Green Giant) 'Harvest Fresh'	1/2 cup	50	12.0	0.0
(Green Giant) in butter sauce	1/2 cup	80	14.0	2.0
(Stokely) in butter sauce 'Singles'	4 oz	90	16.0	1.0
Tiny				
(Birds Eye) tender, 'Deluxe'	3.3 oz	60	11.0	0.0
(Freshlike)	3.3 oz	60	11.0	0.0
(Frosty Acres)	3.3 oz	60	11.0	0.0
(Seabrook)	3.3 oz	60	11.0	0.0
(Veg•All)	3.3 oz	60	11.0	0.0
PEAS, PIGEON				
immature seeds, boiled, drained	1/2 cup	85	15.0	1.0
immature seeds, raw	10 seeds	5	1.0	0.1
raw, in pods	1 lb	296	52.0	3.6
red gram, mature seeds, boiled	1/2 cup	102	19.5	0.3
red gram, mature seeds, raw	1/2 cup	350	64.0	1.5
shelled, boiled, drained	4 oz	126	22.1	1.5
shelled, raw	1 oz	39	6.8	0.5
shelled, raw, approx .1 oz	10 peas	5	1.0	0.1
Dried				
shelled, mature, boiled	4 oz	137	26.4	0.4
shelled, mature, boiled	1/2 cup	102	19.5	0.3
shelled, mature, raw	1/2 cup	350	64.0	1.5
shelled, mature, raw	1 oz	97	17.8	0.4
PEAS, PURPLE HULL				
(Allens) canned 'Fresh'	1/2 cup	100	16.0	<1.0
(Frosty Acres) frozen	3.3 oz	130	23.0	0.0
PEAS, SNAP				
(Birds Eye) carrots, water chestnuts	3.2 oz	50	11.0	0.0
(Birds Eye) 'Deluxe'	2.6 oz	45	9.0	0.0
(Green Giant) 'Harvest Fresh'	1/2 cup	30	8.0	0.0
(Green Giant) 'Sugar Snap' frozen	1/2 cup	30	8.0	0.0
PEAS, SNOW, 'Deluxe' *(Birds Eye)*	3 oz	35	6.0	0.0

Food Name	Serv. Size	Total Cal.	Carbs GMS	Fat GMS
PEAS, WHITE ACRE, canned *(Allens)*	1/2 cup	90	14.0	<1.0
PEAS AND CARROTS, CANNED				
regular pack, solid and liquid	1/2 cup	49	10.9	0.4
special dietary pack, solid and liquid	1/2 cup	49	10.9	0.4
w/liquid	4 oz	43	9.6	0.3
w/liquid, low-sodium	4 oz	43	9.6	0.3
(A&P) early/June 'No Salt Added'	1/2 cup	60	12.0	<1.0
(A&P) mixed sizes	1/2 cup	60	12.0	<1.0
(Del Monte) w/liquid	1/2 cup	50	10.0	0.0
(Finast)	1/2 cup	55	9.0	0.0
(Freshlike)	1/2 cup	50	12.0	0.0
(Freshlike) water pack, w/o salt	1/2 cup	50	12.0	0.0
(Freshlike) water pack, w/o sugar, salt	1/2 cup	50	12.0	0.0
(Kohl's)	1/2 cup	50	20.0	<1.0
(Pathmark)	1/2 cup	60	18.0	1.0
(S&W)	1/2 cup	50	9.0	0.0
(S&W Nutradiet)	1/2 cup	35	7.0	0.0
(Stokely)	1/2 cup	50	9.0	0.0
(Stokely) 'No Salt or Sugar Added'	1/2 cup	45	8.0	0.0
(Veg•All)	1/2 cup	50	12.0	0.0
PEAS AND CARROTS, FROZEN				
boiled, drained	10-oz pkg	133	28.1	1.2
boiled, drained	4 oz	54	11.5	0.5
boiled, drained	1/2 cup	38	8.1	0.3
unprepared	10-oz pkg	151	31.7	1.3
unprepared	1/2 cup	37	7.8	0.3
(A&P)	3.3 oz	60	11.0	<1.0
(A&P) sweet peas	1/2 cup	80	13.0	<1.0
(Freshlike)	3.3 oz	60	11.0	0.0
(Frosty Acres)	3.3 oz	60	11.0	0.0
(Seabrook)	3.3 oz	60	11.0	0.0
(Southern)	3.5 oz	64	11.7	0.0
(Veg•All)	3.3 oz	60	11.0	0.0
PEAS AND ONIONS, CANNED				
solid and liquid	1/2 cup	31	5.1	0.2
w/liquid	4 oz	58	9.7	0.4
(Freshlike) sweet peas, tiny onions	1/2 cup	60	12.0	0.0
(Green Giant) pearl onions, w/liquid	1/2 cup	50	11.0	0.0
(S&W) tiny pearl onions, w/liquid	1/2 cup	60	10.0	1.0
PEAS AND ONIONS, FROZEN				
boiled, drained	4 oz	51	9.8	0.2
boiled, drained	1/2 cup	41	7.8	0.2
unprepared	10-oz pkg	199	38.4	0.9

Food Name	Serv. Size	Total Cal.	Carbs GMS	Fat GMS
unprepared	1/2 cup	48	9.3	0.2
(Birds Eye) pearl onions 'Cheese Sauce Combinations'	5 oz	140	17.0	5.0
(Birds Eye) pearl onions 'Combination Vegetables'	3.3 oz	70	13.0	0.0
(Freshlike)	3.3 oz	70	13.0	0.0
(Frosty Acres) pearl onions	3.3 oz	70	13.0	0.0
(Seabrook)	3.3 oz	70	13.0	0.0
(Veg•All)	3.3 oz	70	13.0	0.0
PECAN, SHELLED				
chopped *(Fisher)*	1 oz	190	5.0	19.0
dried, chopped	1 cup	794	21.7	80.5
dried, ground	1 cup	634	17.3	64.3
dried, halves	1 cup	721	19.7	73.1
dried, halves, pieces, or chips *(Planters)*	1 oz	190	5.0	20.0
dried, 31 large or 20 medium halves	1 oz	190	5.2	19.2
dry-roasted	1 oz	187	6.3	18.4
ground *(Fisher)*	1 oz	190	5.0	19.0
honey-roasted *(Planters)*	1 oz	200	8.0	18.0
oil-roasted	1 cup	753	17.6	78.3
oil-roasted, 15 halves	1 oz	195	4.6	20.2
raw *(Fisher)*	1 oz	190	5.0	19.0
raw, chips *(Planters)*	1 oz	190	5.0	20.0
raw, halves *(Planters)*	1 oz	190	5.0	20.0
raw, pieces *(Planters)*	1 oz	190	5.0	20.0
PECAN FLOUR	1 oz	93	14.4	0.4
PECTIN, unsweetened, dry mix	.5 oz	39	10.9	0.0
PEPITAS				
In shell				
dried	1 lb	1817	59.8	153.9
roasted, whole	1 cup	285	34.4	12.4
roasted, whole, approx 85 seeds	1 oz	127	15.3	5.5
Shelled				
dried	1 cup	747	24.6	63.3
dried, approx 142 kernels	1 oz	154	5.1	13.0
roasted	1 cup	1184	30.5	95.6
roasted	1 oz	148	3.8	12.0
salted	1 lb	2021	243.8	88.0
salted	1 cup	285	34.4	12.4
salted	1 oz	127	15.3	5.5
PEPPER, BANANA, hot rings *(Vlasic)*	1 oz	4	1.0	0.0
PEPPER, BELL. See PEPPER, SWEET.				
PEPPER, CHERRY				
hot *(Progresso)*	1/2 cup	190	3.0	20.0
hot *(Vlasic)*	1 oz	10	2.0	0.0

Food Name	Serv. Size	Total Cal.	Carbs GMS	Fat GMS
hot, pickled *(Progresso)*	1/2 cup	130	3.0	12.0
mild *(Vlasic)*	1 oz	8	2.0	0.0
PEPPER, CHILI				
green, raw, approx 1.6 oz	1 med	18	4.3	0.1
green, raw, chopped	1/2 cup	30	7.1	0.2
green, raw, trimmed	1 oz	11	2.7	0.1
green, raw, untrimmed	1 lb	134	31.3	0.7
red, raw, approx 1.6 oz	1 med	18	4.3	0.1
red, raw, chopped	1/2 cup	30	7.1	0.2
red, raw, trimmed	1 oz	11	2.7	0.1
red, raw, untrimmed	1 lb	134	31.3	0.7
Canned				
green, chopped *(Old El Paso)*	2 tbsp	8	2.0	<1.0
green, diced *(Rosarita)*	1.058 oz	6	1.4	0.1
green, diced, w/liquid *(Del Monte)*	1/2 cup	20	5.0	0.0
green, whole *(Old El Paso)*	1 pepper	8	1.0	<1.0
green, whole *(Rosarita)*	1.235 oz	4	1.1	0.1
green, whole, diced, sliced, or strips *(Ortega)*	1 oz	10	3.0	0.0
green, whole, w/liquid *(Del Monte)*	1/2 cup	20	5.0	0.0
green and red, seeded, chopped, w/liquid	1/2 cup	17	4.2	0.1
green and red, seeded, w/liquid	4 oz	28	6.9	0.1
hot, green, pods, w/o seeds, solid and liquid, chopped	1/2 cup	17	4.2	0.1
hot, green and red, seeded, w/liquid, approx 2.6 oz	1 med	18	4.5	0.1
PEPPER, GREEN. See PEPPER, SWEET.				
PEPPER, GROUND				
black	1 oz	72	18.4	0.9
black	1 tbsp	16	4.2	0.2
black	1 tsp	5	1.4	0.1
black *(Durkee)*	1 tsp	8	0.0	tr
black *(Laurel Leaf)*	1 tsp	8	0.0	tr
black *(Spice Islands)*	1 tsp	9	1.5	0.2
cayenne/red	1 oz	90	16.1	4.9
cayenne/red	1 tbsp	17	3.0	0.9
cayenne/red	1 tsp	6	1.0	0.3
cayenne/red *(Durkee)*	1 tsp	8	0.0	<0.1
cayenne/red *(Laurel Leaf)*	1 tsp	8	0.0	<0.1
cayenne/red *(Spice Islands)*	1 tsp	9	1.1	0.3
chili *(Spice Islands)*	1 tsp	9	1.2	0.3
pizza *(Lawry's)*	1 tsp	2	3.2	0.2
seasoned *(Lawry's)*	1 tsp	9	1.8	0.1
seasoned 'All Pepper' *(Schilling)*	1/4 tsp	1	0.3	0.0
white	1 oz	84	19.5	0.6
white	1 tbsp	21	4.9	0.2

Food Name	Serv. Size	Total Cal.	Carbs GMS	Fat GMS
white	1 tsp	7	1.6	0.1
white *(Durkee)*	1 tsp	9	0.0	tr
white *(Laurel Leaf)*	1 tsp	9	0.0	tr
white *(Spice Islands)*	1 tsp	9	1.5	0.2
PEPPER, JALAPEÑO				
diced *Ortega)*	1 oz	10	3.0	0.0
diced *(Rosarita)*	1.058 oz	5	0.8	0.2
for nachos *(La Victoria)*	14 pieces	5	1.0	0.0
for nachos *(La Victoria)*	1 tbsp	2	1.0	<1.0
hot, diced *(Ortega)*	1 oz	8	2.0	0.0
hot 'Mexican' *(Vlasic)*	1 oz	8	2.0	0.0
hot, tiny, Mexican *(Vlasic)*	1 oz	6	2.0	0.0
hot, whole *(Ortega)*	1 oz	8	2.0	0.0
marinated *(La Victoria)*	1.5 pieces	10	2.0	0.0
marinated *(La Victoria)*	1 tbsp	4	1.0	<1.0
nacho sliced *(Rosarita)*	1.058 oz	4	1.0	0.1
sliced, w/liquid *(Del Monte)*	1/2 cup	30	6.0	1.0
whole *(Old El Paso)*	2 peppers	14	1.0	1.0
whole *(Ortega)*	1 oz	10	3.0	0.0
whole *(Rosarita)*	1.34 oz	6	1.3	0.2
whole, w/escabeche *(Rosarita)*	1.164 oz	8	1.4	0.2
whole, w/liquid *(Del Monte)*	1/2 cup	30	6.0	1.0
PEPPER, PEPPERONCINI				
mild, Greek, salad *(Vlasic)*	1 oz	4	1.0	0.0
Tuscan *(Progresso)*	1/2 cup	20	7.0	0.0
PEPPER, PICCALILLI *(Progresso)*	1/2 cup	190	4.0	20.0
PEPPER, SWEET/bell pepper/green pepper/red pepper/yellow pepper				
boiled, drained	4 oz	32	7.6	0.2
boiled, drained, approx 2.6 oz	1 med	20	4.9	0.2
boiled, drained, chopped	1/2 cup	19	4.6	0.1
raw, approx 3.2 oz	1 med	20	4.8	0.1
raw, chopped	1/2 cup	14	3.2	0.1
raw *(Dole)*	1 med	25	5.0	1.0
raw, trimmed	1 oz	8	1.8	0.1
raw, untrimmed	1 lb	99	23.9	0.7
Canned				
roasted *(Progresso)*	1/2 cup	20	5.0	<1.0
solid and liquid, halves	1/2 cup	13	2.7	0.2
'Sweet Pepper Mementos' *(Heinz)*	1 oz	6	1.0	0.0
w/liquid	4 oz	20	4.4	0.3
Freeze-dried				
	1 oz	89	19.5	0.9
	1/4 cup	5	1.1	0.1

Food Name	Serv. Size	Total Cal.	Carbs GMS	Fat GMS
Frozen				
boiled, drained, chopped	4 oz	20	4.4	0.2
chopped, unprepared	10-oz pkg	57	12.6	0.6
chopped, unprepared	1 oz	6	1.3	0.1
green (Seabrook)	1 oz	6	1.0	0.0
red (Seabrook)	1 oz	8	1.0	0.0
PEPPER DILL SEASONING (Golden Dipt)	2 grams	8	1.0	0.0
PEPPER STEAK DINNER				
(Armour) frozen, beef 'Classics Lite'	11.25 oz	220	29.0	4.0
(Healthy Choice) frozen	11 oz	260	40.0	5.0
(LaChoy)	3.81 oz	36	7.4	0.2
(Le Menu) frozen	11.5 oz	370	36.0	13.0
PEPPER STEAK DINNER MIX				
(LaChoy) 'Dinner Classics'	1/5 pkg	35	9.0	<1.0
(LaChoy) 'Dinner Classics' prepared	3/4 cup	180	9.0	9.0
PEPPER STEAK ENTRÉE				
pork and beef	1 oz	141	0.8	12.5
pork and beef, approx .2 oz	1 slice	27	0.2	2.4
(Budget Gourmet) frozen, w/rice	10 oz	300	39.0	9.0
(Dining Lite) frozen	9 oz	260	33.0	6.0
(Healthy Choice) frozen	9.5 oz	250	36.0	4.0
(LaChoy) frozen, w/rice & vegetables 'Fresh & Lite'	10 oz	280	33.0	8.0
(Stouffer's) frozen, green, w/rice, 1 pkg	10.5 oz	310	35.0	10.0
(Top Shelf) Oriental, microwave bowl	1 serving	290	25.0	10.0
(Tyson) frozen 'Gourmet Selection'	11.25 oz	330	38.0	11.0
(Ultra Slim Fast) beef, and parsley rice	12 oz	270	36.0	4.0
PEPPERONI				
(Hickory Farms)	1 oz	140	1.0	13.0
(Hormel)				
'Chunk'	1 oz	140	0.0	12.0
'Leoni Brand'	1 oz	130	0.0	12.0
'Perma-Fresh'	2 slices	80	0.0	7.0
'Rosa'	1 oz	140	0.0	13.0
'Rosa Grande'	1 oz	140	0.0	13.0
(JM) approx .5 oz	8 slices	70	1.0	6.0
PEPPERS AND ONIONS (Quincy's)	4 oz	80	8.0	5.0
PERCH				
frozen (Booth)	4 oz	100	0.0	1.0
frozen (SeaPak)	4 oz	100	0.0	2.0
frozen, fillet, battered (Van de Kamp's)	2 pieces	310	18.0	21.0
mixed species, dry-heat cooked	4 oz	133	0.0	1.3
mixed species, dry-heat cooked	3 oz	99	0.0	1.0
mixed species, raw	1 lb	413	0.0	4.2

Food Name	Serv. Size	Total Cal.	Carbs GMS	Fat GMS
mixed species, raw	3 oz	77	0.0	0.8
mixed species, raw	1 oz	26	0.0	0.3
PERSIMMON				
Japanese , dried	1 oz	78	20.8	0.2
Japanese, fresh, trimmed	1 oz	20	5.3	0.1
Japanese, fresh, untrimmed	1 lb	268	70.8	0.7
Japanese, raw, 2.5-inch diam	1 med	118	31.2	0.3
native, fresh, trimmed	1 oz	36	9.5	0.1
native, fresh, untrimmed	1 lb	472	124.6	1.5
native, raw, trimmed, approx 1.1 oz	1 med	32	8.4	0.1
PE-TSAI. See CABBAGE, NAPA.				
PHEASANT				
breast meat only, raw	1 oz	38	0.0	0.9
leg meat only, raw	1 oz	38	0.0	1.2
meat and skin, raw	1 oz	51	0.0	2.6
meat only, raw	1 oz	38	0.0	1.0
PHYLLO DOUGH				
1 sheet	1 oz	85	14.9	1.7
1 sheet (Apollo)	1 oz	80	18.0	.4
PICKLES				
BREAD AND BUTTER				
chunks 'Old-Fashion' (Vlasic)	1 oz	25	6.0	0.0
'Deli' (Vlasic)	1 oz	25	6.0	0.0
fresh	2 slices	11	2.7	0.0
one slice (Claussen)	.4 oz	7	1.7	tr
slices	1 cup	124	30.4	0.3
slices (Claussen)	1 oz	20	4.7	0.1
slices, approx 2/3 oz (Mrs. Fanning's)	2 slices	16	3.0	0.0
slices 'Cucumber Slices' (Heinz)	1 oz	25	6.0	0.0
'Sweet Butter Chips' (Vlasic)	1 oz	30	7.0	0.0
'Sweet Butter Stix' (Vlasic)	1 oz	18	5.0	0.0
DILL				
	1 lb	81	18.7	0.9
	1 oz	5	1.2	0.1
baby (Heinz)	1 oz	4	1.0	0.0
baby (Vlasic)	1 oz	4	1.0	0.0
chips (Heinz)	1 oz	4	1.0	0.0
chunks, snack (Vlasic)	1 oz	4	1.0	0.0
chunks, zesty, snacks (Vlasic)	1 oz	4	1.0	0.0
crunchy (Vlasic)	1 oz	4	1.0	0.0
crunchy, half salt (Vlasic)	1 oz	4	1.0	0.0
crunchy, zesty (Vlasic)	1 oz	4	1.0	0.0
gherkins (Vlasic)	1 oz	4	1.0	0.0

Food Name	Serv. Size	Total Cal.	Carbs GMS	Fat GMS
halves 'Deli' *(Vlasic)*	1 oz	4	1.0	0.0
halves 'Deli Style' *(Heinz)*	1 oz	4	1.0	0.0
hamburger chips, half salt *(Vlasic)*	1 oz	2	1.0	0.0
hamburger slices *(Heinz)*	1 oz	2	0.0	0.0
low sodium	1 lb	81	18.7	0.9
low sodium	1 oz	5	1.2	0.1
no garlic *(Claussen)*	1 oz	6	1.0	0.1
no garlic, 1 piece *(Claussen)*	2.9 oz	17	2.8	0.3
'Original' *(Vlasic)*	1 oz	4	1.0	0.0
'Polish Snack Chunks' *(Vlasic)*	1 oz	4	1.0	0.0
spears *(Claussen)*	1 oz	4	0.5	0.1
spears, half salt *(Vlasic)*	1 oz	4	1.0	0.0
spears, kosher *(Heinz)*	1 oz	4	1.0	0.0
spears, kosher *(Vlasic)*	1 oz	4	1.0	0.0
spears, no garlic *(Vlasic)*	1 oz	4	1.0	0.0
spears, 1 piece *(Claussen)*	1.1 oz	4	0.6	0.1
spears, Polish style *(Heinz)*	1 oz	4	1.0	0.0
spears, zesty *(Vlasic)*	1 oz	4	1.0	0.0
whole *(Featherweight)*	1 piece	4	1.0	0.0
whole 'Genuine' *(Heinz)*	1 oz	2	0.0	0.0
whole, kosher *(Heinz)*	1 oz	4	1.0	0.0
whole, Polish style *(Heinz)*	1 oz	4	1.0	0.0
whole, processed *(Heinz)*	1 oz	2	0.0	0.0
HOT AND SPICY, garden, mixed *(Vlasic)*	1 oz	4	1.0	0.0
KOSHER. See also DILL.				
chips, 'Old Fashioned' *(Heinz)*	1 oz	4	1.0	0.0
halves *(Claussen)*	1 oz	4	0.5	0.1
halves 'Old Fashioned Deli Halves' *(Heinz)*	1 oz	4	1.0	0.0
halves, 2.3 oz *(Claussen)*	1 piece	9	1.3	0.2
slices *(Claussen)*	1 oz	3	0.5	0.1
slices, .3 oz *(Claussen)*	1 piece	1	0.2	tr
SOUR				
	1 lb	48	10.2	0.9
	1 oz	3	0.6	0.1
low sodium	1 lb	48	10.2	0.9
low sodium	1 oz	3	0.6	0.1
whole *(Claussen)*	1 oz	3	0.5	0.1
whole 'Old Fashioned' *(Heinz)*	1 oz	4	1.0	0.0
whole, 1 piece *(Claussen)*	2.5 oz	9	1.3	0.2
SWEET				
	1 lb	529	144.3	1.2
	1 oz	33	9.0	0.1
cubes, salad *(Heinz)*	1 oz	30	7.0	0.0

Food Name	Serv. Size	Total Cal.	Carbs GMS	Fat GMS
'Cucumber Stix' (Heinz)	1 oz	25	6.0	0.0
gherkins (Heinz)	1 oz	35	8.0	0.0
gherkins, midget (Heinz)	1 oz	35	8.0	0.0
half salt 'Sweet Butter Chips' (Vlasic)	1 oz	30	7.0	0.0
low sodium	1 lb	529	144.3	1.2
low sodium	1 med	41	11.1	0.1
low sodium	1 oz	33	9.0	0.1
low sodium	1 slice	7	1.9	0.0
low sodium, mixed (Heinz)	1 oz	40	9.0	0.0
low sodium, 3 inches long, approx 1.2 oz	1 large	41	11.1	0.1
sliced (Featherweight)	3-4 slices	24	6.0	0.0
sliced (Heinz)	1 oz	35	8.0	0.0
sliced 'Cucumber Slices' (Heinz)	1 oz	20	5.0	0.0
whole, 3 inches long, approx 1.2 oz	1 large	41	11.1	0.1
PICKLING SPICE (Tone's)	1 tsp	10	1.2	0.6

PIE

APPLE

Fresh

Food Name	Serv. Size	Total Cal.	Carbs GMS	Fat GMS
(Entenmann's) homestyle	2.1 oz	140	21.0	7.0
(McMillin's)	4 oz	430	51.0	23.0

Frozen

Food Name	Serv. Size	Total Cal.	Carbs GMS	Fat GMS
(Amy's Kitchen)	8 oz	282	42.0	12.0
(Banquet) 'Family Size' 3 1/3 oz	1/6 pie	250	37.0	11.0
(Mrs. Smith's) 'Pie In Minutes' 8-inch pie	1/8 pie	210	29.0	9.0
(Pet-Ritz)	1/16 pie	330	53.0	12.0
(Sara Lee) apple streusel 'Free & Light'	1/8 pie	170	36.0	2.0
(Sara Lee) Dutch apple 'Homestyle' 9-inch pie	1/10 pie	300	45.0	12.0
(Sara Lee) 'Homestyle' 9-inch pie	1/10 pie	280	42.0	12.0
(Sara Lee) 'Homestyle High' 10-inch pie	1/10 pie	400	46.0	23.0
(Weight Watchers) 3.5 oz	1/2 pkg	200	39.0	5.0

BANANA CREAM

Frozen

Food Name	Serv. Size	Total Cal.	Carbs GMS	Fat GMS
(Banquet) 2 1/3 oz	1/6 pie	180	21.0	10.0
(Pet-Ritz) 2 1/3 oz	1/6 pie	170	22.0	9.0
BERRY, fresh (McMillin's)	4 oz	430	52.0	23.0
BLACKBERRY, frozen (Banquet) 'Family Size' 3 1/3 oz	1/6 pie	270	40.0	11.0

BLUEBERRY

Frozen

Food Name	Serv. Size	Total Cal.	Carbs GMS	Fat GMS
(Banquet) 'Family Size' 3 1/3 oz	1/6 pie	270	40.0	11.0
(Mrs. Smith's) 'Pie In Minutes' 8-inch pie	1/8 pie	220	32.0	9.0
(Pet-Ritz)	1/6 pie	370	50.0	12.0
(Sara Lee) 'Homestyle' 9-inch pie	1/10 pie	300	45.0	12.0
BOSTON CREAM, frozen (Weight Watchers)	3 oz	160	34.0	4.0

Food Name	Serv. Size	Total Cal.	Carbs GMS	Fat GMS
CHERRY				
Fresh *(McMillin's)*	4 oz	430	51.0	24.0
Frozen				
(Banquet) 'Family Size' 3 1/3 oz	1/6 pie	250	36.0	11.0
(Mrs. Smith's) 'Pie In Minutes' 8-inch pie	1/8 pie	220	32.0	9.0
(Pet-Ritz)	1/6 pie	300	48.0	12.0
(Sara Lee) cherry streusel 'Free & Light'	1/10 pie	160	34.0	2.0
(Sara Lee) 'Homestyle' 9-inch pie	1/10 pie	270	37.0	13.0
CHOCOLATE				
Fresh *(McMillin's)* chocolate pudding	4 oz	420	54.0	21.0
Frozen				
(Banquet) chocolate cream, 2 1/3 oz	1/6 pie	190	24.0	10.0
(Pet Ritz) chocolate cream, 2 1/3 oz	1/6 pie	190	27.0	8.0
(Weight Watchers) chocolate mocha 'Sweet Celebrations' 2.75 oz	1/2 pkg	160	23.0	5.0
COCONUT				
Fresh *(McMillin's)* coconut pudding	4 oz	450	50.0	26.0
Frozen				
(Banquet) cream, 2 1/3 oz	1/6 pie	190	22.0	11.0
(Pet Ritz) cream, 2 1/3 oz	1/6 pie	190	27.0	8.0
COCONUT CUSTARD, fresh *(Entenmann's)*	1.8 oz	140	16.0	8.0
EGG CUSTARD, frozen *(Pet-Ritz)*	1/6 pie	200	28.0	8.0
LEMON				
Fresh *(McMillin's)*	4 oz	450	52.0	25.0
Frozen				
(Banquet) cream, 2 1/3 oz	1/6 pie	170	23.0	9.0
(Mrs. Smith's) meringue, 8-inch pie	1/8 pie	210	38.0	5.0
(Pet Ritz) cream, 2 1/3 oz	1/6 pie	190	26.0	9.0
MINCE				
Frozen				
(Banquet) mincemeat 'Family Size' 3 1/3 oz	1/6 pie	260	38.0	11.0
(Pet-Ritz)	1/6 pie	280	48.0	9.0
(Sara Lee) 'Homestyle' 9-inch pie	1/10 pie	300	43.0	13.0
NEAPOLITAN CREAM, frozen, *(Pet Ritz)* 2 1/3 oz	1/6 pie	180	17.0	10.0
PEACH				
Fresh *(McMillin's)*	4 oz	430	52.0	24.0
Frozen				
(Banquet) 'Family Size' 3 1/3 oz	1/6 pie	245	35.0	11.0
(Mrs. Smith's) 'Pie In Minutes' 8-inch pie	1/8 pie	210	29.0	9.0
(Pet-Ritz)	1/6 pie	320	51.0	12.0
(Sara Lee) 'Homestyle' 9-inch pie	1/10 pie	280	41.0	12.0

Food Name	Serv. Size	Total Cal.	Carbs GMS	Fat GMS
PECAN				
Frozen				
(Mrs. Smith's) 'Pie In Minutes' 8-inch pie	1/8 pie	330	51.0	13.0
(Sara Lee) 'Homestyle' 9-inch pie	1/10 pie	400	56.0	18.0
PUMPKIN				
Frozen				
(Banquet) 'Family Size' 3 1/3 oz	1/6 pie	200	29.0	8.0
(Mrs. Smith's) 'Pie In Minutes' 8-inch pie	1/8 pie	190	30.0	6.0
(Pet Ritz) pumpkin custard	1/6 pie	250	39.0	9.0
(Sara Lee) 'Homestyle' 9-inch pie	1/10 pie	240	34.0	10.0
RASPBERRY, frozen (Sara Lee) 'Homestyle' 9-inch pie	1/10 pie	280	39.0	13.0
STRAWBERRY				
Fresh (McMillin's)	4 oz	400	50.0	20.0
Frozen				
(Banquet) strawberry cream, 2 1/3 oz	1/6 pie	170	22.0	9.0
(Pet Ritz) strawberry cream, 2 1/3 oz	1/6 pie	170	20.0	9.0
SWEET POTATO, frozen (Pet-Ritz)	1/6 pie	150	21.0	7.0
PIE, SNACK				
APPLE				
(Break Cake) 'Fried Pie' 4.5 oz	2 pies	430	63.0	18.0
(Drake's) approx 2 oz	1 piece	210	29.0	10.0
(Hostess)	1 piece	430	60.0	20.0
(Hostess) French apple	1 piece	430	60.0	20.0
(Little Debbie) Dutch apple, 2.17 oz	1 piece	230	42.0	8.0
(Little Debbie) Dutch apple, 2.5 oz	1 piece	270	48.0	8.0
(Tastykake) 4 oz	1 piece	296	46.0	12.3
(Tastycake) French apple, 4.2 oz	1 piece	353	63.0	10.7
BANANA CREAM (Tastycake) 4.2 oz	1 piece	382	53.9	16.1
BLACKBERRY (Hostess)	1 piece	420	59.0	18.0
BLUEBERRY				
(Hostess)	1 piece	420	59.0	18.0
(Tastykake) 4 oz	1 piece	308	55.0	9.4
BLUEBERRY APPLE (Drake's) approx 2 oz	1 piece	210	30.0	10.0
CHERRY				
(Break Cake) 'Fried Pie' 4.5 oz	2 pies	410	64.0	16.0
(Hostess)	1 piece	460	65.0	20.0
(Tastykake) 4 oz	1 piece	298	48.8	9.7
CHERRY APPLE (Drake's) approx 2 oz	1 piece	220	30.0	10.0
CHOCOLATE PUDDING				
(Hostess) chocolate pudding	1 piece	490	76.0	19.0
(Tastycake) chocolate pudding, 4.2 oz	1 piece	443	68.3	16.2
COCONUT CREME (Tastykake) 4 oz	1 piece	377	46.0	20.2

Food Name	Serv. Size	Total Cal.	Carbs GMS	Fat GMS
LEMON				
(Break Cake) 'Fried Pie' 4.5 oz	2 pies	490	66.0	23.0
(Drake's) approx 2 oz	1 piece	210	27.0	11.0
(Hostess)	1 piece	440	60.0	20.0
(Tastykake) 4 oz	1 piece	319	48.1	13.2
LEMON-LIME (Tastykake) 4 oz	1 piece	310	54.1	8.8
MARSHMALLOW BANANA				
(Little Debbie) 3 oz	1 piece	360	60.0	12.0
(Little Debbie) 1.4 oz	1 piece	170	28.0	6.0
MARSHMALLOW CHOCOLATE				
(Little Debbie) 3 oz	1 piece	370	59.0	13.0
(Little Debbie) 1.4 oz	1 piece	170	28.0	6.0
MISSISSIPPI MUD (Pepperidge Farm) frozen 'American Collection'	1 ramekin	310	23.0	23.0
OATMEAL CREME				
(Little Debbie) 1.33 oz	1 piece	160	25.0	6.0
(Little Debbie) 2.75 oz	1 piece	350	51.0	14.0
PEACH				
(Hostess)	1 piece	420	60.0	19.0
(Tastykake) 4 oz	1 piece	310	54.1	8.8
PECAN				
(Little Debbie) 1.83 oz	1 piece	170	37.0	2.0
(Little Debbie) 3 oz	1 piece	280	60.0	3.0
PINEAPPLE CHEESE (Tastykake) 4.2 oz	1 piece	343	53.9	13.2
PUMPKIN (Tastykake) 4 oz	1 piece	324	46.5	14.2
RAISIN CREME				
(Little Debbie) 2.5 oz	1 piece	290	47.0	10.0
(Little Debbie) 1.17 oz	1 piece	140	21.0	6.0
STRAWBERRY				
(Hostess)	1 piece	410	56.0	19.0
(Tastykake) 4 oz	1 piece	342	57.4	11.4
PIE CRUST				
Mix				
(Betty Crocker) dry	1/16 pkg	120	10.0	8.0
(Flako) prepared	1 serving	247	24.4	15.0
(General Mills) dry	1/16 pkg	120	10.0	8.0
(Krusteaz) 9-inch pie	1/8 shell	90	10.0	5.0
(Nabisco) chocolate cookie crumbs 'Oreo' dry	2 tbsp	80	13.0	3.0
(Nabisco) graham crumbs 'Honey Maid' dry	2 1/2 tbsp	70	13.0	2.0
(Nabisco) wafer crumbs 'Nilla' dry	2 tbsp	70	12.0	2.0
(Pillsbury) dry	1/8 pkg	200	20.0	13.0
Shell				
(Mrs. Smith's) 8-inch pie	1/8 shell	80	8.0	5.0

Food Name	Serv. Size	Total Cal.	Carbs GMS	Fat GMS
(Mrs. Smith's) 9-inch pie	1/8 shell	90	10.0	5.0
(Mrs. Smith's) 9 5/8-inch pie	1/8 shell	120	12.0	7.0
(Oronoque) deep dish, 9-inch pie	1/6 shell	130	11.0	9.0
(Oronoque) regular, 9-inch pie	1/6 shell	120	9.0	8.0
(Pet-Ritz)	1/6 shell	110	11.0	7.0
(Pet-Ritz) all vegetable shortening	1/6 shell	110	10.0	8.0
(Pet-Ritz) deep dish, 1 oz	1/6 shell	130	12.0	8.0
(Pet-Ritz) deep dish, whole-grain	1/6 shell	130	14.0	8.0
(Pet-Ritz) graham cracker	1/6 shell	110	8.0	6.0
(Pet-Ritz) 9 5/8-inch pie	1/6 shell	170	15.0	11.0
(Pet-Ritz) tart	3-inch shell	150	12.0	10.0
(Pet-Ritz) vegetable shortening, deep dish	1/6 shell	140	12.0	9.0
(Pillsbury) 'All Ready' 2-crust pie	1/8 shell	240	24.0	15.0
Stick (Betty Crocker)	1/8 stick	120	10.0	8.0

PIE FILLING . See also PUDDING/PIE FILLING MIX.
(NOTE: All pie fillings are canned unless otherwise noted.)

APPLE

Food Name	Serv. Size	Total Cal.	Carbs GMS	Fat GMS
(Comstock)	3.5 oz	120	30.0	0.0
(Comstock) 'Lite'	3.5 oz	80	20.0	0.0
(Lucky Leaf)	4 oz	120	30.0	0.0
(Lucky Leaf) apple turnover, diced	4 oz	120	30.0	0.0
(Lucky Leaf) 'Deluxe'	4 oz	120	35.0	0.0
(Lucky Leaf) 'Plus'	4 oz	121	30.2	0.0
(Musselman's)	4 oz	120	30.0	0.0
(Musselman's) apple turnover, diced	4 oz	120	30.0	0.0
(Musselman's) 'Deluxe'	4 oz	120	35.0	0.0
(Musselman's) 'Plus'	4 oz	121	30.2	0.0
(Pathmark) 'No Frills'	4 oz	130	33.0	0.0
(White House)	3.5 oz	121	29.0	1.0

APRICOT

Food Name	Serv. Size	Total Cal.	Carbs GMS	Fat GMS
(Comstock)	3.5 oz	110	29.0	0.0
(Lucky Leaf)	4 oz	150	39.0	0.0
(Musselman's)	4 oz	150	39.0	0.0
BANANA (Comstock)	3.5 oz	110	22.0	2.0

BLACKBERRY

Food Name	Serv. Size	Total Cal.	Carbs GMS	Fat GMS
(Lucky Leaf)	4 oz	120	31.0	0.0
(Lucky Leaf) 'Plus'	4 oz	121	30.1	0.0
(Musselman's)	4 oz	120	31.0	0.0
(Musselman's) 'Plus'	4 oz	121	30.1	0.0

BLUEBERRY

Food Name	Serv. Size	Total Cal.	Carbs GMS	Fat GMS
(Comstock)	3.5 oz	110	28.0	0.0
(Comstock) 'Lite'	3.5 oz	75	17.0	0.0
(Lucky Leaf) cultivated	4 oz	120	31.0	0.0

Food Name	Serv. Size	Total Cal.	Carbs GMS	Fat GMS
(Lucky Leaf) 'Plus'	4 oz	145	35.2	0.0
(Musselman's) cultivated	4 oz	120	31.0	0.0
(Musselman's) 'Plus'	4 oz	145	35.2	0.0
(White House)	3.5 oz	118	28.0	1.0
BOYSENBERRY				
(Lucky Leaf)	4 oz	120	31.0	0.0
(Musselman's)	4 oz	120	31.0	0.0
CHERRY				
(Comstock)	3.5 oz	110	28.0	0.0
(Comstock) 'Lite'	3.5 oz	75	19.0	0.0
(Lucky Leaf)	4 oz	120	29.0	0.0
(Musselman's)	4 oz	120	29.0	0.0
(Musselman's) 'Plus'	4 oz	108	26.0	0.2
(Pathmark) 'No Frills'	4 oz	130	33.0	0.0
(White House)	3.5 oz	141	33.0	1.0
CHOCOLATE *(Comstock)*	3.5 oz	130	26.0	3.0
COCONUT *(Comstock)*	3.5 oz	120	22.0	3.0
GOOSEBERRY				
(Lucky Leaf)	4 oz	180	45.0	0.0
(Musselman's)	4 oz	180	45.0	0.0
LEMON				
(Comstock)	3.5 oz	140	34.0	1.0
(Lucky Leaf)	4 oz	200	48.0	2.0
(Lucky Leaf) 'French'	4 oz	180	42.0	1.0
(Musselman's)	4 oz	200	48.0	2.0
(Musselman's) 'French'	4 oz	180	42.0	1.0
MINCEMEAT				
(Comstock)	3.5 oz	150	39.0	1.0
(Lucky Leaf)	4 oz	190	48.0	1.0
(Musselman's)	4 oz	190	48.0	1.0
(None Such)	1/3 cup	200	48.0	1.0
(None Such) condensed	1/4 pkg	220	50.0	2.0
(None Such) w/brandy and rum	1/3 cup	220	48.0	2.0
(S&W) w/brandy, 'Old Fashioned'	4 oz	234	55.6	2.3
PEACH				
(Comstock)	3.5 oz	110	26.0	0.0
(Lucky Leaf)	4 oz	150	37.0	0.0
(Lucky Leaf) 'Plus'	4 oz	113	27.4	0.0
(Musselman's)	4 oz	150	37.0	0.0
(Musselman's) 'Plus'	4 oz	113	27.4	0.0
(White House)	3.5 oz	117	28.0	1.0
PINEAPPLE				
(Comstock)	3.5 oz	100	28.0	0.0

Food Name	Serv. Size	Total Cal.	Carbs GMS	Fat GMS
(Lucky Leaf)	4 oz	110	30.0	0.0
(Musselman's)	4 oz	110	30.0	0.0
PUMPKIN				
(Comstock)	3.5 oz	100	24.0	0.0
(Libby's)	1 cup	260	64.0	0.3
(Lucky Leaf)	4 oz	170	33.0	4.0
(Musselman's)	4 oz	170	33.0	4.0
(Stokely)	1/2 cup	170	44.0	0.0
RAISIN				
(Comstock)	3.5 oz	120	32.0	0.0
(Lucky Leaf)	4 oz	130	34.0	1.0
(Musselman's)	4 oz	130	34.0	1.0
RASPBERRY, BLACK				
(Lucky Leaf)	4 oz	190	43.0	0.0
(Musselman's)	4 oz	190	43.0	0.0
RASPBERRY, RED				
(Lucky Leaf)	4 oz	190	46.0	0.0
(Musselman's)	4 oz	190	46.0	0.0
STRAWBERRY				
(Comstock)	3.5 oz	100	25.0	0.0
(Lucky Leaf)	4 oz	120	30.0	0.0
(Lucky Leaf) 'Plus'	4 oz	138	33.5	0.0
(Musselman's)	4 oz	120	30.0	0.0
(Musselman's) 'Plus'	4 oz	138	33.5	0.0
STRAWBERRY-RHUBARB				
(Lucky Leaf) strawberry-rhubarb	4 oz	120	31.0	0.0
(Musselman's) strawberry-rhubarb	4 oz	120	31.0	0.0
PIE MIX				
BANANA CREAM				
(Jell-O) 'No Bake' dry	1 pkg	140	25.0	5.0
(Jell-O) 'No Bake' prepared	1/8 pie	240	27.0	14.0
BOSTON CREAM				
(Betty Crocker) 'Classic' dry	1/8 pkg	230	48.0	4.0
(Betty Crocker) 'Classic' prepared w/egg and 2% milk	1/8 pkg	270	50.0	6.0
(Jell-O) mousse 'No Bake' dry	1 pkg	160	22.0	7.0
(Jell-O) mousse 'No Bake' prepared	1/8 pie	260	25.0	17.0
CHOCOLATE				
(Royal) chocolate mint 'No-Bake' prepared	1/8 pie	260	25.0	15.0
(Royal) mousse 'No-Bake' prepared	1/8 pie	230	27.0	12.0
COCONUT CREAM				
(Jell-O) 'No Bake' dry	1 pkg	160	25.0	7.0
(Jell-O) 'No Bake' prepared	1/8 pie	260	27.0	16.0
KEY LIME *(Royal)* dry	1 serving	50	13.0	0.0

Food Name	Serv. Size	Total Cal.	Carbs GMS	Fat GMS
LEMON				
(Royal) dry	1 serving	50	13.0	0.0
(Royal) lemon meringue 'No Bake' prepared	1/8 pie	310	50.0	11.0
PUMPKIN				
(Jell-O) 'No Bake' dry	1 pkg	140	28.0	3.0
(Jell-O) 'No Bake' prepared	1/8 pie	250	31.0	13.0
(Libby's) prepared	1/6 pie	390	53.0	17.0
VANILLA CREME				
(Lucky Leaf) prepared	4 oz	150	32.0	3.0
(Musselman's) prepared	4 oz	150	32.0	3.0
PIGEON. See SQUAB.				
PIGNOLIA. See PINE NUT.				
PIG'S EAR				
frozen, raw	1 oz	66	0.0	4.3
frozen, simmered	4 oz	188	0.0	12.2
PIG'S FEET				
pickled (Penrose)	6 oz	220	2.0	15.0
pickled, cured	1 lb	921	0.1	73.2
pickled, cured	1 oz	58	0.0	4.6
raw	1 oz	75	0.0	5.3
simmered	5 oz	275	0.0	17.6
PIG'S HEART				
braised	1 cup	215	0.6	7.3
braised	4 oz	168	0.5	5.7
raw	1 oz	33	0.4	1.2
PIG'S JOWL, raw	1 oz	186	0.0	19.7
PIG'S KNUCKLES, pickled (Penrose)	6 oz	290	1.0	21.0
PIG'S TAIL				
raw	1 oz	107	0.0	9.5
simmered	3 oz	337	0.0	30.4
PIG'S TONGUE				
braised	3 oz	230	0.0	15.8
cured, '8-lb can' (Hormel)	3 oz	190	0.0	13.0
raw	1 oz	64	0.0	4.9
PIKE, NORTHERN				
dry-heat cooked	3 oz	96	0.0	0.8
raw	1 lb	401	0.0	3.1
raw	3 oz	75	0.0	0.6
raw	1 oz	25	0.0	0.2
PIKE, WALLEYE				
dry-heat cooked	3 oz	101	0.0	1.3
raw	1 lb	420	0.0	5.5
raw	3 oz	79	0.0	1.0

Food Name	Serv. Size	Total Cal.	Carbs GMS	Fat GMS
raw	1 oz	26	0.0	0.3
PILAF DINNER, CANNED				
oat bran, w/garden vegetables 'Fast Menu' (Health Valley)	7.5 oz	210	31.0	7.0
PILAF MIX				
lentil, approx 1/2 cup cooked or 1 oz dry (Casbah)	1 serving	100	20.0	0.0
three-grain, w/herbs, prepared w/salted butter (Quick Pilaf)	1/2 cup	142	24.0	4.0
three-grain, w/herbs, prepared w/o butter (Quick Pilaf)	1/2 cup	110	24.0	0.6
PILI NUT, CANARY TREE				
dried	1 cup	863	4.8	95.5
dried, 15 kernels	1 oz	204	1.1	22.6
dried, in shell	1 lb	619	3.4	68.5
PIMIENTO, CAN OR JAR				
	2 oz	13	2.9	0.2
	1 tbsp	3	0.6	<.1
all varieties, drained (Dromedary)	1 oz	10	2.0	0.0
PIMIENTO SPREAD (Price's)	1 oz	80	2.0	6.0
PIÑA COLADA. See ALCOHOLIC BEVERAGES.				
PINE NUT/Colorado pinyon pine nut/Italian stone pine nut/pignolia/pinocchio/piñon				
whole	1 oz	161	5.5	17.3
whole	1 tbsp	52	1.4	5.1
whole	10 kernels	6	0.2	0.6
PINEAPPLE				
candied, approx 1/2 cup	4-oz pkg	357	90.4	0.5
raw, diced pieces	1 cup	76	19.2	0.7
raw, 3 1/2-inch diam	1 slice	41	10.4	0.4
raw, 3 1/2-inch diam, 3/4-inch thick (Del Monte)	2 slices	90	24.0	0.0
trimmed	1 oz	14	3.5	0.1
untrimmed	1 lb	117	29.2	1.0
untrimmed (Dole)	2 slices	90	21.0	1.0
PINEAPPLE, CANNED				
chunks	1/2 cup	75	19.6	0.1
chunks (A&P)	1/2 cup	70	18.0	<1.0
chunks, unsweetened 'Hawaiian' (Pathmark)	1/2 cup	70	18.0	0.0
crushed (A&P)	1/2 cup	70	18.0	<1.0
crushed (Empress)	1/2 cup	70	18.0	0.0
crushed, unsweetened 'Hawaiian' (Pathmark)	1/2 cup	70	18.0	0.0
'Fruit Pak' (Mott's)	3.75 oz	86	21.0	0.0
in extra heavy syrup	4 oz	94	24.4	0.1
in extra heavy syrup, chunks	1/2 cup	109	28.0	0.1
in extra heavy syrup, chunks, w/liquid	1 cup	216	55.9	0.3
in extra heavy syrup, crushed	1/2 cup	109	28.0	0.1
in extra heavy syrup, w/1.25 tbsp liquid	1 slice	48	12.5	0.1

Food Name	Serv. Size	Total Cal.	Carbs GMS	Fat GMS
in heavy syrup	4 oz	88	22.9	0.1
in heavy syrup, chunks (A&P)	1/2 cup	90	23.0	<1.0
in heavy syrup, chunks 'Hawaiian' (Pathmark)	1/2 cup	90	23.0	0.0
in heavy syrup, chunks, tidbits, or crushed	1/2 cup	100	25.8	0.1
in heavy syrup, chunks or crushed, w/liquid	1 cup	199	51.5	0.3
in heavy syrup, crushed (A&P)	1/2 cup	90	23.0	<1.0
in heavy syrup, slices (A&P)	2 slices	90	23.0	<1.0
in heavy syrup, slices 'Hawaiian' (Pathmark)	1/2 cup	90	23.0	0.0
in heavy syrup, slices '100% Hawaiian' (S&W)	2 slices	90	23.0	0.0
in heavy syrup, w/1.25 tbsp liquid	1 slice	45	11.7	0.1
in juice	4 oz	68	17.8	0.1
in juice, all cuts (Dole)	1/2 cup	70	17.5	0.5
in juice, chunks (Del Monte)	1/2 cup	70	18.0	0.0
in juice, chunks or tidbits, w/liquid	1 cup	150	39.2	0.2
in juice, crushed (Del Monte)	1/2 cup	70	18.0	0.0
in juice, slices (A&P)	2 slices	70	18.0	<1.0
in juice, slices (Del Monte)	1/2 cup	70	18.0	0.0
in juice, slices (Featherweight)	1/2 cup	70	18.0	0.0
in juice, slices '100% Hawaiian' (S&W)	1/2 cup	70	17.0	0.0
in juice, tidbits (Del Monte)	1/2 cup	70	18.0	0.0
in juice, w/1.25 tbsp liquid	1 slice	35	9.1	0.1
in light syrup	1/2 cup	66	16.9	0.1
in light syrup	4 oz	59	15.3	0.1
in light syrup, w/liquid	1 cup	131	33.9	0.3
in light syrup, w/1.75 tbsp liquid	1 slice	30	7.8	0.1
in pineapple juice (Dole)	1/2 cup	70	18.0	<1.0
in pineapple syrup (Dole)	1/2 cup	90	23.0	0.0
in syrup, all cuts (Del Monte)	1/2 cup	90	23.0	0.0
in syrup, all cuts (Dole)	1/2 cup	95	24.8	0.2
in water	4 oz	36	9.4	0.1
in water, tidbits	1/2 cup	40	10.2	0.1
in water, tidbits, w/liquid	1 cup	79	20.4	0.2
in water, w/1.25 tbsp liquid	1 slice	19	4.8	0.1
spears, approx 3.1 oz (Del Monte)	2 spears	50	14.0	0.0
spears or slices, unsweetened 'Hawaiian' (Pathmark)	1/2 cup	70	18.0	0.0
tidbits	1/2 cup	75	19.6	0.1
unsweetened, slices (S&W Nutradiet)	1/2 cup	60	15.0	0.0
PINEAPPLE, FROZEN				
sweetened, chunks	1/2 cup	104	27.1	0.1
sweetened, chunks	4 oz	96	25.2	0.1
PINEAPPLE CITRUS DRINK				
'Thirst Quencher Light' (Gatorade)	8 oz	25	7.0	0.0

Food Name	Serv. Size	Total Cal.	Carbs GMS	Fat GMS
PINEAPPLE COCKTAIL JUICE				
w/banana 'Orchard Tropicals' (Welch's) bottled	6 oz	100	24.0	0.0
w/banana 'Orchard Tropicals' (Welch's) boxed	8.45 oz	140	34.0	0.0
w/banana 'Orchard Tropicals' (Welch's) frozen	6 oz	100	24.0	0.0
w/grapefruit juice (Ocean Spray)	6 oz	110	26.0	0.0
PINEAPPLE COCONUT JUICE (Knudsen & Sons)	8 oz	110	24.0	0.0
PINEAPPLE DRINK				
frozen 'Bright & Early Pineapple' prepared (Bright & Early)	6 oz	90	23.0	0.0
w/grapefruit juice (Tropicana)	6 oz	100	24.0	<1.0
w/grapefruit juice	6 oz	90	21.6	0.2
w/grapefruit juice (Del Monte)	6 oz	90	24.0	0.0
w/grapefruit juice (Pathmark)	6 oz	80	21.0	0.0
w/grapefruit juice 'Single Serve' (Tropicana)	10 oz	159	39.0	0.0
w/grapefruit juice 'Twister' (Tropicana)	8 oz	125	32.0	0.0
w/pink grapefruit juice (Del Monte)	6 oz	90	24.0	0.0
PINEAPPLE GRAPEFRUIT JUICE				
canned	1 cup	117	29.0	0.3
canned	1 oz	15	3.6	0.0
PINEAPPLE JUICE				
Can, bottle, or box				
	6 oz	104	25.8	0.2
(Dole)	6 oz	103	25.4	0.2
(Knudsen & Sons)	8 oz	110	25.0	0.0
(Minute Maid)	6 oz	90	23.0	0.0
(Mott's)	9.5 oz	169	42.0	0.0
50% juice (J. Hungerford)	9.03 oz	123	30.8	0.0
float (Knudsen & Sons)	8 oz	130	31.0	0.0
'Hawaiian' (Pathmark)	6 oz	100	25.0	0.0
'No Frills Unsweetened' (Pathmark)	6 oz	100	25.0	0.0
'100%' (Veryfine)	8 oz	125	31.0	0.0
100% juice (J. Hungerford)	9.03 oz	124	31.3	0.0
regular (J. Hungerford)	9.03 oz	114	28.6	0.0
'Unsweetened' (Del Monte)	6 oz	100	25.0	0.0
'Unsweetened' (IGA)	6 oz	100	25.0	0.0
'Unsweetened' (S&W)	6 oz	100	25.0	0.0
unsweetened, w/added ascorbic acid	1 cup	140	34.4	0.2
unsweetened, w/added ascorbic acid	1 oz	18	4.3	0.0
unsweetened, w/o added ascorbic acid	1 cup	140	34.4	0.2
unsweetened, w/o added ascorbic acid	1 oz	18	4.3	0.0
Frozen or chilled				
(Dole)	6 oz	90	22.0	0.0
(Minute Maid)	6 oz	90	23.0	0.0
concentrate (Dole) diluted	6 oz	100	25.0	na

Food Name	Serv. Size	Total Cal.	Carbs GMS	Fat GMS
unsweetened concentrate, diluted	1 cup	130	31.9	0.1
unsweetened concentrate, diluted	1 oz	16	4.0	0.0
unsweetened concentrate, undiluted	6 oz	387	95.7	0.2
w/grapefruit juice *(Dole)*	6 oz	90	23.0	na
w/grapefruit juice '100% Pure' *(Tropicana)*	8 oz	120	29.3	0.0
w/pink grapefruit juice *(Dole)*	6 oz	101	25.4	0.1
PINEAPPLE NECTAR *(Libby's)*	6 oz	110	27.0	0.0
PINEAPPLE ORANGE DRINK				
	6 oz	96	22.2	0.0
(Del Monte)	6 oz	90	24.0	0.0
(Veryfine)	8 oz	130	32.0	0.0
PINEAPPLE ORANGE JUICE				
(Dole)	6 oz	100	23.0	na
chilled, carton *(Dole)*	6 oz	90	22.0	0.0
chilled, w/banana, carton *(Dole)*	6 oz	100	23.0	0.0
chilled, w/guava, carton *(Dole)*	6 oz	100	21.0	0.0
frozen, can *(Dole)*	6 oz	90	22.0	0.0
frozen, w/banana, can *(Dole)*	6 oz	90	21.0	0.0
frozen, w/guava, can *(Dole)*	6 oz	100	22.0	0.0
frozen or chilled *(Minute Maid)*	6 oz	90	23.0	0.0
w/banana *(Dole)*	6 oz	90	23.0	0.1
PINEAPPLE PASSION JUICE				
frozen, can, w/banana *(Dole)*	6 oz	100	21.0	0.0
frozen, carton, w/banana *(Dole)*	6 oz	100	21.0	0.0
PINEAPPLE TOPPING				
	1 cup	860	225.8	0.3
	2 tbsp	106	27.9	0.0
(Kraft)	1 tbsp	50	13.0	0.0
(Smucker's)	2 tbsp	130	32.0	0.0
PINK BEAN				
boiled	4 oz	169	31.6	0.6
mature seeds, boiled	1/2 cup	125	23.4	0.4
mature seeds, raw	1/2 cup	360	67.4	1.2
raw	1 oz	97	18.2	0.3
PINOCCHIO. See PINE NUT.				
PIÑON. See PINE NUT.				
PINTO BEAN				
(Allens)	1/2 cup	105	18.0	<1.0
boiled	4 oz	155	29.1	0.6
boiled *(A&P)*	1 cup	230	42.0	1.0
mature seeds, boiled	1/2 cup	116	21.8	0.4
mature seeds, raw	1/2 cup	326	60.9	1.1
raw	1 oz	96	18.0	0.3

Food Name	Serv. Size	Total Cal.	Carbs GMS	Fat GMS
raw *(Arrowhead Mills)*	2 oz	200	36.0	1.0
raw, dry *(Evans)*	1 cup	660	121.0	2.0
sprouted, mature seeds, boiled, drained	4 oz	25	4.6	0.4
sprouted, mature seeds, raw	1 lb	280	52.6	4.1
sprouted, mature seeds, raw	1 oz	18	3.3	0.3
Canned				
(Bush's Best)	1/2 cup	60	15.0	0.0
(Gebhardt)	4 oz	197	35.7	0.5
(Green Giant)	1/2 cup	90	20.0	1.0
(Joan of Arc)	1/2 cup	90	20.0	1.0
(Old El Paso)	1/2 cup	100	19.0	0.0
(Progresso)	1/2 cup	110	21.0	<1.0
baked style, and Great Northern, w/pork *(Luck's)*	7.25 oz	200	29.0	5.0
baked style, w/pork, 15-oz can *(Luck's)*	7.5 oz	220	30.0	6.0
baked style, w/pork, 29-oz can *(Luck's)*	7.25 oz	220	30.0	6.0
mature seeds	1/2 cup	94	17.5	0.4
organic, very low sodium, no salt added *(Eden Foods)*	1/2 cup	70	17.0	<1.0
organic, w/liquid *(Eden Foods)*	1/2 cup	110	20.0	<1.0
picante style *(Green Giant)*	1/2 cup	100	21.0	1.0
picante style *(Joan of Arc)*	1/2 cup	100	21.0	1.0
w/liquid	4 oz	88	16.5	0.4
Frozen				
	10-oz pkg	484	92.3	1.4
(Seabrook)	3.2 oz	160	29.0	0.0
boiled, drained	4 oz	184	35.0	0.5
immature seeds, boiled, drained, 10-oz pkg	1/3 pkg	152	29.0	0.5
immature seeds, unprepared, 10-oz pkg	1/3 pkg	160	30.6	0.5
PIROGIES, FROZEN				
pasta pocket, potato and American cheese filled *(Mrs. T's)*	1 pocket	70	10.0	2.0
pasta pocket, potato and cheddar cheese filled *(Mrs. T's)*	1 pocket	60	11.0	<1.0
pasta pocket, potato and onion filled *(Mrs. T's)*	1 pocket	50	10.0	<1.0
pasta pocket, sauerkraut filled *(Mrs. T's)*	1 pocket	50	9.0	<1.0
PISTACHIO BUTTER, roasted *(Maranatha Natural)*	2 tbsp	170	7.0	13.0
PISTACHIO NUT				
In shell				
dried	1 lb	1309	56.3	109.7
dried *(Dole)*	1 oz	90	3.0	7.0
dried *(Fisher)*	1 oz	170	7.0	14.0
dried *(Fisher)* red tint	1 oz	170	7.0	14.0
dry-roasted	1 lb	1429	64.9	124.5
dry-roasted, salted	1 lb	1429	64.9	124.5
Shelled				
dried	1 cup	739	31.8	61.9

Food Name	Serv. Size	Total Cal.	Carbs GMS	Fat GMS
dried, approx 47 kernels	1 oz	164	7.1	13.7
dry-roasted	1 cup	776	35.2	67.6
dry-roasted	1 oz	172	7.8	15.0
dry-roasted (Dole)	1 oz	163	7.0	14.0
dry-roasted (Planters)	1 oz	170	6.0	15.0
dry-roasted, natural (Planters)	1 oz	170	6.0	14.0
dry-roasted, red tint (Planters)	1 oz	170	6.0	14.0
PITA BREAD. See BREAD.				
PITANGA/Surinam cherry				
raw	1 cup	57	13.0	0.7
raw, trimmed	1/2 cup	29	6.5	0.3
raw, trimmed	1 oz	9	2.1	0.1
raw, trimmed, approx .3 oz	1 med	2	0.5	0.0
raw, untrimmed	1 lb	132	29.9	1.6
PIZZA, FRENCH BREAD, FROZEN				
Canadian style bacon, 1 pkg (Stouffer's)	5.5 oz	370	40.0	15.0
cheese (Healthy Choice)	5.6 oz	300	48.0	3.0
cheese (Lean Cuisine)	5 1/8 oz	300	38.0	9.0
cheese (Pappalo's)	1 piece	360	40.0	15.0
cheese, microwave (Oven Lovin')	1 serving	350	40.0	14.0
cheese 'Microwave' (Pillsbury)	1 piece	370	41.0	15.0
cheese, 1 pkg (Stouffer's)	5 1/8 oz	350	40.0	14.0
cheese 'Zap' (Banquet)	4.5 oz	310	41.0	10.0
combination (Pappalo's)	1 piece	430	41.0	21.0
combination, microwave (Oven Lovin')	1 serving	420	41.0	21.0
deluxe (Healthy Choice)	6.25 oz	330	41.0	8.0
deluxe (Lean Cuisine)	6 1/8 oz	350	40.0	11.0
deluxe, 1 pkg (Stouffer's)	6 1/8 oz	420	40.0	19.0
deluxe 'Zap' (Banquet)	4.8 oz	330	39.0	13.0
double cheese, 1 pkg (Stouffer's)	5 7/8 oz	420	43.0	18.0
hamburger, 1 pkg (Stouffer's)	6 oz	410	39.0	18.0
Italian turkey sausage (Healthy Choice)	6.45 oz	320	42.0	7.0
pepperoni (Healthy Choice)	6.25 oz	320	41.0	8.0
pepperoni (Lean Cuisine)	5 1/4 oz	340	41.0	11.0
pepperoni (Pappalo's)	1 piece	410	41.0	20.0
pepperoni, microwave (Oven Lovin')	1 serving	410	40.0	21.0
pepperoni 'Microwave' (Pillsbury)	1 piece	430	45.0	19.0
pepperoni, 1 pkg (Stouffer's)	5 3/4 oz	400	39.0	19.0
pepperoni 'Zap' (Banquet)	4.5 oz	350	36.0	16.0
pepperoni and mushroom (Stouffer's)	6 oz	410	40.0	19.0
sausage (Lean Cuisine)	6 oz	350	42.0	10.0
sausage (Pappalo's)	1 piece	410	41.0	18.0
sausage (Stouffer's)	6 oz	430	40.0	21.0

Food Name	Serv. Size	Total Cal.	Carbs GMS	Fat GMS
sausage, microwave *(Oven Lovin')*	1 serving	400	41.0	20.0
sausage 'Microwave' *(Pillsbury)*	1 piece	410	48.0	16.0
sausage and pepperoni *(Stouffer's)*	6.25 oz	460	41.0	23.0
sausage combo, and pepperoni 'Microwave' *(Pillsbury)*	1 piece	450	47.0	21.0
three cheese *(Lean Cuisine)*	5.5 oz	330	38.0	10.0
vegetable deluxe *(Stouffer's)*	6.5 oz	420	41.0	20.0

PIZZA, FROZEN
(Banquet)

Food Name	Serv. Size	Total Cal.	Carbs GMS	Fat GMS
pepperoni 'Pizza Pie'	6-oz pie	470	45.0	27.0
sausage 'Pizza Pie'	6-oz pie	500	48.0	29.0
sausage and pepperoni 'Pizza Pie'	6-oz pie	470	43.0	27.0
(Celeste)				
cheese	1/4 pie	315	28.0	17.0
cheese 'Pizza for One'	1 pie	500	48.0	25.0
deluxe	1/4 pie	380	29.0	22.0
deluxe 'Pizza for One'	1 pie	580	51.0	32.0
four cheese, original 'Pizza for One'	1 pie	540	47.0	30.0
four cheese, zesty 'Pizza for One'	1 pie	550	45.0	31.0
pepperoni	1/4 pie	370	29.0	21.0
pepperoni 'Pizza for One'	1 pie	545	50.0	30.0
sausage	1/4 pie	375	30.0	22.0
sausage 'Pizza for One'	1 pie	570	49.0	32.0
suprema	1/4 pie	380	29.0	24.0
suprema 'Pizza for One'	1 pie	680	54.0	39.0
vegetable 'Pizza for One'	1 pie	490	44.0	26.0
(Jeno's)				
combination 'Crisp 'N Tasty'	1/2 pizza	280	27.0	15.0
pepperoni 'Crisp 'N Tasty'	1/2 pizza	280	28.0	15.0
pepperoni 'Pizza Pocket'	1 serving	370	35.0	20.0
sausage 'Crisp 'N Tasty'	1/2 pizza	280	27.0	15.0
sausage 'Pizza Pocket'	1 serving	360	35.0	19.0
sausage and pepperoni 'Pizza Pocket'	1 serving	360	35.0	20.0
supreme 'Pizza Pocket'	1 serving	370	36.0	19.0
(Oven Lovin')				
cheese, microwave	1/2 pie	250	24.0	12.0
combination, microwave	1/2 pie	310	26.0	18.0
pepperoni, microwave	1/2 pie	300	25.0	17.0
sausage, microwave	1/2 pie	290	26.0	16.0
supreme, microwave	1/2 pie	310	27.0	18.0
(Pappalo's)				
pepperoni, 9 inch, traditional crust	1/2 pie	390	47.0	14.0
pepperoni, 12 inch, traditional crust	1/4 pie	350	40.0	11.0
pepperoni, pan pizza	1/6 pie	350	40.0	11.0

Food Name	Serv. Size	Total Cal.	Carbs GMS	Fat GMS
sausage, 9 inch, traditional crust	1/2 pie	380	47.0	13.0
sausage, 12 inch, traditional crust	1/4 pie	350	39.0	12.0
sausage, pan pizza	1/5 pie	350	39.0	11.0
sausage and pepperoni, 9 inch, traditional crust	1/2 pie	390	45.0	15.0
sausage and pepperoni, 12 inch, traditional crust	1/4 pie	360	40.0	12.0
sausage and pepperoni, pan pizza	1/5 pie	360	40.0	12.0
supreme, 9 inch, traditional crust	1/2 pie	400	46.0	16.0
supreme, 12 inch, traditional crust	1/4 pie	350	38.0	12.0
supreme, pan pizza	1/5 pie	340	37.0	12.0
three cheese, 9 inch, traditional crust	1/2 pie	350	47.0	11.0
three cheese, 12 inch, traditional crust	1/4 pie	310	41.0	7.0
three cheese, pan pizza	1/5 pie	310	39.0	8.0
(Pepperidge Farm)				
cheese, croissant pastry	1 pie	430	41.0	23.0
deluxe, croissant pastry	1 pie	440	43.0	23.0
pepperoni, croissant pastry	1 pie	420	43.0	22.0
(Tombstone)				
bacon, Canadian style, 'Original' 12 inch	3.6 oz	230	23.0	10.0
bacon cheeseburger, 'Special Order' 12 inch	4.7 oz	330	29.0	16.0
cheese, microwave, 7 inch	7.7 oz	500	45.0	24.0
cheese, 'Original' 9 inch	5.6 oz	380	40.0	17.0
cheese, 'Original' 12 inch	3.4 oz	230	23.0	10.0
cheese, w/hamburger, 'Original' 12 inch	3.7 oz	250	23.0	12.0
cheese, w/Italian sausage 'Italian Style Thincrust'	3.2 oz	220	15.0	13.0
cheese, w/pepperoni 'Italian Style Thincrust'	3 oz	230	15.0	14.0
cheese, w/pepperoni, 'Original' 12 inch	3.6 oz	260	23.0	14.0
cheese, w/sausage, mushrooms, 'Original' 12 inch	3.8 oz	240	23.0	11.0
cheese, w/sausage, 'Original' 12 inch	3.7 oz	240	23.0	11.0
cheese and hamburger, 'Original' 9 inch	6.3 oz	440	41.0	21.0
cheese and pepperoni, microwave, 7 inch	7.5 oz	550	38.0	32.0
cheese and pepperoni, 'Original' 9 inch	6.3 oz	480	40.0	26.0
cheese and sausage, 'Original' 9 inch	6.3 oz	420	41.0	19.0
chicken, 'Light' 8 inch	4.5 oz	240	28.0	8.0
chicken deluxe 'Light' approx 1/2 pizza	3.7 oz	180	23.0	4.0
deluxe, 'Original' 9 inch	7.0 oz	440	41.0	20.0
deluxe, 'Original' 12 inch	3.9 oz	240	23.0	11.0
four cheese 'Special Order'	4.3 oz	300	28.0	14.0
four meat 'Special Order'	4.6 oz	320	28.0	15.0
four meat, 'Special Order' 9 inch	3.9 oz	280	24.0	14.0
Italian sausage, microwave, 7 inch	8.0 oz	550	38.0	32.0
Italian sausage 'Special Order'	4.5 oz	300	28.0	13.0
pepperoni, 'Double Top' w/double cheese, 12 inch	4.8 oz	360	24.0	20.0
pepperoni 'Light' 8 inch	4.0 oz	250	27.0	10.0

Food Name	Serv. Size	Total Cal.	Carbs GMS	Fat GMS
pepperoni 'Special Order'	4.4 oz	320	28.0	16.0
pepperoni 'Special Order' 9 inch	3.7 oz	280	24.0	14.0
pepperoni and sausage, 'Original' 9 inch	6.6 oz	490	40.0	26.0
ranchero deluxe 'Mexican Style Thincrust'	3.4 oz	230	16.0	13.0
sausage, 'Double Top' w/double cheese, 12 inch	4.8 oz	330	24.0	16.0
sausage, w/pepperoni, 'Original' 12 inch	3.7 oz	260	23.0	13.0
sausage and pepperoni, 'Double Top' w/double cheese, 12 inch	4.8 oz	340	24.0	18.0
sausage and pepperoni, microwave, 7 inch	8 oz	570	39.0	32.0
supreme 'Italian Style Thincrust'	3.38 oz	230	16.0	14.0
supreme, 'Light' 8 inch	4.6 oz	250	26.0	9.0
supreme, 'Light' 12 inch	4.5 oz	250	29.0	9.0
supreme, microwave, 7 inch	8.5 oz	550	40.0	31.0
supreme, 'Original' 12 inch	3.8 oz	270	24.0	14.0
supreme 'Special Order'	4.4 oz	320	29.0	15.0
supreme, 'Special Order' 9 inch	4.0 oz	280	24.0	14.0
taco, microwave, 7 inch	8.4 oz	590	41.0	34.0
three sausage, 'Special Order' 9 inch	3.8 oz	260	24.0	12.0
vegetable, 'Light' 8 inch	4.4 oz	240	30.0	8.0
vegetable, 'Light' 12 inch	4.3 oz	230	30.0	7.0
(Totino's)				
Canadian bacon 'Party Pizza'	1/2 pie	330	42.0	13.0
cheese 'Pan Pizza'	1/6 pie	290	35.0	10.0
cheese 'Party Pizza'	1/2 pie	290	40.0	10.0
cheese 'Party Pizza Family Size'	1/3 pie	320	43.0	11.0
combination 'Party Pizza'	1/2 pie	370	43.0	17.0
combination 'Party Pizza Family Size'	1/3 pie	400	47.0	18.0
hamburger 'Party Pizza'	1/2 pie	350	37.0	17.0
pepperoni 'Pan Pizza'	1/6 pie	330	35.0	15.0
pepperoni 'Party Pizza'	1/2 pie	380	41.0	19.0
pepperoni 'Party Pizza Family Size'	1/3 pie	410	44.0	20.0
sausage 'Pan Pizza'	1/6 pie	320	35.0	13.0
sausage 'Party Pizza'	1/2 pie	370	44.0	17.0
sausage 'Party Pizza Family Size'	1/3 pie	410	48.0	18.0
sausage and pepperoni 'Pan Pizza'	1/6 pie	330	35.0	15.0
PIZZA CRUST, 'All Ready' *(Pillsbury)*	1/8 crust	90	16.0	1.0
PIZZA CRUST MIX				
deep dish, prepared w/water, crust only *(Martha White)*	1 slice	110	23.0	<1.0
'Pouch Mix' *(Gold Medal)*	1/6 pkg	110	22.0	1.0
'Pouch Mix' *(Robin Hood)*	1/6 pkg	110	22.0	1.0
'Quick & Easy' *(Chef Boyardee)*	1/6 pkg	150	26.0	2.0
regular, prepared w/water, crust only *(Martha White)*	1 slice	100	19.0	2.0

Food Name	Serv. Size	Total Cal.	Carbs GMS	Fat GMS
PIZZA DINNER, FROZEN				
cheese *(Kid Cuisine)*	6.85 oz	380	57.0	12.0
cheese 'Mega Meal' *(Kid Cuisine)*	9.7 oz	430	75.0	7.0
hamburger *(Kid Cuisine)*	6.85 oz	330	50.0	10.0
PIZZA ENTRÉE, FROZEN				
cheese *(Weight Watchers)*	6.03 oz	300	36.0	7.0
deluxe combination 'Lowfat' *(Weight Watchers)*	7.32 oz	320	36.0	9.0
hamburger 'Looney Tunes Wile E. Coyote' *(Tyson)*	6 oz	310	40.0	11.0
pepperoni 'Looney Tunes Foghorn Leghorn' *(Tyson)*	6.35 oz	400	57.0	13.0
pepperoni 'Lowfat' *(Weight Watchers)*	6.08 oz	320	36.0	8.0
supreme, hand held 'Aussie Pie' *(Mrs. Paterson's)*	5.5 oz	470	44.0	27.0
PIZZA MIX				
cheese 'Complete' *(Chef Boyardee)*	1/4 pkg	230	36.0	6.0
cheese, kit *(Contadina)*	4.94 oz	320	41.0	10.0
cheese '2 Complete' *(Chef Boyardee)*	1/8 pkg	210	31.0	5.0
pepperoni 'Complete' *(Chef Boyardee)*	1/4 pkg	250	31.0	9.0
pepperoni, kit *(Contadina)*	4.94 oz	370	38.0	16.0
pepperoni '2 Complete' *(Chef Boyardee)*	1/8 pkg	210	31.0	7.0
plain *(Chef Boyardee)*	1/4 pkg	180	32.0	3.0
sausage *(Chef Boyardee)*	1/4 pkg	270	34.0	10.0
PIZZA ROLL, FROZEN				
cheese, approx 6 rolls *(Jeno's)*	3 oz	240	23.0	12.0
combination *(Jeno's)*	3 oz	220	26.0	9.0
hamburger, approx 6 rolls *(Jeno's)*	3 oz	240	21.0	13.0
pepperoni, approx 6 rolls *(Jeno's)*	3 oz	220	26.0	9.0
pepperoni and cheese, approx 6 rolls *(Jeno's)*	3 oz	230	22.0	13.0
pepperoni and cheese 'Microwave' 6 rolls *(Jeno's)*	3 oz	240	23.0	13.0
sausage *(Jeno's)*	3 oz	210	26.0	7.0
sausage and cheese 'Microwave' approx 6 rolls *(Jeno's)*	3 oz	250	24.0	13.0
sausage and pepperoni, approx 6 rolls *(Jeno's)*	3 oz	230	22.0	13.0
PLANTAIN				
cooked	4 oz	132	35.3	0.2
cooked, sliced	1 cup	179	48.0	0.3
raw, approx 9.7 oz	1 med	218	57.1	0.7
raw, sliced	1 cup	181	47.2	0.6
raw, trimmed	1 oz	35	9.0	0.1
raw, trimmed, approx 9.7 oz	1 med	218	57.1	0.7
raw, untrimmed	1 lb	360	94.0	1.1
PLUM				
pitted	1 oz	16	3.7	0.2
raw, sliced	1 cup	91	21.5	1.0
raw, 2 1/8-inch diam	1 med	36	8.6	0.4
untrimmed *(Dole)*	2 pieces	70	17.0	1.0

Food Name	Serv. Size	Total Cal.	Carbs GMS	Fat GMS
w/pits	1 lb	235	55.5	2.6
PLUM, JAPANESE				
peeled and seeded	1 oz	13	3.4	0.1
raw, approx .6 oz	1 med	5	1.2	<.1
untrimmed	1 lb	132	34.1	0.6
PLUM, PURPLE, CANNED				
halves or whole, unpeeled (S&W Nutradiet)	1/2 cup	52	13.0	0.0
in extra heavy syrup	1/2 cup	133	34.3	0.1
in extra heavy syrup, pitted	4 oz	115	29.8	0.1
in extra heavy syrup, unpeeled, halves (S&W)	1/2 cup	135	35.0	0.0
in extra heavy syrup, unpeeled, whole (S&W)	1/2 cup	135	35.0	0.0
in extra heavy syrup, w/liquid	1 cup	264	68.7	0.3
in extra heavy syrup, w/2.75 tbsp liquid	3 plums	134	35.0	0.1
in heavy syrup	1/2 cup	115	30.0	0.1
in heavy syrup (Stokely)	1/2 cup	130	30.0	0.1
in heavy syrup, pitted	4 oz	101	26.4	0.1
in heavy syrup, w/liquid	1 cup	230	60.0	0.3
in heavy syrup, w/2.75 tbsp liquid	3 plums	118	30.9	0.1
in juice	1/2 cup	73	19.1	<.1
in juice, pitted	4 oz	66	17.2	<.1
in juice, whole (Featherweight)	1/2 cup	80	18.0	0.0
in light syrup	1/2 cup	79	20.5	0.1
in light syrup (Stokely)	1/2 cup	100	16.0	0.0
in light syrup, pitted	4 oz	71	18.5	0.1
in water	1/2 cup	51	13.7	<.1
in water, pitted	4 oz	46	12.5	<.1
POHA. See CAPE GOOSEBERRY.				
POI				
fresh	1/2 cup	134	32.7	0.2
fresh	1 oz	32	7.7	<.1
POKEBERRY SHOOTS				
boiled, drained	4 oz	23	3.5	0.5
boiled, drained	1/2 cup	16	2.5	0.3
raw	1/2 cup	18	3.0	0.3
raw, trimmed	4 oz	26	4.2	0.5
POLENTA MIX, prepared (Fantastic Foods)	1/2 cup	106	18.0	2.0
POLISH SAUSAGE				
	1 oz	92	0.5	8.1
link, 10 inches long x 1 1/4 inch diam, 8 oz	1 large	739	3.7	65.2
(Hillshire Farm) 'Links'	2 oz	190	2.0	17.0
(Hormel)	2 links	170	0.0	14.0
(OHSE)	1 oz	80	1.0	7.0
(OHSE) hot	1 oz	70	3.0	5.0

Food Name	Serv. Size	Total Cal.	Carbs GMS	Fat GMS
(Pilgrim's Pride)	3 oz	131	2.3	7.7
POLLACK, ALASKAN				
baked	4 oz	128	0.0	1.3
broiled	4 oz	128	0.0	1.3
microwaved	4 oz	128	0.0	1.3
raw	1 lb	365	0.0	3.6
raw	1 oz	23	0.0	0.2
POLLACK, ATLANTIC				
raw	1 lb	416	0.0	4.4
raw	3 oz	78	0.0	0.8
raw	1 oz	26	0.0	0.3
POLLACK, WALLEYE				
baked	4 oz	128	0.0	1.3
broiled	4 oz	128	0.0	1.3
dry-heat cooked	3 oz	96	0.0	1.0
microwaved	4 oz	128	0.0	1.3
raw	1 lb	365	0.0	3.6
raw	3 oz	69	0.0	0.7
raw	1 oz	23	0.0	0.2
POLLYFISH. See PARROTFISH.				
POMEGRANATE/Chinese apple				
raw, approx 3 3/8-inch diam	1 med	105	26.4	0.5
trimmed	1 oz	19	4.9	0.1
untrimmed	1 lb	172	43.6	0.8
POMEGRANATE JUICE *(Knudsen & Sons)*	8 oz	85	21.0	0.0
POMELO/pumelo				
raw, approx 5 1/2-inch diam, 2.4 lbs	1 med	228	58.6	0.2
sections	1/2 cup	36	9.1	<.1
trimmed	1 oz	11	2.7	<.1
untrimmed	1 lb	95	24.4	0.1
POMFRET				
raw	1 lb	663	0.0	36.4
raw	1 oz	41	0.0	2.3
POMPANO, FLORIDA				
baked	4 oz	239	0.0	13.8
broiled	4 oz	239	0.0	13.8
dry-heat cooked	3 oz	179	0.0	10.3
microwaved	4 oz	239	0.0	13.8
raw	1 lb	745	0.0	42.9
raw	1 oz	46	0.0	2.7

Food Name	Serv. Size	Total Cal.	Carbs GMS	Fat GMS

POPCORN

(NOTE: All popcorn is popped unless otherwise noted.)

(Bachman)

	Serv. Size	Total Cal.	Carbs GMS	Fat GMS
cheese flavor	.5 oz	90	7.0	6.0
'Lite'	.5 oz	50	10.0	1.0
regular	.5 oz	80	7.0	6.0
white cheddar cheese flavor	.5 oz	70	7.0	4.0
(Bearitos)				
cheese flavor 'Organic'	1 oz	137	13.2	8.0
'Organic 50% Less Oil'	.5 oz	70	9.0	3.0
'Organic Lite'	1 oz	132	14.7	6.9
'Organic No Salt'	1 oz	108	21.7	0.8
'Organic Traditional'	1 oz	140	12.0	9.2
(Bonnie Lee)				
w/oil and salt	1 oz	172	20.0	8.0
w/o oil and salt	1 oz	109	20.0	1.0
(Cape Cod) white cheddar cheese flavor	.5 oz	80	6.0	5.0
(Clover Club) white cheddar cheese flavor	.5 oz	70	6.0	5.0
(Cracker Jack) caramel coated, w/peanuts	1 oz	120	22.0	3.0
(Estee) caramel coated	1 oz	140	25.0	3.0
(Frito Lay)				
cheese flavor	.5 oz	80	7.0	5.0
regular	.5 oz	70	9.0	3.0
(Jiffy Pop)				
butter flavor 'Pan Popcorn'	4 cups	130	16.0	6.0
'Pan Popcorn'	4 cups	130	16.0	6.0
(Jolly Time)				
white, air-popped	3 cups	60	15.0	<1.0
white, w/o salt	4 cups	75	20.0	1.0
yellow, air-popped	3 cups	60	14.0	<1.0
yellow, w/o salt	4 cups	75	19.0	1.0
(Keebler)				
honey caramel 'Pop Deluxe'	1 oz	120	22.0	3.0
white cheddar cheese flavor	1 oz	140	13.0	10.0
(Kettle Poppins)				
lightly salted	.5 oz	70	9.0	2.5
white cheddar	.5 oz	70	9.0	2.5
(Laura Scudder)				
'Tender Baby White Corn'	.5 oz	80	6.0	6.0
white cheddar cheese flavor	.5 oz	70	6.0	5.0
(Nature's Choice)				
caramel, original	1 oz	108	25.0	1.0
caramel, w/peanuts	1 oz	114	23.0	1.0

Food Name	Serv. Size	Total Cal.	Carbs GMS	Fat GMS
(Orville Redenbacher)				
caramel 'Ready-to-Eat'	1 oz	112	22.4	3.5
hot air 'Gourmet' prepared	3 cups	40	10.0	<1.0
original 'Gourmet' prepared	3 cups	80	10.0	4.0
white 'Gourmet'	3 cups	80	10.0	4.0
white cheddar cheese 'Ready-to-Eat'	1.058 oz	139	16.5	8.6
(Pops-Rite)				
white, w/o salt, air popped	1 oz	100	20.0	2.0
white, w/o salt, oil popped	1 oz	220	20.0	15.0
yellow, w/o salt, air popped	1 oz	100	21.0	2.0
yellow, w/o salt, oil popped	1 oz	220	21.0	15.0
(Smartfood) white cheddar cheese flavor	.5 oz	80	7.0	5.0
(Ultra Slim Fast) butter flavor 'Lite 'N Tasty'	.5 oz	60	10.0	2.0
(Vic's)				
caramel, lite 'Gourmet'	1/2 cup	60	10.0	2.0
white, lite 'Gourmet'	1 cup	35	6.0	2.0
white cheddar cheese, lite 'Gourmet'	2/3 cup	40	4.0	2.0
yellow cheddar cheese, lite 'Gourmet'	2/3 cup	40	4.0	2.0
(Weight Watchers)				
butter	.66-oz pkg	90	13.0	3.0
caramel	.9-oz pkg	100	23.0	1.0
'Lightly Salted'	.66-oz pkg	80	12.0	4.0
white cheddar cheese flavor	.66-oz pkg	100	10.0	6.0
(Wise)				
butter flavor, 1 cup	.5 oz	80	7.0	5.0
'Tender Baby White Corn'	.5 oz	80	6.0	6.0
'Tender Eating Baby Popcorn'	.5 oz	70	4.0	6.0
white cheddar cheese flavor	.5 oz	70	6.0	5.0
POPCORN, FROZEN				
(Orville Redenbacher)				
butter flavor 'Gourmet' microwave	3 cups	100	11.0	6.0
natural 'Gourmet' microwave	3 cups	100	11.0	6.0
(Pillsbury)				
butter flavor	3 cups	210	20.0	13.0
'Original'	3 cups	210	20.0	13.0
'Salt-Free'	3 cups	170	23.0	7.0
POPCORN, MICROWAVE				
(NOTE: All microwave popcorn is popped unless otherwise noted.)				
(Betty Crocker)				
butter flavor 'Pop•Secret'	1/4 bag	120	13.0	8.0
butter flavor 'Pop•Secret By Request'	1/3 bag	60	12.0	1.0
butter flavor 'Pop•Secret Light'	1/4 bag	90	13.0	4.0
butter flavor 'Pop•Secret Pop Qwiz'	1 bag	110	11.0	7.0

Food Name	Serv. Size	Total Cal.	Carbs GMS	Fat GMS
butter flavor, salt-free 'Pop•Secret'	1/4 bag	120	13.0	7.0
butter flavor, singles 'Pop•Secret'	1 bag	250	27.0	16.0
butter flavor, singles 'Pop•Secret Light'	1 bag	180	28.0	8.0
cheese flavor 'Pop•Secret'	1/3 bag	170	15.0	11.0
natural 'Pop•Secret'	1/4 bag	120	13.0	8.0
natural 'Pop•Secret By Request'	1/3 bag	60	12.0	1.0
natural 'Pop•Secret Light'	1/4 bag	90	13.0	4.0
natural 'Pop•Secret Pop Qwiz'	1 bag	110	11.0	7.0
natural, singles 'Pop•Secret Light'	1 bag	170	26.0	7.0
(Featherweight)				
butter flavor 'Low Salt'	3 cups	100	14.0	3.0
'Natural Low Salt'	3 cups	80	14.0	1.0
(Jiffy Pop)				
butter flavor	4 cups	140	17.0	7.0
natural	4 cups	140	17.0	7.0
(Jolly Time)				
butter flavor	3 cups	90	13.0	5.0
butter flavor, light	3 cups	60	12.0	2.0
cheddar flavor	3 cups	155	17.0	10.0
natural	3 cups	120	15.0	7.0
natural, light	3 cups	70	13.0	2.0
(Orville Redenbacher)				
butter flavor 'Gourmet'	3 cups	100	11.0	6.0
butter flavor, light 'Gourmet'	3 cups	70	8.0	3.0
butter flavor, light, snack size	3 cups	70	11.0	3.0
butter flavor, salt-free 'Gourmet'	3 cups	100	11.0	6.0
butter flavor 'Smart•Pop'	3 cups	50	11.0	1.0
butter flavor, snack size	3 cups	100	11.0	6.0
butter toffee flavor 'Gourmet'	2 1/2 cups	210	26.0	12.0
caramel flavor 'Gourmet'	2 1/2 cups	240	29.0	14.0
cheddar cheese flavor 'Gourmet'	3 cups	130	14.0	8.0
natural 'Gourmet'	3 cups	100	11.0	6.0
natural, light 'Gourmet'	3 cups	70	8.0	3.0
natural, salt-free 'Gourmet'	3 cups	100	11.0	6.0
red herb and garlic flavor, 2 tbsp unpopped	1.27 oz	150	15.4	10.7
sour cream 'n onion flavor 'Gourmet'	3 cups	160	12.0	12.0
zesty butter flavor 'Reddenbutter' 2 tbsp unpopped	1.27 oz	148	15.9	10.2
(Pillsbury)				
butter flavor	3 cups	210	20.0	13.0
'Original'	3 cups	210	20.0	13.0
(Planters)				
butter flavor	3 cups	140	13.0	10.0
natural	3 cups	140	14.0	9.0

Food Name	Serv. Size	Total Cal.	Carbs GMS	Fat GMS
(Pop Weavers)				
butter flavor	4 cups	140	20.0	8.0
'Natural'	4 cups	140	20.0	8.0
(Pops-Rite)				
butter flavor	3 cups	90	13.0	5.0
'Natural'	3 cups	90	13.0	5.0
(Weight Watchers)	1-oz pkg	100	22.0	1.0
POPCORN OIL				
(Orville Redenbacher) popping	1 tbsp	120	0.0	14.0
(Planters)	1 tbsp	120	0.0	14.0
(Wesson) buttery flavor popping oil	1 tbsp	120	0.0	13.5
(Wesson) popping and topping oil 'Food Service'	1 tbsp	122	0.0	13.5
POPCORN SEASONING				
(McCormick/Schilling) 'Parsley Patch'	1 tsp	10	3.0	0.1
POPPY SEED				
whole	1 oz	151	6.7	12.6
whole	1 tbsp	47	2.1	3.9
whole	1 tsp	15	0.7	1.3
whole *(Durkee)*	1 tsp	15	0.0	<0.1
whole *(Laurel Leaf)*	1 tsp	15	0.0	<0.1
whole *(Spice Islands)*	1 tsp	13	0.8	0.9
POPPY SEED OIL				
	1 cup	1927	0.0	218.0
	1 oz	251	0.0	28.4
	1 tbsp	120	0.0	13.6
PORK. See also HAM, CANNED; HAM, CURED; HAM, FRESH; HAM PATTY.				
(NOTE: TRIMMED = Lean; separable fat removed. UNTRIMMED = Separable fat not removed.				
BACKFAT				
wholesale cuts, raw	1 lb	3683	0.0	402.3
wholesale cuts, raw	1 oz	230	0.0	25.1
BACKRIB				
Untrimmed				
raw	1 lb	1279	0.0	107.0
raw	1 oz	80	0.0	6.7
raw 'Gourmet' *(JM)*	5.5 oz	220	0.0	18.0
roasted	3 oz	315	0.0	25.1
BELLY				
wholesale cuts, raw	1 lb	2350	0.0	240.5
wholesale cuts, raw	1 oz	147	0.0	15.0
BOSTON BUTT				
Trimmed				
cured, medium fat, chopped, roasted	1 cup	340	0.0	19.3
cured, medium fat, roasted	9.8 oz	678	0.0	38.5

Food Name	Serv. Size	Total Cal.	Carbs GMS	Fat GMS
BRAINS				
braised	3 oz	117	0.0	8.1
in milk gravy *(Armour)*	2.75 oz	110	1.0	8.0
raw	1 oz	36	0.0	2.6
CENTER LOIN				
Trimmed				
braised	3 oz	172	0.0	7.1
broiled	3 oz	172	0.0	6.9
chopped, braised	1 cup	381	0.0	19.2
chopped, broiled	1 cup	323	0.0	14.7
chopped, roasted	1 cup	336	0.0	18.3
pan-fried	3 oz	197	0.0	8.9
pan-fried in vegetable oil	4 oz	302	0.0	14.0
raw	1 oz	45	0.0	2.0
roasted	3 oz	169	0.0	7.7
Untrimmed				
braised	3 oz	210	0.0	12.0
broiled	3 oz	204	0.0	11.1
chopped, braised	1 cup	496	0.0	35.5
chopped, broiled	1 cup	442	0.0	30.9
chopped, pan-fried in vegetable oil	1 cup	372	0.0	22.3
chopped, roasted	1 cup	427	0.0	30.5
pan-fried	3 oz	235	0.0	14.1
pan-fried in vegetable oil	4 oz	425	0.0	34.6
raw	1 oz	80	0.0	6.2
roasted	3 oz	199	0.0	11.4
CENTER RIB				
Trimmed				
braised	3 oz	175	0.0	8.0
broiled	3 oz	186	0.0	8.3
chopped, braised	1 cup	388	0.0	20.2
chopped, broiled	1 cup	361	0.0	20.9
chopped, pan-fried in vegetable oil	1 cup	360	0.0	21.4
chopped, roasted	1 cup	343	0.0	19.3
pan-fried	3 oz	185	0.0	9.2
pan-fried in vegetable oil	4 oz	291	0.0	17.4
raw	1 lb	676	0.0	27.3
roasted	3 oz	190	0.0	9.5
Untrimmed				
braised	3 oz	213	0.0	12.8
broiled	3 oz	224	0.0	13.2
chopped, braised	1 cup	514	0.0	38.0
chopped, broiled	1 cup	480	0.0	36.9

Food Name	Serv. Size	Total Cal.	Carbs GMS	F G
chopped, pan-fried in vegetable oil	1 cup	546	0.0	46
chopped, roasted	1 cup	445	0.0	33
pan-fried	3 oz	225	0.0	14
pan-fried in vegetable oil	4 oz	442	0.0	37
raw	1 oz	82	0.0	6
roasted	3 oz	217	0.0	13
CHITTERLINGS				
raw	1 oz	71	0.1	6
simmered	3 oz	258	0.0	24
CHOP, BONELESS, 'America's Cut' *(JM)*	6 oz	330	0.0	20.
COMPOSITE CUTS				
Trimmed				
loin and shoulder, cooked	3 oz	179	0.0	8
loin and shoulder, raw	1 lb	653	0.0	26
loin and shoulder, raw	1 oz	41	0.0	1.
retail cuts, cooked	3 oz	232	0.0	14.
retail cuts, raw	1 lb	980	0.0	67.
retail cuts, raw	1 oz	61	0.0	4
roasted	3 oz	180	0.0	8.
Untrimmed				
loin and shoulder, cooked	3 oz	214	0.0	12
loin and shoulder, raw	1 lb	907	0.0	58.
loin and shoulder, raw	1 oz	57	0.0	3.
raw	1 lb	1030	0.0	74.
raw	1 oz	64	0.0	4.
KIDNEYS				
braised	1 cup	211	0.0	6.
braised	3 oz	128	0.0	4.
raw	1 oz	28	0.0	0.
LIVER				
braised	3 oz	140	3.2	3.
fried	3 oz	205	2.1	9.
raw	1 oz	38	0.7	1.
LOIN				
Trimmed				
blade, braised	3 oz	191	0.0	11.
blade, broiled	3 oz	199	0.0	11.
blade, chopped, braised	1 cup	438	0.0	28.
blade, chopped, broiled	1 cup	420	0.0	30.
blade, chopped, roasted	1 cup	391	0.0	27.
blade, pan-fried	3 oz	205	0.0	12.
blade, pan-fried in vegetable oil	4 oz	321	0.0	22.
blade, raw	1 lb	712	0.0	37.

Food Name	Serv. Size	Total Cal.	Carbs GMS	Fat GMS
blade, roasted	3 oz	210	0.0	12.6
country-style ribs, braised	3 oz	199	0.0	11.6
country-style ribs, raw	1 lb	712	0.0	37.4
country-style ribs, raw	1 oz	45	0.0	2.3
country-style ribs, roasted	3 oz	210	0.0	12.6
whole, braised	3 oz	173	0.0	7.8
whole, broiled	3 oz	178	0.0	8.3
whole, chopped, braised	1 cup	382	0.0	20.4
whole, chopped, broiled	1 cup	360	0.0	21.4
whole, chopped, roasted	1 cup	336	0.0	19.5
whole, raw	1 oz	44	0.0	2.1
whole, roasted	3 oz	178	0.0	8.2
whole or half, center cut, boneless *(JM)*	3 oz	190	0.0	13.0
Untrimmed				
blade, braised	3 oz	275	0.0	21.6
blade, broiled	3 oz	272	0.0	21.1
blade, chopped, braised	1 cup	574	0.0	47.7
blade, chopped, broiled	1 cup	550	0.0	47.4
blade, chopped, roasted	1 cup	510	0.0	42.6
blade, pan-fried	3 oz	291	0.0	23.6
blade, pan-fried in vegetable oil	4 oz	469	0.0	41.9
blade, raw	1 lb	1293	0.0	109.4
blade, roasted	3 oz	275	0.0	20.9
country-style ribs, braised	3 oz	252	0.0	18.3
country-style ribs, raw	1 lb	1093	0.0	84.9
country-style ribs, raw	1 oz	68	0.0	5.3
country-style ribs, roasted	3 oz	279	0.0	21.5
whole, braised	4 oz	417	0.0	31.6
whole, broiled	3 oz	206	0.0	11.8
whole, chopped, braised	1 cup	515	0.0	39.1
whole, chopped, broiled	1 cup	484	0.0	38.1
whole, chopped, roasted	1 cup	447	0.0	34.0
whole, raw	1 lb	898	0.0	57.1
whole, roasted	3 oz	211	0.0	12.4
LUNGS				
braised	3 oz	84	0.0	2.6
raw	1 oz	24	0.0	0.8
PANCREAS				
braised	3 oz	186	0.0	9.2
raw	1 oz	56	0.0	3.8
SHOULDER				
Trimmed				
arm picnic, braised	3 oz	211	0.0	10.4

Food Name	Serv. Size	Total Cal.	Carbs GMS	Fat GMS
arm picnic, chopped, braised	1 cup	347	0.0	17.
arm picnic, chopped, roasted	1 cup	319	0.0	17.
arm picnic, raw	1 lb	635	0.0	27.
arm picnic, raw	1 oz	40	0.0	1.
arm picnic, roasted	3 oz	194	0.0	10.
Boston blade, braised	3 oz	232	0.0	13.
Boston blade, broiled	3 oz	193	0.0	10.
Boston blade, chopped, braised	1 cup	412	0.0	24.
Boston blade, chopped, broiled	1 cup	384	0.0	25.
Boston blade, chopped, roasted	1 cup	358	0.0	23.
Boston blade, raw	1 oz	47	0.0	2.
Boston blade, roasted	3 oz	197	0.0	12.
whole, chopped, roasted	1 cup	341	0.0	21.0
whole, raw	1 lb	671	0.0	32.
whole, raw	1 oz	42	0.0	2.
whole, roasted	3 oz	195	0.0	11.
whole, roasted, diced	1 cup	310	0.0	18.
Untrimmed				
arm picnic, roasted	3 oz	269	0.0	20.
Boston blade, braised	3 oz	271	0.0	18.
Boston blade, broiled	3 oz	220	0.0	14.
Boston blade, chopped, braised	1 cup	519	0.0	40.
Boston blade, chopped, broiled	1 cup	490	0.0	39.
Boston blade, raw	1 lb	989	0.0	71.
Boston blade, roasted	3 oz	229	0.0	16.
whole, chopped, roasted	1 cup	456	0.0	36.
whole, diced, roasted	1 cup	394	0.0	28.
whole, raw	1 lb	1070	0.0	81.
whole, raw	1 oz	67	0.0	5.
whole, roasted	3 oz	248	0.0	18.
SIRLOIN				
Trimmed				
boneless, braised	3 oz	149	0.0	5.
boneless, broiled	3 oz	164	0.0	5.
boneless, raw	1 lb	581	0.0	19.
boneless, roasted	3 oz	168	0.0	7.
braised	3 oz	167	0.0	7.
broiled	3 oz	181	0.0	8.
chopped, braised	1 cup	365	0.0	18.
chopped, broiled	1 cup	340	0.0	19.0
chopped, roasted	1 cup	330	0.0	18.
raw	1 oz	43	0.0	1.
raw, approx 3.1 oz	1 chop	133	0.0	5.

Food Name	Serv. Size	Total Cal.	Carbs GMS	Fat GMS
roasted	3 oz	184	0.0	8.8
Untrimmed				
boneless, braised	3 oz	161	0.0	7.1
boneless, broiled	3 oz	177	0.0	7.3
boneless, raw	1 lb	658	0.0	28.6
boneless, roasted	3 oz	176	0.0	8.0
braised	3 oz	208	0.0	12.8
broiled	3 oz	220	0.0	13.7
chopped, braised	1 cup	493	0.0	36.0
chopped, broiled	1 cup	463	0.0	35.4
chopped, roasted	1 cup	407	0.0	28.6
raw	1 oz	78	0.0	6.3
roasted	3 oz	222	0.0	13.6
SPARERIBS				
Untrimmed				
braised	3 oz	337	0.0	25.8
raw	1 lb	1297	0.0	107.0
raw	1 oz	81	0.0	6.7
raw 'Gourmet' *(JM)*	4.5 oz	250	0.0	22.0
SPLEEN				
braised	3 oz	127	0.0	2.7
raw	1 oz	28	0.0	0.7
STOMACH, raw	1 oz	45	0.0	2.7
TENDERLOIN				
Trimmed				
boneless *(JM)*	3 oz	120	0.0	5.0
broiled	3 oz	159	0.0	5.4
chopped or diced, roasted	1 cup	232	0.0	6.7
raw	1 lb	544	0.0	15.5
raw	1 oz	34	0.0	1.0
roasted	3 oz	139	0.0	4.1
Untrimmed				
broiled	3 oz	171	0.0	6.9
raw	1 lb	617	0.0	24.5
raw	1 oz	39	0.0	1.5
roasted	3 oz	147	0.0	5.1
TOP LOIN				
Trimmed				
braised	3 oz	172	0.0	7.3
broiled	3 oz	173	0.0	6.6
chopped, braised	1 cup	388	0.0	20.2
chopped, broiled	1 cup	361	0.0	20.9
chopped, pan-fried in vegetable oil	1 cup	360	0.0	21.4

Food Name	Serv. Size	Total Cal.	Carbs GMS	Fa G
chopped, roasted	1 cup	343	0.0	19
pan-fried	3 oz	191	0.0	8
pan-fried in vegetable oil	4 oz	291	0.0	17
raw	1 oz	46	0.0	2
roast, boneless, raw	1 lb	640	0.0	24
roast, boneless, raw	1 oz	40	0.0	1.
roasted	3 oz	165	0.0	6.
Untrimmed				
braised	3 oz	198	0.0	10.
broiled	3 oz	195	0.0	9
chopped, braised	1 cup	533	0.0	40.
chopped, broiled	1 cup	504	0.0	40.
chopped, pan-fried in vegetable oil	1 cup	549	0.0	46.
chopped, roasted	1 cup	462	0.0	35.
pan-fried	3 oz	218	0.0	12.
pan-fried in vegetable oil	3 oz	337	0.0	28
raw	1 oz	86	0.0	7
roast, boneless, raw	1 lb	866	0.0	52.
roast, boneless, raw	1 oz	54	0.0	3.
roasted	3 oz	192	0.0	9.
PORK, CANNED				
	1 oz	95	0.6	8.
approx .75 oz	1 slice	70	0.4	6.
(Hormel)	3 oz	240	2.0	21.
(Hormel) chopped	3 oz	200	2.0	16.
PORK, CURED				
blade roll, untrimmed, diced, roasted	1 cup	402	0.5	32.
blade roll, untrimmed, diced, unheated	1 cup	377	0.0	30.
blade roll, untrimmed, roasted	4 oz	325	0.4	26.
blade roll, untrimmed, unheated	1 oz	76	0.0	6.
boneless, blade roll, untrimmed, roasted	3 oz	244	0.3	20.
boneless, blade roll, untrimmed, unheated	1 oz	76	0.0	6.
PORK, GROUND				
cooked	3 oz	252	0.0	17.
raw	1 oz	75	0.0	6.
(JM)	3 oz	190	0.0	14.
PORK, SALT, cured, raw	1 oz	212	0.0	22.
PORK DINNER, FROZEN, chow mein 'Bi-Pack' *(LaChoy)*	8.642 oz	87	10.3	3.2
PORK ENTRÉE				
Canned				
chow mein 'Bi-Pack' *(LaChoy)*	3/4 cup	80	7.0	3.
sweet and sour *(LaChoy)*	3/4 cup	250	48.0	4.

Food Name	Serv. Size	Total Cal.	Carbs GMS	Fat GMS
Frozen				
barbecued back ribs 'Pork Classics' *(John Morrell)*	4.75 oz	240	8.0	17.0
barbecued chops, center cut 'Pork Classics' *(John Morrell)*	4.5 oz	230	7.0	9.0
barbecued loin, thin sliced 'Pork Classics' *(John Morrell)*	3 oz	150	5.0	6.0
barbecued spare ribs 'Pork Classics' *(John Morrell)*	4.5 oz	250	7.0	18.0
barbecued tenderloin 'Pork Classics' *(John Morrell)*	3 oz	130	3.0	5.0
breaded, steak *(Hormel)*	3 oz	220	11.0	15.0
patty, deluxe 'Looney Tunes Porky Pig' *(Tyson)*	6.5 oz	370	48.0	14.0
sweet and sour *(Chun King)*	13 oz	400	78.0	5.0
PORK FAT				
separable fat from fully cooked ham, roasted	1 oz	167	0.0	17.5
separable fat from fully cooked ham, unheated	1 oz	164	<.1	17.4
separable fat from ham and arm picnic, roasted	3 oz	502	0.0	52.6
separable fat from ham and arm picnic, roasted	1 oz	168	0.0	17.5
separable fat from ham and arm picnic, unheated	1 oz	164	0.0	17.4
PORK RIND SNACK				
(Baken-ets)	1 oz	160	2.0	10.0
(Baken-ets) hot 'n spicy	1 oz	150	1.0	9.0
PORK SEASONING AND COATING MIX				
'Bag 'n Season' *(Schilling)*	1 pkg	103	23.6	0.4
POT ROAST DINNER/ENTRÉE, FROZEN				
homestyle *(Right Course)*	9.25 oz	220	22.0	7.0
homestyle, w/browned potatoes *(Stouffer's)*	8 7/8 oz	280	24.0	11.0
Yankee *(Budget Gourmet)*	11 oz	380	22.0	21.0
Yankee *(Healthy Choice)*	11 oz	260	36.0	4.0
Yankee *(Le Menu)*	10 oz	330	27.0	13.0
Yankee 'Classics' *(Armour)*	10 oz	310	26.0	12.0
POT ROAST SEASONING MIX				
'Bag 'n Season' *(Schilling)*	1 pkg	55	8.5	0.6
'Seasoning Blends' *(Lawry's)*	1 pkg	122	25.0	0.7
POTATO				
Baked				
in skin	4 oz	124	28.6	0.1
in skin, pulp only	4 oz	105	24.4	0.1
in skin, skin only	2 oz	112	26.1	0.1
pulp	1/2 cup	57	13.1	0.1
Boiled				
in skin	2 oz	44	9.8	0.1
in skin, pulp only	4 oz	99	22.8	0.1
in skin, pulp only	1/2 cup	68	15.7	0.1
in skin, pulp only, approx 2.5-inch diam	1 potato	118	27.4	0.1
pulp only	4 oz	98	22.7	0.1
pulp only	1/2 cup	67	15.6	0.1

Food Name	Serv. Size	Total Cal.	Carbs GMS	Fat GMS
pulp only, approx 2.5-inch diam	1 potato	116	27.0	0.1
Hash brown, cooked in vegetable oil	4 oz	237	24.2	15.8
Microwaved				
in skin	4 oz	119	27.4	0.1
in skin, pulp only	4 oz	113	26.4	0.1
in skin, pulp only	1/2 cup	78	18.2	0.1
in skin, skin only	2 oz	75	16.8	0.1
Raw				
peeled	1 oz	22	5.1	<.1
pulp only, diced	1/2 cup	59	13.5	0.1
skin only	2 oz	33	7.1	0.1
unpeeled	1 lb	269	61.2	0.3
POTATO, CANNED				
(Stokely)	1/2 cup	50	11.0	0.0
(Veg•All)	1/2 cup	60	13.0	0.0
approx 1.2 oz	1 potato	21	4.8	0.1
diced (Bush's Best)	1/2 cup	40	8.0	0.0
diced (Taylor's Brand)	1 cup	90	25.0	0.0
drained	4 oz	68	15.4	0.2
drained	1/2 cup	54	12.3	0.2
drained, approx 1-inch diam	1 potato	21	4.8	0.1
new, extra small, whole (S&W)	1/2 cup	45	9.0	0.0
new, small, whole (IGA)	1/2 cup	45	9.0	0.0
new, whole, drained (Hunt's)	4 oz	70	15.0	<1.0
sliced (Bush's Best)	1/2 cup	40	8.0	0.0
sliced (Taylor's Brand)	1 cup	90	25.0	0.0
sliced, w/liquid (Del Monte)	1/2 cup	45	10.0	0.0
white, diced (Allens)	1/2 cup	45	10.0	<1.0
white, double diced (Allens)	1/2 cup	45	10.0	<1.0
white, sliced (A&P)	1/2 cup	45	11.0	<1.0
white, sliced (Allens)	1/2 cup	45	10.0	<1.0
white, sliced 'No Salt Added' (Pathmark)	1 cup	100	20.0	0.0
white, small, sliced (Finast)	1/2 cup	55	13.0	0.0
white, small, whole (Finast)	1/2 cup	55	13.0	0.0
white, whole (A&P)	1/2 cup	45	11.0	<1.0
white, whole 'No Salt Added' (Pathmark)	1 cup	100	20.0	0.0
whole (Bush's Best)	1/2 cup	40	8.0	0.0
whole, w/liquid	1 cup	120	26.0	0.5
whole, w/liquid	1/2 cup	60	13.0	0.2
whole, w/liquid (Del Monte)	1/2 cup	45	10.0	0.0
w/liquid	4 oz	45	9.8	0.2
POTATO, FINNISH YELLOW, raw (Frieda's)	3.5 oz	100	22.0	na

Food Name	Serv. Size	Total Cal.	Carbs GMS	Fat GMS
POTATO, FREEZE-DRIED				
hash brown, prepared *(Mountain House)*	1 cup	150	36.0	0.0
POTATO, FROZEN				
fried	9 oz	419	63.8	16.5
fried, cottage cut, heated in oven	4 oz	247	38.6	9.3
fried, partially fried in oil, heated in oven	4 oz	252	38.4	9.9
fried, partially fried in oil, heated in oven	1.75 oz	111	17.0	4.4
hash brown, prepared in vegetable oil	4 oz	247	31.9	13.0
hash brown, w/butter sauce, prepared	4 oz	202	27.4	10.0
puffs, partially fried in oil, prepared	4 oz	252	34.6	12.2
whole, peeled	10 oz	221	49.6	0.5
whole, peeled, boiled, drained	4 oz	74	16.5	0.1
(A&P)				
fried, crinkle cut	3.5 oz	140	25.0	4.0
fried, regular	3.5 oz	140	25.0	4.0
fried, shoestring	3.5 oz	170	24.0	6.0
fried, steak fries	3.5 oz	140	24.0	4.0
hash brown	3.5 oz	80	17.0	0.0
morsels	3.5 oz	140	23.0	4.0
(Heinz)				
fried, crinkle cut 'Deep Fries'	3 oz	150	22.0	6.0
fried 'Deep Fries'	3 oz	160	23.0	6.0
fried, shoestring 'Deep Fries'	3 oz	200	25.0	10.0
hash brown, w/butter and onions 'Deep Fries'	3 oz	110	14.0	7.0
(MicroMagic)				
fried	3 oz	290	40.0	13.0
fried, skinny	3 oz	350	49.0	15.0
sticks 'Tater Sticks'	4 oz	390	43.0	22.0
(Ore-Ida)				
fried, cottage cut	3 oz	120	19.0	5.0
fried 'Country Style Dinner Fries'	3 oz	110	19.0	3.0
fried, crinkle cut 'Golden Crinkles'	3 oz	120	19.0	4.0
fried, crinkle cut 'Lites'	3 oz	90	16.0	2.0
fried, crinkle cut, microwave	3.5 oz	180	26.0	8.0
fried, crinkle cut 'Pixie Crinkles'	3 oz	140	21.0	6.0
fried 'Crisp Crowns'	3 oz	160	20.0	9.0
fried 'Crispers!'	3 oz	230	25.0	15.0
fried, French, extra crispy 'Nacho Crispers'	3 oz	180	21.0	10.0
fried, French 'Fast Fries'	3 oz	150	23.0	7.0
fried 'Golden Fries'	3 oz	120	19.0	4.0
fried 'Lites'	3 oz	90	16.0	2.0
fried, shoestring	3 oz	140	21.0	6.0
fried, shoestring 'Lites'	3 oz	90	15.0	4.0

Food Name	Serv. Size	Total Cal.	Carbs GMS	Fat GMS
fried, wedges 'Home Style Potato Wedges'	3 oz	100	17.0	3.0
fried, w/onions 'Crispy Crowns'	3 oz	170	20.0	9.0
hash brown 'Golden Patties'	2.5 oz	140	15.0	8.0
hash brown, microwave	2 oz	130	12.0	8.0
hash brown, shredded	3 oz	70	15.0	<1.0
hash brown 'Southern Style'	3 oz	70	16.0	<1.0
hash brown, w/cheddar 'Cheddar Browns'	3 oz	90	13.0	2.0
mashed, natural butter flavor, prepared w/2% milk	1/2 cup	170	23.0	5.0
mashed, natural butter flavor, unprepared	2.25 oz	100	14.0	3.0
puffs, bacon flavored 'Tater Tots'	3 oz	140	19.0	6.0
puffs 'Tater Tots'	3 oz	140	19.0	7.0
puffs 'Tater Tots' microwave	4 oz	200	29.0	9.0
puffs, w/onion 'Tater Tots'	3 oz	140	19.0	6.0
whole, small	3 oz	70	16.0	<1.0
(Quick 'n Crispy)				
fried, crinkle cut	4 oz	370	44.0	19.0
fried, shoestring	4 oz	390	48.0	20.0
fried, thin cuts	4 oz	370	44.0	19.0
wedges	4 oz	280	36.0	13.0
(Seabrook)				
diced and hash-shred	4 oz	80	19.0	0.0
fried	3 oz	120	20.0	4.0
fried, cottage cut	2.8 oz	110	17.0	4.0
fried, crinkle cut	3 oz	120	20.0	4.0
fried, shoestring	3 oz	140	20.0	6.0
white, whole, boiled	3.2 oz	60	13.0	0.0
(Southern) white, whole	3.5 oz	69	15.0	0.1
POTATO CHIPS AND SNACKS				
(Allens)				
barbecue flavor	1 oz	150	14.0	9.0
hot flavor	1 oz	150	14.0	9.0
potato sticks, shoestring, canned	1 oz	140	16.0	8.0
potato sticks, shoestring, canned 'No Salt'	1 oz	140	16.0	8.0
regular flavor	1 oz	160	14.0	10.0
(Bachman)				
'Kettle Cooked'	1 oz	140	16.0	8.0
pasta snack chip 'Pastapazazz'	1 oz	150	15.0	9.0
'Ridge'	1 oz	160	14.0	10.0
'Ruffled'	1 oz	160	14.0	10.0
Saratoga-style 'Kettle Cooked'	1 oz	140	16.0	8.0
sour cream and onion flavor	1 oz	150	14.0	9.0
'Unsalted'	1 oz	160	14.0	10.0
vinegar flavor	**1 oz**	**150**	**15.0**	**9.0**

Food Name	Serv. Size	Total Cal.	Carbs GMS	Fat GMS
(Barbara's Bakery)				
herb and garlic flavor 'True Blues'	1 oz	140	15.0	9.0
ripple	1 oz	150	14.0	10.0
'True Blues'	1 oz	150	15.0	10.0
(Barrel O'Fun)	1 oz	150	14.0	10.0
(Cape Cod)				
dill and sour cream flavor	1 oz	150	16.0	8.0
dill and sour cream flavor 'No Salt'	1 oz	150	16.0	8.0
'No Salt Added'	1 oz	150	16.0	8.0
regular flavor	1 oz	150	16.0	8.0
'Waves'	1 oz	150	16.0	8.0
(Cottage Fries) 'No Salt Added'	1 oz	160	14.0	11.0
(Eagle)				
barbecue flavor 'Extra Crunchy'	1 oz	150	16.0	8.0
barbecue flavor 'Extra Crunchy Louisiana'	1 oz	150	16.0	8.0
barbecue flavor 'Thins'	1 oz	150	15.0	10.0
'Eagle Thins'	1 oz	150	15.0	10.0
'Extra Crunchy'	1 oz	150	16.0	8.0
'Idaho Russet'	1 oz	150	16.0	8.0
'Ridged Thins'	1 oz	150	15.0	10.0
sour cream and onion flavor 'Ridged'	1 oz	150	15.0	10.0
(Eden Foods)				
brown rice chips	1 oz	130	19.0	5.0
sea vegetable chips	1 oz	130	22.0	5.0
wasabi snack chips	1 oz	130	22.0	4.0
(Featherweight) 'Low Salt'	1 oz	160	14.0	11.0
(Flavor Tree) sour cream and onion flavor potato sticks	1/4 cup	127	12.5	8.3
(Funyuns) rings, onion flavor, approx 11 rings	1 oz	140	18.0	6.0
(Great Snackers)				
barbecue flavor	1 serving	60	8.0	3.0
cheddar cheese flavor	1 serving	60	8.0	3.0
sour cream and onion flavor	.5 oz	70	10.0	3.0
toasted onion flavor	1 serving	60	8.0	3.0
(Hain)				
carrot chip	1 oz	150	16.0	9.0
carrot chip, barbecue	1 oz	140	16.0	8.0
carrot chip 'No Salt Added'	1 oz	150	16.0	7.0
(Health Valley)				
'Country'	1 oz	160	15.0	10.0
'Country Dip'	1 oz	160	15.0	10.0
'Country Dip No Salt Added'	1 oz	160	15.0	10.0
'Country Natural No Salt Added'	1 oz	160	15.0	10.0
'Country No Salt Added'	1 oz	160	15.0	10.0

Food Name	Serv. Size	Total Cal.	Carbs GMS	Fat GMS
'Country Ripple'	1 oz	160	15.0	10.0
'Country Ripple No Salt Added'	1 oz	160	15.0	10.0
'Natural'	1 oz	160	15.0	10.0
(Keebler)				
original flavor, lightly seasoned	1 oz	140	18.0	7.0
sour cream and onion flavor	1 oz	140	17.0	7.0
(Kettle Chips)				
jalapeño jack flavor	1 oz	150	15.0	9.0
lightly salted	1 oz	150	15.0	9.0
New York cheddar flavor	1 oz	150	15.0	9.0
no salt	1 oz	150	15.0	9.0
organically grown, w/sea salt	1 oz	150	15.0	9.0
salsa w/mesquite flavor	1 oz	150	15.0	9.0
sea salt and vinegar flavor	1 oz	150	15.0	9.0
yogurt and green onion flavor	1 oz	150	15.0	9.0
(King Kold)				
au gratin flavor	1 oz	150	15.0	8.0
barbecue flavor 'BBQ'	1 oz	140	16.0	8.0
dill flavor	1 oz	150	16.0	8.0
onion-garlic flavor	1 oz	150	15.0	9.0
regular flavor	1 oz	150	16.0	9.0
'Rip-L'	1 oz	150	16.0	9.0
sour cream and onion flavor	1 oz	150	15.0	10.0
(Lay's)				
barbecue flavor, approx 15-20 chips	1 oz	150	15.0	9.0
barbecue flavor 'Kansas City Style' approx 15-20 chips	1 oz	150	15.0	9.0
Cajun flavor 'Crunch Tators Amazin Cajun'	1 oz	150	17.0	8.0
cheddar cheese flavor, approx 15-20 chips	1 oz	150	14.0	10.0
'Flamin' Hot' approx 15-20 chips	1 oz	150	15.0	9.0
jalapeño flavor 'Crunch Tators Hoppin' Jalapeño'	1 oz	140	18.0	7.0
mesquite flavor 'Crunch Tators Mighty Mesquite'	1 oz	150	17.0	8.0
original flavor, approx 15-20 chips	1 oz	150	15.0	10.0
original flavor 'Crunch Tators' approx 16 chips	1 oz	150	17.0	8.0
salt and vinegar flavor, approx 15-20 chips	1 oz	150	14.0	10.0
sour cream and onion flavor, approx 15-20 chips	1 oz	160	15.0	10.0
tangy ranch flavor, approx 15-20 chips	1 oz	160	15.0	10.0
'Unsalted'	1 oz	150	15.0	10.0
(Louise's)				
mesquite barbecue flavor, fat-free	1 oz	100	23.0	<1.0
original flavor, fat-free	1 oz	100	23.0	<1.0
vinegar and salt flavor, fat-free	1 oz	100	23.0	<1.0
(Mr. Phipps)				
tater crisps, barbecue flavor	.5 oz	60	10.0	2.0

Food Name	Serv. Size	Total Cal.	Carbs GMS	Fat GMS
tater crisps, sour cream and onion flavor	.5 oz	60	10.0	2.0
(Munchos) plain, approx 16 chips	1 oz	160	15.0	10.0
(Nabisco)				
baked, cheddar cheese flavor, cracker chips 'Zings'	.5 oz	70	9.0	3.0
baked, ranch flavor, cracker chips 'Zings'	.5 oz	70	9.0	3.0
cracker chips, baked 'Zings'	.5 oz	70	10.0	3.0
(O'Boisies)				
regular flavor	1 oz	150	16.0	9.0
sour cream and onion flavor	1 oz	150	15.0	9.0
(Planters)				
potato sticks	1 oz	160	15.0	10.0
potato sticks, barbecue flavor	1 oz	160	15.0	10.0
(Poore Brothers)				
barbecue flavor	1 oz	150	15.0	10.0
Cajun flavor	1 oz	140	16.0	8.0
dill pickle flavor	1 oz	140	16.0	8.0
grilled steak and onion flavor	1 oz	140	15.0	8.0
jalapeño flavor	1 oz	140	16.0	9.0
Parmesan and garlic flavor	1 oz	140	16.0	9.0
regular flavor	1 oz	140	17.0	8.0
salt and vinegar flavor	1 oz	140	15.0	9.0
unsalted	1 oz	140	17.0	8.0
(Pringle's)				
barbecue flavor 'Light'	1 oz	150	17.0	8.0
cheese flavor 'Cheez-ums'	1 oz	170	12.0	13.0
French onion flavor 'Idaho Rippled'	1 oz	170	13.0	12.0
'Idaho Rippled'	1 oz	170	13.0	12.0
'Light'	1 oz	150	17.0	8.0
ranch flavor 'Light'	1 oz	150	17.0	8.0
'Regular'	1 oz	170	12.0	13.0
sour cream and onion flavor	1 oz	170	13.0	12.0
taco and cheddar flavor 'Idaho Rippled'	1 oz	170	13.0	12.0
(Ray's)				
taro chips, salted	1 oz	139	20.0	6.0
taro chips, unsalted	1 oz	139	20.0	6.0
(Ruffles)				
barbecue flavor	1 oz	150	16.0	9.0
Cajun flavor 'Cajun Spice'	1 oz	150	15.0	10.0
cheddar and sour cream flavor	1 oz	150	16.0	9.0
'Choice' 40% less fat, approx 16 chips	1 oz	130	18.0	6.0
'Light Choice' 1/3 less fat	1 oz	130	19.0	6.0
mesquite barbecue flavor 'Mesquite Grille'	1 oz	160	14.0	10.0
ranch flavor	1 oz	160	15.0	10.0

Food Name	Serv. Size	Total Cal.	Carbs GMS	Fat GMS
regular flavor	1 oz	150	15.0	10.0
sour cream and onion flavor	1 oz	150	15.0	9.0
(Schlotzsky's) barbecue, deli style	1 oz	150	17.0	6.0
(Snacktime)				
jalapeño flavor 'Krunchers!'	1 oz	150	16.0	9.0
'Krunchers!'	1 oz	150	16.0	9.0
mesquite barbecue flavor 'Krunchers!'	1 oz	150	16.0	9.0
(Spicer's)				
barbecue wheat flavor, for weight control	1 oz	100	12.0	5.0
natural flavor, for weight control	1 oz	100	11.0	4.0
sour cream and onion flavor, for weight control	1 oz	100	12.0	4.0
(Sun Chips)				
multi-grain snacks, French onion flavor	1 oz	140	18.0	7.0
multi-grain snacks, harvest cheddar flavor	1 oz	140	18.0	7.0
multi-grain snacks, original flavor	1 oz	150	18.0	8.0
(Tato Skins)				
potato skins, baked	1 oz	150	17.0	8.0
potato skins, cheese and bacon flavor,	1 oz	150	17.0	8.0
potato skins, sour cream and chives flavor	1 oz	150	17.0	8.0
(Westbrae)				
no salt	1 oz	150	16.0	8.0
'Ripple'	1 oz	150	16.0	8.0
salted	1 oz	160	15.0	10.0
(Wise)				
barbecue flavor	1 oz	150	14.0	10.0
barbecue flavor 'Ridgies'	1 oz	150	14.0	10.0
hot flavor	1 oz	160	14.0	11.0
'New York Deli'	1 oz	160	14.0	11.0
onion-garlic flavor	1 oz	150	14.0	10.0
'Plain'	1 oz	150	14.0	10.0
'Ridgies'	1 oz	150	14.0	10.0
'Ridgies Super Crispy'	1 oz	150	14.0	10.0
rings, onion flavor	1 oz	130	21.0	5.0
'Rippled'	1 oz	150	14.0	10.0
sour cream and onion flavor 'Ridgies'	1 oz	160	14.0	11.0
(Zapp's)				
Cajun flavor 'Lite Kettle'	1 oz	150	16.0	8.0
Cajun flavor 'Original Kettle'	1 oz	150	16.0	8.0
jalapeño flavor 'Original Kettle'	1 oz	150	16.0	8.0
'Lite Kettle'	1 oz	150	16.0	8.0
'Lite Kettle No Salt Added'	1 oz	150	16.0	8.0
mesquite barbecue flavor 'Lite Kettle'	1 oz	150	16.0	8.0
mesquite barbecue flavor 'Original Kettle'	1 oz	150	16.0	8.0

Food Name	Serv. Size	Total Cal.	Carbs GMS	Fat GMS
'Original Kettle'	1 oz	150	16.0	8.0
'Original Kettle No Salt Added'	1 oz	150	16.0	8.0
sour cream and onion flavor 'Lite Kettle'	1 oz	150	16.0	8.0
POTATO DISH, CANNED, au gratin *(Pantry Express)*	1/2 cup	120	17.0	5.0
POTATO DISH, FROZEN				
au gratin 'Family Side Dish' *(Freezer Queen)*	4 oz	100	19.0	2.0
au gratin 'For One' *(Birds Eye)*	5.5 oz	240	24.0	13.0
au gratin 'One Serving' *(Green Giant)*	5.5 oz	200	20.0	10.0
au gratin, side dish *(Stouffer's)*	5.75 oz	170	17.0	9.0
baked, butter 'Twice Baked' *(Ore-Ida)*	5 oz	200	27.0	9.0
baked, cheddar cheese 'Twice Baked' *(Ore-Ida)*	5 oz	190	28.0	7.0
baked, ranch 'Twice Baked' *(Ore-Ida)*	5 oz	180	28.0	6.0
baked, sour cream and chives 'Twice Baked' *(Ore-Ida)*	5 oz	180	28.0	6.0
baked, stuffed w/cheddar cheese *(Oh Boy!)*	6 oz	142	23.0	4.0
baked, stuffed w/cheese flavored topping *(Green Giant)*	5 oz	200	33.0	6.0
baked, stuffed w/real bacon *(Oh Boy!)*	6 oz	116	18.0	3.0
baked, stuffed w/sour cream and chives *(Green Giant)*	5 oz	230	31.0	10.0
baked, stuffed w/sour cream and chives *(Oh Boy!)*	6 oz	129	18.0	5.0
baked, topped w/salsa and cheese *(Ore-Ida)*	5.6 oz	160	25.0	4.0
cheddared, 'Side Dish' *(Budget Gourmet)*	5.5 oz	230	22.0	13.0
cheddared, w/broccoli 'Side Dish' *(Budget Gourmet)*	5 oz	130	18.0	4.0
fried, 'Country Style Dinner Fries' *(Ore-Ida)*	3 oz	110	19.0	3.0
fried, w/onions 'Crispy Crowns' *(Ore-Ida)*	3 oz	170	20.0	9.0
garden casserole, low-fat, 'Quick Meals' *(Healthy Choice)*	9.25 oz	180	23.0	4.0
hash brown, w/butter and onions, 'Deep Fries' *(Heinz)*	3 oz	110	14.0	7.0
hash brown, w/cheddar, 'Cheddar Browns' *(Ore-Ida)*	3 oz	90	13.0	2.0
nacho, 'Side Dish' *(Budget Gourmet)*	5 oz	180	14.0	10.0
new, in sour cream sauce, 'Side Dish' *(Budget Gourmet)*	5 oz	120	15.0	6.0
'O'Brien' *(Ore-Ida)*	3 oz	60	14.0	<1.0
puffs, w/bacon-flavored vegetable protein, 'Tater Tots' *(Ore-Ida)*	3 oz	140	19.0	6.0
puffs, w/onion, 'Tater Tots' *(Ore-Ida)*	3 oz	140	19.0	6.0
scalloped, side dish *(Stouffer's)*	5.75 oz	130	16.0	6.0
shredded, w/cheese sauce and vegetables, 'Singles' *(Stokely)*	4.5 oz	130	15.0	6.0
sliced, w/cheddar cheese sauce and bacon, 'Singles' *(Stokely)*	4.5 oz	150	24.0	5.0
three cheese, 'Side Dish' *(Budget Gourmet)*	5.75 oz	230	25.0	11.0
wedges, hot and spicy, 'Texas Crispers' *(Ore-Ida)*	3 oz	180	19.0	10.0
w/broccoli and cheese flavor sauce, 'One Serving' *(Green Giant)*	5.5 oz	130	19.0	5.0
w/broccoli and cheese sauce, 'Family Side Dish' *(Freezer Queen)*	5.5 oz	140	25.0	3.0

Food Name	Serv. Size	Total Cal.	Carbs GMS	Fat GMS
POTATO DISH, MICROWAVE				
au gratin, 'Microwave Shelf Pack' (Green Giant)	1/2 cup	120	17.0	5.0
scalloped, microwave cup (Lunch Bucket)	7.5 oz	160	20.0	7.0
scalloped, w/ham, micro cup (Hormel)	7.5 oz	260	21.0	16.0
POTATO DISH MIX				
and cheese, au gratin, 'Potatoes & Cheese' (Kraft) prepared	1/2 cup	130	19.0	5.0
and cheese, broccoli au gratin (Kraft) prepared	1/2 cup	150	20.0	5.0
broccoli au gratin 'Potato Medleys' (Betty Crocker) dry	1/5 pkg	110	22.0	1.0
broccoli au gratin 'Potato Medleys' (Betty Crocker) prepared w/margarine and 2% milk	1/2 cup	140	23.0	4.0
cheddar, w/mushrooms 'Potato Medleys' (Betty Crocker) dry	1/5 pkg	110	22.0	1.0
cheddar, w/mushrooms 'Potato Medleys' (Betty Crocker) prepared w/margarine and whole milk	1/2 cup	140	23.0	4.0
scalloped, w/broccoli 'Potato Medleys' (Betty Crocker) dry	1/5 pkg	100	19.0	2.0
scalloped, w/broccoli 'Potato Medleys' (Betty Crocker) prepared	1/2 cup	140	21.0	5.0
scalloped, w/green beans and mushrooms (Betty Crocker) dry	1/5 pkg	110	20.0	2.0
scalloped, w/green beans and mushrooms (Betty Crocker) prepared	1/2 cup	140	21.0	5.0
'SpudFlakes' (Martha White) prepared w/2% milk	1/3 cup	120	15.0	6.0
w/cheese, scalloped, and ham (Kraft) prepared	1/2 cup	150	20.0	5.0
w/cheese, scalloped 'Potatoes & Cheese' (Kraft) prepared	1/2 cup	140	20.0	5.0
w/cheese, sour cream and chive (Kraft) prepared	1/2 cup	150	20.0	5.0
w/two cheeses 'Potatoes & Cheese' (Kraft) prepared	1/2 cup	130	19.0	4.0
POTATO ENTRÉE, FROZEN				
baked, chicken divan (Weight Watchers)	11.25 oz	280	38.0	7.0
baked, homestyle turkey (Weight Watchers)	11.25 oz	230	27.0	7.0
baked, vegetable primavera (Weight Watchers)	11.15 oz	320	49.0	9.0
baked, w/broccoli and cheddar (Lean Cuisine)	10 3/8 oz	290	37.0	9.0
baked, w/broccoli and cheese (Weight Watchers)	10.5 oz	270	43.0	6.0
baked, w/broccoli and ham (Weight Watchers)	11.5 oz	240	30.0	5.0
baked, w/cheese sauce and broccoli 'Light & Healthy' (Budget Gourmet)	10.5 oz	300	40.0	10.0
baked, w/sour cream (Lean Cuisine)	10 3/8 oz	230	38.0	5.0
POTATO FLOUR				
	1/2 cup	316	71.9	0.7
	1 oz	100	22.7	0.2

Food Name	Serv. Size	Total Cal.	Carbs GMS	Fat GMS
POTATO MIX				
AU GRATIN				
(Betty Crocker) prepared w/margarine and skim milk	1/2 cup	150	21.0	5.0
(Fantastic Foods) prepared w/whole milk	1/2 cup	156	25.0	4.0
(Fantastic Foods) prepared w/whole milk and salted butter	1/2 cup	196	25.0	8.0
(French's) tangy, prepared	1/2 cup	130	20.0	5.0
(General Mills) dry	1/6 pkg	100	20.0	1.0
(General Mills) homestyle, w/broccoli, dry	1/6 pkg	90	18.0	1.0
(General Mills) homestyle, w/broccoli, prepared w/margarine and 2% milk	1/2 cup	140	19.0	6.0
(General Mills) prepared w/margarine and 2% milk	1/2 cup	150	21.0	6.0
(Idahoan) prepared	1/2 cup	130	18.0	5.0
(Pillsbury) 'Specialty' tangy, dry	1/6 pkg	90	19.0	1.0
(Pillsbury) tangy, prepared w/butter and whole milk	1/2 cup	140	20.0	6.0
CASSEROLE (French's) cheddar and bacon, prepared	1/2 cup	130	18.0	5.0
COUNTRY STYLE				
(Fantastic Foods) prepared	1/2 cup	85	19.0	0.3
(Fantastic Foods) prepared w/salted butter	1/2 cup	118	19.0	4.0
HASH BROWN				
(Betty Crocker) w/onions, prepared	1/6 pkg	110	24.0	1.0
(Betty Crocker) w/onions, prepared w/margarine	1/2 cup	160	24.0	6.0
(General Mills)	1/6 pkg	110	24.0	<1.0
(General Mills) prepared w/margarine	1/2 cup	160	24.0	6.0
(Idahoan) herb and butter, dry	1/6 pkg	90	16.0	2.0
(Idahoan) prepared w/unsalted butter	1/2 cup	140	18.0	7.0
(Idahoan) 'Quick One-Pan' prepared	1/2 cup	140	18.0	7.0
JULIENNE				
(General Mills) dry	1/6 pkg	90	17.0	1.0
(General Mills) prepared w/margarine and 2% milk	1/2 cup	130	19.0	5.0
MASHED				
(Betty Crocker) bacon and cheddar 'Twice Baked' dry	1/6 pkg	110	19.0	2.0
(Betty Crocker) bacon and cheddar 'Twice Baked' prepared	1/2 cup	210	21.0	11.0
(Betty Crocker) butter, herbed 'Twice Baked' dry	1/6 pkg	100	18.0	2.0
(Betty Crocker) butter, herbed 'Twice Baked' prepared	1/2 cup	220	20.0	13.0
(Betty Crocker) cheddar, mild, w/onion 'Twice Baked' dry	1/6 pkg	100	18.0	2.0
(Betty Crocker) cheddar, mild, w/onion 'Twice Baked' prepared	1/2 cup	190	19.0	11.0
(Betty Crocker) cheddar cheese 'Potato Buds' dry	1/12 pkg	110	20.0	2.0
(Betty Crocker) cheddar cheese 'Potato Buds' prepared	1/2 cup	180	21.0	9.0
(Betty Crocker) cheddar cheese 'Potato Buds' reduced fat recipe, dry	1/12 pkg	140	21.0	5.0

Food Name	Serv. Size	Total Cal.	Carbs GMS	Fat GMS
(Betty Crocker) 'Potato Buds' prepared	1/2 cup	130	17.0	6.0
(Betty Crocker) 'Potato Buds' prepared w/o added salt	1/2 cup	130	17.0	6.0
(Country Store) prepared	1/3 cup	70	16.0	0.0
(General Mills) American cheese, homestyle, dry	1/6 pkg	100	20.0	1.0
(General Mills) American cheese, homestyle, prepared w/margarine and 2% milk	1/2 cup	150	21.0	6.0
(General Mills) cheddar and bacon, dry	1/6 pkg	100	20.0	1.0
(General Mills) cheddar and bacon, prepared w/margarine and 2% milk	1/2 cup	150	21.0	6.0
(General Mills) cheddar cheese, homestyle, dry	1/6 pkg	90	19.0	1.0
(General Mills) cheddar cheese, homestyle, prepared w/margarine and 2% milk	1/2 cup	150	21.0	6.0
(Hungry Jack) 'Flakes' prepared	1/2 cup	140	17.0	7.0
(Idahoan) cheddar, spicy, dry	1/6 pkg	90	17.0	1.0
(Idahoan) cheddar, spicy, prepared	1/2 cup	140	21.0	5.0
(Pillsbury) cheddar and bacon 'Specialty' dry	1/6 pkg	90	18.0	1.0
(Pillsbury) cheddar and bacon 'Specialty' prepared w/butter and whole milk	1/2 cup	140	19.0	6.0
SCALLOPED				
(Betty Crocker) cheesy, dry	1/6 pkg	90	19.0	1.0
(Betty Crocker) cheesy, prepared	1/2 cup	140	20.0	5.0
(Betty Crocker) dry	1/6 pkg	90	19.0	1.0
(Betty Crocker) prepared	1/2 cup	140	20.0	5.0
(Betty Crocker) sour cream and chives, dry	1/6 pkg	100	19.0	2.0
(Betty Crocker) sour cream and chives, prepared	1/2 cup	140	21.0	5.0
(Betty Crocker) w/ham, dry	1/5 pkg	100	20.0	1.0
(Betty Crocker) w/ham, prepared	1/2 cup	160	22.0	6.0
(French's) creamy Italian, prepared	1/2 cup	120	19.0	3.0
(French's) crispy top, w/savory onion mix, prepared	1/2 cup	140	20.0	5.0
(French's) real cheese, prepared	1/2 cup	140	19.0	5.0
(French's) sour cream and chives, prepared	1/2 cup	150	19.0	7.0
(General Mills) dry	1/6 pkg	90	19.0	1.0
(General Mills) prepared w/margarine and 2% milk	1/2 cup	140	20.0	5.0
(General Mills) smoky cheddar, dry	1/6 pkg	100	20.0	1.0
(General Mills) smoky cheddar, prepared w/margarine and 2% milk	1/2 cup	140	21.0	5.0
(General Mills) sour cream and chive	1/6 pkg	100	19.0	2.0
(General Mills) sour cream and chive, prepared w/margarine and 2% milk	1/2 cup	150	20.0	6.0
(General Mills) w/ham, dry	1/5 pkg	100	20.0	1.0
(General Mills) w/ham, prepared w/margarine and 2% milk	1/2 cup	170	22.0	7.0
(Idahoan) prepared	1/2 cup	140	20.0	5.0
(Idahoan) prepared w/o added salt, w/unsalted butter	1/2 cup	140	16.0	7.0

Food Name	Serv. Size	Total Cal.	Carbs GMS	Fat GMS
(Idahoan) sour cream and chives, dry	1/6 pkg	90	15.0	2.0
(Idahoan) sour cream and chives, prepared	1/2 cup	130	18.0	5.0
(Pillsbury) sour cream and chives 'Specialty,' dry	1/6 pkg	100	18.0	2.0
(Pillsbury) sour cream and chives, 'Specialty,' prepared w/butter and whole milk	1/2 cup	150	20.0	6.0
STUFFED				
(Betty Crocker) sour cream and chives 'Twice Baked,' dry	1/6 pkg	90	17.0	2.0
(Betty Crocker) sour cream and chives 'Twice Baked' prepared	1/2 cup	200	19.0	11.0
WESTERN				
(Arrowhead Mills) flakes	2 oz	140	44.0	0.0
(Barbara's Bakery) dry	4 oz	389	89.0	1.0
(French's) creamy, prepared	1/2 cup	130	20.0	4.0
(General Mills) cheesy homestyle, dry	1/6 pkg	100	19.0	2.0
(General Mills) cheesy homestyle, prepared w/margarine and 2% milk	1/2 cup	150	20.0	6.0
(General Mills) potato buds, dry	1/8 pkg	70	16.0	0.0
(General Mills) potato buds, prepared	1/2 cup	130	17.0	6.0
(General Mills) potato buds, prepared w/o salt	1/2 cup	130	17.0	6.0
(Hungry Jack) flakes	13.3 oz	70	16.0	0.0
(Hungry Jack) flakes, prepared w/margarine, 2% milk, and water	1/2 cup	130	17.0	6.0
(Hungry Jack) flakes, prepared w/margarine, 2% milk, salt, and water	1/2 cup	130	17.0	6.0
(Idaho) granules	13.3 oz	60	14.0	0.0
(Idaho) granules, prepared	1/2 cup	130	16.0	6.0
(Idaho) granules, prepared w/margarine, 2% milk, and water	1/2 cup	120	16.0	5.0
(Idaho) granules, prepared w/margarine, 2% milk, salt, and water	1/2 cup	120	16.0	5.0
(Idaho Spuds) flakes	13.3 oz	70	15.0	0.0
(Idaho Spuds) flakes, prepared	1/2 cup	140	17.0	7.0
(Idaho Spuds) flakes, prepared w/margarine, 2% milk, and water	1/2 cup	130	16.0	6.0
(Idaho Spuds) flakes, prepared w/margarine, 2% milk, salt, and water	1/2 cup	130	16.0	6.0
(Idahoan) dry	1/3 cup	80	18.0	0.0
(Idahoan) 'Complete' dry	1/3 cup	100	19.0	2.0
(Pillsbury) cheesy 'Specialty' dry	1/6 pkg	100	19.0	2.0
(Pillsbury) cheesy 'Specialty,' prepared w/butter and whole milk	1/2 cup	150	20.0	6.0
(Pillsbury) creamy white sauce, 'Specialty,' dry	1/6 pkg	100	19.0	2.0

Food Name	Serv. Size	Total Cal.	Carbs GMS	Fat GMS
POTATO PANCAKE				
(Idaho) 3-inch diam each, prepared	3 cakes	90	16.0	2.0
(Kosher Empire) frozen, triangle, latkes w/onions	2 oz	77	13.0	2.4
(Pillsbury) 'Specialty'	1/8 pkg	70	16.0	0.0
(Pillsbury) 'Specialty' prepared w/water and egg, 3-inch diam each	3 cakes	90	16.0	2.0
POTATO SALAD, CANNED				
(Joan of Arc) German	1/2 cup	120	23.0	3.0
(Joan of Arc) homestyle	1/2 cup	340	32.0	22.0
(Read) German	1/2 cup	120	23.0	3.0
(Read) homestyle	1/2 cup	340	32.0	22.0
POTATO SALAD SEASONING (Tone's)	1 tsp	5	0.3	0.2
POTATO STARCH (Featherweight)	1 cup	620	154.0	1.0
POTATO STICKS. See POTATO CHIPS AND SNACKS.				
POTTED MEAT SPREAD. See also LUCHEON MEAT, CANNED; SANDWICH SPREAD.				
beef	1 cup	558	0.0	43.2
chicken	1 cup	558	0.0	43.2
turkey	1 cup	558	0.0	43.2
(Hormel)	1 oz	53	2.0	4.0
(Hormel)	1 tbsp	30	0.0	2.0
(Libby's)	1.83 oz	110	0.0	9.0
POULTRY SEASONING				
dry	1 oz	87	18.6	2.1
dry	1 tbsp	11	2.4	0.3
dry	1 tsp	5	1.0	0.1
PRESERVES. See also FRUIT SPREAD; JAM; JELLY; MARMALADE.				
APPLE BUTTER				
(Bama)	2 tsp	25	6.0	0.0
(Knudsen & Sons) organic	2 tbsp	25	6.0	0.0
(Lucky Leaf)	4 oz	200	49.0	1.0
(Musselman's)	4 oz	200	49.0	1.0
(Smucker's) 'Autumn Harvest'	1 tsp	12	3.0	0.0
(Smucker's) cider	1 tsp	12	3.0	0.0
(Smucker's) natural	1 tsp	12	3.0	0.0
(Smucker's) 'Simply Fruit'	1 tsp	16	4.0	0.0
(Smucker's) spiced	1 tsp	12	3.0	0.0
(Tap'n Apple)	1 oz	45	13.2	<.1
(White House)	1 oz	50	12.0	0.0
APRICOT				
(Knott's Berry Farm)	1 tsp	18	4.0	0.0
(Polaner)	2 tsp	35	9.0	0.0
APRICOT-PINEAPPLE				
(Knott's Berry Farm)	1 tsp	18	4.0	0.0

Food Name	Serv. Size	Total Cal.	Carbs GMS	Fat GMS
(Knudsen & Sons)	2 tsp	35	8.0	<1.0
BING CHERRY (Knott's Berry Farm)	1 tsp	18	4.0	0.0
BLACK CHERRY (Knudsen & Sons)	2 tsp	35	8.0	<1.0
BLACKBERRY				
(Knott's Berry Farm) seedless	1 tsp	18	4.0	0.0
(Knudsen & Sons)	2 tsp	35	8.0	<1.0
(Knudsen & Sons) organic	2 tsp	25	7.0	<1.0
(Polaner) seedless	2 tsp	35	9.0	0.0
BLUEBERRY				
(Knott's Berry Farm)	1 tsp	18	4.0	0.0
(Knudsen & Sons)	2 tsp	35	8.0	<1.0
(Knudsen & Sons) organic	2 tsp	25	7.0	<1.0
(Polaner)	2 tsp	35	9.0	0.0
BOYSENBERRY				
(Knott's Berry Farm)	1 tsp	18	4.0	0.0
(Knudsen & Sons)	2 tsp	35	8.0	<1.0
CONCORD GRAPE (Knudsen & Sons)	2 tsp	35	8.0	<1.0
KADOTA FIG (Knott's Berry Farm)	1 tsp	18	4.0	0.0
PEACH				
(Bama)	2 tsp	30	8.0	0.0
(Knudsen & Sons)	2 tsp	35	8.0	<1.0
(Polaner)	2 tsp	35	9.0	0.0
PINEAPPLE (Polaner)	2 tsp	35	9.0	0.0
RED CHERRY (Knott's Berry Farm)	1 tsp	18	4.0	0.0
RED RASPBERRY				
(Knott's Berry Farm) seedless	1 tsp	18	4.0	0.0
(Knudsen & Sons)	2 tsp	35	8.0	<1.0
(Knudsen & Sons) organic	2 tsp	25	7.0	<1.0
(Polaner)	2 tsp	35	9.0	0.0
(Polaner) seedless	2 tsp	35	9.0	0.0
(Smucker's) natural ingredients	1 tsp	18	4.0	0.0
STRAWBERRY				
(Bama)	2 tsp	30	8.0	0.0
(Knott's Berry Farm) pure, seedless	1 tsp	18	4.0	0.0
(Knudsen & Sons)	2 tsp	35	8.0	<1.0
(Knudsen & Sons) organic	2 tsp	25	7.0	<1.0
(Polaner)	2 tsp	35	9.0	0.0
(Smucker's) natural ingredients	1 tsp	18	4.0	0.0
PRETZELS				
(A & Eagle)	1 oz	110	22.0	2.0
(Bachman) 'Nutzels'	1 oz	110	21.0	2.0
(Bachman) 'Petite'	1 oz	110	21.0	2.0
(Bachman) 'Petite Sodium Free'	1 oz	110	21.0	2.0

Food Name	Serv. Size	Total Cal.	Carbs GMS	Fat GMS
(Estee) 'Unsalted'	5 pretzels	25	5.0	<1.0
(Featherweight) 'Low Salt'	20 pretzels	110	23.0	1.0
(Mister Salty) 'Juniors'	1 oz	110	22.0	2.0
(Pepperidge Farm) 'Goldfish'	1 oz	110	20.0	3.0
(Rokeach) 'Baldies Unsalted'	1 oz	110	20.0	0.0
(Rold Gold) 'Tiny Tim'	1 oz	110	23.0	1.0
BAVARIAN				
(Barbara's Bakery) 1 oz	2 pretzels	110	21.0	<1.0
(Barbara's Bakery) no salt added, 1 oz	2 pretzels	110	21.0	<1.0
(Rold Gold) 1 oz	3 pretzels	120	22.0	2.0
BEER *(Quinlan)*	1 oz	110	21.6	1.4
BRAIDS *(Keebler)* 'Butter Pretzels'	1 oz	110	21.0	1.0
CHEDDAR *(Combos)*	10 nuggets	143	19.5	5.8
CHIPS				
'Mr. Phipps' *(Nabisco)* lightly salted, .5 oz	8 chips	60	11.0	1.0
'Mr. Phipps' *(Nabisco)* original, .5 oz	8 chips	60	10.0	1.0
'Mr. Phipps' *(Nabisco)* sesame, .5 oz	8 chips	60	10.0	2.0
DUTCH STYLE				
	7.5-oz pkg	831	161.7	9.6
	1 pretzel	62	12.1	0.7
(Estee) 'Unsalted'	2 pretzels	110	23.0	<1.0
(Mister Salty) 1 oz	2 pretzels	110	22.0	1.0
(Rokeach)	1 oz	110	24.0	0.0
(Rokeach) 'Unsalted'	1 oz	110	20.0	0.0
HARD				
(Bachman)	1 oz	110	23.0	<1.0
(Bachman) unsalted	1 oz	110	23.0	<1.0
plain, made w/unenriched flour, salted	10 twists	322	31.7	20.8
plain, made w/unenriched flour, unsalted	10 twists	229	47.5	2.1
plain, salted	10 twists	229	47.5	2.1
plain, unsalted	10 twists	229	47.5	2.1
whole wheat	2 oz	205	46.0	1.5
HONEYSWEET *(Barbara's Bakery)* 1 oz	2 pretzels	110	21.0	<1.0
KNOTS *(Keebler)* 'Butter Pretzels'	1 oz	110	21.0	1.0
LOGS				
(Bachman)	1 oz	110	21.0	2.0
(Quinlan)	1 oz	103	21.5	0.8
MINIS				
(Barbara's Bakery) 1 oz	17 pretzels	110	21.0	<1.0
(Barbara's Bakery) no salt added, 1 oz	17 pretzels	110	21.0	<1.0
(Mister Salty) 1 oz	22 pretzels	110	21.0	1.0
NINE-GRAIN *(Barbara's Bakery)* 1 oz	2 pretzels	110	21.0	<1.0
OAT BRAN *(Quinlan)*	1 oz	115	21.8	1.5

Food Name	Serv. Size	Total Cal.	Carbs GMS	Fat GMS
PARTY				
(Delicious)	1 oz	110	23.0	1.0
(Rokeach) 'Party Cannister'	1 oz	110	23.0	1.0
RICE BRAN, 'No-Salt' (Quinlan)	1 oz	101	19.5	2.3
RINGS				
(Bachman)	1 oz	110	21.0	2.0
(Mister Salty)	1 oz	110	21.0	2.0
(Mister Salty) butter flavor	1 oz	110	21.0	2.0
RODS				
(Bachman)	1 oz	110	21.0	2.0
(Rold Gold)	1 oz	110	22.0	2.0
(Seyfert's) butter flavor	1 oz	110	21.0	1.0
STICKS				
(Delicious)	1 oz	110	23.0	1.0
(Mister Salty)	1 oz	110	22.0	1.0
(Mister Salty) butter flavor	1 oz	110	22.0	1.0
(Mister Salty) fat-free	1 oz	110	23.0	<1.0
(Mister Salty) very thin, 1 oz	92 sticks	110	22.0	3.0
(Pepperidge Farm) 'Snack Sticks'	8 sticks	120	23.0	3.0
(Quinlan)	1 oz	105	22.3	0.6
(Rold Gold)	1 oz	110	23.0	1.0
THINS				
(Bachman)	1 oz	110	21.0	2.0
(Bachman) 'Thin'n Light'	1 oz	110	21.0	2.0
(Quinlan)	1 oz	104	22.0	0.6
(Quinlan) tiny	1 oz	109	21.2	1.5
(Quinlan) tiny 'No-Salt'	1 oz	115	22.4	1.6
(Quinlan) 'Ultra Thins'	1 oz	106	22.5	0.6
(Rold Gold) baked, 33% less sodium 'Fat Free'	1 oz	110	23.0	0.0
TREATS (Bachman)	1 oz	110	21.0	2.0
TWISTS				
(Bachman)	1 oz	110	21.0	2.0
(Delicious)	1 oz	110	23.0	1.0
(Mister Salty) .5 oz	5 twists	110	21.0	2.0
(Mister Salty) fat-free, 1 oz	9 twists	110	23.0	<1.0
(Rold Gold) thin, 1 oz	10 twists	110	23.0	1.0
(Rold Gold) tiny, 1 oz	15 twists	110	23.0	1.0
(Ultra Slim Fast)	1 oz	100	21.0	1.0
PRICKLY PEAR				
raw, trimmed	1 oz	12	2.7	0.1
raw, trimmed, approx 4.8 oz	1 fruit	42	9.9	0.5
raw, untrimmed	1 lb	140	32.6	1.7

PROSCIUTTO. See LUNCHEON MEAT, HAM.

Food Name	Serv. Size	Total Cal.	Carbs GMS	Fat GMS
PRUNE				
dehydrated	4 oz	384	101.0	0.8
dehydrated, cooked	4 oz	128	33.7	0.3
Canned				
in heavy syrup, w/liquid	1 cup	246	65.1	0.5
in heavy syrup, w/liquid	1/2 cup	123	32.5	0.2
in heavy syrup, w/2 tbsp liquid	5 fruits	90	23.9	0.2
pitted, in heavy syrup, w/liquid	4 oz	119	31.5	0.2
PRUNE, DRIED				
pitted	1 cup	385	101.0	0.8
pitted	4 oz	271	71.1	0.6
pitted, approx 3 oz	10 fruits	201	52.7	0.4
pitted, cooked, stewed, sweetened	4 oz	141	37.3	0.2
pitted, cooked, stewed, unsweetened	4 oz	121	31.8	0.3
(Del Monte)	2 oz	120	31.0	0.0
(Del Monte) 'Moist Pak'	2 oz	120	30.0	0.0
(Del Monte) pitted	2 oz	140	35.0	0.0
(Dole)	2 oz	140	36.0	1.0
(Mariani) pitted, premium	1/4 cup	140	36.0	0.3
(SunSweet)	2 oz	120	32.0	0.0
(SunSweet) pitted	2 oz	140	36.0	0.0
PRUNE JUICE				
	6 oz	136	33.5	0.1
(Del Monte) 'Unsweetened'	6 oz	120	33.0	0.0
(J. Hungerford) 100% juice	9.03 oz	178	43.9	0.0
(Knudsen & Sons) organic	8 oz	170	42.0	0.0
(Lucky Leaf)	6 oz	150	36.0	0.0
(Mott's)	6 oz	130	32.0	0.0
(Mott's) country style	6 oz	130	32.0	0.0
(Pathmark) 'All Natural'	6 oz	120	30.0	0.0
(Pathmark) w/prune pulp 'Homestyle'	6 oz	130	32.0	0.0
(S&W) 'Unsweetened'	6 oz	120	31.0	0.0
(SunSweet)	6 oz	130	33.0	0.0
PRUNE WHIP				
cold	1 cup	203	48.0	0.3
hot	1 cup	140	33.2	0.2
PUDDING, FROZEN				
butterscotch (Rich's)	3 oz	130	18.0	6.0
chocolate (Rich's)	3 oz	140	18.0	7.0
vanilla (Rich's)	3 oz	130	18.0	6.0
PUDDING, READY-TO-SERVE				
ALMOND (Rice Dream) 'Dream Pudding,' non-dairy, low fat	4 oz	150	31.0	2.0

Food Name	Serv. Size	Total Cal.	Carbs GMS	Fat GMS
BANANA				
(Del Monte) 'Pudding Cup'	5 oz	180	30.0	5.0
(Lucky Leaf)	4 oz	150	24.0	5.0
(Musselman's)	4 oz	150	24.0	5.0
(Rice Dream) 'Dream Pudding,' non-dairy, fat-free	4 oz	120	30.0	0.0
(Snack Pack)	4.25 oz	145	22.0	6.0
(Snack Pack)	4 oz	158	25.0	5.7
BUTTERSCOTCH				
(Crowley)	4.5 oz	150	27.0	3.0
(Del Monte) 'Pudding Cup'	5 oz	180	31.0	5.0
(Featherweight)	1/2 cup	100	21.0	1.0
(Lucky Leaf)	4 oz	170	26.0	7.0
(Musselman's)	4 oz	170	26.0	7.0
(Rice Dream) 'Dream Pudding,' non-dairy, fat-free	4 oz	120	30.0	0.0
(Snack Pack)	4.25 oz	170	27.0	6.0
(Snack Pack)	4 oz	153	23.6	5.7
(Swiss Miss)	4 oz	156	24.1	5.6
(Ultra Slim Fast) 'Lite 'N Tasty'	4 oz	100	21.0	<1.0
(White House)	3.5 oz	113	20.0	3.0
BUTTERSCOTCH-CHOCOLATE-VANILLA SWIRL *(Jell-O)*	4 oz	180	28.0	5.0
CARAMELLO *(Hershey's)*	4 oz	180	28.0	6.0
CAROB *(Rice Dream)* 'Dream Pudding' non-dairy, fat-free	4 oz	130	31.0	0.0
CHOCOLATE				
(Crowley)	4.5 oz	190	29.0	3.0
(Del Monte) 'Pudding Cup'	5 oz	190	31.0	6.0
(Del Monte) 'Pudding Snack Light'	4.25 oz	100	19.0	1.0
(Estee)	1/2 cup	70	12.0	<1.0
(Featherweight)	1/2 cup	100	21.0	1.0
(Hershey's)	4 oz	180	29.0	5.0
(Jell-O) 'Free'	4 oz	100	24.0	0.0
(Jell-O) 'Light Pudding Snacks'	4 oz	100	21.0	2.0
(Jell-O) 'Pudding Snacks'	5.5 oz	230	38.0	8.0
(Jell-O) 'Pudding Snacks'	4 oz	170	28.0	6.0
(Lucky Leaf)	4 oz	180	27.0	7.0
(Musselman's)	4 oz	180	27.0	7.0
(Pathmark) 'No Frills'	5 oz	200	30.0	8.0
(Rice Dream) 'Dream Pudding,' non-dairy, fat-free	4 oz	170	39.0	0.0
(Snack Pack)	4.25 oz	160	28.0	5.0
(Snack Pack)	4 oz	161	24.6	5.9
(Snack Pack) fat-free	4 oz	96	21.2	0.4
(Snack Pack) 'Light'	4 oz	100	20.1	2.0
(Swiss Miss)	4 oz	166	25.8	5.7
(Swiss Miss) fat-free	4 oz	99	22.3	0.4

Food Name	Serv. Size	Total Cal.	Carbs GMS	Fat GMS
(Swiss Miss) 'Light'	4 oz	100	20.1	(mq)
(Swiss Miss) sundae	4 oz	220	36.0	7.0
(White House)	3.5 oz	120	22.0	4.0
CHOCOLATE FUDGE				
(Del Monte) 'Pudding Cup'	5 oz	190	31.0	6.0
(Jell-O) 'Light Pudding Snacks'	4 oz	100	22.0	1.0
(Jell-O) 'Pudding Snacks'	4 oz	170	28.0	6.0
(Lucky Leaf)	4 oz	180	25.0	8.0
(Musselman's)	4 oz	180	25.0	8.0
(Snack Pack)	4.25 oz	165	27.0	6.0
(Snack Pack)	4 oz	158	23.9	5.9
(Swiss Miss)	4 oz	175	27.9	5.6
(Swiss Miss) fat-free	4 oz	103	23.3	0.3
(Swiss Miss) 'Light'	4 oz	100	20.0	1.0
CHOCOLATE FUDGE-MILK CHOCOLATE SWIRL *(Jell-O)*	4 oz	170	28.0	6.0
CHOCOLATE-ALMOND *(Hershey's)*	4 oz	180	29.0	6.0
CHOCOLATE-CARAMEL SWIRL				
(Jell-O) 'Pudding Snacks'	4 oz	170	28.0	6.0
(Snack Pack)	4 oz	165	25.3	5.9
(Snack Pack) 4 pack	4 oz	170	27.0	6.0
(Swiss Miss)	4 oz	165	25.3	5.9
CHOCOLATE-MARSHMALLOW				
(Snack Pack)	4.25 oz	165	26.0	6.0
(Snack Pack)	4 oz	155	23.4	5.9
CHOCOLATE-MINT SWIRL *(Jell-O)* 'Free'	4 oz	100	24.0	0.0
CHOCOLATE-PEANUT BUTTER SWIRL				
(Snack Pack)	4 oz	169	25.7	6.3
(Snack Pack) 4 pack	4 oz	170	26.0	7.0
CHOCOLATE-VANILLA SWIRL				
(Hershey's) 'Kisses'	4 oz	180	29.0	6.0
(Hershey's) 'Kisses Free'	4 oz	100	22.0	0.0
(Jell-O) combo 'Light Pudding Snacks'	4 oz	100	21.0	2.0
(Jell-O) 'Free'	4 oz	100	24.0	0.0
(Jell-O) 'Pudding Snacks'	5.5 oz	240	39.0	8.0
(Jell-O) 'Pudding Snacks'	4 oz	170	28.0	6.0
CHOCOLATE-VANILLA-CHOCOLATE SWIRL *(Swiss Miss)*	4 oz	172	26.6	6.0
COCONUT				
(Rice Dream) 'Dream Pudding,' non-dairy, low fat	4 oz	150	32.0	2.0
LEMON				
(Rice Dream) 'Dream Pudding,' non-dairy, fat-free	4 oz	120	30.0	0.0
(Snack Pack)	4.25 oz	150	30.0	4.0
(Snack Pack)	4 oz	138	28.0	2.8
(White House)	3.5 oz	152	37.0	1.0

Food Name	Serv. Size	Total Cal.	Carbs GMS	Fat GMS
MILK CHOCOLATE				
(Jell-O) 'Pudding Snacks'	4 oz	170	29.0	6.0
(Snack Pack)	4 oz	166	26.4	5.9
(Snack Pack) 4 pack	4 oz	160	26.0	6.0
(Swiss Miss)	4 oz	166	26.4	2.9
MILK CHOCOLATE-CHOCOLATE FUDGE SWIRL (Jell-O)	4 oz	170	28.0	6.0
RICE				
(Crowley)	4.5 oz	125	22.0	2.0
(Lucky Leaf)	4 oz	120	20.0	3.0
(Musselman's)	4 oz	120	20.0	3.0
(White House)	3.5 oz	111	20.0	3.0
S'MORES SWIRL				
(Snack Pack)	4 oz	154	24.7	5.6
(Snack Pack) 4 pack	4 oz	150	25.0	6.0
TAPIOCA				
(Crowley)	4.5 oz	135	27.0	1.0
(Del Monte) 'Pudding Cup'	5 oz	180	30.0	4.0
(Jell-O) 'Pudding Snacks'	4 oz	170	27.0	4.0
(Lucky Leaf)	4 oz	140	20.0	6.0
(Musselman's)	4 oz	140	20.0	6.0
(Snack Pack)	4.25 oz	160	28.0	4.0
(Snack Pack)	4 oz	151	22.9	5.7
(Snack Pack) fat-free	4 oz	94	20.7	0.4
(Snack Pack) 'Light'	4 oz	100	18.1	2.0
(Swiss Miss)	4 oz	138	23.6	3.9
(Swiss Miss) fat-free	4 oz	99	22.0	0.3
(Swiss Miss) 'Light'	4 oz	100	18.1	2.0
(White House)	3.5 oz	131	19.0	6.0
VANILLA				
(Crowley)	4.5 oz	140	26.0	3.0
(Del Monte) 'Pudding Cup'	5 oz	180	32.0	5.0
(Del Monte) 'Pudding Snack Light'	4.25 oz	100	19.0	1.0
(Estee)	1/2 cup	70	12.0	<1.0
(Featherweight)	1/2 cup	100	20.0	2.0
(Jell-O) 'Free'	4 oz	100	23.0	0.0
(Jell-O) 'Light Pudding Snacks'	4 oz	100	20.0	2.0
(Jell-O) 'Pudding Snacks'	5.5 oz	250	38.0	9.0
(Jell-O) 'Pudding Snacks'	4 oz	180	28.0	7.0
(Lucky Leaf)	4 oz	170	25.0	7.0
(Musselman's)	4 oz	170	25.0	7.0
(Pathmark) 'No Frills'	5 oz	200	28.0	8.0
(Snack Pack)	4.25 oz	170	28.0	6.0
(Snack Pack)	4 oz	158	25.0	5.7

Food Name	Serv. Size	Total Cal.	Carbs GMS	Fat GMS
(Snack Pack) fat-free	4 oz	93	20.8	0.4
(Swiss Miss)	4 oz	156	24.1	5.6
(Swiss Miss) fat-free	4 oz	98	22.1	0.4
(Swiss Miss) 'Light'	4 oz	100	18.1	2.0
(Swiss Miss) sundae	4 oz	175	26.5	6.8
(Ultra Slim Fast) 'Lite 'N Tasty'	4 oz	100	21.0	<1.0
(White House)	3.5 oz	111	20.0	3.0
VANILLA-CHOCOLATE SWIRL (Jell-O) 'Pudding Snacks'	4 oz	180	28.0	6.0
PUDDING MIX. See also PUDDING/PIE FILLING MIX.				
BANANA				
(Jell-O) 'Instant' prepared	1/2 cup	160	28.0	4.0
(Jell-O) 'Instant Sugar-free' prepared w/2% milk	1/2 cup	80	11.0	2.0
BANANA CREAM				
(Jell-O) 'Microwave' prepared	1/2 cup	150	25.0	4.0
(Royal) 'Instant' prepared	1/2 cup	180	29.0	5.0
(Royal) prepared	1/2 cup	160	27.0	4.0
BUTTER ALMOND (Royal) toasted 'Instant' prepared	1/2 cup	170	30.0	4.0
BUTTER PECAN (Jell-O) 'Instant' prepared	1/2 cup	170	28.0	5.0
BUTTERSCOTCH				
(D-Zerta) low calorie, prepared w/skim milk	1/2 cup	70	12.0	0.0
(Featherweight) 'Instant' prepared	1/2 cup	100	19.0	0.0
(Featherweight) prepared	1/2 cup	12	3.0	0.0
(Jell-O) 'Instant' prepared	1/2 cup	160	28.0	4.0
(Jell-O) 'Instant Sugar-free' prepared w/2% milk	1/2 cup	90	12.0	2.0
(Jell-O) 'Microwave' prepared	1/2 cup	170	28.0	4.0
(Jell-O) prepared	1/2 cup	170	30.0	4.0
(Royal) 'Instant' prepared	1/2 cup	180	29.0	5.0
(Royal) 'Instant Sugar-free' prepared w/2% milk	1/2 cup	100	16.0	2.0
(Royal) prepared	1/2 cup	160	27.0	4.0
CHOCOLATE				
(D-Zerta) low calorie, prepared w/skim milk	1/2 cup	60	11.0	0.0
(Featherweight) 'Instant' prepared	1/2 cup	110	22.0	0.0
(Featherweight) prepared	1/2 cup	12	3.0	0.0
(Jell-O) 'Cook 'n Serve Sugar-free' prepared w/skim milk	1/2 cup	70	13.0	3.0
(Jell-O) 'Cook 'n Serve Sugar-free' prepared w/2% milk	1/2 cup	90	13.0	3.0
(Jell-O) 'Instant' prepared	1/2 cup	180	31.0	4.0
(Jell-O) 'Instant Sugar-free' prepared w/2% milk	1/2 cup	90	13.0	3.0
(Jell-O) 'Microwave' prepared	1/2 cup	170	28.0	5.0
(Jell-O) prepared	1/2 cup	160	28.0	4.0
(Royal) dark and sweet, prepared	1/2 cup	180	33.0	4.0
(Royal) 'Instant' prepared	1/2 cup	190	35.0	4.0
(Royal) 'Instant Sugar-free' prepared w/2% milk	1/2 cup	110	17.0	3.0
(Royal) prepared	1/2 cup	180	33.0	4.0

Food Name	Serv. Size	Total Cal.	Carbs GMS	Fat GMS
(Weight Watchers) 'Instant' prepared w/skim milk	1/2 cup	90	18.0	1.0
CHOCOLATE FUDGE				
(Jell-O) 'Instant' prepared	1/2 cup	180	31.0	5.0
(Jell-O) 'Instant Sugar-free' prepared w/2% milk	1/2 cup	100	14.0	3.0
(Jell-O) prepared	1/2 cup	160	28.0	4.0
CHOCOLATE-CHOCOLATE CHIP *(Royal)* prepared	1/2 cup	190	35.0	4.0
CHOCOLATE-MINT *(Royal)* 'Instant' prepared	1/2 cup	190	35.0	4.0
COCONUT, TOASTED *(Royal)* 'Instant' prepared	1/2 cup	170	30.0	4.0
COCONUT CREAM *(Jell-O)* 'Instant' prepared	1/2 cup	180	27.0	6.0
EGG				
(Jell-O) custard 'Americana' prepared	1/2 cup	160	23.0	5.0
(Royal) custard, prepared	1/2 cup	150	22.0	5.0
FLAN				
(Jell-O) prepared	1/2 cup	150	26.0	4.0
(Royal) w/caramel sauce, prepared	1/2 cup	150	22.0	5.0
FRENCH VANILLA				
(Jell-O) 'Instant' prepared	1/2 cup	160	28.0	4.0
(Jell-O) prepared	1/2 cup	170	30.0	4.0
KEY LIME *(Royal)* prepared	1/2 cup	160	30.0	3.0
LEMON				
(Featherweight) custard, prepared	1/2 cup	40	8.0	0.0
(French's) prepared	1/2 cup	110	22.0	1.0
(Jell-O) 'Instant' prepared	1/2 cup	170	29.0	4.0
(Royal) 'Instant' prepared	1/2 cup	180	29.0	5.0
(Royal) prepared	1/2 cup	160	30.0	3.0
MILK CHOCOLATE				
(Jell-O) 'Instant' prepared	1/2 cup	180	31.0	5.0
(Jell-O) 'Microwave' prepared	1/2 cup	160	27.0	5.0
(Jell-O) prepared	1/2 cup	160	28.0	4.0
PISTACHIO				
(Jell-O) 'Instant' prepared	1/2 cup	170	28.0	5.0
(Jell-O) 'Instant Sugar-free' prepared w/2% milk	1/2 cup	90	12.0	3.0
(Royal) nut 'Instant' prepared	1/2 cup	170	30.0	4.0
RASPBERRY *(Salada)* pudding and pie glaze, prepared	1/2 cup	130	32.0	0.0
RICE *(Jell-O)* 'Americana' prepared	1/2 cup	170	30.0	4.0
STRAWBERRY *(Salada)* pudding and pie glaze, prepared	1/2 cup	130	32.0	0.0
VANILLA				
(D-Zerta) low calorie, prepared w/skim milk	1/2 cup	70	12.0	0.0
(Featherweight) custard, prepared	1/2 cup	40	8.0	0.0
(Featherweight) 'Instant' prepared	1/2 cup	100	19.0	0.0
(Featherweight) prepared	1/2 cup	12	3.0	0.0
(Jell-O) 'Cook 'n Serve Sugar-free' prepared w/skim milk	1/2 cup	60	11.0	2.0
(Jell-O) 'Cook 'n Serve Sugar-free' prepared w/2% milk	1/2 cup	80	11.0	2.0

Food Name	Serv. Size	Total Cal.	Carbs GMS	Fat GMS
(Jell-O) 'Instant' prepared	1/2 cup	170	29.0	4.0
(Jell-O) 'Instant Sugar-free' prepared w/2% milk	1/2 cup	90	12.0	2.0
(Jell-O) 'Microwave' prepared	1/2 cup	160	26.0	4.0
(Jell-O) prepared	1/2 cup	160	26.0	4.0
(Jell-O) tapioca 'Americana' prepared	1/2 cup	160	27.0	4.0
(Royal) 'Instant' prepared	1/2 cup	180	29.0	5.0
(Royal) 'Instant Sugar-free' prepared w/2% milk	1/2 cup	100	16.0	2.0
(Royal) prepared	1/2 cup	160	27.0	4.0
(Royal) tapioca, prepared	1/2 cup	160	27.0	4.0
PUDDING/PIE FILLING MIX. See also PUDDING MIX.				
BANANA (Jell-O) instant, sugar-free, prepared w/2% milk	1/2 cup	80	11.0	2.0
BANANA CREAM				
(Jell-O) instant, prepared	1/2 cup	160	28.0	4.0
(Jell-O) microwave, prepared	1/2 cup	150	25.0	4.0
(Jell-O) prepared, w/o crust	1/6 pie	100	17.0	3.0
(Royal) dry	1 serving	80	20.0	0.0
(Royal) instant, dry	1 serving	90	22.0	0.0
BUTTER PECAN (Jell-O) instant, prepared	1/2 cup	170	28.0	5.0
BUTTERSCOTCH				
(D-Zerta) reduced calorie, prepared	1/2 cup	70	12.0	0.0
(Jell-O) instant, prepared	1/2 cup	160	28.0	4.0
(Jell-O) instant, sugar-free, prepared w/2% milk	1/2 cup	90	12.0	2.0
(Jell-O) microwave, prepared	1/2 cup	170	28.0	4.0
(Jell-O) prepared	1/2 cup	170	30.0	4.0
(Nabisco) 'My•T•Fine' prepared	1/2 cup	90	22.0	0.0
(Royal) instant, dry	1 serving	90	22.0	0.0
(Royal) prepared	1/2 cup	90	23.0	0.0
CHERRY-VANILLA (Royal) instant, dry	1 serving	90	23.0	0.0
CHOCOLATE				
(D-Zerta) reduced calorie, prepared	1/2 cup	60	11.0	0.0
(Jell-O) instant, prepared	1/2 cup	180	31.0	4.0
(Jell-O) instant, sugar-free, prepared w/2% milk	1/2 cup	90	13.0	3.0
(Jell-O) microwave, prepared	1/2 cup	170	28.0	5.0
(Jell-O) prepared	1/2 cup	160	28.0	4.0
(Jell-O) sugar-free, prepared w/2% milk	1/2 cup	90	13.0	3.0
(Nabisco) 'My•T•Fine' prepared	1/2 cup	100	23.0	0.0
(Royal) dark and sweet, instant, dry	1 serving	110	25.0	0.0
(Royal) dark and sweet, prepared	1/2 cup	90	22.0	0.0
(Royal) instant, dry	1 serving	110	27.0	0.0
(Royal) instant, sugar-free, prepared	1/2 cup	50	11.0	0.0
(Royal) prepared	1/2 cup	90	22.0	0.0
CHOCOLATE FUDGE				
(Jell-O) instant, prepared	1/2 cup	180	31.0	5.0

Food Name	Serv. Size	Total Cal.	Carbs GMS	Fat GMS
(Jell-O) instant, sugar-free, prepared w/2% milk	1/2 cup	100	14.0	3.0
(Jell-O) prepared	1/2 cup	160	28.0	4.0
(Nabisco) 'My•T•Fine' prepared	1/2 cup	100	24.0	0.0
CHOCOLATE-ALMOND				
(Nabisco) 'My•T•Fine' prepared	1/2 cup	100	23.0	1.0
(Royal) instant, prepared	1/2 cup	120	26.0	1.0
CHOCOLATE-CHOCOLATE CHIP *(Royal)* instant, dry	1 serving	110	26.0	1.0
CHOCOLATE-PEANUT BUTTER CHIP *(Royal)* instant, dry	1 serving	110	26.0	1.0
COCONUT, TOASTED *(Royal)* instant, prepared	1/2 cup	100	20.0	2.0
COCONUT CREAM				
(Jell-O) instant, prepared	1/2 cup	180	27.0	6.0
(Jell-O) prepared, w/o crust	1/6 pie	110	16.0	4.0
EGG *(Royal)* custard, prepared	1/2 cup	60	16.0	0.0
FLAN				
(Jell-O) prepared	1/2 cup	150	26.0	4.0
(Royal) caramel custard, prepared	1/2 cup	60	15.0	0.0
FRENCH VANILLA				
(Jell-O) instant, prepared	1/2 cup	160	28.0	4.0
(Jell-O) prepared	1/2 cup	170	30.0	4.0
LEMON				
(Jell-O) instant, prepared	1/2 cup	170	29.0	4.0
(Nabisco) 'My•T•Fine' dry	1 serving	90	22.0	0.0
(Royal) instant, dry	1 serving	90	23.0	0.0
MILK CHOCOLATE				
(Jell-O) instant, prepared	1/2 cup	180	31.0	5.0
(Jell-O) microwave, prepared	1/2 cup	160	27.0	5.0
(Jell-O) prepared	1/2 cup	160	28.0	4.0
PISTACHIO				
(Jell-O) instant, prepared	1/2 cup	170	28.0	5.0
(Jell-O) instant, sugar-free, prepared w/2% milk	1/2 cup	90	12.0	3.0
(Royal) instant, dry	1 serving	90	22.0	1.0
STRAWBERRY *(Royal)* instant, dry	1 serving	100	24.0	0.0
TAPIOCA *(Nabisco)* 'My•T•Fine' dry	1 serving	80	19.0	0.0
VANILLA				
(D-Zerta) reduced calorie, w/aspartame, prepared	1/2 cup	70	12.0	0.0
(Jell-O) instant, prepared	1/2 cup	170	29.0	4.0
(Jell-O) instant, sugar-free, prepared w/2% milk	1/2 cup	90	12.0	2.0
(Jell-O) microwave, prepared	1/2 cup	160	26.0	4.0
(Jell-O) prepared	1/2 cup	160	26.0	4.0
(Jell-O) sugar-free, w/aspartame, prepared w/2% milk	1/2 cup	80	11.0	2.0
(Nabisco) 'My•T•Fine' prepared	1/2 cup	90	22.0	0.0
(Royal) instant, dry	1 serving	90	23.0	0.0
VANILLA-CHOCOLATE CHIP *(Royal)* instant, dry	1 serving	90	22.0	1.0

Food Name	Serv. Size	Total Cal.	Carbs GMS	Fat GMS
PUERTO RICAN CHERRY. See CHERRY, PUERTO RICAN.				
PUFF PASTRY, FROZEN				
sheet *(Pepperidge Farm)*	1/4 sheet	260	22.0	17.0
shell, mini *(Pepperidge Farm)*	1 shell	50	4.0	4.0
shell, patty *(Pepperidge Farm)*	1 shell	210	16.0	15.0
shell, ready to bake	1 shell	259	21.2	17.9
shell, ready to bake	1 oz	156	12.8	10.8
PUMELO. See POMELO.				
PUMPKIN				
boiled, drained	4 oz	23	5.5	0.1
boiled, drained, mashed	1/2 cup	24	6.0	0.1
raw, 1-inch cubes	1/2 cup	15	3.8	0.1
raw, trimmed	1 oz	7	1.8	<.1
raw, untrimmed	1 lb	83	20.6	0.3
PUMPKIN, CANNED				
	1/2 cup	41	9.9	0.3
w/winter squash	4 oz	39	9.2	0.3
(Del Monte)	1/2 cup	35	9.0	0.0
(Libby's)	1/2 cup	42	10.1	0.4
(Libby's) solid pack	1/2 cup	42	10.1	0.4
(Stokely)	1/2 cup	40	10.0	0.0
PUMPKIN FLOWER				
boiled, drained	4 oz	17	3.7	0.1
boiled, drained	1/2 cup	10	2.2	0.1
raw	1 cup	5	1.1	0.0
raw, trimmed	1 oz	4	0.9	<.1
raw, trimmed	1/2 cup	3	0.5	<.1
raw, untrimmed	1 lb	23	5.2	0.1
PUMPKIN LEAF				
boiled, drained	4 oz	24	3.8	0.2
boiled, drained	1/2 cup	7	1.2	0.1
raw	1/2 cup	4	0.5	0.1
raw, trimmed	1 oz	5	0.7	0.1
raw, untrimmed	1 lb	36	4.3	0.7
PUMPKIN PIE SPICE				
dried	1 tbsp	19	3.9	0.7
dried	1 tsp	6	1.2	0.2
PUMPKIN SEED				
dried	1 lb	1817	59.8	153.9
roasted	1 lb	2021	243.8	88.0
roasted	1 cup	285	34.4	12.4
roasted, approx 85 seeds	1 oz	127	15.3	5.5
w/squash seeds, roasted	1 cup	285	34.4	12.4

Food Name	Serv. Size	Total Cal.	Carbs GMS	Fat GMS
w/squash seeds, roasted	1 oz	127	15.3	5.5
PUMPKIN SEED, SHELLED				
dried	1 cup	747	24.6	63.3
dried, approx 142 kernels	1 oz	154	5.1	13.0
roasted	1 cup	1184	30.5	95.6
roasted	1 oz	148	3.8	12.0
w/squash seed kernels, dried	1 cup	747	24.6	63.3
w/squash seed kernels, dried, approx 142 kernels	1 oz	154	5.1	13.0
w/squash seed kernels, roasted	1 cup	1185	30.5	95.6
w/squash seed kernels, roasted	1 oz	149	3.8	12.0
PUNCH. See also FRUIT PUNCH; and individual listings.				
(J. Hungerford)	9.03 oz	133	33.4	0.0
(Squeezit) 'Mean Green Puncher'	6.75 oz	100	25.0	0.0
(Squeezit) 'Rockin Red Puncher'	6.75 oz	110	28.0	0.0
PURPLESAURUS REX DRINK MIX				
(Kool-Aid) sugar-free, w/NutraSweet, prepared	8 oz	4	0.0	0.0
(Kool-Aid) sugar-sweetened, prepared	8 oz	80	21.0	0.0
(Kool-Aid) unsweetened, prepared w/sugar	8 oz	100	25.0	0.0
(Kool-Aid) unsweetened, prepared w/o sugar	8 oz	2	0.0	0.0
PURSLANE/pussley				
boiled, drained	4 oz	20	4.0	0.2
boiled, drained	1/2 cup	10	2.1	0.1
raw	1 cup	7	1.5	0.0
raw, trimmed	1 oz	5	1.0	<.1
raw, trimmed	1/2 cup	4	0.7	<.1
raw, untrimmed	1 lb	56	11.8	0.3

Q

Food Name	Serv. Size	Total Cal.	Carbs GMS	Fat GMS
QUAIL/bobwhite				
breast meat only, raw	1 oz	35	0.0	0.8
meat and skin, raw	1 oz	54	0.0	3.4
raw	1 oz	34	0.0	0.9
QUAIL GIBLETS, raw	3.5 oz	176	6.7	6.2
QUICHE				
(Nancy's) Classic French, Monterey jack and swiss,				
w/bacon	1 quiche	520	30.0	37.0
(Nancy's) French baked, broccoli, cheddar	1 quiche	490	33.0	33.0
QUINCE				
raw, trimmed	1 med	52	14.1	0.1
raw, trimmed	1 oz	16	4.3	<.1

Food Name	Serv. Size	Total Cal.	Carbs GMS	Fat GMS
raw, untrimmed	1 lb	158	42.3	0.3
QUINOA, WHOLE GRAIN				
dry	1/2 cup	318	58.6	4.9
dry	1 oz	106	19.5	1.6
dry *(Ancient Harvest)*	1/4 cup	159	28.0	2.0
dry *(Eden Foods)*	2 oz	200	38.0	4.0
dry *(Quinoa)*	1/4 cup	159	28.0	2.0
steam-rolled, flakes *(Ancient Harvest)*	1/3 cup	105	23.0	1.0
steam-rolled, flakes *(Quinoa)*	1/3 cup	105	23.0	1.0
QUINOA FLOUR, WHOLE GRAIN				
non-gluten *(Ancient Harvest)*	1/4 cup	132	24.0	2.0
non-gluten *(Quinoa)*	1/4 cup	132	24.0	2.0
QUINOA PASTA. See PASTA.				
QUINOA SEED *(Arrowhead Mills)*	2 oz	200	35.0	3.0

R

Food Name	Serv. Size	Total Cal.	Carbs GMS	Fat GMS
RABBIT				
Domesticated				
raw	1 lb	617	0.0	25.2
raw	1 oz	38	0.0	1.5
roasted	3 oz	167	0.0	6.8
roasted, diced	1 cup	216	0.0	8.8
stewed	3 oz	175	0.0	7.2
stewed, diced	1 cup	288	0.0	11.8
Wild				
raw	1 lb	517	0.0	10.5
raw	1 oz	32	0.0	0.7
stewed	3 oz	147	0.0	3.0
stewed, diced	1 cup	242	0.0	4.9
RACCOON				
roasted	3 oz	217	0.0	12.3
roasted, diced	1 cup	357	0.0	20.3
RADICCHIO				
raw	1 med	2	0.4	0.0
raw, shredded	1/2 cup	5	0.9	0.1
RADISH				
fresh *(Dole)*	7 med	20	3.0	0.0
raw, sliced	1/2 cup	10	2.1	0.3
raw, 1 inch long, 3/4-inch diam	10 radishes	8	1.6	0.2
raw, trimmed	1 oz	5	1.0	0.2

Food Name	Serv. Size	Total Cal.	Carbs GMS	Fat GMS
raw, untrimmed	1 lb	68	14.6	2.2
RADISH, BLACK/winter radish				
raw, trimmed	1 lb	77	16.3	0.5
raw, trimmed	1 oz	5	1.0	<.1
RADISH, ORIENTAL. See DAIKON.				
RADISH, WHITE ICICLE				
raw	1 med	2	0.5	0.0
raw, sliced	1/2 cup	7	1.3	0.1
raw, trimmed	1 oz	4	0.7	<.1
raw, untrimmed	1 lb	41	7.7	0.3
RADISH, WINTER. See RADISH, BLACK.				
RADISH LEAVES, trimmed	1 oz	15	2.8	0.1
RADISH SEED				
sprouted	1 lb	186	13.9	11.5
sprouted	1 oz	12	0.9	0.7
sprouted, raw	1/2 cup	8	0.7	0.5
RAG GOURD. See GOURD, DISHCLOTH.				
RAINBOW PUNCH (Kool-Aid) 'Koolers'	8.45 oz	130	36.0	0.0
RAINBOW PUNCH MIX				
(Kool-Aid) sugar-sweetened	8 oz	80	21.0	0.0
(Kool-Aid) unsweetened, prepared w/sugar	8 oz	100	25.0	0.0
(Kool-Aid) unsweetened, prepared w/o sugar	8 oz	2	0.0	0.0
RAINBOW SMELT. See SMELT, RAINBOW.				
RAISIN				
Dark				
seedless	1 cup packed	495	130.6	0.8
seedless	1 cup	435	114.7	0.7
seedless	1 oz	85	22.4	0.1
seedless (Cinderella) Thompson	1/2 cup	250	66.0	0.0
seedless (Dole)	1/2 cup	260	63.0	0.0
seedless (Finast)	.5 oz	45	11.0	0.0
seedless (Sun•Maid)	1/2 cup	290	69.0	0.0
seedless (Sun•Maid) California sun-dried, 100% natural	1/2 cup	250	68.0	0.0
w/seeds	1 cup packed	488	129.5	0.9
w/seeds	1 cup	429	113.8	0.8
w/seeds	1 oz	84	22.2	0.2
w/seeds (Sun•Maid) Muscat	1/2 cup	270	67.0	1.0
Golden				
seedless	1 lb	1368	360.7	2.1
seedless	1 cup packed	498	131.2	0.8
seedless	1 cup	438	115.3	0.7
seedless	1 oz	86	22.5	0.1
seedless (Del Monte) natural	3 oz	250	68.0	0.0

Food Name	Serv. Size	Total Cal.	Carbs GMS	Fat GMS
seedless *(Dole)*	1/2 cup	260	63.0	0.0
w/seed *(Del Monte)*	3 oz	260	68.0	0.0
w/seed *(Dole)*	1/2 cup	250	66.0	0.0
w/seed *(Sun•Maid)* California	1/2 cup	250	68.0	0.0
RASPBERRY/bramble				
trimmed	1 pint	153	36.1	1.7
trimmed	1 cup	60	14.2	0.7
trimmed	1 oz	14	3.3	0.2
untrimmed	1 lb	215	50.4	2.4
untrimmed	1 pint	154	36.1	1.7
Canned				
red, in heavy syrup	4 oz	103	26.5	0.1
red, in heavy syrup, solid and liquid	1/2 cup	116	29.9	0.2
Frozen				
red, in light syrup *(Birds Eye)* 'Quick Thaw Pouch'	5 oz	100	25.0	1.0
red, sweetened, unthawed	10 oz	293	74.3	0.5
red, sweetened, unthawed	1 cup	258	65.4	0.4
sweetened	10 oz	291	74.3	0.5
sweetened	1/2 cup	128	32.7	0.2
sweetened	4 oz	117	29.7	0.2
RASPBERRY DRINK, W/CRANBERRY				
(A&P)	6 oz	110	27.0	<1.0
(Finast)	6 oz	110	27.0	0.0
(Pathmark)	6 oz	110	27.0	0.0
(Pathmark) 'Sodium Free'	6 oz	110	27.0	0.0
RASPBERRY JUICE				
(Apple & Eve) w/cranberry	6 oz	90	21.0	0.0
(Dole) blend 'Pure & Light Country Raspberry'	6 oz	87	24.0	0.2
(Santa Cruz Natural) red, organic	8 oz	120	28.0	<1.0
(Smucker's) red 'Naturally 100%'	8 oz	120	30.0	0.0
RASPBERRY JUICE COCKTAIL				
(Welch's) 'Orchard,' bottled	10 oz	160	40.0	0.0
RASPBERRY JUICE FLOAT *(Knudsen & Sons)*	8 oz	130	31.0	0.0
RASPBERRY LEMONADE				
(Knudsen & Sons)	8 oz	110	28.0	0.0
(Santa Cruz Natural) organic	8 oz	60	20.0	<1.0
(Santa Cruz Natural) 'Sparkling' organic	8 oz	85	20.0	<1.0
RASPBERRY NECTAR *(Knudsen & Sons)*	8 oz	120	30.0	0.0
RASPBERRY PUNCH MIX				
(Kool-Aid) sugar-sweetened, prepared	8 oz	80	20.0	0.0
(Kool-Aid) unsweetened, prepared w/sugar	8 oz	100	25.0	0.0
(Kool-Aid) unsweetened, prepared w/o sugar	8 oz	2	0.0	0.0
RASPBERRY SYRUP *(Knudsen & Sons)*	1 oz	75	18.0	<1.0

Food Name	Serv. Size	Total Cal.	Carbs GMS	Fat GMS
RASPBERRY TOPPING, fat-free *(Smucker's)* 'Light'	2 tbsp	55	14.0	0.0
RASPBERRY-PEACH JUICE *(Knudsen & Sons)*	8 oz	115	28.0	0.0
RAVIOLI ENTRÉE				
CANNED				
Beef				
(Chef Boyardee) 'Sir Chomps'	7.5 oz	170	32.0	3.0
(Chef Boyardee) w/meat sauce 'Smurfs'	7.5 oz	230	38.0	5.0
(Estee)	7.5 oz	230	25.0	11.0
(Finast) w/sauce	7.5 oz	250	33.0	10.0
(Franco-American) w/meat sauce 'RavioliO's'	7.5 oz	250	35.0	8.0
(Nalley's)	7.5 oz	180	30.0	3.0
(Pathmark) bite size, w/tomato sauce 'No Frills'	7.5 oz	180	28.0	4.0
(Pathmark) w/tomato sauce 'No Frills'	7.5 oz	180	28.0	4.0
Cheese				
(Buitoni) w/sauce	7.5 oz	190	27.0	6.0
(Chef Boyardee) 'Sir Chomps'	7.5 oz	170	38.0	1.0
(Pathmark) w/tomato sauce 'No Frills'	7.5 oz	185	27.0	6.0
Chicken				
(Buitoni) meat, w/sauce	7.5 oz	180	28.0	4.0
(Chef Boyardee)	7.5 oz	180	29.0	4.0
(Chef Boyardee) mini	7.5 oz	220	29.0	8.0
FROZEN				
(Celentano)	6.5 oz	380	50.0	11.0
(Celentano) mini	4 oz	250	39.0	5.0
Cheese				
(Amy's Kitchen) organic	1 cup	215	26.0	5.0
(Buitoni)	4 oz	360	31.0	8.0
(Healthy Choice) baked	9 oz	250	44.0	2.0
(Kid Cuisine) mini	8.75 oz	250	52.0	2.0
(Lean Cuisine) w/tomato sauce	8.5 oz	240	30.0	8.0
(Smart Ones) Florentine	8.5 oz	130	22.0	1.0
(Ultra Slim Fast)	12 oz	330	60.0	3.0
(Weight Watchers) baked	9 oz	240	27.0	6.0
MICROWAVE				
(Kid's Kitchen) mini microwave cup	7.5 oz	230	34.0	6.0
Beef				
(Chef Boyardee)	7.5 oz	190	31.0	4.0
(Chef Boyardee) 'Main Meals' microwave cup	10.5 oz	290	52.0	4.0
(Hormel) w/tomato sauce micro cup	7.5 oz	247	28.0	11.0
(Libby's) w/sauce 'Diner' microwave cup	7.75 oz	240	35.0	5.0
Cheese, w/meat sauce *(Chef Boyardee)*	7.5 oz	200	37.0	3.0
REFRIGERATED				
(Contadina) w/beef 'Fresh'	3 oz	270	30.0	11.0

Food Name	Serv. Size	Total Cal.	Carbs GMS	Fat GMS
(Contadina) w/cheese 'Fresh'	3 oz	270	30.0	11.0
(DiGiorno) w/Italian herb cheese, cooked	1 cup	280	35.0	10.0
(DiGiorno) w/Italian sausage, cooked	1 cup	270	34.0	9.0
RAZZLEBERRY JUICE *(Knudsen & Sons)*	8 oz	90	21.0	0.0
RED BEAN, CANNED				
(A&P)	1/2 cup	120	23.0	<1.0
(Allens)	1/2 cup	115	20.0	<1.0
(Bush's Best)	1/2 cup	70	17.0	0.0
(Green Giant)	1/2 cup	90	19.0	1.0
(Joan of Arc)	1/2 cup	90	19.0	1.0
(Van Camp's)	1 cup	194	38.0	0.6
Small				
(B&M) baked style	8 oz	223	36.0	5.0
(Hunt's)	4.48 oz	89	18.9	0.5
RED CABBAGE. See CABBAGE, RED.				
RED CURRY BASE *(A Taste of Thai)*	1 tbsp	20	1.0	1.5
RED PERCH. See OCEAN PERCH, ATLANTIC.				
REDFISH. See OCEAN PERCH, ATLANTIC.				
REDHEAD. See SHEEPSHEAD.				
REFRIED BEANS, CANNED				
	1/2 cup	135	23.3	1.4
	4 oz	121	21.0	1.2
(Del Monte)	1/2 cup	130	20.0	2.0
(Gebhardt)	4 oz	130	20.0	2.0
(Little Pancho)	1/2 cup	80	15.0	0.0
(Old El Paso)	1/4 cup	55	8.0	<1.0
(Rosarita)	4.5 oz	109	19.8	2.8
NO-FAT *(Rosarita)*	4.5 oz	92	19.5	0.5
ORGANIC				
(Bearitos)	1 oz	30	4.8	0.5
(Bearitos) no salt	1 oz	29	4.7	0.5
(Bearitos) spicy	1 oz	31	4.9	0.6
SPICY				
(Del Monte)	1/2 cup	130	20.0	2.0
(Old El Paso)	1/4 cup	35	5.0	1.0
(Rosarita)	4.5 oz	109	19.9	2.6
VEGETARIAN				
(Old El Paso) spicy	1/4 cup	70	15.0	1.0
(Rosarita)	4.5 oz	118	20.9	2.3
(Rosarita) spicy	4 oz	120	19.0	2.0
(Rosarita) w/canola oil	4 oz	100	18.0	2.0
(Rosarita) w/soybean oil	4 oz	100	18.0	2.0
W/BACON *(Rosarita)*	4.5 oz	116	18.7	3.1

Food Name	Serv. Size	Total Cal.	Carbs GMS	Fat GMS
W/CHEESE *(Old El Paso)*	1/4 cup	36	4.0	1.0
W/GREEN CHILIES				
(Little Pancho)	1/2 cup	80	15.0	0.0
(Old El Paso)	1/4 cup	49	8.0	<1.0
(Rosarita)	4.5 oz	110	19.7	2.9
W/JALAPEÑO *(Gebhardt)*	4.5 oz	106	19.0	3.0
W/NACHO CHEESE *(Rosarita)*	4.5 oz	122	20.6	3.1
W/ONION *(Rosarita)*	4.5 oz	114	20.8	2.8
W/SAUSAGE *(Old El Paso)*	1/4 cup	180	8.0	8.0
REFRIED BEANS, DRIED *(Rosarita)*	1/3 cup	123	20.5	4.5
REFRIED BEANS ENTRÉE *(Chi-Chi's)*	7.5 oz	250	29.0	11.0
REFRIED BEANS MIX				
(Fantastic Foods) instant, prepared w/o added ingredients	1/2 cup	157	28.0	2.0
(Fantastic Foods) instant, prepared w/2 tbsp salted butter	1/2 cup	207	28.0	8.0
RELISH. See also specific listings.				
CHOWCHOW				
sour, w/cauliflower, onion, mustard	1 cup	70	9.8	3.1
sweet, w/cauliflower, onion, mustard	1 cup	284	66.2	2.2
CRANBERRY-ORANGE				
canned	1/2 cup	246	63.8	0.1
canned	4 oz	202	52.4	0.1
DILL *(Vlasic)*	1 oz	2	1.0	0.0
HAMBURGER				
pickle	1/2 cup	157	42.1	0.7
pickle	1 tbsp	19	5.2	0.1
(Heinz)	1 oz	40	9.0	0.0
HOT DOG				
pickle	1/2 cup	111	28.5	0.6
pickle	1 tbsp	14	3.5	0.1
(Heinz)	1 oz	35	8.0	0.0
(Vlasic)	1 oz	40	8.0	1.0
INDIA				
(Heinz)	1 oz	35	9.0	0.0
(Vlasic)	1 oz	30	8.0	0.0
JALAPEÑO *(Old El Paso)*	2 tbsp	16	4.0	0.0
PICCALILLI				
(Claussen)	1 oz	26	5.6	0.3
(Heinz)	1 oz	30	7.0	0.0
(Vlasic) hot	1 oz	35	8.0	0.0
PICKLE				
sweet	1/2 cup	159	42.8	0.6
sweet	1 tbsp	20	5.3	0.1
(Claussen)	1 tbsp	14	2.9	0.2

Food Name	Serv. Size	Total Cal.	Carbs GMS	Fat GMS
SWEET				
. . . .	1 tbsp	21	5.1	0.1
chopped	1 cup	338	83.3	1.5
chopped	1 tbsp	21	5.1	0.1
finely cut	1 cup	338	83.3	1.5
finely cut	1 tbsp	21	5.1	0.1
(Heinz)	1 oz	35	9.0	0.0
(Vlasic)	1 oz	30	8.0	0.0
RENNIN, enzyme tablet, unsweetened	1 tablet	1	0.2	0.0
RHUBARB				
frozen	1/2 cup	14	3.5	0.1
frozen	4 oz	24	5.8	0.1
frozen, sweetened, cooked	4 oz	132	35.4	0.1
frozen, sweetened, cooked	1/2 cup	139	37.4	0.1
raw, diced	1/2 cup	13	2.8	0.1
raw, trimmed	1 oz	6	1.3	0.1
raw, untrimmed	1 lb	71	15.4	0.7
RICE, ARBORIO, dry (Colavita)	1 oz	100	22.0	0.0
RICE, BASMATI				
BROWN				
(Arrowhead Mills) long grain, dry	2 oz	200	44.0	1.0
(Fantastic Foods) cooked	1/2 cup	102	22.0	0.5
(Fantastic Foods) cooked, prepared w/1 tbsp salted butter	1/2 cup	115	22.0	2.0
WHITE				
(Fantastic Foods) cooked	1/2 cup	103	23.0	0.0
(Fantastic Foods) cooked, prepared w/1 tbsp salted butter	1/2 cup	116	23.0	1.0
(Texmati) long grain, cooked	1/2 cup	82	31.0	0.0
RICE, BROWN				
(Lundberg Family) cooked	1 cup	232	49.7	1.2
(Minute) instant	1/2 cup	120	25.0	1.0
(Uncle Ben's) precooked, prepared	1/2 cup	90	21.0	1.0
LONG GRAIN				
cooked	1/2 cup	109	22.5	0.9
cooked	4 oz	126	26.0	1.0
cooked (Carolina)	1/2 cup	110	23.0	0.0
cooked (Mahatma)	1/2 cup	110	23.0	0.0
cooked (River)	1/2 cup	110	23.0	0.0
cooked (S&W)	3.5 oz	119	26.0	0.0
cooked (Uncle Ben's)	2/3 cup	130	27.0	1.0
dry	1 oz	105	21.9	0.8
dry	1/2 cup	340	71.1	2.7
dry (Arrowhead Mills)	2 oz	200	44.0	1.0
quick-cooked (S&W)	3.5 oz	110	25.0	0.0

Food Name	Serv. Size	Total Cal.	Carbs GMS	Fat GMS
MEDIUM GRAIN				
cooked	4 oz	127	26.7	0.9
cooked	1/2 cup	110	23.0	0.8
dry	1/2 cup	344	72.4	2.5
dry	1 oz	103	21.6	0.8
dry *(Arrowhead Mills)*	2 oz	200	44.0	1.0
SHORT GRAIN *(Arrowhead Mills)* dry	2 oz	200	44.0	1.0
RICE, GLUTINOUS				
cooked	1/2 cup	116	25.3	0.2
cooked	4 oz	110	23.9	0.2
dry	1/2 cup	120	26.4	0.2
dry	1 oz	105	23.2	0.2
RICE, WHITE				
LONG GRAIN				
cooked	1/2 cup	194	52.3	5.6
cooked	4 oz	111	24.1	0.2
cooked *(Carolina)*	1/2 cup	100	22.0	0.0
cooked *(Finast)*	1/2 cup	115	26.0	0.0
cooked *(Mahatma)*	1/2 cup	110	23.0	0.0
cooked *(River)*	1/2 cup	100	22.0	0.0
cooked *(S&W)*	3.5 oz	106	23.0	0.0
cooked *(Uncle Ben's)*	2/3 cup	130	28.0	1.0
cooked *(Water Maid)*	1/2 cup	100	22.0	0.0
raw, enriched	1/2 cup	336	73.6	0.6
raw, unenriched	1 oz	103	22.7	0.2
In cooking bag				
(Minute)	1/2 cup	90	20.0	0.0
(Success) enriched, cooked	1/2 cup	100	21.0	0.0
(Uncle Ben's)	1/2 cup	90	20.0	<1.0
Parboiled				
cooked	1/2 cup	100	21.8	0.2
cooked	4 oz	129	28.0	3.1
enriched, cooked	1/2 cup	100	21.8	0.2
unenriched, dry	1/2 cup	341	75.2	0.5
(Uncle Ben's) 'Converted'	2/3 cup	120	28.0	<1.0
Precooked or instant				
cooked *(Carolina)* 'Instant'	1/2 cup	110	23.0	0.0
cooked *(Minute)* 'Original'	2/3 cup	120	27.0	0.0
cooked *(Minute)* 'Premium'	2/3 cup	120	27.0	0.0
cooked *(Uncle Ben's)*	2/3 cup	120	27.0	<1.0
dry	1/2 cup	182	40.1	0.1
dry	1 oz	107	23.7	0.1
enriched, cooked	1/2 cup	80	17.4	0.1

Food Name	Serv. Size	Total Cal.	Carbs GMS	Fat GMS
MEDIUM GRAIN				
cooked	1/2 cup	345	76.0	0.5
cooked	4 oz	147	32.4	0.2
dry	1 oz	102	22.5	0.2
enriched, dry	1/2 cup	353	77.8	0.6
unenriched, cooked	1/2 cup	133	29.2	0.2
unenriched, dry	1/2 cup	353	77.8	0.6
SHORT GRAIN				
cooked	1/2 cup	333	73.6	0.5
cooked	4 oz	147	32.6	0.2
dry	1/2 cup	130	28.6	0.2
dry	1 oz	101	22.4	0.1
unenriched, cooked	1/2 cup	133	29.3	0.2
unenriched, dry	1/2 cup	358	79.2	0.5
RICE, WILD				
cooked	4 oz	115	24.2	0.4
cooked	1/2 cup	83	17.5	0.3
cooked *(Fantastic Foods)*	1/2 cup	83	18.0	0.0
dry	1/2 cup	286	59.9	0.9
dry	1 oz	101	21.2	0.3
RICE BEVERAGE				
almond 'Amazake' *(Grainaissance)*	8 oz	198	37.0	4.0
apricot 'Amazake' *(Grainaissance)*	8 oz	158	36.0	0.0
carob 'Lite' *(Rice Dream)*	8 oz	150	32.0	3.0
chocolate flavored *(Rice Dream)*	8 oz	190	44.0	3.0
cocoa-almond 'Amazake' *(Grainaissance)*	8 oz	198	36.0	4.0
mocha java 'Amazake' *(Grainaissance)*	8 oz	178	37.0	2.0
original flavor 'Amazake' *(Grainaissance)*	8 oz	148	34.0	0.0
original flavor 'Horchata' *(Don José)*	8 oz	70	6.0	4.0
sesame 'Amazake' *(Grainaissance)*	8 oz	198	37.0	1.0
strawberry 'Horchata' *(Don José)*	8 oz	70	7.0	3.5
vanilla 'Lite' *(Rice Dream)*	8 oz	120	28.0	2.0
vanilla pecan 'Amazake' *(Grainaissance)*	8 oz	198	37.0	4.0
RICE BRAN				
crude	1 oz	90	14.1	5.9
crude	1/3 cup	88	13.9	5.8
RICE BRAN OIL				
	1 cup	1927	0.0	218.0
	1 oz	251	0.0	28.4
	1 tbsp	120	0.0	13.6
(Hain)	1 tbsp	120	0.0	14.0
RICE CAKE				
(Lundberg Family) sodium-free, all flavors	1 cake	60	14.0	0.5

Food Name	Serv. Size	Total Cal.	Carbs GMS	Fat GMS
(Lundberg Family) very low sodium, all flavors	1 cake	60	14.0	0.5
APPLE CINNAMON				
(Hain) mini	1/2 cup	60	12.0	<1.0
(Quaker)	1 cake	40	9.0	0.0
(Quaker) mini	5 cakes	50	12.0	0.0
BARBEQUE *(Hain)* mini	.5 oz	70	10.0	3.0
BROWN RICE				
buckwheat	1 cake	34	7.2	0.3
buckwheat, unsalted	1 cake	35	7.3	0.3
corn	1 cake	35	7.3	0.3
multi-grain	1 cake	35	7.2	0.3
multi-grain, unsalted	1 cake	34	7.2	0.3
plain	1 cake	35	7.3	0.3
rye	1 cake	35	7.2	0.3
sesame seed	1 cake	35	7.3	0.3
sesame seed, unsalted	1 cake	35	7.2	0.3
unsalted	1 cake	34	7.1	0.3
CARAMEL CORN *(Quaker)* mini	5 cakes	50	12.0	0.0
CAROB COATED				
(Carafection) 'Mint Rice Crisps'	1 oz	139	17.0	7.0
(Carafection) 'Rice Crisps'	1 oz	139	17.0	7.0
CHEESE *(Hain)* mini	5 cakes	60	10.0	2.0
CINNAMON				
(Chico-San) sugar, mini	5 cakes	50	12.0	0.0
(Quaker) crunch, fat-free	1 cake	50	11.0	0.0
CORN *(Quaker)*	1 cake	35	7.4	0.2
DILL *(Lundberg Family)* creamy, mini	5 cakes	60	13.0	<1.0
FIVE-GRAIN *(Hain)*	1 cake	40	8.0	<1.0
HONEY NUT				
(Chico-San) unglazed, mini	4 cakes	60	2.0	1.0
(Hain) mini	.5 oz	60	11.0	<1.0
MUGWORT *(Grainaissance)* bake & serve 'Mochi'	2 oz	140	29.0	1.3
MULTI-GRAIN				
(Chico-San) very low sodium	1 cake	35	8.0	0.0
(Pritikin) sodium-free	1 cake	35	7.0	0.0
(Pritikin) very low sodium	1 cake	35	7.0	0.0
(Quaker)	.32 oz	34	6.9	0.4
NACHO CHEESE				
(Hain) mini	.5 oz	70	10.0	2.0
(Lundberg Family) mini	5 cakes	57	13.0	<1.0
PLAIN				
(Chico-San) original	1 cake	35	8.0	0.0
(Grainaissance) organic bake & serve 'Mochi'	2 oz	140	29.0	1.3

Food Name	Serv. Size	Total Cal.	Carbs GMS	Fat GMS
(Hain)	1 cake	40	8.0	<1.0
(Hain) mini	.5 oz	60	12.0	<1.0
(Hain) mini, unsalted	.5 oz	60	12.0	<1.0
(Hain) unsalted	1 cake	40	8.0	<1.0
(Konriko) 'Original Unsalted'	1 cake	30	7.0	0.0
(Pritikin) sodium-free	1 cake	35	7.0	0.0
(Pritikin) very low sodium	1 cake	35	7.0	0.0
(Quaker)	.32 oz	35	7.1	0.3
(Quaker) lightly salted	1 cake	35	7.0	0.0
(Quaker) unsalted	.32 oz	35	7.2	0.3
RAISIN-CINNAMON *(Grainaissance)* bake & serve 'Mochi'	2 oz	143	30.0	1.2
RANCH				
(Hain) mini	.5 oz	70	9.0	3.0
(Quaker)	1 cake	35	6.5	0.3
SESAME				
(Chico-San) original	1 cake	35	8.0	0.0
(Hain)	1 cake	40	8.0	<1.0
(Hain) unsalted	1 cake	40	8.0	<1.0
(Pritikin) sodium-free	1 cake	35	7.0	0.0
(Pritikin) very low sodium	1 cake	35	7.0	0.0
(Quaker)	.32 oz	35	7.1	0.3
(Westbrae) 'Double Sesame'	.28 oz	30	6.0	<1.0
SESAME-GARLIC				
(Grainaissance) bake & serve 'Mochi'	2 oz	143	28.0	1.9
(Westbrae)	.28 oz	30	6.0	<1.0
TERIYAKI				
(Hain) mini	.5 oz	50	12.0	<1.0
(Westbrae)	.28 oz	30	6.0	<1.0
WHEAT *(Quaker)*	1 cake	34	6.7	0.3
RICE DISH				
CANNED				
Fried *(LaChoy)*	4.903 oz	236	53.4	1.1
Spanish				
(Featherweight)	7.5 oz	140	30.0	0.0
(Heinz)	7.25 oz	150	26.0	5.0
(Old El Paso)	1/2 cup	70	15.0	1.0
(Van Camp's)	1 cup	160	27.0	4.0
FREEZE-DRIED, w/chicken, *(Mountain House)*	1 cup	400	41.0	13.0
FROZEN				
Country style *(Birds Eye)* 'International Rice Recipes'	3.3 oz	90	19.0	0.0
Florentine *(Green Giant)* 'Rice Originals'	1/2 cup	140	22.0	4.0
French style *(Birds Eye)* 'International Rice Recipes'	3.3 oz	110	23.0	0.0

Food Name	Serv. Size	Total Cal.	Carbs GMS	Fat GMS
Fried				
w/chicken *(Chun King)*	8 oz	260	41.0	4.0
w/pork *(Chun King)*	8 oz	270	44.0	6.0
Medley *(Green Giant)* 'Rice Originals'	1/2 cup	100	19.0	1.0
Mexican style, w/chicken *(Lean Cuisine)* 'Lunch Express'	9 1/8 oz	270	43.0	5.0
Oriental, w/vegetables *(Budget Gourmet)* 'Side Dish'	5.75 oz	210	27.0	10.0
Pilaf				
'Rice Originals' *(Green Giant)*	1/2 cup	110	21.0	1.0
w/green beans *(Budget Gourmet)* 'Side Dish'	5.5 oz	240	35.0	9.0
Spanish style *(Birds Eye)* 'International Rice Recipes'	3.3 oz	110	24.0	0.0
White and wild *(Green Giant)* 'Rice Originals'	1/2 cup	130	24.0	2.0
Wild, w/sherry *(Green Giant)* 'Microwave Garden Gourmet'	1 pkg	210	40.0	4.0
W/broccoli				
au gratin *(Birds Eye)* 'For One'	5.75 oz	180	27.0	6.0
in cheese flavored sauce *(Green Giant)*	1/2 cup	120	18.0	4.0
in cheese sauce *(Green Giant)* 'One Serving'	5.5 oz	180	25.0	6.0
'Rice Originals' *(Green Giant)*	1/2 cup	120	18.0	4.0
W/peas and mushrooms in sauce, *(Green Giant)* 'One Serving'	5.5 oz	130	27.0	2.0
W/spinach in cheese sauce *(Green Giant)* 'Italian Blend'	1/2 cup	140	22.0	4.0
RICE DISH MIX				
(Arrowhead Mills)	2 oz	200	43.0	1.0
ALFREDO *(Country Inn)* prepared	1/2 cup	140	23.0	4.0
AMANDINE *(Hain)* '3-Grain Goodness' prepared	1/2 cup	130	17.0	5.0
BEEF BROCCOLI				
(Rice-A-Roni) 'Rice & Sauce'	1/4 pkg	120	24.0	0.0
(Rice-A-Roni) 'Rice & Sauce' prepared	1/2 cup	140	24.0	3.0
BEEF FLAVOR				
(Finast) dry mix	1.3 oz	130	26.0	1.0
(Lipton) 'Rice and Sauce' dry mix	1/2 pkg	120	26.0	<1.0
(Lipton) 'Rice and Sauce' prepared w/1 tbsp butter	1/2 cup	150	26.0	3.0
(Mahatma) prepared	1/2 cup	100	20.0	0.0
(Minute) microwave, family size, dry mix	1 pkg	140	28.0	0.0
(Minute) microwave, family size, prepared w/salted butter	1/2 cup	160	28.0	3.0
(Minute) microwave, single size, dry mix	1 pkg	140	28.0	0.0
(Minute) microwave, single size, prepared w/salted butter	1/2 cup	150	28.0	2.0
(Rice-A-Roni) dry mix	1.13 oz	110	24.0	1.0
(Rice-A-Roni) prepared	1/2 cup	140	24.0	4.0
(Success) prepared	1/2 cup	100	19.0	0.0
W/mushrooms				
(Rice-A-Roni) dry mix	1.27 oz	120	26.0	<1.0
(Rice-A-Roni) prepared	1/2 cup	150	26.0	3.0
W/vermicelli *(Make-It-Easy)* dry mix	1.3 oz	130	28.0	1.0

Food Name	Serv. Size	Total Cal.	Carbs GMS	Fat GMS
BROWN AND WILD				
(Success) prepared	1/2 cup	120	23.0	0.0
(Uncle Ben's) prepared	1/2 cup	130	27.0	1.0
Herb (Arrowhead Mills) 'Quick'	2 oz	140	28.0	1.0
Spanish style (Arrowhead Mills) 'Quick'	2 oz	150	30.0	1.0
Vegetable herb (Arrowhead Mills) 'Quick'	2 oz	150	30.0	1.0
W/mushrooms (Uncle Ben's) prepared	1/2 cup	130	27.0	1.0
CAJUN				
(Lipton) 'Rice and Sauce' dry mix	1/4 pkg	120	26.0	<1.0
(Lipton) 'Rice and Sauce' prepared w/1 tbsp butter	1/2 cup	150	26.0	3.0
CHICKEN FLAVOR				
(Finast) dry mix	1.6 oz	160	31.0	2.0
(Lipton) 'Rice and Sauce' dry mix	1/4 pkg	130	25.0	1.0
(Lipton) 'Rice and Sauce' prepared w/1 tbsp butter	1/2 cup	150	25.0	4.0
(Mahatma) prepared	1/2 cup	100	20.0	0.0
(Minute) microwave, family size, dry mix	1 pkg	130	27.0	1.0
(Minute) microwave, family size prepared w/salted butter	1/2 cup	160	27.0	4.0
(Minute) microwave, single size, dry mix	1 pkg	130	27.0	1.0
(Minute) microwave, single size, prepared w/salted butter	1/2 cup	150	27.0	3.0
(Rice-A-Roni) dry mix	1.13 oz	110	24.0	1.0
(Rice-A-Roni) prepared	1/2 cup	150	24.0	4.0
(Success) prepared	1/2 cup	110	18.0	2.0
Florentine				
(Rice-A-Roni) 'Savory Classics' dry mix	1.12 oz	108	21.7	0.8
(Rice-A-Roni) 'Savory Classics' prepared	1/2 cup	130	22.0	4.0
Honey-lemon, w/broccoli (Suzi Wan) prepared	7.5 oz	370	45.0	11.0
W/broccoli				
(Rice-A-Roni) dry mix	1.23 oz	120	25.0	1.0
(Rice-A-Roni) prepared	1/2 cup	150	25.0	3.0
(Suzi Wan) prepared	1/2 cup	120	23.0	1.0
W/creamy mushroom (Country Inn) prepared	1/2 cup	140	25.0	3.0
W/homestyle vegetables (Country Inn) prepared	1/2 cup	140	25.0	3.0
W/mushroom				
(Country Inn) 'Mushroom Royale' prepared	1/2 cup	120	25.0	1.0
(Rice-A-Roni) dry mix	1.17 oz	130	26.0	1.0
(Rice-A-Roni) prepared	1/2 cup	180	26.0	7.0
W/mushroom stock (Country Inn) prepared	1/2 cup	130	25.0	1.0
W/vegetables				
(Rice-A-Roni) dry mix	1.2 oz	120	25.0	<1.0
(Rice-A-Roni) prepared	1/2 cup	140	25.0	3.0
(Suzi Wan) prepared	1/2 cup	120	24.0	1.0
W/vegetables and vermicelli (Make-It-Easy) dry mix	1.3 oz	130	28.0	1.0

Food Name	Serv. Size	Total Cal.	Carbs GMS	Fat GMS
DRUMSTICK				
(Minute) dry mix	1 pkg	120	25.0	0.0
(Minute) prepared w/salted butter	1/2 cup	150	25.0	4.0
FLORENTINE (Country Inn) prepared	1/2 cup	140	24.0	3.0
FRIED				
(Minute) dry mix	1 pkg	120	25.0	0.0
(Minute) prepared w/oil, w/o salt or butter	1/2 cup	160	25.0	5.0
(Rice-A-Roni) dry mix	1 oz	110	21.0	1.0
(Rice-A-Roni) prepared	1/2 cup	110	21.0	5.0
W/almonds				
(Rice-A-Roni) '1/2 less salt' dry mix	1/5 pkg	120	26.0	1.0
(Rice-A-Roni) '1/2 less salt' prepared	1/2 cup	130	26.0	2.0
JASMINE, soft (A Taste of Thai)	1/4 cup	160	36.0	0.0
HERB				
And butter				
(Lipton) 'Rice and Sauce' prepared w/1 tbsp butter	1/2 cup	150	24.0	5.0
(Rice-A-Roni) dry mix	1 oz	110	22.0	1.0
(Rice-A-Roni) prepared	1/2 cup	130	22.0	4.0
Au gratin				
(Country Inn) prepared	1/2 cup	140	25.0	3.0
(Success) prepared	1/2 cup	100	20.0	0.0
Wild rice and herbs (Arrowhead Mills)	1/4 pkg	140	28.0	1.0
LONG GRAIN AND WILD				
(Lipton) 'Rice and Sauce Original' dry mix	1/4 pkg	120	26.0	<1.0
(Lipton) 'Rice and Sauce Original' prepared w/1 tbsp butter	1/2 cup	150	26.0	3.0
(Mahatma) prepared	1/2 cup	100	20.0	0.0
(Minute) dry mix	1 pkg	120	25.0	0.0
(Minute) prepared w/salted butter	1/2 cup	150	25.0	4.0
(Minute) prepared w/o salt or butter	2/3 cup	120	27.0	0.0
(Near East) prepared	1/2 cup	130	21.0	4.0
(Rice-A-Roni) 'Original' dry mix	1.1 oz	110	23.0	0.0
(Rice-A-Roni) 'Original' prepared	1/2 cup	130	23.0	3.0
(Uncle Ben's) 'Fast Cooking' prepared	1/2 cup	100	21.0	<1.0
(Uncle Ben's) 'Fast Cooking' prepared w/salt and butter	1/2 cup	130	21.0	4.0
(Uncle Ben's) 'Original' prepared w/salt and butter	1/2 cup	120	22.0	2.0
(Uncle Ben's) 'Original' prepared w/o salt or butter	1/2 cup	100	22.0	<1.0
Mexican (Old El Paso) prepared	1/2 cup	140	28.0	2.0
Pilaf				
(Rice-A-Roni) dry mix	1 oz	100	23.0	0.0
(Rice-A-Roni) prepared	1/2 cup	130	23.0	3.0
W/chicken and almonds				
(Rice-A-Roni) dry mix	1.2 oz	120	23.0	1.0

Food Name	Serv. Size	Total Cal.	Carbs GMS	Fa GM
(Rice-A-Roni) prepared	1/2 cup	140	24.0	4.
W/chicken sauce				
(Uncle Ben's) prepared w/salt and butter	1/2 cup	160	27.0	5.
(Uncle Ben's) prepared w/o salt or butter	1/2 cup	140	27.0	2.
ORIENTAL				
(Hain) '3-Grain Goodness' prepared	1/2 cup	120	15.0	5.
(Lipton) dry mix	1/4 pkg	120	26.0	<1.
(Lipton) prepared w/1 tbsp butter	1/2 cup	150	26.0	3.
PILAF				
(Casbah) dry mix	1 oz	90	20.0	0.
(Casbah) prepared	1/2 cup	90	20.0	0.
(Lipton) 'Rice and Sauce'	1/4 pkg	120	25.0	<1.
(Lipton) 'Rice and Sauce' prepared w/1 tbsp margarine	1/2 cup	140	25.0	3.
(Lipton) 'Rice and Sauce' prepared w/2 tbsp butter	1/2 cup	170	25.0	6.
(Near East) prepared	1/2 cup	140	21.0	5.
(Rice-A-Roni) dry mix	1.2 oz	120	25.0	0.
(Rice-A-Roni) prepared	1/2 cup	150	25.0	4.
(Success) prepared	1/2 cup	120	24.0	0.
Beef flavored *(Near East)* prepared	1/2 cup	140	21.0	5.
Brown rice				
(Quick Pilaf) Spanish, prepared w/o salt or butter	1/2 cup	98	21.0	0.
(Quick Pilaf) Spanish, prepared w/2 tbsp salted butter	1/2 cup	136	21.0	5.
(Quick Pilaf) w/miso, prepared w/o salt or butter	1/2 cup	105	21.0	1.
(Quick Pilaf) w/miso, prepared w/2 tbsp salted butter	1/2 cup	145	21.0	5.5
Chicken flavored *(Near East)* prepared	1/2 cup	140	21.0	5.
French				
(Minute) microwave, family size, dry mix	1 pkg	110	24.0	0.
(Minute) microwave, family size, prepared w/salted butter	1/2 cup	130	24.0	3.0
(Minute) microwave, single size, dry mix	1 pkg	110	24.0	0.
(Minute) microwave, single size, prepared w/salted butter	1/2 cup	120	24.0	2.
Garden				
(Rice-A-Roni) 'Savory Classics' dry mix	1.12 oz	113	22.9	0.8
(Rice-A-Roni) 'Savory Classics' prepared	1/2 cup	140	23.0	4.
Lentil *(Near East)* prepared	1/2 cup	170	21.0	7.
Nutted				
(Casbah) dry mix	1 oz	160	30.0	2.0
(Casbah) prepared	1/2 cup	160	30.0	2.
Spanish				
(Casbah) dry mix	1 oz	90	20.0	0.
(Casbah) prepared	1/2 cup	90	20.0	0.0
(Country Inn) w/vegetables, prepared	1/2 cup	120	25.0	1.0
Wheat *(Near East)* Spanish, prepared	1/2 cup	150	21.0	6.

Food Name	Serv. Size	Total Cal.	Carbs GMS	Fat GMS
RIB ROAST				
(Minute) dry mix	1 pkg	120	25.0	0.0
(Minute) prepared w/salted butter	1/2 cup	150	25.0	4.0
RISOTTO				
(Rice-A-Roni) dry mix	1.5 oz	160	32.0	1.0
(Rice-A-Roni) prepared	1/2 cup	200	32.0	6.0
Chicken and cheese (Country Inn) prepared	1/2 cup	120	23.0	2.0
SPANISH STYLE				
(Arrowhead Mills) quick, dry mix	1/4 pkg	150	30.0	1.0
(Lipton) 'Rice and Sauce' dry mix	1/4 pkg	120	26.0	<1.0
(Lipton) 'Rice and Sauce' prepared w/1 tbsp butter	1/2 cup	140	26.0	3.0
(Mahatma) prepared	1/2 cup	100	20.0	0.0
(Near East) prepared	1/2 cup	170	24.0	7.0
(Rice-A-Roni) dry mix	.97 oz	110	22.0	1.0
(Rice-A-Roni) prepared	1/2 cup	150	25.0	4.0
STROGANOFF				
(Rice-A-Roni) dry mix	1.35 oz	150	27.0	3.0
(Rice-A-Roni) prepared	1/2 cup	200	27.0	8.0
SWEET AND SOUR				
(Suzi Wan) 'Dinner Recipe' prepared	7.5 oz	220	48.0	1.0
(Suzi Wan) 'Dinner Recipe' prepared w/o butter	1/2 cup	130	28.0	1.0
(Suzi Wan) 'Dinner Recipe' prepared w/o butter or salt	7.5 oz	340	49.0	5.0
TERIYAKI				
(Suzi Wan) 'Dinner Recipe' prepared	7.5 oz	180	39.0	1.0
(Suzi Wan) 'Dinner Recipe' prepared w/o butter	1/2 cup	120	25.0	1.0
(Suzi Wan) 'Dinner Recipe' prepared w/o butter or salt	7.5 oz	360	39.0	12.0
THREE-FLAVOR (Suzi Wan) prepared	1/2 cup	120	24.0	1.0
W/ASPARAGUS				
Au gratin (Country Inn) prepared	1/2 cup	130	22.0	3.0
W/hollandaise sauce				
(Lipton) w/hollandaise sauce 'Rice & Sauce' dry mix	1/4 pkg	120	25.0	1.0
(Lipton) w/hollandaise sauce 'Rice and Sauce' prepared w/butter	1/2 cup	170	25.0	7.0
(Lipton) w/hollandaise sauce 'Rice and Sauce' prepared w/margarine	1/2 cup	150	25.0	4.0
W/BROCCOLI				
Amandine (Country Inn) prepared	1/2 cup	130	23.0	2.0
Au gratin				
(Country Inn) prepared	1/2 cup	130	22.0	3.0
(Rice-A-Roni) 'Savory Classics' dry mix	1.12 oz	129	20.9	3.4
(Rice-A-Roni) 'Savory Classics' prepared	1/2 cup	180	21.0	9.0
Stir-fry				
(Suzi Wan) prepared w/salt and butter	7.5 oz	370	37.0	15.0

Food Name	Serv. Size	Total Cal.	Carbs GMS	Fa GM!
(Suzi Wan) prepared w/o salt or butter	7.5 oz	200	37.0	3.(
W/cheddar cheese				
(Minute) microwave, dry mix	1 pkg	140	26.0	2.(
(Minute) microwave, prepared w/salted butter	1/2 cup	160	26.0	5.(
W/CAULIFLOWER, AU GRATIN				
(Country Inn) prepared	1/2 cup	130	23.0	3.(
(Rice-A-Roni) 'Savory Classics' dry mix	.5 oz	141	22.7	3.(
(Rice-A-Roni) 'Savory Classics' prepared	1/2 cup	170	23.0	7.(
W/CHEESE				
Cheddar				
(Rice-A-Roni) white, w/herbs, prepared	1 cup	130	52.0	5.(
(Rice-A-Roni) zesty 'Savory Classics' dry mix	1.3 oz	151	24.7	3.8
(Rice-A-Roni) zesty 'Savory Classics' prepared	1/2 cup	180	25.0	7.(
Parmesan				
(Rice-A-Roni) creamy, w/herbs 'Savory Classics' dry mix	1.22 oz	145	22.0	4.2
(Rice-A-Roni) creamy, w/herbs 'Savory Classics' prepared	1/2 cup	170	22.0	7.(
(Ultra Slim Fast) w/chicken flavored sauce, prepared	8 oz	240	56.0	1.(
W/GREEN BEANS, AMANDINE				
(Country Inn) casserole, prepared	1/2 cup	120	23.0	2.(
(Rice-A-Roni) 'Savory Classics' dry mix	1.25 oz	152	22.3	4.8
(Rice-A-Roni) 'Savory Classics' prepared	1/2 cup	210	22.0	11.(
W/MUSHROOMS				
(Country Inn) creamy, w/wild rice, prepared	1/2 cup	140	24.0	3.(
(Lipton) 'Rice and Sauce' dry mix	1/4 pkg	120	26.0	<1.(
(Lipton) 'Rice and Sauce' prepared w/1 tbsp butter	1/2 cup	150	26.0	3.(
W/ORIENTAL STYLE SAUCE *(Ultra Slim Fast)* prepared	8 oz	240	58.0	1.(
W/VEGETABLES				
And cheddar				
(Lipton) dry mix	1/4 pkg	130	26.0	2.(
(Lipton) prepared w/1 tbsp margarine	1/2 cup	160	26.0	5.(
(Lipton) prepared w/2 tbsp butter	1/2 cup	180	26.0	7.(
Medley *(Country Inn)* prepared	1/2 cup	140	28.0	1.(
Spring vegetable and cheese				
(Arrowhead Mills) vegetable herb, dry mix	1/4 pkg	150	30.0	1.(
(Rice-A-Roni) 'Savory Classics' dry mix	1.22 oz	141	22.8	3.5
(Rice-A-Roni) 'Savory Classics' prepared	1/2 cup	170	23.0	7.(
YELLOW				
(Mahatma) prepared	1/2 cup	100	21.0	0.(
(Rice-A-Roni) dry mix	1.16 oz	110	25.0	0.(
(Rice-A-Roni) prepared	1/2 cup	140	25.0	4.(
(Success) prepared	1/2 cup	100	21.0	0.(
RICE FLOUR				
brown	1/2 cup	287	60.4	2.2

Food Name	Serv. Size	Total Cal.	Carbs GMS	Fat GMS
brown	1 oz	103	21.7	0.8
brown *(Arrowhead Mills)*	2 oz	200	44.0	1.0
brown *(Featherweight)*	1 cup	500	113.0	1.0
white	1/2 cup	289	63.3	1.1
white	1 oz	104	22.7	0.4
RICE SEASONING *(Lawry's)* Mexican 'Seasoning Blends'	1 pkg	94	17.0	2.0
RICE SYRUP *(Lundberg Family)* organic 'Sweet Dreams'	1 tbsp	42	10.0	<1.0
RIGATONI. See PASTA.				
RIGATONI ENTRÉE				
(Budget Gourmet) w/broccoli and chicken, in cream sauce, frozen	10.8 oz	290	44.0	7.0
(Chef Boyardee) microwave	7.5 oz	210	31.0	6.0
(Chef Boyardee) 'Special Recipe,' canned	7.5 oz	210	33.0	6.0
(Healthy Choice) w/chicken 'Classics' frozen	12.5 oz	360	50.0	4.0
(Healthy Choice) w/meat sauce, frozen	9.5 oz	260	34.0	6.0
(Lean Cuisine) baked w/meat sauce and cheese, frozen	9.75 oz	250	27.0	8.0
(Stouffer's) w/meat sauce, homestyle, frozen	12 oz	400	49.0	13.0
ROAST BEEF ENTRÉE				
(Libby's) canned, w/gravy	6 oz	210	6.5	8.0
(Top Shelf) frozen, tender	10 oz	240	19.0	6.0
ROAST BEEF HASH				
(Armour) canned	7.5 oz	350	20.0	21.0
(Mary Kitchen) canned	7.5 oz	350	18.0	22.0
(Stouffer's) frozen	10 oz	380	16.0	22.0
ROAST BEEF LUNCHEON MEAT. See LUNCHEON MEAT.				
ROAST BEEF SPREAD, CANNED				
(Hormel)	.5 oz	31	0.0	2.0
(Underwood)	2 1/8 oz	140	<1.0	11.0
(Underwood) 'Light'	2 1/8 oz	90	2.0	6.0
(Underwood) mesquite-smoked	2 1/8 oz	126	<1.0	11.0
ROCK-A-DILE RED DRINK				
(Kool-Aid) 'Kool Bursts'	6.75 oz	110	30.0	0.0
(Kool-Aid) 'Koolers'	8.45 oz	130	34.0	0.0
ROCK-A-DILE RED DRINK MIX				
(Kool-Aid) sugar-free w/NutraSweet, prepared	8 oz	4	0.0	0.0
(Kool-Aid) sugar-sweetened, prepared	8 oz	70	18.0	0.0
(Kool-Aid) unsweetened, prepared w/sugar	8 oz	100	25.0	0.0
(Kool-Aid) unsweetened, prepared w/o sugar	8 oz	2	0.0	0.0
ROCKET. See ARUGULA.				
ROCKFISH, PACIFIC, MIXED SPECIES				
baked, broiled, or microwaved	4 oz	137	0.0	2.3
baked, broiled, or microwaved	3 oz	103	0.0	1.7
raw	1 lb	427	0.0	7.1

Food Name	Serv. Size	Total Cal.	Carbs GMS	Fa GMS
raw	3 oz	80	0.0	1.3
raw	1 oz	27	0.0	0.4
ROE, MIXED SPECIES				
dry-heat cooked	3 oz	173	1.6	7.0
dry-heat cooked	1 oz	58	0.5	2.3
raw	1 lb	635	6.8	29.1
raw	3 oz	119	1.3	5.5
raw	1 oz	39	0.4	1.8
raw	1 tbsp	22	0.2	1.0
ROLL. See also BREAD; BUN; CROISSANT; ENGLISH MUFFIN.				
BUTTER *(Pillsbury)* 'Butterflake' refrigerated	1 roll	140	20.0	5.0
BUTTERMILK *(Wonder)* brown and serve	1 roll	80	13.0	2.0
CRESCENT				
(Pepperidge Farm) 'Deli Classic'	1 roll	110	13.0	6.0
(Pillsbury) refrigerated	1 roll	100	11.0	6.0
CLUB *(Pepperidge Farm)* 'Deli Classic' brown and serve	1 roll	100	19.0	1.0
DINNER				
egg	1-oz roll	87	14.7	1.8
oat bran	1-oz roll	67	11.4	1.3
rye	1-oz roll	81	15.1	1.0
wheat	1-oz roll	77	13.0	1.8
whole wheat	1-oz roll	75	14.5	1.3
(Arnold) 'Dinner Party' 24 per pkg	1 roll	51	9.4	1.2
(Awrey's)	1 roll	60	11.0	1.0
(Awrey's) 'Black Forest'	1 roll	50	10.0	1.0
(Awrey's) cracked wheat	1 roll	50	10.0	1.0
(Awrey's) crusty	1 roll	70	12.0	1.0
(Awrey's) poppy seed	1 roll	59	11.0	1.0
(Awrey's) sesame seed	1 roll	60	11.0	1.0
(Home Pride) wheat	1 roll	70	12.0	1.0
(Home Pride) white	1 roll	80	14.0	2.0
(Pepperidge Farm) country style 'Classic'	1 roll	50	9.0	1.0
(Pepperidge Farm) 'Old Fashioned'	1 roll	50	7.0	2.0
(Pepperidge Farm) 'Party'	1 roll	30	5.0	1.0
(Roman Meal)	1 roll	69	13.0	1.2
(Wonder)	1 roll	80	14.0	1.0
EGG *(Levy's)* 'Old Country Deli'	1-oz roll	146	28.1	2.8
FINGER *(Pepperidge Farm)* w/poppy seeds	1 roll	50	8.0	2.0
49ER				
(Colombo Brand) sour	1.2-oz roll	90	16.4	0.6
(Colombo Brand) sweet	1.2-oz roll	96	15.4	1.8
FRENCH STYLE				
	1 oz	79	14.2	1.2

Food Name	Serv. Size	Total Cal.	Carbs GMS	Fat GMS
(Du Jour) petite, brown and serve	1 roll	230	45.0	2.0
(Francisco) 'International'	1 roll	108	21.3	1.5
(Pepperidge Farm) 'Deli Classic' brown and serve, 3 per pkg	1/2 roll	120	24.0	1.0
(Pepperidge Farm) 'Deli Classic' 9 per pkg	1 roll	100	20.0	1.0
GEM STYLE (Wonder) brown and serve	1 roll	80	13.0	2.0
HARD	1 oz	83	14.9	1.2
HEARTH				
(Brownberry) 'Hearth' assorted	1 roll	124	23.7	2.3
(Pepperidge Farm) 'Hearth' brown and serve	1 roll	50	10.0	1.0
HOAGIE				
(Pepperidge Farm) soft 'Deli Classic'	1 roll	210	34.0	5.0
(Wonder)	1 roll	400	73.0	7.0
ITALIAN (Du Jour) crusty, brown and serve	1 roll	80	16.0	1.0
KAISER				
	1 oz	83	14.9	1.2
(Arnold) 'Francisco'	1 roll	184	35.4	2.9
(Brownberry) 'Hearth'	1 roll	152	29.3	2.8
LUIGI (Colombo Brand) 'Twin Pack'	2-oz roll	146	25.4	1.6
ONION (Levy's) 'Old Country Deli'	1-oz roll	153	30.8	1.9
PAN (Wonder)	1 roll	80	14.0	1.0
PARKER HOUSE				
(Bridgford)	1-oz roll	85	15.8	1.3
(Pepperidge Farm)	1 roll	60	9.0	1.0
POTATO (Pepperidge Farm) 'Hearty Classic'	1 roll	90	14.0	3.0
SANDWICH				
(Arnold) egg 'Dutch'	1 roll	123	21.6	3.3
(Awrey's) oat bran	1 roll	120	22.0	2.0
(Pepperidge Farm) onion, w/poppy seeds	1 roll	150	26.0	3.0
(Pepperidge Farm) potato	1 roll	160	28.0	4.0
(Pepperidge Farm) salad 'Deli Classic'	1 roll	110	16.0	4.0
(Pepperidge Farm) soft 'Family'	1 roll	100	18.0	2.0
(Pepperidge Farm) w/sesame seeds	1 roll	140	23.0	3.0
SOURDOUGH (Pepperidge Farm) French style	1 roll	100	19.0	1.0
STEAK				
(Colombo Brand) sour	2.6-oz roll	200	35.1	2.2
(Colombo Brand) sweet	2.6-oz roll	206	34.2	3.3
TWIST (Pepperidge Farm) golden 'Heat 'n Serve'	1 roll	110	14.0	5.0
ROLL, MIX				
(Dromedary) dry mix	1/8 pkg	209	41.0	2.0
(Dromedary) prepared	2 rolls	239	41.0	5.0
(Krusteaz) prepared	1 roll	150	28.0	3.0
(Pillsbury) prepared	2 rolls	270	25.0	17.0

Food Name	Serv. Size	Total Cal.	Carbs GMS	
(Pillsbury) 'Hot Roll Mix' dry mix	1/16 pkg	100	21.0	0
(Pillsbury) 'Hot Roll Mix' prepared	1 roll	120	21.0	2
ROLL, SWEET. See also BUN, SWEET; DANISH PASTRY.				
APPLE				
(Break Cake) 4.5 oz	2 rolls	380	75.0	5
(Break Cake) multi-pak, 1.4 oz	1 roll	120	24.0	2
APPLE CINNAMON, old fashioned *(Aunt Fanny's)* individual	2 oz	180	34.0	1
CARAMEL NUT *(Aunt Fanny's)* individual	2 oz	190	33.0	6
CHEESE	1 oz	102	12.4	5
CHERRY				
(Break Cake) 4.5 oz	2 rolls	400	79.0	3
(Break Cake) multi-pak, 1.4 oz	1 roll	130	25.0	2
CINNAMON				
(Aunt Fanny's) duos, individual	1.9 oz	180	32.0	5
(Aunt Fanny's) individual	2 oz	190	34.0	5
(Aunt Fanny's) rectangular 11-oz size	2 oz	181	33.0	4
(Awrey's) homestyle	1 roll	240	40.0	7
(Awrey's) swirl 'Grande'	1 roll	340	46.0	16
(Break Cake) 4.5 oz	2 rolls	420	73.0	10
(Break Cake) multi-pak, 1.3 oz	1 roll	120	22.0	3
(Hungry Jack) refrigerated dough w/icing, prepared	2 rolls	290	37.0	14
(Pillsbury) refrigerated dough w/icing, prepared	1 roll	110	17.0	5
CINNAMON NUT *(Break Cake)* 3 oz	2 rolls	330	52.0	11
CINNAMON RAISIN *(Aunt Fanny's)* rectangular 11-oz size	2 oz	181	34.0	3
DIXIE FRUIT ROLL *(Aunt Fanny's)* individual	2 oz	180	34.0	4
PECAN				
(Aunt Fanny's) rectangular 11-oz size	2 oz	184	32.0	4
(Break Cake) multi-pak, 1.3 oz	1 roll	120	22.0	3
RAISIN CINNAMON *(Break Cake)* multi-pak, 1.25 oz	1 roll	120	21.0	3
STRAWBERRY *(Aunt Fanny's)* rectangular 11-oz size	2 oz	190	35.0	4
ROLL, SWEET, FROZEN				
APPLE *(Weight Watchers)* sweet 'Microwave'	1/2 pkg	160	27.0	4
CHEESE *(Weight Watchers)* 'Microwave'	1/2 pkg	180	32.0	4
CINNAMON				
(Pepperidge Farm) 2 per pkg	1 roll	280	34.0	14
(Sara Lee) all butter	2-oz roll	230	31.0	11
(Sara Lee) all butter, w/icing packet	.5-oz pkt	50	12.0	0
(Weight Watchers) glazed	2.1 oz	180	31.0	5
STRAWBERRY *(Weight Watchers)* 'Microwave'	1/2 pkg	170	29.0	5
ROLL DOUGH, FROZEN				
unraised, enriched, 2 x 2 3/8 inches	1 roll	75	13.3	1.
unraised, unenriched, 2 x 2 3/8 inches	1 roll	75	13.3	1
ROMAN BEAN. See CRANBERRY BEAN.				

Food Name	Serv. Size	Total Cal.	Carbs GMS	Fat GMS
ROOT BEER. See SOFT DRINKS AND MIXERS.				
ROOT BEER FLOAT (Skipper's)	1 serving	302	33.0	10.0
ROQUETTE. See ARUGULA.				
ROSE APPLE				
raw	100 gm	25	5.7	0.3
trimmed	1 oz	7	1.6	0.1
untrimmed	1 lb	76	17.3	0.9
ROSE COCO BEAN. See CRANBERRY BEAN.				
ROSEFISH. See OCEAN PERCH, ATLANTIC.				
ROSELLE				
raw, trimmed	1 cup	28	6.4	0.4
trimmed	1 oz	14	3.2	0.2
untrimmed	1 lb	136	31.3	1.8
ROSEMARY				
dried	1 oz	94	18.2	4.3
dried	1 tbsp	11	2.1	0.5
dried	1 tsp	4	0.8	0.2
dried (Durkee)	1 tsp	5	0.0	tr
dried (Laurel Leaf)	1 tsp	5	0.0	tr
dried (Spice Islands)	1 tsp	5	0.8	0.2
ROTINI. See PASTA.				
ROTINI ENTRÉE, FROZEN				
(Green Giant) cheddar 'Microwave Garden Gourmet'	1 pkg	230	32.0	10.0
(Mrs. Paul's) seafood 'Light'	9 oz	240	34.0	6.0
(Weight Watchers) three cheese, w/vegetables	9 oz	270	34.0	8.0
ROTINI ENTRÉE MIX				
(Velveeta) w/cheese and broccoli, dry mix	1/4 box	210	24.0	8.0
(Velveeta) w/cheese and broccoli, prepared	1/2 cup	210	24.0	8.0
RUCULO. See ARUGULA.				
RUGULA. See ARUGULA.				
RUM. See ALCOHOLIC BEVERAGES.				
RUTABAGA				
boiled, drained	4 oz	39	8.8	0.2
boiled, drained, cubed	1/2 cup	33	7.4	0.2
boiled, drained, mashed	1/2 cup	47	10.5	0.3
raw, cubed	1/2 cup	25	5.7	0.1
raw, trimmed	1 oz	10	2.3	0.1
raw, untrimmed	1 lb	140	31.4	0.8
RUTABAGA, CANNED (Allens) diced	1/2 cup	20	4.0	<1.0
RYE				
flakes	1/2 cup	281	58.6	2.1
flakes (Arrowhead Mills)	2 oz	190	42.0	1.0
whole grain	1 cup	567	117.9	4.2

Food Name	Serv. Size	Total Cal.	Carbs GMS	Fat GMS
whole grain	1 oz	95	19.8	0.7
whole grain (Arrowhead Mills)	2 oz	190	42.0	1.0
RYE CAKE (Quaker) 'Grain Cakes'	.32-oz piece	35	6.5	0.3
RYE FLOUR				
dark	1/2 cup	207	44.0	1.7
dark	1 oz	92	19.5	0.8
light	1/2 cup	187	40.9	0.7
light	1 oz	104	22.7	0.4
medium	1/2 cup	181	39.5	0.9
medium	1 oz	100	22.0	0.5
(Arrowhead Mills) whole grain	2 oz	190	39.0	1.0
(Krusteaz)	1 cup	351	73.0	2.0
(Pillsbury) 'Bohemian Style' w/wheat flour	1 cup	400	86.0	1.0
(Pillsbury's Best)	1 cup	400	83.0	2.0
(Robin Hood) stone ground	1 cup	360	86.0	2.0
RYE WHISKEY. See ALCOHOLIC BEVERAGES.				

S

Food Name	Serv. Size	Total Cal.	Carbs GMS	Fat GMS
SABLEFISH/skil				
cooked	3 oz	213	0.0	16.7
raw	1 lb	886	0.0	69.4
raw	3 oz	166	0.0	13.0
raw	1 oz	55	0.0	4.3
raw, approx 6.8 oz	1/2 fillet	376	0.0	29.5
smoked	4 oz	291	0.0	22.8
smoked	3 oz	218	0.0	17.1
SACCHARIN. See SUGAR, ALTERNATIVE.				
SAFFLOWER OIL				
'Hi-Oleic' (Hain)	1 tbsp	120	0.0	14.0
high oleic (Spectrum Naturals)	1 tbsp	120	0.0	14.0
high oleic, unrefined (Spectrum Naturals)	1 tbsp	120	0.0	14.0
linoleic	1/2 cup	964	0.0	109.0
linoleic	1 tbsp	120	0.0	13.6
oleic	1/2 cup	964	0.0	109.0
oleic	1 tbsp	120	0.0	13.6
organic, unrefined (Spectrum Naturals)	1 tbsp	120	0.0	14.0
over 70% oleic	1 cup	1927	0.0	218.0
over 70% oleic	1 tbsp	124	0.0	14.0
SAFFLOWER SEED, dried, kernels	1 oz	147	9.7	10.9
SAFFLOWER SEED MEAL, partially defatted	1 oz	97	13.8	0.7

Food Name	Serv. Size	Total Cal.	Carbs GMS	Fat GMS
SAFFRON				
dried	1 oz	88	18.5	1.7
dried	1 tbsp	7	1.4	0.1
dried	1 tsp	2	0.5	0.0
SAGE				
ground	1 oz	89	17.2	3.6
ground	1 tbsp	6	1.2	0.3
ground	1 tsp	2	0.4	0.1
ground *(Durkee)*	1 tsp	3	0.0	tr
ground *(Laurel Leaf)*	1 tsp	3	0.0	tr
ground *(Spice Islands)*	1 tsp	4	0.6	0.1
SALAD DRESSING				
BACON *(Kraft)* creamy 'Reduced Calorie'	1 tbsp	30	2.0	2.0
BACON AND TOMATO				
(Estee)	1 tbsp	8	1.0	<1.0
(Kraft)	1 tbsp	70	1.0	7.0
(Kraft) 'Reduced Calorie'	1 tbsp	30	2.0	2.0
BLUE CHEESE				
	1 cup	1235	18.1	128.1
	1 tbsp	77	1.1	8.0
(Ayla's Organics) fat free	2 tbsp	30	4.0	0.0
(Estee)	1 tbsp	8	1.0	<1.0
(Featherweight) 'Neu Bleu'	1 tbsp	4	1.0	0.0
(Hidden Valley Ranch) 'Lowfat'	1 tbsp	10	3.0	0.0
(Kraft) chunky	1 tbsp	60	2.0	6.0
(Kraft) chunky 'Reduced Calorie'	1 tbsp	30	2.0	2.0
(Kraft) 'Free'	1 tbsp	16	4.0	0.0
(Lawry's) 'Classic'	1 tbsp	186	1.9	2.0
(Litehouse) country, dressing and dip, refrigerated	1 tbsp	76	0.0	8.0
(Litehouse) 'Lite' dressing and dip, refrigerated	1 tbsp	33	1.0	3.0
(Litehouse) 'Original' dressing and dip, refrigerated	1 tbsp	77	0.0	8.0
(Roka)	1 tbsp	60	1.0	6.0
(Roka) 'Reduced Calorie'	1 tbsp	16	1.0	1.0
(S&W Nutradiet)	1 tbsp	25	2.0	2.0
(Skipper's) premium	1 pouch	222	4.0	23.0
(T. Marzetti)	1 tbsp	90	1.0	9.0
(T. Marzetti) chunky, refrigerated	1 tbsp	78	1.0	8.0
(T. Marzetti) 'Lite' refrigerated	1 tbsp	45	0.0	5.0
(Wish-Bone) chunky	1 tbsp	75	0.7	7.9
(Wish-Bone) chunky 'Lite'	1 tbsp	40	1.5	3.7
(Wish-Bone) chunky, lite 'Food Service'	.5 oz	40	1.0	4.0
(Wish-Bone) 'Healthy Sensation!'	.5 oz	20	4.0	na

Food Name	Serv. Size	Total Cal.	Carbs GMS	Fat GMS
BUTTERMILK				
(Hain) 'Old Fashioned'	1 tbsp	70	(mq)	7.0
(Hollywood) 'Old Fashion'	1 tbsp	75	1.0	8.0
(Kraft) creamy	1 tbsp	80	1.0	8.0
(Kraft) creamy 'Reduced Calorie'	1 tbsp	30	1.0	3.0
(Seven Seas) 'Buttermilk Recipe'	1 tbsp	80	1.0	8.0
(T. Marzetti) and herbs	1 tbsp	95	0.0	10.0
(T. Marzetti) bacon, refrigerated	1 tbsp	93	0.0	10.0
(T. Marzetti) blue cheese, refrigerated	1 tbsp	90	1.0	10.0
CAESAR				
(Estee)	2 tbsp	8	<1.0	<1.0
(Hain) creamy	1 tbsp	60	1.0	6.0
(Hain) creamy 'Low Salt'	1 tbsp	60	1.0	6.0
(Hollywood)	1 tbsp	70	2.0	7.0
(Kraft) golden	1 tbsp	70	1.0	7.0
(Lawry's) 'Classic'	1 tbsp	130	1.0	13.5
(Litehouse) dressing and dip, refrigerated	1 tbsp	57	0.0	6.0
(T. Marzetti)	1 tbsp	80	1.0	8.0
(T. Marzetti) house	1 tbsp	75	<1.0	8.0
(T. Marzetti) refrigerated	1 tbsp	75	0.0	8.0
(Weight Watchers)	1 tbsp	4	1.0	0.0
(Wish-Bone)	1 tbsp	77	0.9	8.0
(Wish-Bone) w/olive oil 'Lite'	.5 oz	30	1.0	3.0
CALIFORNIA FRENCH				
(Catalina) nonfat 'Free'	1 tbsp	16	3.0	0.0
(T. Marzetti)	1 tbsp	90	5.0	6.0
(T. Marzetti) 'Fat-Free'	1 tbsp	16	4.0	0.0
(T. Marzetti) 'Light'	1 tbsp	40	3.0	3.0
CELERY SEED				
(T. Marzetti) and onion	1 tbsp	75	9.0	6.0
(T. Marzetti) refrigerated	1 tbsp	72	5.0	5.0
CHEESE				
(Featherweight)	1 tbsp	20	1.0	2.0
(Hain) vinaigrette	1 tbsp	55	0.0	6.0
(Hollywood)	1 tbsp	80	2.0	8.0
CHINESE VINEGAR				
(Lawry's) w/sesame and ginger 'Classic'	1 tbsp	145	2.4	15.0
CITRUS (Hain) tangy 'Canola'	1 tbsp	50	1.0	5.0
CREAMY				
(Estee)	1 tbsp	4	1.0	0.0
(Hain)	1 tbsp	80	0.0	8.0
(Hain) 'No Salt Added'	1 tbsp	80	1.0	8.0
(Hollywood)	1 tbsp	90	2.0	9.0

Food Name	Serv. Size	Total Cal.	Carbs GMS	Fat GMS
(Kraft) no oil 'Reduced Calorie'	1 tbsp	4	1.0	0.0
(Kraft) 'Reduced Calorie'	1 tbsp	25	1.0	2.0
(Kraft) w/real sour cream	1 tbsp	50	1.0	5.0
(Kraft) zesty	1 tbsp	50	1.0	5.0
(Kraft) zesty 'Reduced Calorie'	1 tbsp	20	1.0	2.0
(Lawry's) w/Parmesan cheese 'Classic'	1 oz	156	4.5	15.1
(Life) egg-free 'All Natural'	1 tbsp	39	2.0	4.0
(Pathmark)	1 tbsp	70	1.0	7.0
(Pathmark) zesty	1 tbsp	70	1.0	8.0
(Pathmark) zesty 'Reduced Calorie'	1 tbsp	6	1.0	0.0
(Rancher's Choice)	1 tbsp	90	1.0	10.0
(Rancher's Choice) 'Reduced Calorie'	1 tbsp	30	1.0	3.0
(S&W Nutradiet)	1 tbsp	10	1.0	1.0
(S&W Nutradiet) no oil	1 tbsp	2	0.0	0.0
(Seven Seas)	1 tbsp	70	1.0	7.0
(Wish-Bone)	1 tbsp	56	1.5	5.5
(Wish-Bone) 'Lite'	1 tbsp	26	2.0	2.0
(Weight Watchers) 'Single Serve' 1 packet	1 tbsp	9	2.0	0.0
CUCUMBER				
(Featherweight) creamy	1 tbsp	4	1.0	0.0
(Hain) dill, creamy	1 tbsp	80	0.0	8.0
(Kraft) creamy	1 tbsp	70	1.0	8.0
(Kraft) creamy 'Reduced Calorie'	1 tbsp	25	1.0	2.0
(Weight Watchers) creamy	1 tbsp	18	4.0	0.0
DIJON				
(Estee) creamy	1 tbsp	8	<1.0	<1.0
(Featherweight) creamy	1 tbsp	20	1.0	2.0
(Great Impressions) mustard	1 tbsp	57	0.3	6.1
(Hain) vinaigrette	1 tbsp	50	0.0	5.0
(Hollywood) vinaigrette	1 tbsp	60	2.0	6.0
(Wish-Bone) vinaigrette 'Classic'	1 tbsp	60	1.0	6.1
(Wish-Bone) vinaigrette 'Lite Classic'	1 tbsp	30	1.1	2.8
DILL				
(Ayla's Organics) creamy, fat free	2 tbsp	15	3.0	0.0
(Nasoya) creamy 'Vegi-Dressing'	1 tbsp	40	1.0	3.0
FRENCH				
(Ayla's Organics) fat free	2 tbsp	10	3.0	0.0
(Catalina)	1 tbsp	60	4.0	5.0
(Catalina) 'Reduced Calorie'	1 tbsp	18	3.0	1.0
(Estee)	1 tbsp	4	1.0	0.0
(Estee) creamy	2 tbsp	10	2.0	0.0
(Featherweight)	1 tbsp	14	3.0	0.0
(Great Impressions) w/green pepper, low calorie	1 tbsp	64	4.1	5.2

Food Name	Serv. Size	Total Cal.	Carbs GMS	Fat GMS
(Hain) creamy	1 tbsp	60	1.0	6.0
(Hain) spicy mustard 'Canola'	1 tbsp	50	1.0	5.0
(Hollywood) creamy	1 tbsp	70	2.0	7.0
(Kraft)	1 tbsp	60	2.0	6.0
(Kraft) 'Miracle'	1 tbsp	70	3.0	6.0
(Kraft) nonfat 'Free'	1 tbsp	20	4.0	0.0
(Kraft) 'Reduced Calorie'	1 tbsp	20	3.0	1.0
(Litehouse) country herb, dressing and marinade, refrigerated	1 tbsp	54	2.0	5.0
(Pathmark) creamy	1 tbsp	60	2.0	6.0
(Pathmark) 'Reduced Calorie'	1 tbsp	20	3.0	1.0
(Pritikin) style, fat-free, sodium-free	1 tbsp	10	3.0	0.0
(S&W Nutradiet)	1 tbsp	18	3.0	0.0
(Seven Seas) creamy	1 tbsp	60	2.0	6.0
(Seven Seas) 'French! Light'	1 tbsp	35	2.0	3.0
(T. Marzetti) country	1 tbsp	72	4.0	6.0
(T. Marzetti) 'Frenchette'	1 tbsp	10	3.0	0.0
(T. Marzetti) honey, refrigerated	1 tbsp	74	5.0	6.0
(T. Marzetti) honey blue, refrigerated	1 tbsp	70	5.0	6.0
(T. Marzetti) honey 'Lite' refrigerated	1 tbsp	48	5.0	3.0
(T. Marzetti) 'Light'	1 tbsp	16	3.0	1.0
(Ultra Slim Fast) 'Cholesterol Free'	1 tbsp	20	4.0	<1.0
(Weight Watchers) low-calorie	1 tbsp	10	2.0	0.0
(Wish-Bone) creamy, garlic	1 tbsp	55	1.8	5.3
(Wish-Bone) 'Deluxe'	1 tbsp	60	2.3	5.4
(Wish-Bone) 'Deluxe Food Service'	1 tbsp	61	2.4	5.6
(Wish-Bone) garlic	1 tbsp	55	1.8	5.3
(Wish-Bone) 'Healthy Sensation!'	.5 oz	20	4.0	na
(Wish-Bone) 'Lite'	1 tbsp	31	2.1	2.5
(Wish-Bone) 'Lite Sweet 'n Spicy'	1 tbsp	18	3.2	0.5
(Wish-Bone) low-calorie 'Lite'	1 tbsp	30	1.9	2.5
(Wish-Bone) red, low-calorie 'Lite'	1 tbsp	17	3.2	0.4
(Wish-Bone) style 'Lite'	.5 oz	18	3.0	na
(Wish-Bone) style, lite 'Food Service'	.5 oz	30	2.0	3.0
(Wish-Bone) sweet 'n spicy	.5 oz	70	3.0	6.0
(Wish-Bone) sweet 'n spicy 'Lite'	.5 oz	18	4.0	na
FRUIT SALAD				
(Great Impressions) orange marmalade	1 tbsp	87	5.4	7.1
(Knott's Berry Farm)	1 tbsp	50	3.0	5.0
GARLIC				
(Ayla's Organics) and onion, fat free	2 tbsp	10	2.0	0.0
(Ayla's Organics) creamy, fat free	2 tbsp	30	4.0	0.0
(Estee) creamy	1 tbsp	2	0.0	0.0

Food Name	Serv. Size	Total Cal.	Carbs GMS	Fat GMS
(Hain) and sour cream	1 tbsp	70	0.0	7.0
(Kraft) creamy	1 tbsp	50	1.0	5.0
(Life) w/tofu 'All Natural' dressing and dip	1 tbsp	70	1.4	7.1
(Nasoya) herb 'Vegi-Dressing'	1 tbsp	40	1.0	3.0
(Pritikin) and herb, fat-free, sodium-free	1 tbsp	6	2.0	0.0
(T. Marzetti) Italian, refrigerated	1 tbsp	81	1.0	9.0
(Wish-Bone) creamy	1 tbsp	74	0.5	8.0
(Wish-Bone) Sierra	.5 oz	80	1.0	8.0
GINGER PLUM VINAIGRETTE				
(Simply Delicious) 'Un-Dressing'	1 tbsp	36	1.0	4.0
HERB				
(Featherweight)	1 tbsp	6	1.0	0.0
(Featherweight) garden	1 tbsp	25	2.0	2.0
(Hain) savory 'No Salt Added'	1 tbsp	90	0.0	10.0
(Marie's) vinaigrette, fat-free 'Lite & Zesty'	1 tbsp	16	4.0	0.0
(Pritikin) vinaigrette, fat-free, sodium-free	1 tbsp	8	2.0	0.0
(Seven Seas) and spice 'Viva'	1 tbsp	60	1.0	6.0
(Seven Seas) and spice 'Viva Herbs & Spices! Light'	1 tbsp	30	1.0	3.0
(Simply Delicious) garlic vinaigrette 'Un-Dressing'	1 tbsp	43	1.0	4.0
(Wish-Bone) creamy 'Classics'	1 tbsp	70	1.2	7.3
HOMESTYLE				
(Dorothy Lynch)	1 tbsp	55	5.0	3.8
(Dorothy Lynch) 'Reduced Calorie'	1 tbsp	30	7.0	<1.0
HONEY AND SESAME *(Hain)*	1 tbsp	60	2.0	5.0
HONEY MUSTARD				
(Knott's Berry Farm) 'Peggy Jane's'	1 tbsp	60	2.0	6.0
(Litehouse) dressing and dip, refrigerated	1 tbsp	67	2.0	7.0
(Simply Delicious) vinaigrette 'Un-Dressing'	1 tbsp	41	2.0	4.0
(T. Marzetti) Dijon	1 tbsp	67	3.0	6.0
(T. Marzetti) Dijon, refrigerated	1 tbsp	68	3.0	6.0
(Wish-Bone) Dijon 'Healthy Sensation!'	1 tbsp	25	5.0	0.0
ITALIAN				
(Ayla's Organics) fat free	2 tbsp	10	2.0	0.0
(Estee)	2 tbsp	4	1.0	0.0
(Featherweight)	1 tbsp	4	1.0	0,0
(Hain) 'Canola'	1 tbsp	50	1.0	5.0
(Hain) 'Traditional'	1 tbsp	80	0.0	8.0
(Hain) 'Traditional No Salt Added'	1 tbsp	60	1.0	6.0
(Hollywood)	1 tbsp	90	1.0	9.0
(Kraft) 'Deliciously Light'	1 tbsp	35	1.0	3.0
(Kraft) house	1 tbsp	60	1.0	6.0
(Kraft) house 'Reduced Calorie'	1 tbsp	30	1.0	2.0
(Kraft) nonfat 'Free'	1 tbsp	6	1.0	0.0

Food Name	Serv. Size	Total Cal.	Carbs GMS	Fat GMS
(Kraft) oil-free 'Reduced Calorie'	1 tbsp	4	1.0	0.0
(Kraft) 'Presto'	1 tbsp	70	1.0	7.0
(Kraft) zesty	1 tbsp	50	1.0	5.0
(Kraft) zesty 'Reduced Calorie'	1 tbsp	20	1.0	2.0
(Marie's) vinaigrette, fat-free 'Lite & Zesty'	1 tbsp	16	4.0	0.0
(Nasoya) 'Vegi-Dressing'	1 tbsp	40	1.0	3.0
(Ott's)	1 tbsp	80	0.2	9.1
(Pritikin) fat-free, sodium-free	1 tbsp	8	2.0	0.0
(Seven Seas) 'Free Viva'	1 tbsp	4	1.0	0.0
(Seven Seas) 'Viva'	1 tbsp	50	1.0	5.0
(Seven Seas) 'Viva Italian! Light'	1 tbsp	30	1.0	3.0
(Skipper's) gourmet	1 pouch	140	2.0	15.0
(Skipper's) lo-cal	1 pouch	17	2.0	1.0
(T. Marzetti) 'Fat-Free'	1 tbsp	5	1.0	0.0
(T. Marzetti) 'Frenchette'	1 tbsp	6	2.0	0.0
(T. Marzetti) gusto	1 tbsp	58	0.0	8.0
(T. Marzetti) 'Light'	1 tbsp	35	1.0	3.0
(T. Marzetti) w/olive oil	1 tbsp	60	1.0	7.0
(Ultra Slim Fast) 'Cholesterol Free'	1 tbsp	6	1.0	<1.0
(Wish-Bone)	1 tbsp	46	1.5	4.5
(Wish-Bone) blended	.5 oz	35	1.0	4.0
(Wish-Bone) 'Food Service'	.5 oz	45	2.0	5.0
(Wish-Bone) 'Healthy Sensation!'	1 tbsp	6	1.0	0.0
(Wish-Bone) 'Lite'	1 tbsp	7	0.9	0.3
(Wish-Bone) lite 'Food Service'	.5 oz	6	1.0	na
(Wish-Bone) 'Robusto'	1 tbsp	47	1.8	4.5
(Weight Watchers) style	1 tbsp	6	1.0	0.0
(Weight Watchers) style 'Single Serve' 1 packet	.75 oz	8	2.0	0.0
ITALIAN, CREAMY				
(Estee)	2 tbsp	14	2.0	<1.0
(Kraft)	1 tbsp	60	1.0	6.0
(Kraft) 'Deliciously Light'	1 tbsp	25	1.0	2.0
(Kraft) 'Reduced Calorie'	1 tbsp	25	1.0	2.0
(Kraft) w/real sour cream	1 tbsp	50	1.0	5.0
(Litehouse) dressing and dip, refrigerated	1 tbsp	60	0.0	6.0
(Seven Seas) 'Viva Creamy Italian! Light'	1 tbsp	45	1.0	4.0
(T. Marzetti)	1 tbsp	80	1.0	8.0
(Weight Watchers)	1 tbsp	12	3.0	0.0
(Weight Watchers) whipped	1 tbsp	50	2.0	5.0
(Wish-Bone)	.5 oz	60	1.0	6.0
(Wish-Bone) 'Food Service'	.5 oz	25	4.0	na
(Wish-Bone) 'Lite'	.5 oz	25	4.0	na

Food Name	Serv. Size	Total Cal.	Carbs GMS	Fat GMS
LEMON TAHINI VINAIGRETTE				
(Simply Delicious) 'Un-Dressing'	1 tbsp	43	1.0	4.0
LIME CILANTRO VINAIGRETTE				
(Simply Delicious) 'Un-Dressing'	1 tbsp	41	1.0	4.0
MAYONNAISE TYPE. See also MAYONNAISE.				
(A&P)	1 tbsp	70	2.0	7.0
(Bama)	1 tbsp	50	3.0	4.0
(Finast)	1 tbsp	70	2.0	7.0
(Kraft) 'Miracle Whip'	1 tbsp	70	2.0	7.0
(Kraft) 'Miracle Whip Light'	1 tbsp	40	3.0	3.0
(Kraft) nonfat 'Miracle Whip Free'	1 tbsp	15	3.0	0.0
(P&Q)	1 tbsp	50	3.0	5.0
(Pathmark) 'No Frills'	1 tbsp	50	3.0	5.0
(Spin Blend)	1 tbsp	60	3.0	5.0
(Spin Blend) cholesterol free	1 tbsp	40	2.0	4.0
(Weight Watchers) whipped	1 tbsp	45	3.0	4.0
(Weight Watchers) whipped, fat-free	1 tbsp	12	4.0	0.0
(Weight Watchers) whipped, light	1 tbsp	50	1.0	5.0
(Weight Watchers) whipped, low-sodium	1 tbsp	50	1.0	5.0
OIL AND VINEGAR				
W/balsamic vinegar *(Great Impressions)*	1 tbsp	67	2.3	6.5
W/olive oil				
(Kraft)	1 tbsp	70	1.0	8.0
(Wish-Bone) Italian 'Classic'	1 tbsp	34	1.7	3.0
(Wish-Bone) 'Lite Classic'	.5 oz	20	2.0	2.0
(Wish-Bone) vinaigrette	1 tbsp	28	1.8	2.3
(Wish-Bone) vinaigrette 'Lite'	1 tbsp	16	1.9	0.9
W/red wine vinegar				
(Estee)	1 tbsp	2	0.0	0.0
(Featherweight)	1 tbsp	6	1.0	0.0
(Great Impressions)	1 tbsp	64	2.5	6.1
(Kraft)	1 tbsp	60	4.0	4.0
(Pathmark)	1 tbsp	70	2.0	7.0
(Seven Seas) 'Free'	1 tbsp	6	1.0	0.0
(Seven Seas) 'Viva'	1 tbsp	70	1.0	7.0
(Seven Seas) 'Viva Red Wine!'	1 tbsp	45	1.0	4.0
W/Cabernet *(Lawry's)* 'Classics'	1 tbsp	138	4.9	13.7
W/white wine vinegar *(Great Impressions)*	1 tbsp	63	0.8	6.6
ONION AND CHIVES				
(Kraft) creamy	1 tbsp	70	1.0	7.0
(Wish-Bone) 'Lite'	1 tbsp	37	1.6	3.3
ORIENTAL STYLE *(Featherweight)*	1 tbsp	20	1.0	2.0
PARMESAN *(Hidden Valley Ranch)* Italian 'Lowfat'	1 tbsp	16	3.0	1.0

Food Name	Serv. Size	Total Cal.	Carbs GMS	Fat GMS
PARMESAN PEPPERCORN				
(T. Marzetti)	1 tbsp	81	<1.0	9.0
(T. Marzetti) refrigerated	1 tbsp	85	1.0	9.0
PEPPERCORN				
(Litehouse) dressing and dip, refrigerated	1 tbsp	67	0.0	7.0
(Simply Delicious) pink, vinaigrette 'Un-Dressing'	1 tbsp	40	1.0	4.0
(T. Marzetti) cracked, refrigerated	1 tbsp	62	0.0	7.0
(Weight Watchers) creamy	1 tbsp	8	2.0	0.0
POPPYSEED				
(Great Impressions)	1 tbsp	131	8.0	11.0
(Hain) 'Rancher's'	1 tbsp	60	0.0	7.0
(Knott's Berry Farm) 'Peggy Jane's'	1 tbsp	60	4.0	5.0
(Litehouse) dressing and dip, refrigerated	1 tbsp	65	3.0	6.0
(T. Marzetti)	1 tbsp	72	5.0	6.0
(T. Marzetti) refrigerated	1 tbsp	65	5.0	5.0
POTATO SALAD (T. Marzetti)	1 tbsp	80	3.0	7.0
RANCH				
(Hidden Valley Ranch) honey Dijon 'Lowfat'	1 tbsp	20	3.0	1.0
(Hidden Valley Ranch) original 'Light'	1 tbsp	40	2.0	4.0
(Kraft) nonfat 'Free'	1 tbsp	16	3.0	0.0
(Litehouse) country, dressing and dip, refrigerated	1 tbsp	61	1.0	7.0
(Litehouse) dressing and dip, refrigerated	1 tbsp	59	1.0	6.0
(Litehouse) jalapeño, dressing and dip, refrigerated	1 tbsp	60	1.0	6.0
(Litehouse) 'Lite' dressing and dip, refrigerated	1 tbsp	35	1.0	3.0
(Pritikin) fat-free, sodium-free	1 tbsp	16	4.0	0.0
(Seven Seas) 'Buttermilk Recipe Ranch! Light'	1 tbsp	50	1.0	5.0
(Seven Seas) 'Free'	1 tbsp	16	4.0	0.0
(Seven Seas) 'Viva'	1 tbsp	80	1.0	8.0
(Seven Seas) 'Viva Ranch! Light'	1 tbsp	50	2.0	5.0
(Skipper's) house	1 pouch	188	2.0	20.0
(T. Marzetti)	1 tbsp	90	0.0	2.0
(T. Marzetti) buttermilk, refrigerated	1 tbsp	93	0.0	10.0
(T. Marzetti) buttermilk 'Lite' refrigerated	1 tbsp	45	1.0	5.0
(T. Marzetti) Caesar	1 tbsp	95	1.0	10.0
(T. Marzetti) 'Fat-Free'	1 tbsp	12	3.0	0.0
(T. Marzetti) garden	1 tbsp	100	1.0	10.0
(T. Marzetti) honey Dijon	1 tbsp	89	1.0	9.0
(T. Marzetti) honey Dijon, refrigerated	1 tbsp	79	1.0	8.0
(T. Marzetti) 'Light'	1 tbsp	40	2.0	4.0
(T. Marzetti) Parmesan, refrigerated	1 tbsp	86	1.0	9.0
(T. Marzetti) peppercorn	1 tbsp	85	1.0	9.0
(T. Marzetti) peppercorn 'Fat-Free'	1 tbsp	14	3.0	0.0
(T. Marzetti) style	1 tbsp	90	5.0	6.0

Food Name	Serv. Size	Total Cal.	Carbs GMS	Fat GMS
(Weight Watchers) creamy	1 tbsp	25	6.0	0.0
(Weight Watchers) creamy 'Single Serve'	1 pkt	35	8.0	0.0
(Wish-Bone)	1 tbsp	78	1.1	8.3
(Wish-Bone) 'Food Service'	.5 oz	80	1.0	8.0
(Wish-Bone) 'Healthy Sensation!'	1 tbsp	16	3.0	0.0
(Wish-Bone) 'Lite'	1 tbsp	42	2.5	3.5
RED WINE VINAIGRETTE				
(Wish-Bone)	1 tbsp	51	4.2	3.8
(Wish-Bone) 'Lite'	.5 oz	20	2.0	2.0
ROMANO				
(T. Marzetti) cheese Italian	1 tbsp	80	0.0	8.0
(T. Marzetti) cheese Italian, refrigerated	1 tbsp	77	<1.0	8.0
RUSSIAN				
(Ayla's Organics) fat free	2 tbsp	10	3.0	0.0
(Featherweight)	1 tbsp	6	1.0	0.0
(Kraft)	1 tbsp	60	4.0	5.0
(Kraft) creamy	1 tbsp	60	2.0	5.0
(Kraft) 'Reduced Calorie'	1 tbsp	30	4.0	1.0
(Kraft) w/pure honey, low-calorie	1 tbsp	60	4.0	5.0
(S&W Nutradiet)	1 tbsp	25	4.0	1.0
(Weight Watchers) whipped	1 tbsp	50	2.0	5.0
(Wish-Bone)	1 tbsp	46	6.0	2.5
(Wish-Bone) 'Food Service'	1 tbsp	47	6.0	2.5
(Wish-Bone) 'Lite'	1 tbsp	22	3.9	0.6
SAN FRANCISCO *(Lawry's)* w/Romano cheese 'Classic'	1 oz	136	2.0	14.0
SANTA FE *(Wish-Bone)*	.5 oz	70	1.0	7.0
SESAME SEED				
(Ayla's Organics) toasted, fat free	2 tbsp	20	3.0	0.0
(Nasoya) garlic 'Vegi-Dressing'	1 tbsp	40	1.0	3.0
(Wish-Bone) vinaigrette 'Food Service'	.5 oz	35	3.0	2.0
SOUR CREAM				
(Crowley) nondairy	1 oz	40	1.0	4.0
(Friendship) 'Sour Treat'	1 oz	36	2.0	3.0
SOUR CREAM AND CHIVES				
(Litehouse) vinaigrette, refrigerated	1 tbsp	63	1.0	7.0
SPINACH SALAD *(T. Marzetti)* refrigerated	1 tbsp	35	2.0	3.0
SWEET AND SAUCY *(T. Marzetti)*	1 tbsp	65	4.0	5.0
SWEET AND SOUR				
(T. Marzetti)	1 tbsp	72	5.0	6.0
(T. Marzetti) 'Fat-Free'	1 tbsp	20	5.0	0.0
(T. Marzetti) 'Light'	1 tbsp	45	5.0	3.0
(T. Marzetti) refrigerated	1 tbsp	72	5.0	6.0
SWISS CHEESE VINAIGRETTE *(Hain)*	1 tbsp	60	0.0	7.0

Food Name	Serv. Size	Total Cal.	Carbs GMS	Fat GMS
THOUSAND ISLAND				
(Estee)	1 tbsp	8	2.0	0.0
(Featherweight)	1 tbsp	18	3.0	0.0
(Hain)	1 tbsp	50	0.0	5.0
(Hollywood)	1 tbsp	60	3.0	6.0
(Kraft)	1 tbsp	60	2.0	5.0
(Kraft) and bacon	1 tbsp	60	2.0	6.0
(Kraft) nonfat 'Free'	1 tbsp	20	5.0	0.0
(Kraft) 'Reduced Calorie'	1 tbsp	20	3.0	1.0
(Litehouse) dressing and dip, refrigerated	1 tbsp	65	1.0	7.0
(S&W Nutradiet)	1 tbsp	25	2.0	2.0
(Seven Seas) creamy	1 tbsp	50	2.0	5.0
(Seven Seas) 'Thousand Island! Light'	1 tbsp	30	3.0	2.0
(Skipper's)	1 pouch	160	8.0	14.0
(T. Marzetti)	1 tbsp	74	2.0	7.0
(T. Marzetti) 'Fat-Free'	1 tbsp	17	4.0	0.0
(T. Marzetti) 'Frenchette'	1 tbsp	20	3.0	0.0
(T. Marzetti) 'Light'	1 tbsp	35	3.0	3.0
(T. Marzetti) refrigerated	1 tbsp	82	6.0	5.0
(Ultra Slim Fast) 'Cholesterol Free'	1 tbsp	18	4.0	<1.0
(Weight Watchers) whipped	1 tbsp	50	2.0	5.0
(Wish-Bone)	1 tbsp	63	3.1	5.6
(Wish-Bone) 'Food Service'	1 tbsp	40	2.6	3.2
(Wish-Bone) 'Healthy Sensation!'	.5 oz	20	4.0	na
(Wish-Bone) 'Lite'	1 tbsp	36	1.9	3.0
(Wish-Bone) lite 'Food Service'	.5 oz	20	4.0	na
TOMATO				
(Featherweight) zesty	1 tbsp	2	0.0	0.0
(Hain) vinaigrette, garden 'Canola'	1 tbsp	60	1.0	6.0
(Weight Watchers) vinaigrette	1 tbsp	8	2.0	0.0
VEGETABLE (T. Marzetti) dressing and dip, refrigerated	1 tbsp	88	1.0	10.0
VINTAGE (Lawry's) w/sherry wine 'Classic'	1 tbsp	110	2.5	10.5
WHITE WINE				
(Lawry's) w/Chardonnay 'Classic'	1 tbsp	153	2.7	15.7
(Marie's) fat-free 'Lite & Zesty'	1 tbsp	20	5.0	0.0
SALAD DRESSING MIX				
BACON (Lawry's) dry mix	1 pkg	65	9.1	0.8
BLUE CHEESE				
(Hain) 'No Oil' prepared	1 tbsp	14	1.0	1.0
(Hidden Valley Ranch) dry mix	1 pkg	112	19.0	2.0
(Weight Watchers) dry mix	1 tbsp	8	1.0	0.0
BLUE CHEESE AND HERBS (Good Seasons) dry mix	1 pkg	4	1.0	0.0

Food Name	Serv. Size	Total Cal.	Carbs GMS	Fat GMS
BUTTERMILK				
(Hain) 'No Oil' prepared	1 tbsp	11	1.0	<1.0
(Hidden Valley Ranch) original recipe, dry mix, .4 oz	1 pkg	25	na	0.0
(Good Seasons) 'Farm Style' dry mix	1 pkg	4	1.0	0.0
CAESAR				
(Lawry's) dry mix	1 pkg	75	8.7	3.1
(Hain) 'No Oil' prepared	1 tbsp	6	1.0	<1.0
CHEESE AND GARLIC				
(Good Seasons) dry mix	1 pkg	4	1.0	0.0
(Hain) 'No Oil' prepared	1 tbsp	6	1.0	<1.0
DILL *(Good Seasons)* 'Classic' dry mix	1 tbsp	2	0.0	0.0
FRENCH				
(Hain) 'No Oil' prepared	1 tbsp	12	3.0	0.0
(Weight Watchers) style, dry mix	1 tbsp	3	1.0	0.0
GARLIC AND HERBS *(Good Seasons)* dry mix	1 pkg	4	1.0	0.0
HERB				
(Good Seasons) 'Classic' dry mix	1 pkg	2	0.0	0.0
(Hain) 'No Oil' prepared	1 tbsp	2	1.0	0.0
(Hidden Valley Ranch) creamy, dry mix	1 pkg	76	16.0	0.0
HONEY MUSTARD *(Good Seasons)* dry mix	1 tbsp	6	1.0	0.0
ITALIAN				
(Good Seasons) dry mix	1 pkg	2	1.0	0.0
(Good Seasons) 'Lite' prepared	1 tbsp	25	1.0	3.0
(Good Seasons) mild	1 tbsp	70	1.0	8.0
(Good Seasons) 'No Oil' prepared	1 tbsp	6	2.0	0.0
(Good Seasons) zesty, dry mix	1 pkg	2	1.0	0.0
(Good Seasons) zesty 'Lite' prepared	1 tbsp	25	1.0	3.0
(Hain) 'No Oil' prepared	1 tbsp	2	1.0	0.0
(Lawry's) dry mix	1 pkg	45	9.3	0.2
(Lawry's) w/cheese, dry mix	1 pkg	74	11.6	2.1
(Weight Watchers) dry mix	1 tbsp	2	0.0	0.0
ITALIAN, CREAMY *(Weight Watchers)* dry mix	1 tbsp	3	1.0	0.0
ITALIAN CHEESE				
(Good Seasons) dry mix	1 pkg	4	1.0	0.0
(Good Seasons) 'Lite' prepared	1 tbsp	25	1.0	3.0
LEMON AND HERBS *(Good Seasons)* dry mix	1 pkg	2	1.0	0.0
PEPPERCORN				
(Hidden Valley Ranch) original recipe, prepared	1 tbsp	58	1.0	3.0
RANCH				
(Good Seasons) dry mix	1 pkg	4	1.0	0.0
(Good Seasons) 'Lite' prepared	1 tbsp	30	2.0	2.0
(Hidden Valley Ranch) 'Original' dry mix	1 pkg	93	18.0	1.0
(Hidden Valley Ranch) reduced calorie, dry mix	1 pkg	98	17.0	2.0

Food Name	Serv. Size	Total Cal.	Carbs GMS	Fat GMS
(Hidden Valley Ranch) w/bacon, dry mix	1.2 oz	118	1.0	2.0
RUSSIAN (Weight Watchers) dry mix	1 tbsp	4	1.0	0.0
SPICY PEANUT (A Taste of Thai) dry mix	1 tbsp	40	6.0	1.5
THOUSAND ISLAND				
(Hain) 'No Oil' prepared	1 tbsp	12	3.0	0.0
(Weight Watchers) dry mix	1 tbsp	4	1.0	0.0
SALAD MIX. See also PASTA DISH MIX; PASTA SALAD MIX.				
(Saco Foods) 'Easy Caesar' unprepared	.75 oz	98	7.0	7.0
SALAD SEASONING (Schilling) 'Salad Supreme'	1 tsp	11	0.5	0.1
SALAD TOPPING				
(Salad Nibbler) crouton topping, buttermilk ranch	1 oz	128	13.0	5.0
(Salad Nibbler) crouton topping, seasoned cheddar	1 oz	129	13.0	6.0
(Special Edition) sesame salad nuggets	1 tbsp	35	3.0	2.5
(Special Edition) sesame salad nuggets, garlic and cheese	1 tbsp	40	3.0	2.5
SALAMI. See LUNCHEON MEAT.				
SALISBURY STEAK DINNER. See BEEF DINNER, FROZEN.				
SALISBURY STEAK ENTRÉE. See BEEF ENTRÉE, FROZEN; BEEF ENTRÉE, PACKAGED.				
SALMON, ALTERNATIVE, smoked (Mox Lox)	1.5 oz	25	3.0	<1.0
SALMON, ATLANTIC				
Farmed				
dry-heat cooked	3 oz	175	0.0	10.5
raw	3 oz	156	0.0	9.2
Wild				
dry-heat cooked	3 oz	155	0.0	6.9
raw	3 oz	121	0.0	5.4
SALMON, CANNED				
CHUM				
(Bumble Bee)	1 cup	306	0.0	11.4
(Bumble Bee) w/liquid	3.5 oz	160	0.0	8.0
COHO (Deming's) boiled	1/2 cup	140	0.0	5.0
MIXED (Libby's) skinless, boneless	3.25 oz	110	1.0	4.0
PINK				
Alaska, w/liquid (Deming's)	1/2 cup	140	0.0	6.0
chunk, skinless, boneless, in spring water				
(Chicken of the Sea)	2 oz	60	0.0	2.0
chunk, skinless, boneless, w/liquid (Deming's)	3.25 oz	120	0.0	5.0
skinless, boneless, w/liquid (Bumble Bee)	3.5 oz	120	0.0	5.0
solids, w/bone and liquid	3 oz	118	0.0	5.1
w/liquid	4 oz	158	0.0	6.9
w/liquid (Bumble Bee)	1 cup	310	0.0	13.0
w/liquid (Bumble Bee)	3.5 oz	160	0.0	8.0
w/liquid (Del Monte)	1/2 cup	160	0.0	7.0
w/liquid (Featherweight)	2 oz	70	0.0	3.0

Food Name	Serv. Size	Total Cal.	Carbs GMS	Fat GMS
w/liquid *(Libby's)*	7.75 oz	310	0.0	13.0
SOCKEYE				
(Bumble Bee)	1 cup	376	0.0	20.5
(Libby's)	7.75 oz	380	0.0	21.0
Alaska *(Deming's)*	1/2 cup	170	0.0	9.0
Alaska, med *(Deming's)*	1/2 cup	150	0.0	7.0
blueback *(Rubinstein's)*	1/2 cup	170	0.0	9.0
blueback *(S&W Nutradiet)*	1/2 cup	188	0.0	11.0
blueback 'Fancy' *(S&W)*	1/2 cup	190	0.0	10.0
skinless, boneless, w/liquid *(Bumble Bee)*	3.5 oz	130	0.0	6.0
solids, w/bone, drained	3 oz	130	0.0	6.2
solids, w/bone, drained, w/o salt	3 oz	130	0.0	6.2
w/liquid *(Bumble Bee)*	3.5 oz	180	0.0	10.0
w/liquid *(Del Monte)*	1/2 cup	180	0.0	9.0
SALMON, CHINOOK/king/lox/smoked				
dry-heat cooked	3 oz	196	0.0	11.4
raw	1 lb	816	0.0	47.4
raw	3 oz	153	0.0	8.9
raw, approx 7 oz	1/2 fillet	356	0.0	20.7
smoked	3 oz	99	0.0	3.7
smoked, lox	4 oz	133	0.0	4.9
smoked, lox	3 oz	99	0.0	3.7
SALMON, CHUM/dog/keta				
dry-heat cooked	3 oz	131	0.0	4.1
raw	1 lb	544	0.0	17.1
raw	3 oz	102	0.0	3.2
raw	1 oz	34	0.0	1.1
raw, approx 7 oz	1/2 fillet	238	0.0	7.5
raw, fillet portions *(Peter Pan Seafoods)*	3.5 oz	120	na	3.8
raw, sides, w/pinbone, *(Peter Pan Seafoods)*	3.5 oz	120	na	3.8
raw, solids, w/bone, drained, w/o salt	3 oz	120	0.0	4.7
raw, steaks *(Peter Pan Seafoods)*	3.5 oz	120	na	3.8
SALMON, COHO/silver				
Farmed				
dry-heat cooked	3 oz	151	0.0	7.0
raw	3 oz	136	0.0	6.5
Wild				
dry-heat cooked	3 oz	118	0.0	3.7
moist-heat cooked	3 oz	156	0.0	6.4
raw	1 lb	662	0.0	27.0
raw	3 oz	124	0.0	5.0
raw	1 oz	41	0.0	1.7
raw, approx 7 oz	1/2 fillet	289	0.0	11.7

Food Name	Serv. Size	Total Cal.	Carbs GMS	Fat GMS
SALMON, DOG. See SALMON, CHUM.				
SALMON, FROZEN, steak, w/o seasoning mix *(SeaPak)*	8-oz pkg	270	0.0	9.0
SALMON, HUMPBACK. See SALMON, PINK.				
SALMON, KETA. See SALMON, CHUM.				
SALMON, KING. See SALMON, CHINOOK.				
SALMON, PINK/humpback				
dry-heat cooked	3 oz	127	0.0	3.8
raw	1 lb	527	0.0	15.6
raw	3 oz	99	0.0	2.9
raw	1 oz	33	0.0	1.0
SALMON, RED. See SALMON, SOCKEYE.				
SALMON, REDEYE. See SALMON, SOCKEYE.				
SALMON, SILVER. See SALMON, COHO.				
SALMON, SMOKED. See SALMON, CHINOOK.				
SALMON, SOCKEYE/red/redeye				
dry-heat cooked	4 oz	245	0.0	12.4
dry-heat cooked	3 oz	184	0.0	9.3
raw	1 lb	763	0.0	38.8
raw	3 oz	143	0.0	7.3
raw	1 oz	48	0.0	2.4
raw, approx 7 oz	1/2 fillet	333	0.0	17.0
SALSA. See also SAUCE.				
(Hot Cha Cha) 'Texas'	1 oz	6	2.5	0.0
(La Victoria) 'Brava'	1 tbsp	6	1.0	<1.0
(La Victoria) 'Casera'	1 tbsp	4	1.0	<1.0
(La Victoria) 'Supreme'	2 tbsp	10	2.0	0.0
(La Victoria) 'Victoria'	1 tbsp	4	1.0	<1.0
BURRITO *(Del Monte)*	1/4 cup	20	4.0	0.0
EXTRA CHUNKY *(Rosarita)* 'de Mexico Style'	2 tbsp	30	7.0	<1.0
GREEN CHILI				
(Del Monte) mild	1/4 cup	20	3.0	0.0
(Hain) hot	1/4 cup	22	4.0	0.0
(La Victoria)	2 tbsp	10	2.0	0.0
(Nabisco) hot	1 tbsp	6	2.0	0.0
(Nabisco) medium 'Green Chile Salsa'	1 tbsp	6	1.0	0.0
(Nabisco) mild 'Green Chile Salsa'	1 tbsp	8	2.0	0.0
(Old El Paso) 'Thick 'n Chunky'	2 tbsp	3	1.0	0.0
(Ortega) hot	1 oz	10	2.0	0.0
(Ortega) medium	1 oz	8	2.0	0.0
(Ortega) mild	1 oz	8	2.0	0.0
(Rosarita) mild	1.093 oz	7	1.5	0.1
(Territorial House)	.5 oz	4	<1.0	<1.0

Food Name	Serv. Size	Total Cal.	Carbs GMS	Fat GMS
HOT				
(Chi-Chi's)	1 oz	8	2.0	2.0
(Enrico's) 'Chunky Style'	2 tbsp	8	2.0	0.0
(Enrico's) 'Chunky Style No Salt Added'	2 tbsp	8	2.0	0.0
(Old El Paso) 'Thick 'n Chunky'	2 tbsp	6	1.0	<1.0
(Pablo's) 'Deli Style'	1 oz	10	2.0	0.0
(Rosarita) chunky	3 tbsp	25	6.0	<1.0
JALAPEÑO				
(La Victoria) green	1 tbsp	4	1.0	<1.0
(La Victoria) red	1 tbsp	6	1.0	<1.0
MEDIUM				
(Chi-Chi's)	1 oz	7	2.0	2.0
(Litehouse) 'Zesty'	1 tbsp	4	1.0	0.0
(Old El Paso) 'Thick 'n Chunky'	2 tbsp	6	1.0	<1.0
(Ortega) thick and chunky	1 tbsp	4	1.0	0.0
(Pace) 'Thick & Chunky'	2 tbsp	4	<1.0	<1.0
(Rosarita) chunky	3 tbsp	25	6.0	<1.0
(Rosarita) 'Traditional'	1.093 oz	7	1.6	0.1
MILD				
(Chi-Chi's)	1 oz	7	2.0	2.0
(Enrico's) 'Chunky Style'	2 tbsp	8	2.0	0.0
(Enrico's) 'Chunky Style No Salt Added'	2 tbsp	8	2.0	0.0
(Hain)	1/2 cup	20	4.0	0.0
(Hunt's) 'Homestyle'	1.093 oz	27	6.2	0.2
(Old El Paso) 'Thick 'n Chunky'	2 tbsp	6	1.0	<1.0
(Pablo's) 'Deli Style'	1 oz	10	2.0	0.0
(Pace) and dip, mild 'Chunky'	2 tbsp	4	<1.0	<1.0
(Pace) 'Thick & Chunky'	2 tbsp	4	<1.0	<1.0
(Rosarita) 'Casa Mamita'	1.129 oz	7	1.2	0.1
(Rosarita) chunky	3 tbsp	25	6.0	<1.0
(Rosarita) roasted	1.093 oz	10	1.7	0.3
(Rosarita) 'Traditional'	1.093 oz	7	1.4	0.1
OMELETTE *(La Victoria)*	1 tbsp	6	1.0	<1.0
PICANTE				
(Del Monte) hot	1/2 cup	20	4.0	0.0
(Del Monte) hot and chunky	1/4 cup	15	3.0	0.0
(La Victoria) medium	2 tbsp	5	1.0	0.0
(La Victoria) mild	2 tbsp	10	2.0	0.0
(LàCasita) mild, chunky	2 oz	16	4.0	0.0
(Old El Paso) hot	2 tbsp	10	2.0	<1.0
(Old El Paso) medium	2 tbsp	10	2.0	<1.0
(Old El Paso) mild	2 tbsp	10	2.0	<1.0
(Ortega)	1 oz	10	2.0	0.0

Food Name	Serv. Size	Total Cal.	Carbs GMS	Fat GMS
(Rosarita)	1.093 oz	7	1.3	0.1
RANCHERA				
(La Victoria)	1 tbsp	6	1.0	<1.0
(Ortega)	1 oz	12	3.0	0.0
ROJA *(Del Monte)* mild	1/4 cup	20	4.0	0.0
TACO				
(Nabisco) 'Hot Thick and Smooth'	1 tbsp	8	2.0	0.0
(Nabisco) 'Medium Thick and Smooth'	1 tbsp	8	2.0	0.0
(Nabisco) 'Mild Thick and Smooth'	1 tbsp	8	2.0	0.0
(Ortega) hot	1 oz	10	2.0	0.0
(Ortega) mild	1 oz	10	2.0	0.0
(Rosarita) medium, chunky	3 tbsp	25	6.0	<1.0
(Rosarita) mild	2 oz	27	6.1	0.1
(Rosarita) mild, chunky	3 tbsp	25	6.0	<1.0
TOMATILLO				
(Rosarita) green 'de Mexico Style'	2 tbsp	20	4.0	<1.0
(Rosarita) medium	1.093 oz	8	1.8	0.2
TRADITIONAL *(Rosarita)* 'de Mexico Style'	2 tbsp	12	3.0	0.0
VERDE *(Old El Paso)* 'Thick 'n Chunky'	2 tbsp	10	2.0	<1.0
VERY LOW SODIUM *(Pritikin)*	1/4 cup	25	5.0	0.0
SALSIFY/oyster plant/vegetable oyster				
boiled, drained	4 oz	77	17.4	0.2
boiled, drained, sliced	1/2 cup	46	10.5	0.1
raw, sliced	1/2 cup	55	12.5	0.1
raw, trimmed	1 oz	23	5.3	0.1
raw, untrimmed	1 lb	325	73.4	0.8
SALSIFY, BLACK/scorzonera				
raw	1 lb	372	84.4	0.1
raw	1 oz	23	5.3	tr
SALT				
iodized *(Morton)*	1 tsp	0	0.0	0.0
kosher *(Morton)*	1 tsp	0	0.0	0.0
mixture 'Lite Salt' *(Morton)*	1 tsp	<1	tr	0.0
non-iodized *(Morton)*	1 tsp	0	0.0	0.0
plain	1 cup	0	0.0	0.0
plain	1 tbsp	0	0.0	0.0
plain	1 tsp	0	0.0	0.0
sea *(Hain)*	1 tsp	0	0.0	0.0
SALT, ALTERNATIVE				
Plain				
(Estee) 'Salt-It'	1/8 tsp	0	0.0	0.0
(Featherweight)	1/4 tsp	0	0.0	0.0
(Lawry's) 'Salt-Free'	1 tsp	10	1.8	0.2

Food Name	Serv. Size	Total Cal.	Carbs GMS	Fat GMS
(Morton)	1 tsp	<1	0.1	0.0
Seasoned				
(Estee) 'Seasoned Salt-It'	1/8 tsp	0	0.0	0.0
(Featherweight)	1/4 tsp	0	0.0	0.0
(Health Valley) all-purpose 'Instead of Salt'	1 tsp	11	1.5	0.5
(Lawry's) 'Salt-Free'	1 tsp	3	0.6	<.1
(Morton)	1 tsp	2	0.5	<.1
SALT PORK, cured *(Hormel)*	2 oz	320	0.0	33.0
SALT SEASONING				
(Lawry's)	1 tsp	4	0.6	0.1
(Lawry's) 'Hot 'n Spicy'	1 tsp	3	1.5	0.1
(Lawry's) 'Lite'	1 tsp	8	1.7	<.1
(Morton)	1 tsp	4	<1.0	<.1
(Morton) 'Nature's Seasons'	1 tsp	3	<1.0	<.1
(Schilling)	1 tsp	4	0.6	na
(Schilling) 'Salt 'n Spice'	1 tsp	3	0.6	na
SANDWICH				
BEEF				
(Hot Pockets) frozen, pocket, and cheddar	5 oz	370	36.0	17.0
(Lean Pockets) frozen, pocket, and broccoli	1 pkg	250	30.0	8.0
(Manwich) extra thick and chunky, prepared	1 sandwich	330	36.0	13.0
(Manwich) Mexican, prepared	1 sandwich	310	30.0	13.0
(Manwich) original, prepared	1 sandwich	320	31.0	13.0
(Manwich) 'Sloppy Joe' prepared	1 sandwich	310	31.0	13.0
(Tyson) frozen, barbecue, microwave	1 sandwich	200	29.0	2.7
CANADIAN BACON				
(Quick Meal) muffin, w/egg and cheese	4.5 oz	250	29.0	8.0
CHEESEBURGER				
(Kid Cuisine) frozen	6.25 oz	400	47.0	19.0
(Kid Cuisine) frozen, double 'Mega Meal'	9.1 oz	480	55.0	20.0
(MicroMagic) frozen	4.75 oz	450	29.0	25.0
CHICKEN				
(Banquet) patties, breast meat 'Microwave'	4 oz	310	31.0	14.0
(BestFresh) breast, teriyaki, charbroiled	1 sandwich	490	45.0	20.0
(BestFresh) w/cucumber yogurt dressing	1 sandwich	390	38.0	15.0
(Hot Pockets) frozen, pocket, and cheddar	5 oz	310	38.0	11.0
(Kid Cuisine)	8.2 oz	470	61.0	17.0
(Lean Pockets) frozen, pocket, Oriental	1 pkg	250	35.0	6.0
(Lean Pockets) frozen, pocket, Parmesan	1 pkg	270	35.0	6.0
(Lean Pockets) frozen, pocket, white meat only 'Fajita'	1 sandwich	250	36.0	6.0
(Lean Pockets) frozen, pocket, white meat only, glazed 'Supreme'	1 sandwich	240	35.0	7.0
(MicroMagic) frozen	4.5 oz	390	42.0	16.0

Food Name	Serv. Size	Total Cal.	Carbs GMS	Fat GMS
(Quick Meal)	4.3 oz	320	40.0	11.0
(Quick Meal) biscuit	4.2 oz	310	36.0	13.0
(Quick Meal) grilled	4.7 oz	300	35.0	9.0
(Tyson) boneless, grilled	3.5 oz	200	25.0	5.0
(Tyson) breast, boneless, grilled	3.5 oz	150	2.0	8.0
(Tyson) frozen, barbecue 'Microwave'	4 oz	230	27.0	6.0
(Tyson) frozen, breast 'Microwave'	3.5 oz	275	27.0	12.0
(Tyson) frozen, mini 'Microwave'	3.5 oz	230	39.0	5.0
(Ultimate 200) grilled	4 oz	200	22.0	5.0
EGG				
(Jimmy Dean) frozen, w/egg and cheese	1 biscuit	300	28.0	16.0
(Jimmy Dean) frozen, w/ham and cheese	1 biscuit	240	26.0	10.0
(Jimmy Dean) w/sausage and cheese	1 biscuit	390	28.0	27.0
(Swanson) frozen, w/beefsteak and cheese 'Great Starts'	4.9 oz	360	27.0	20.0
(Swanson) frozen, w/Canadian bacon and cheese 'Great Starts'	5.2 oz	420	37.0	22.0
(Swanson) frozen, w/Canadian bacon and cheese 'Great Starts'	4.1 oz	290	25.0	15.0
(Swanson) frozen, w/sausage and cheese 'Great Starts'	5.5 oz	460	35.0	28.0
ENGLISH MUFFIN *(Weight Watchers)*	4 oz	240	29.0	8.0
FISH FILLET *(Quick Meal)*	5.2 oz	430	56.0	16.0
HAM AND CHEESE				
(Hot Pockets) frozen, pocket	5 oz	360	36.0	16.0
(Owens) refrigerated 'Border Breakfasts'	2 oz	150	14.0	6.0
(Swanson) refrigerated, bagel 'Great Starts'	3 oz	240	28.0	8.0
(Ultimate 200) frozen, pocket	4 oz	200	24.0	6.0
(Weight Watchers) bagel	3 oz	210	28.0	6.0
HAMBURGER *(MicroMagic)* frozen	4 oz	350	26.0	18.0
HOT DOG				
(Kid Cuisine)	6.7 oz	450	27.0	19.0
(Kid Cuisine) 'Mega Meal'	8.25 oz	500	52.0	25.0
OMELET				
(Weight Watchers) 'Classic'	3.84 oz	210	22.0	7.0
(Weight Watchers) 'Garden'	3.60 oz	210	28.0	6.0
PIZZA				
(Amy's Kitchen) frozen, pocket, cheese calzone, organic	4.5 oz	313	41.0	9.0
(Hot Pockets) frozen, pocket, pepperoni	5 oz	380	40.0	17.0
(Hot Pockets) frozen, pocket, sausage	5 oz	360	40.0	16.0
(Lean Pockets) frozen, pocket 'Deluxe'	1 pkg	280	34.0	9.0
(Lean Pockets) frozen, pocket, sausage and pepperoni 'Deluxe'	1 sandwich	300	37.0	11.0
(Ultimate 200) pocket 'Deluxe'	4 oz	200	25.0	5.0

Food Name	Serv. Size	Total Cal.	Carbs GMS	Fat GMS
PORK *(Quick Meal)* barbecue	4.3 oz	350	40.0	14.0
RIB *(Swanson)* hot, smothered	10.25 oz	340	50.0	10.0
SAUSAGE				
(Jimmy Dean) refrigerated, microwave	1 sandwich	160	10.0	11.0
(Owens) refrigerated, biscuit 'Border Breakfasts'	2 oz	210	14.0	14.0
(Owens) refrigerated, biscuit, smoked 'Border Breakfasts'	2 oz	200	15.0	6.0
(Owens) refrigerated, biscuit, w/egg and cheese 'Border Breakfasts'	2.5 oz	250	15.0	15.0
(Quick Meal) biscuit	3.7 oz	350	29.0	22.0
(Quick Meal) biscuit, w/cheese	4.3 oz	420	31.0	27.0
(Quick Meal) biscuit, w/egg	4.5 oz	350	30.0	21.0
(Quick Meal) muffin, w/egg and cheese	5.1 oz	76	5.0	4.0
(Swanson) frozen, biscuit, w/egg 'Great Starts'	4.7 oz	410	36.0	22.0
(Weight Watchers) frozen, biscuit 'Microwave'	3 oz	220	19.0	11.0
SUBMARINE *(BestFresh)* 'Deluxe'	1 sandwich	790	59.0	44.0
TURKEY				
(BestFresh) smoked	1 sandwich	580	49.0	26.0
(Healthy Deli) w/corned beef 'Doubledecker'	1 oz	30	0.6	0.7
(Healthy Deli) w/ham 'Doubledecker'	1 oz	30	0.8	0.9
(Hot Pockets) pocket, frozen, w/ham and cheese	5 oz	320	37.0	11.0
(Lean Pockets) pocket, frozen, w/broccoli and cheese	1 sandwich	260	32.0	9.0
VEGETABLE				
(Ken & Robert's) pocket, barbecue style 'Truly Amazing'	5 oz	320	50.0	10.0
(Ken & Robert's) pocket, broccoli cheddar 'Truly Amazing'	5 oz	275	37.0	9.0
(Ken & Robert's) pocket, Greek style 'Truly Amazing'	5 oz	270	35.0	10.0
(Ken & Robert's) pocket, Indian style 'Truly Amazing'	5 oz	300	41.0	12.0
(Ken & Robert's) pocket, Oriental style 'Truly Amazing'	5 oz	295	40.8	12.0
(Ken & Robert's) pocket, pizza style 'Truly Amazing'	5 oz	315	42.0	12.0
(Ken & Robert's) pocket, Tex Mex style 'Truly Amazing'	5 oz	310	43.0	11.0
SANDWICH SEASONING MIX, dry *(Manwich)*	.25 oz	20	5.0	<1.0
SANDWICH SPREAD. See also LUCHEON MEAT, CANNED; POTTED MEAT SPREAD.				
'Chub' *(Oscar Mayer)*	1 oz	67	4.3	4.7
pork and beef	1 oz	67	3.4	4.9
pork and beef	1 tbsp	35	1.8	2.6
SAPODILLA				
approx 7.5 oz	1 med	141	33.9	1.9
pulp	1 cup	200	48.1	2.7
trimmed	1 oz	24	5.7	0.3
untrimmed	1 lb	300	72.5	4.0
SAPOTE/marmalade plum				
trimmed	1 oz	38	9.6	0.2
trimmed, approx 11.2 oz	1 med	301	76.0	1.4
untrimmed	1 lb	431	108.7	1.9

Food Name	Serv. Size	Total Cal.	Carbs GMS	Fat GMS
SARDINE				
ATLANTIC				
in soybean oil, drained	3.75-oz can	191	0.0	10.5
in soybean oil, drained	2 oz	118	0.0	6.5
in soybean oil, drained, approx .8 oz	2 med	50	0.0	2.8
BRISLING, w/liquid (Underwood)	3.75-oz can	260	1.0	20.0
MAINE				
in mustard sauce, drained (Beach Cliff)	3 oz	227	4.0	18.0
in soybean oil, drained (Beach Cliff)	3 oz	240	0.0	20.0
in tomato sauce, drained (Beach Cliff)	3 oz	210	0.0	17.0
in water, drained (Beach Cliff)	3 oz	230	1.0	18.0
MIXED				
'Kippered Snacks' (Brunswick)	3.5 oz	185	1.0	14.0
in mustard sauce (Underwood)	3.75 oz	220	2.0	16.0
in oil (Featherweight)	1 7/8 oz	130	1.0	10.0
in soya oil, drained (Underwood)	3.75 oz	230	1.0	18.0
in Tabasco sauce, drained (Underwood)	3 oz	220	1.0	16.0
in tomato sauce (Del Monte)	1/2 cup	360	45.0	12.0
in tomato sauce (Underwood)	3.75 oz	220	2.0	16.0
in water (Featherweight)	1 7/8 oz	95	1.0	7.0
NORWAY				
in mild sardine oil, drained (Empress)	3.75-oz can	260	1.0	20.0
in mild sardine oil, w/liquid (Empress)	3.75-oz can	460	1.0	42.0
NORWEGIAN BRISLING (S&W)	1.5 oz	130	0.0	10.0
PACIFIC				
in tomato sauce, drained	13 oz	659	0.0	44.3
in tomato sauce, drained	2 oz	101	1.0	6.8
in tomato sauce, drained, approx 1.3 oz	1 med	68	0.0	4.6
SAUCE. See also APPLESAUCE; BARBECUE SAUCE; CRANBERRY SAUCE; SALSA; TOMATO SAUCE.				
ALFREDO SAUCE				
(Betty Crocker) 'Recipe Sauces'	4 oz	190	8.0	17.0
(Contadina)	4 oz	350	6.0	34.0
(Contadina) 'Fresh' refrigerated	6 oz	540	10.0	53.0
(Contadina) 'Light' refrigerated	3.33 oz	150	7.0	10.0
(DiGiorno) reduced fat 'Lighter Varieties'	1/4 cup	180	15.0	11.0
(DiGiorno) refrigerated	2 oz	200	2.0	20.0
(Progresso) 'Authentic Pasta Sauces'	1/2 cup	340	6.0	30.0
APPLE-APRICOT SAUCE				
(Lucky Leaf/Musselman's) 'Fruit n' Sauce'	4 oz	90	22.0	0.0
APPLE-CHERRY SAUCE				
(Lucky Leaf/Musselman's) 'Fruit n' Sauce'	4 oz	100	24.0	0.0

Food Name	Serv. Size	Total Cal.	Carbs GMS	Fat GMS
APPLE-CRANBERRY SAUCE				
(Lucky Leaf/Musselman's) 'Fruit n' Sauce'	4 oz	80	19.0	0.0
APPLE-PEACH SAUCE				
(Lucky Leaf/Musselman's) 'Fruit n' Sauce'	4 oz	90	22.0	0.0
APPLE-PINEAPPLE SAUCE				
(Lucky Leaf/Musselman's) 'Fruit n' Sauce'	4 oz	110	26.0	0.0
APPLE-STRAWBERRY SAUCE				
(Lucky Leaf/Musselman's) 'Fruit n' Sauce'	4 oz	100	24.0	0.0
BASIL-HERB SAUCE (Golden Dipt) 'Nature Bay'	2 grams	8	1.0	0.0
BEARNAISE SAUCE (Great Impressions)	2 tbsp	192	0.2	21.0
BEEF SAUCE				
(Ragu) barbecue 'Beef Tonight'	4 oz	70	15.0	<1.0
(Ragu) skillet lasagna 'Beef Tonight'	4 oz	60	9.0	1.0
(Ragu) Stroganoff 'Beef Tonight'	4 oz	130	6.0	12.0
BOLOGNESE SAUCE				
(Contadina)	5 oz	130	0.0	7.0
(Contadina) 'Fresh' refrigerated	7.5 oz	230	12.0	11.0
(Progresso) 'Authentic Pasta Sauces'	1/2 cup	150	12.0	8.0
BROWN GRAVY SAUCE (LaChoy)	3.139 oz	284	68.5	0.1
BROWNING SAUCE (Gravymaster)	1 tsp	12	2.4	tr
CACCIATORE SAUCE (Recipe Sauces)	3.9 oz	40	9.0	<1.0
CARBONARA SAUCE (DiGiorno) refrigerated	2 oz	200	3.0	19.0
CHARDONNAY SAUCE (Golden Dipt) 'Nature Bay'	1 oz	60	1.0	6.0
CHEDDAR CHEESE SAUCE				
(J. Hungerford) 'Stadium'	2.011 oz	80	6.0	5.0
(Lucky Leaf/Musselman's)	4 oz	220	12.0	18.0
(Lucky Leaf/Musselman's) aged	4 oz	240	11.0	20.0
(Lucky Leaf/Musselman's) aged, mild	4 oz	200	9.0	18.0
(Lucky Leaf/Musselman's) aged, sharp	4 oz	230	6.0	17.0
CHEESE SAUCE				
(Snow's) Welsh rarebit	1/2 cup	170	10.0	11.0
(White House) aged	3.5 oz	213	10.0	18.0
CHICKEN SAUCE				
(Ragu) cacciatore 'Chicken Tonight'	4 oz	70	12.0	2.0
(Ragu) country French 'Chicken Tonight'	4 oz	140	6.0	12.0
(Ragu) creamy, primavera 'Chicken Tonight'	4 oz	90	9.0	6.0
(Ragu) creamy, w/mushrooms 'Chicken Tonight'	4 oz	110	5.0	10.0
(Ragu) herbed, w/wine 'Chicken Tonight'	4 oz	100	13.0	4.0
(Ragu) honey mustard, light 'Chicken Tonight'	4 oz	50	12.0	<1.0
(Ragu) sweet and sour 'Chicken Tonight'	4 oz	80	19.0	0.0
(Ragu) sweet and spicy, light 'Chicken Tonight'	4 oz	50	10.0	<1.0
CHILI SAUCE				
(Chef Boyardee) hot dog, w/beef	1 oz	30	4.0	1.0

Food Name	Serv. Size	Total Cal.	Carbs GMS	Fat GMS
(Del Monte) tomato	1/4 cup	70	17.0	0.0
(El Molino) green, mild	2 tbsp	10	2.0	0.0
(Featherweight)	1 tbsp	8	2.0	0.0
(Gebhardt) hot dog	2 tbsp	20	2.0	1.0
(Heinz)	1 oz	30	7.0	0.0
(Hunt's)	1.199 oz	35	8.0	0.1
(Las Palmas) red	1/2 cup	25	3.0	1.0
(Manwich) 'Chili Fixin's'	5.3 oz	110	20.0	<1.0
(S&W) 'Chili Makin's'	1/2 cup	100	20.0	1.0
(Wolf Brand) hot dog	1.25 oz	44	4.4	2.3
CHOCOLATE SAUCE *(Chocolate Mountain)*	2 tbsp	120	20.0	4.0
CLAM SAUCE				
Red				
(Buitoni)	5 oz	190	28.0	6.0
(Contadina) 'Fresh' refrigerated	7.5 oz	120	15.0	4.0
(Ferrara)	4 oz	70	8.0	2.0
(Progresso)	1/2 cup	70	7.0	3.0
White				
(Contadina) 'Fresh' refrigerated	6 oz	290	13.0	23.0
(Ferrara)	4 oz	80	4.0	5.0
(Progresso)	1/2 cup	110	1.0	8.0
COCKTAIL SAUCE				
(Del Monte)	1/4 cup	70	17.0	0.0
(Estee)	1 tbsp	10	2.0	<1.0
(Golden Dipt) extra hot	1 tbsp	20	5.0	0.0
(Golden Dipt) regular	1 tbsp	20	5.0	0.0
(Great Impressions)	1 tbsp	21	4.7	0.1
(Great Impressions) 'Brandy Glow'	1 tbsp	68	1.6	6.7
(Great Impressions) 'Low Salt'	1 tbsp	21	4.8	0.1
(Sauceworks)	1 tbsp	14	3.0	0.0
(Skipper's)	1 tbsp	20	5.0	0.0
(Stokely)	1 tbsp	18	5.0	0.0
CRANBERRY-ORANGE SAUCE				
(Ocean Spray) crushed, for chicken 'Cran•Fruit'	2 oz	90	23.0	0.0
CRANBERRY-RASPBERRY SAUCE				
(Ocean Spray) crushed, for chicken 'Cran•Fruit'	2 oz	90	23.0	0.0
CREOLE SAUCE				
(Enrico's) Cajun 'Light'	4 oz	76	9.0	2.8
(Golden Dipt) cooking sauce	1 oz	20	2.0	1.0
DIABLO SAUCE *(Escoffier)*	1 tbsp	20	4.0	0.0
DIJONAISSE SAUCE *(Golden Dipt)* cooking sauce	1 oz	52	2.0	4.0
ENCHILADA SAUCE				
(Gebhardt)	3 tbsp	25	3.0	1.0

Food Name	Serv. Size	Total Cal.	Carbs GMS	Fat GMS
(La Victoria)	1 cup	80	10.0	5.0
(Rosarita)	3 oz	20	4.0	0.0
Green (Old El Paso)	2 tbsp	11	3.0	0.0
Hot				
(Del Monte)	1/2 cup	45	11.0	0.0
(El Molino)	2 tbsp	16	2.0	1.0
(Las Palmas)	1/2 cup	25	3.0	1.0
(Old El Paso)	1/4 cup	30	4.0	1.0
(Ortega)	1 oz	12	3.0	0.0
Mild				
(Del Monte)	1/2 cup	45	11.0	0.0
(Old El Paso)	1/4 cup	25	4.0	1.0
(Ortega)	1 oz	12	3.0	0.0
(Rosarita)	2.5 oz	25	3.0	1.0
FAJITA SAUCE (Tio Sancho) 'Skillet Sauce'	1 oz	14	1.8	0.5
FORESTIERA SAUCE (Contadina) 'Fresh' refrigerated	7.5 oz	270	15.0	9.0
FOUR CHEESE SAUCE				
(Contadina)	4 oz	300	7.0	27.0
(Contadina) 'Fresh' refrigerated	6 oz	470	8.0	45.0
(DiGiorno) refrigerated	2 oz	170	3.0	16.0
FRENCH WHITE SAUCE (Golden Dipt) cooking sauce	1 oz	55	3.0	4.0
GARLIC-CHILI PEPPER SAUCE (A Taste of Thai)	1 tbsp	10	2.0	0.0
GARLIC-HERB SAUCE (Golden Dipt) 'Nature Bay'	2 grams	8	1.0	0.0
GUAVA SAUCE, cooked	1/2 cup	43	11.3	0.2
HERB AND GARLIC SAUCE (Lawry's) w/lemon juice	1/4 cup	36	3.8	0.4
HOLLANDAISE SAUCE (Great Impressions)	2 tbsp	192	0.3	21.0
HONEY SOY SAUCE				
(Golden Dipt) cooking sauce	1 oz	90	5.0	8.0
(Golden Dipt) 'Nature Bay'	1 oz	90	5.0	8.0
HORSERADISH SAUCE				
(Great Impressions)	1 tbsp	74	1.4	7.6
(Heinz)	1 tbsp	74	2.0	7.4
(Life) strong 'All Natural'	1/2 tbsp	7	<1.0	<1.0
(Sauceworks)	1 tbsp	50	2.0	5.0
HOT DOG SAUCE (Just Rite)	2 oz	60	6.0	3.0
HOT PEPPER SAUCE				
(Gebhardt) 'Louisiana Style'	1/2 tsp	0	(tr)	0.0
(Tabasco)	1/4 tsp	<1	<1.0	tr
HOT SAUCE (Gebhardt)	1/2 tsp	<1	<1.0	<1.0
JALAPEÑO CHEESE SAUCE				
(Pablo's) 'Deli Style'	1 oz	59	4.0	4.0
(White House)	3.5 oz	193	10.0	16.0

Food Name	Serv. Size	Total Cal.	Carbs GMS	Fat GMS
LEMON BUTTER-DILL SAUCE				
(Golden Dipt) cooking sauce	1 oz	110	5.0	10.0
LEMON-DILL SAUCE (Golden Dipt) 'Nature Bay'	1 oz	110	3.0	11.0
LOBSTER SAUCE (Progresso) rock	1/2 cup	120	11.0	8.0
MARINARA SAUCE				
(Angela Mia)	4.409 oz	47	9.0	1.5
(Buitoni)	1/2 cup	70	11.0	3.0
(DiGiorno) refrigerated	5 oz	110	12.0	6.0
(Millina's Finest) organic, fat-free	4 oz	48	9.0	0.5
(Millina's Finest) Zinfandel, organic, fat-free	4 oz	44	9.0	0.5
(Pathmark) 'All Natural'	1/2 cup	80	12.0	2.0
(Pathmark) 'No Frills'	1/2 cup	80	12.0	3.0
(Prego)	4 oz	100	10.0	6.0
(Progresso)	1/2 cup	90	9.0	5.0
(Progresso) 'Authentic Pasta Sauces'	1/2 cup	110	10.0	6.0
(Rokeach)	3 oz	60	9.0	2.0
(Westbrae)	4 oz	40	7.0	<1.0
(Westbrae) w/mushrooms	4 oz	50	7.0	29.0
MESQUITE SAUCE (Lawry's) w/lime juice	1/4 cup	24	3.0	0.4
MUSHROOM SAUCE (Quincy's)	3 oz	27	5.0	<1.0
NACHO CHEESE SAUCE				
(J. Hungerford)	2.011 oz	120	7.0	9.0
(J. Hungerford) 'Stadium'	2.011 oz	80	6.0	5.0
(Kaukauna)	1 oz	80	4.0	6.0
(Lucky Leaf)	4 oz	220	11.0	18.0
(Musselman's)	4 oz	220	11.0	18.0
(Pablo's) 'Deli Style'	1 oz	59	4.0	4.0
(White House)	3.5 oz	193	10.0	16.0
NEWBURG SAUCE (Snow's) w/sherry	1/3 cup	120	10.0	8.0
ORANGE SAUCE (LaChoy) Mandarin	1 tbsp	24	6.1	tr
ORANGE-DIJON SAUCE (Golden Dipt) 'Nature Bay'	1 oz	110	6.0	9.0
OREGANO-HERB SAUCE (Golden Dipt) 'Nature Bay'	2 grams	6	1.0	0.0
PARMIGIANA SAUCE (Betty Crocker) 'Recipe Sauces'	3.9 oz	50	9.0	1.0
PASTA SAUCE/spaghetti sauce				
(Angela Mia)	4.409 oz	49	10.6	0.5
(Campbell's) 'Homestyle'	4 oz	40	10.0	0.0
(Enrico's) 'All Natural'	4 oz	60	9.0	1.0
(Hunt's) 'Homestyle'	4 oz	60	10.0	2.0
(Hunt's) 'Olde Country'	4 oz	60	8.0	2.0
(Progresso)	1/2 cup	110	13.0	5.0
(Ragu) 'Old World Style'	4 oz	80	9.0	4.0
(Ragu) 'Slow Cooked Homestyle'	4 oz	110	15.0	5.0
(Ragu) 'Thick & Hearty'	4 oz	100	15.0	3.0

Food Name	Serv. Size	Total Cal.	Carbs GMS	Fat GMS
Garden				
(Prego) combination	4 oz	80	14.0	2.0
(Pritikin) chunky	1/2 cup	50	11.0	0.0
(Ragu) harvest 'Todays Recipe'	4 oz	50	8.0	1.0
Garlic and herb				
(Healthy Choice)	4 oz	40	9.0	<1.0
(Hunt's) 'Classic'	4.409 oz	58	9.5	2.1
(Hunt's) 'Light'	4.409 oz	39	7.3	0.8
(Hunt's) 'Olde Country'	4.409 oz	63	8.9	2.7
Garlic and onion				
(Campbell's) extra	4 oz	50	12.0	<1.0
(Del Monte)	1/2 cup	70	10.0	2.0
(Healthy Choice) chunky	4 oz	40	10.0	0.0
(Prego)	4 oz	110	16.0	4.0
Italian				
(Campbell's)	4 oz	50	12.0	0.0
(Healthy Choice) vegetable, chunky	4 oz	40	9.0	0.0
(Hunt's) vegetable 'Olde Country'	4.409 oz	64	9.0	2.6
(Pastorelli) 'Italian Chef'	4 oz	81	11.0	3.0
(Ragu) 'Fresh Italian'	4 oz	90	13.0	3.0
(Ragu) garden combination 'Chunky Gardenstyle'	4 oz	110	15.0	5.0
Meat				
(Chef Boyardee) w/ground beef 'Jars'	4 oz	90	14.0	3.0
(Hunt's)	4.444 oz	65	10.9	2.3
(Hunt's) 'Homestyle'	4.409 oz	56	6.9	2.6
(Hunt's) 'Light'	4.409 oz	45	7.9	1.2
(Hunt's) 'Olde Country'	4.409 oz	56	7.2	2.6
(Ragu) 'Homestyle'	4 oz	110	15.0	5.0
Meat flavor				
(Chef Boyardee)	3.75 oz	80	11.0	3.0
(Chef Boyardee) 'Original'	3.75 oz	120	13.0	6.0
(Contadina) 'Original Recipe'	1/2 cup	100	17.2	3.2
(Del Monte)	1/2 cup	70	9.0	2.0
(Hunt's)	4 oz	70	12.0	2.0
(P&Q)	1/2 cup	70	11.0	2.0
(Pathmark) 'All Natural'	1/2 cup	80	11.0	3.0
(Pathmark) 'No Frills'	1/2 cup	90	11.0	5.0
(Prego)	4 oz	140	20.0	6.0
(Progresso)	1/2 cup	110	13.0	5.0
(Weight Watchers)	1/3 cup	50	9.0	1.0
Meatless				
(Chef Boyardee) 'Jars'	4 oz	60	11.0	1.0
(P&Q)	1/2 cup	70	14.0	1.0

Food Name	Serv. Size	Total Cal.	Carbs GMS	Fat GMS
(Pathmark) 'All Natural'	1/2 cup	70	11.0	2.0
(Pathmark) 'No Frills'	1/2 cup	80	11.0	3.0
Mushroom				
(Campbell's)	4 oz	50	11.0	<1.0
(Campbell's) 'Healthy Request'	4 oz	50	11.0	<1.0
(Contadina) 'Original Recipe'	1/2 cup	90	17.5	2.3
(Del Monte)	1/2 cup	70	11.0	2.0
(Healthy Choice) chunky	4 oz	45	10.0	0.0
(Hunt's)	4.444 oz	65	10.9	2.3
(Hunt's) 'Homestyle'	4.409 oz	56	6.9	2.6
(Hunt's) 'Light'	4.409 oz	39	7.3	0.8
(Hunt's) 'Olde Country'	4.409 oz	53	7.0	2.7
(Prego) w/extra spice 'Extra Chunky'	4 oz	100	17.0	3.0
(Ragu) chunky 'Todays Recipe'	4 oz	50	8.0	1.0
(Ragu) 'Homestyle'	4 oz	110	15.0	2.0
(Ragu) super 'Chunky Gardenstyle'	4 oz	110	15.0	5.0
(Ragu) 'Thick & Hearty'	4 oz	100	15.0	3.0
Mushroom and green pepper				
(Enrico's) 'All Natural'	4 oz	60	9.0	1.0
(Enrico's) 'All Natural No Salt Added'	4 oz	60	9.0	1.0
(Prego) 'Extra Chunky'	4 oz	100	14.0	4.0
(Ragu) 'Chunky Gardenstyle'	4 oz	110	15.0	5.0
Mushroom and onion				
(Prego) 'Extra Chunky'	4 oz	100	13.0	4.0
(Ragu) 'Chunky Gardenstyle'	4 oz	110	15.0	5.0
Mushroom and tomato				
(DiGiorno) w/plum tomatoes, refrigerated	5 oz	100	20.0	1.0
(Millina's Finest) organic, fat-free	4 oz	45	9.0	0.5
(Prego) 'Extra Chunky'	4 oz	110	14.0	5.0
Mushroom flavor				
(Chef Boyardee)	3.75 oz	60	11.0	1.0
(Chef Boyardee) 'Jars'	4 oz	70	11.0	2.0
(Chef Boyardee) 'Original'	3.75 oz	80	13.0	3.0
(Enrico's)	4 oz	60	9.0	1.0
(Enrico's) w/fresh mushrooms	4 oz	60	9.0	1.0
(Featherweight)	4 oz	60	11.0	1.0
(Hunt's)	4 oz	70	12.0	2.0
(P&Q)	1/2 cup	70	14.0	1.0
(Pathmark) 'All Natural'	1/2 cup	70	11.0	2.0
(Prego)	4 oz	130	20.0	5.0
(Progresso)	1/2 cup	110	13.0	5.0
(Weight Watchers)	1/3 cup	40	9.0	0.0

Food Name	Serv. Size	Total Cal.	Carbs GMS	Fat GMS
No salt added				
(Eden Foods) organic	4 oz	80	14.0	2.0
(Enrico's) 'All Natural No Salt Added'	4 oz	60	9.0	1.0
(Prego) 'No Salt Added'	4 oz	110	11.0	6.0
Original (Pritikin)	1/2 cup	60	14.0	1.0
Parmesan, 'Classic' (Hunt's)	4.409 oz	50	7.8	2.1
Primavera				
(Progresso) creamy 'Authentic Pasta Sauces'	1/2 cup	190	8.0	17.0
(Westbrae)	4 oz	60	7.0	3.0
(Westbrae) no salt	4 oz	40	7.0	0.0
Sausage and green pepper (Prego) 'Extra Chunky'	4 oz	160	19.0	8.0
Sicilian (Progresso) 'Authentic Pasta Sauces'	1/2 cup	30	2.0	2.5
Sweet pepper and onion (Millina's Finest) organic, fat-free	4 oz	41	7.0	0.5
Three cheese (Prego)	4 oz	100	17.0	2.0
Tomato and basil				
(Hunt's) 'Classic'	4.409 oz	48	7.5	2.1
(Millina's Finest) organic, fat-free	4 oz	46	9.0	0.5
Tomato and herb				
(Ragu) 'Homestyle'	4 oz	110	15.0	5.0
(Ragu) 'Ragu Fine Italian'	4 oz	90	13.0	3.0
(Ragu) 'Today's Recipe'	4 oz	50	8.0	1.0
Tomato chunks (Hunt's) 'Chunky Style'	4 oz	50	12.0	<1.0
Tomato-based				
(Prego) and basil	4 oz	100	18.0	2.0
(Prego) and onion 'Extra Chunky'	4 oz	110	14.0	5.0
Tomatoes, garlic, and onion (Ragu) 'Chunky Gardenstyle'	4 oz	110	15.0	5.0
Traditional				
(Contadina) 'Original Recipe'	1/2 cup	90	17.0	2.3
(Del Monte)	1/2 cup	70	11.0	2.0
(Healthy Choice)	4 oz	40	9.0	<1.0
(Hunt's) 'Homestyle'	4.409 oz	56	3.9	2.6
(Hunt's) 'Light'	4.409 oz	39	7.3	0.8
(Hunt's) 'Olde Country'	4.409 oz	53	7.0	2.7
(Hunt's) 'Traditional'	4 oz	70	12.0	2.0
Zinfandel wine (Sutter Home)	1/2 cup	100	11.0	5.0
PEPPER STEAK SAUCE (Betty Crocker) 'Recipe Sauces'	3.8 oz	50	8.0	2.0
PEPPER-DILL SAUCE (Golden Dipt) 'Nature Bay'	2 grams	8	1.0	0.0
PESTO SAUCE				
(Contadina) refrigerated 'Fresh'	2.33 oz	350	6.0	34.0
(DiGiorno) refrigerated	2.3 oz	340	5.0	32.0
PICANTE SAUCE				
(Estee)	2 tbsp	8	2.0	0.0
(Gebhardt)	1 tbsp	4	1.0	0.0

Food Name	Serv. Size	Total Cal.	Carbs GMS	Fat GMS
(Wise)	2 tbsp	12	3.0	0.0
All varieties				
(Old El Paso)	2 tbsp	8	2.0	<1.0
(Old El Paso) 'Chunky'	2 tbsp	7	2.0	0.0
Extra mild *(Pace)* 'Thick & Chunky'	2 tsp	3	0.5	0.1
Hot				
(Chi-Chi's)	1 oz	10	2.0	2.0
(Guiltless Gourmet)	1 oz	8	1.0	0.0
(Pace) 'Thick & Chunky'	2 tsp	3	0.5	0.1
(Rosarita) chunky	3 tbsp	18	4.0	<1.0
(Rosarita) zesty jalapeño	1.093 oz	8	1.7	0.2
Medium				
(Chi-Chi's)	1 oz	8	2.0	2.0
(Guiltless Gourmet)	1 oz	8	1.0	0.0
(Pace) 'Thick & Chunky'	2 tsp	3	0.5	0.1
(Rosarita) chunky	3 tbsp	16	4.0	(mq)
(Rosarita) zesty jalapeño	1.093 oz	9	1.7	0.2
Mild				
(Azteca)	1 tbsp	4	1.0	0.0
(Chi-Chi's)	1 oz	9	2.0	2.0
(Guiltless Gourmet)	1 oz	8	1.0	0.0
(Hunt's) 'Homestyle'	1.093 oz	11	2.1	0.2
(Pace) 'Thick & Chunky'	2 tsp	3	0.5	0.1
(Rosarita)	3.5 oz	45	9.0	<1.0
(Rosarita) chunky	3 tbsp	25	5.0	<1.0
(Rosarita) zesty jalapeño	1.093 oz	8	1.7	0.1
PIZZA SAUCE				
(Angela Mia)	2.222 oz	27	5.2	0.6
(Angela Mia) super heavy 'Premium Choice'	2.258 oz	28	5.8	0.5
(Chef Boyardee) w/cheese	2.63 oz	70	7.0	4.0
(Chef Boyardee) w/cheese 'Jars'	3.88 oz	90	10.0	6.0
(Contadina) original 'Quick & Easy'	1/4 cup	30	5.0	1.0
(Contadina) 'Pizza Squeeze'	1/4 cup	30	5.0	1.0
(Contadina) w/Italian cheese	1/4 cup	30	5.0	1.0
(Contadina) w/pepperoni	1/4 cup	40	5.0	2.0
(Eden Foods) and pasta sauce, organic	4 oz	80	10.0	3.0
(Enrico's) 'Homemade Style All Natural'	4 oz	60	9.0	1.0
(Enrico's) 'Homemade Style All Natural No Salt'	4 oz	60	9.0	1.0
(Hunt's)	2.363 oz	32	4.9	1.1
(Hunt's)	2.222 oz	21	3.8	0.5
(Pastorelli) 'Italian Chef'	4 oz	90	12.0	3.0
(Pizza Quick)	3 tbsp	35	3.0	2.0
(Pizza Quick) traditional	1.7 oz	35	3.0	2.0

Food Name	Serv. Size	Total Cal.	Carbs GMS	Fat GMS
PLUM SAUCE *(LaChoy)* tangy	1 oz	45	10.8	0.1
RIB SAUCE *(Dip 'n Joy)* 'Saucy Rib'	1 oz	60	14.0	0.0
RIGOLLETO SAUCE *(DiGiorno)* refrigerated	5 oz	110	9.0	8.0
ROBERT SAUCE *(Escoffier)* 'Sauce Robert'	1 tbsp	20	5.0	0.0
SANDWICH SAUCE				
(Hormel) 'Not-so-Sloppy Sloppy Joe'	2.24 oz	70	16.0	1.0
(Libby's) 'Sloppy Joe'	2.5 oz	45	10.0	<1.0
(Manwich)	2.5 oz	40	10.0	0.0
(Manwich) bold	2.222 oz	62	13.1	1.1
(Manwich) extra thick and chunky	2.5 oz	60	15.0	<1.0
(Manwich) Mexican	2.258 oz	26	5.0	0.2
(Manwich) Mexican 'Sloppy Joe'	2.5 oz	35	9.0	<1.0
(Manwich) thick and chunky	2.293 oz	44	8.6	0.5
SEAFOOD COCKTAIL SAUCE *(Heinz)*	1/4 cup	60	13.0	0.0
SEAFOOD SAUCE				
(Great Impressions) Creole	1 tbsp	21	4.7	0.1
(Great Impressions) dipping	1 tbsp	17	2.2	0.7
(Great Impressions) dipping, Polynesian	1 tbsp	38	9.5	<1.0
SEASONING SAUCE *(A Taste of Thai)*	1 tbsp	15	1.0	0.0
SHOYU. See SOY SAUCE.				
SHRIMP SAUCE *(Tone's)* 'Craboil'	1 tsp	10	1.2	0.6
SOY SAUCE				
shoyu	1 tbsp	9	1.5	tr
shoyu, low-sodium	1 tbsp	9	1.5	tr
tamari	1 tbsp	11	1.0	<.1
(Eden Foods) shoyu, organic	1/2 tsp	2	0.0	0.0
(Eden Foods) shoyu, organic, reduced sodium	1/2 tsp	2	0.0	0.0
(Kikkoman)	1 tbsp	10	0.9	tr
(Kikkoman) 'Lite'	1 tbsp	11	1.3	tr
(LaChoy)	1 tsp	<1	0.3	0.0
(LaChoy) 'Lite'	1 tsp	<1	0.3	0.0
(Westbrae) mild	1/2 tsp	2	1.0	0.0
(Westbrae) organic	1/2 tsp	2	1.0	0.0
(Westbrae) tamari	1/2 tsp	2	1.0	0.0
(Westbrae) wheat-free	1/2 tsp	3	1.0	0.0
SPAGHETTI SAUCE. See PASTA SAUCE.				
STEAK SAUCE				
(A.1.)	1 tbsp	18	4.0	0.0
(A.1.) bold	1 tbsp	18	4.0	0.0
(Heinz) '57'	1 tbsp	16	4.0	0.0
(Heinz) hickory smoke '57'	1 tbsp	16	4.0	0.0
(Heinz) traditional	1 tbsp	12	2.6	0.0
(Hunt's)	1 tbsp	10	2.3	0.1

Food Name	Serv. Size	Total Cal.	Carbs GMS	Fat GMS
(Lea & Perrins)	1 oz	40	10.0	<1.0
STIR-FRY SAUCE				
(Kikkoman)	1 tsp	6	2.3	tr
(LaChoy) Mandarin	4.48 oz	71	15.6	0.2
(LaChoy) sweet and sour	4.797 oz	146	34.8	0.1
(LaChoy) Szechwan	4.55 oz	73	16.0	0.2
(Lawry's)	1/4 cup	120	19.6	3.8
STROGANOFF SAUCE (Betty Crocker) 'Recipe Sauces'	4 oz	60	6.0	4.0
SWEET AND SOUR SAUCE				
(A Taste of Thai) tangy, hot	2 tbsp	30	8.0	0.0
(Betty Crocker) 'Recipe Sauces'	4.1 oz	130	32.0	0.0
(Contadina)	1/2 cup	150	32.0	3.0
(Great Impressions) Hawaiian	2 tbsp	102	25.5	0.0
(Great Impressions) hot	2 tbsp	102	25.5	0.0
(Great Impressions) regular	2 tbsp	102	25.5	0.0
(Hickory Farms) Hawaiian	2 tbsp	102	25.5	0.0
(Hickory Farms) regular	2 tbsp	102	25.5	0.0
(Kikkoman)	1 tbsp	18	4.0	0.0
(LaChoy)	1 tbsp	30	7.0	na
(LaChoy) duck sauce	1 tbsp	26	6.9	tr
(Lawry's)	1/4 cup	549	11.7	7.5
(Sauceworks)	1 tbsp	25	5.0	0.0
SZECHUAN SAUCE (LaChoy) hot and spicy	1 oz	48	12.0	0.2
TACO SAUCE				
(Estee)	2 tbsp	14	3.0	0.0
(Hain) and dip	4 tbsp	25	5.0	1.0
(Lawry's) 'Sauce'n Seasoner'	1/4 cup	40	7.6	0.6
(Old El Paso)	2 tbsp	15	3.0	0.0
(Rosarita)	.1764 oz	2	0.4	0.0
Chunky (Lawry's)	1/4 cup	22	4.0	0.4
Green (La Victoria)	1 tbsp	0	1.0	0.0
Hot				
(Chi-Chi's)	1 oz	18	4.0	2.0
(Del Monte)	1/4 cup	15	4.0	0.0
(Old El Paso)	2 tbsp	10	2.0	<1.0
(Ortega)	1 oz	12	3.0	0.0
Medium				
(Heinz)	1 tbsp	6	1.0	0.0
(Old El Paso)	2 tbsp	10	2.0	<1.0
Mild				
(Del Monte)	1/2 cup	15	4.0	0.0
(Enrico's) 'No Salt Added'	2 tbsp	14	3.0	0.0
(Heinz)	1 tbsp	6	1.0	0.0

Food Name	Serv. Size	Total Cal.	Carbs GMS	Fat GMS
(Old El Paso)	2 tbsp	10	2.0	<1.0
(Ortega)	1 oz	12	3.0	0.0
Red				
(El Molino) mild	2 tbsp	10	2.0	0.0
(La Victoria)	1 tbsp	5	1.0	0.0
Thick, chunky (Chi-Chi's)	1 oz	12	3.0	2.0
Western style (Ortega)	1 oz	8	2.0	0.0
TAMARI SAUCE. See SOY SAUCE.				
TARTAR SAUCE				
(Best Foods)	1 tbsp	70	0.0	8.0
(Best Foods) reduced fat	1 tbsp	30	3.0	2.0
(Golden Dipt)	1 tbsp	70	2.0	7.0
(Golden Dipt) 'Lite'	1 tbsp	50	4.0	4.0
(Great Impressions)	1 tbsp	86	1.2	9.0
(Heinz)	2 tbsp	140	4.0	14.0
(Hellmann's)	1 tbsp	70	0.0	8.0
(Kraft) nonfat 'Free'	1 tbsp	10	3.0	0.0
(Life) egg-free 'All Natural'	1 tbsp	38	<1.0	4.0
(Sauceworks)	1 tbsp	50	2.0	5.0
(Sauceworks) natural lemon and herb flavor	1 tbsp	70	0.0	8.0
(Skipper's)	1 tbsp	65	0.0	7.0
(Weight Watchers)	1 tbsp	35	3.0	3.0
TERIYAKI SAUCE				
(Betty Crocker) 'Recipe Sauces'	3.9 oz	60	13.0	<1.0
(Golden Dipt) ginger marinade	1 oz	120	12.0	7.0
(Kikkoman)	1 tbsp	15	2.7	tr
(Kikkoman) 'Baste & Glaze'	1 tbsp	27	6.0	tr
(LaChoy)	1/2 tsp	5	1.0	<1.0
(LaChoy) basting sauce	1/2 tsp	2	<1.0	<1.0
(LaChoy) 'Lite'	1/2 tsp	5	1.0	<1.0
(LaChoy) 'Sauce and Marinade'	1 oz	30	5.0	0.0
(LaChoy) stir-fry sauce	4.621 oz	105	24.3	0.1
(LaChoy) thick and rich	1 oz	41	9.4	0.1
(Lawry's) barbecue marinade	1/8 cup	82	13.7	1.1
(Lawry's) w/pineapple juice	1/4 cup	72	11.0	0.4
VEGETABLE SAUCE				
(Contadina) refrigerated, garden 'Light'	.5 oz	50	10.0	0.0
WORCESTERSHIRE SAUCE				
(French's) regular	1 tbsp	10	2.0	0.0
(French's) smoky	1 tbsp	10	2.0	0.0
(Heinz)	1 tsp	0	0.0	0.0
(Lea & Perrins)	1 tsp	5	1.0	<1.0
(Lea & Perrins) white wine	1 tsp	4	1.0	<1.0

Food Name	Serv. Size	Total Cal.	Carbs GMS	Fat GMS
(Life) 'All Natural'	1/2 tbsp	5	1.0	<1.0
SAUCE MIX				
ALFREDO SAUCE				
(French's) 'Pasta Toss' dry mix	2 tsp	25	2.0	2.0
(Lawry's) 'Pasta Alfredo' dry mix	1 pkg	226	19.2	13.3
BEARNAISE SAUCE dry mix	.9-oz pkg	90	14.8	2.2
BEEF SAUTÉ SAUCE *(Lipton)* golden, dry mix	1/6 pkg	120	24.0	2.0
CHEESE SAUCE				
(French's) prepared	1/4 cup	80	7.0	4.0
(McCormick/Schilling) dry mix	1/4 pkg	35	3.5	1.5
(McCormick/Schilling) nacho, dry mix	1/4 pkg	42	4.5	1.5
CHICKEN SAUCE				
(Lawry's) southwest 'Seasoning Blends' dry mix	1 pkg	71	16.0	0.3
(McCormick/Schilling) cacciatore 'Sauce Blends' dry mix	1 pkg	132	28.0	4.8
(McCormick/Schilling) Creole 'Sauce Blends' dry mix	1 pkg	140	24.0	4.8
(McCormick/Schilling) curry 'Sauce Blends' dry mix	1 pkg	152	24.0	5.6
(McCormick/Schilling) Dijon 'Sauce Blends' dry mix	1 pkg	156	20.0	6.8
(McCormick/Schilling) mesquite marinade 'Sauce Blends' dry mix	1 pkg	132	24.0	3.0
(McCormick/Schilling) teriyaki 'Sauce Blends' dry mix	1 pkg	172	28.0	3.6
CURRY SAUCE, prepared	1/2 cup	135	12.9	7.4
HOLLANDAISE SAUCE *(McCormick/Schilling)* dry mix	1/4 pkg	51	3.5	3.8
LEMON BUTTER SAUCE *(Weight Watchers)* dry mix	1 tbsp	6	1.0	0.0
MUSHROOM SAUCE dry mix	1-oz pkg	99	15.5	2.7
PASTA SAUCE				
(Estee) prepared w/margarine and skim milk	4 oz	60	9.0	1.0
(Featherweight) prepared w/margarine and skim milk	4 oz	60	11.0	1.0
(French's) cheese and garlic 'Pasta Toss' dry mix	2 tsp	25	2.0	2.0
(French's) Italian 'Pasta Toss' dry mix	2 tsp	25	2.0	2.0
(French's) Italian style, prepared	5/8 cup	100	15.0	4.0
(French's) Romanoff 'Pasta Toss' dry mix	2 tsp	30	1.0	2.0
(French's) w/mushrooms, prepared	5/8 cup	100	13.0	4.0
(Lawry's) 'Rich & Thick' dry mix	1 pkg	147	28.1	2.2
(Lawry's) w/imported mushrooms, dry mix	1 pkg	143	26.0	1.5
(McCormick/Schilling) dry mix	1/4 pkg	32	6.0	0.3
(Prego) prepared w/margarine and skim milk	4 oz	130	20.0	5.0
(Ragu) prepared w/margarine and skim milk	4 oz	80	9.0	4.0
PEANUT SAUCE *(A Taste of Thai)* dry mix	2 tbsp	25	4.0	0.5
PESTO SAUCE *(French's)* 'Pasta Toss' dry mix	2 tsp	20	1.0	1.0
SANDWICH SAUCE *(Manwich)* dry mix	.2469 oz	22	5.3	0.1
SEAFOOD SAUCE *(Progresso)* prepared	1/2 cup	110	12.0	6.0
SOUR CREAM SAUCE *(McCormick/Schilling)* dry mix	1/4 pkg	44	4.0	2.8

Food Name	Serv. Size	Total Cal.	Carbs GMS	Fat GMS
STROGANOFF SAUCE				
(Lawry's) dry mix	1 pkg	123	25.5	0.3
(Natural Touch) prepared	4 oz	90	10.0	3.0
SWEET AND SOUR SAUCE, dry mix	2-oz pkg	220	54.5	0.1
TACO SAUCE (Tio Sancho) 'Dinner Kit' dry mix	2-oz pkg	62	13.4	0.2
TERIYAKI SAUCE dry mix	1.6-oz pkg	130	27.6	0.9
WHITE SAUCE prepared	1/2 cup	121	10.7	6.7
SAUERKRAUT, CANNED				
(A&P)	1/2 cup	20	5.0	<1.0
(Allens) w/liquid, shredded	1/2 cup	21	5.0	<1.0
(Bush's Best) 'Bavarian Kraut'	1/2 cup	60	15.0	0.0
(Bush's Best) 'Kraut' deli style	1/2 cup	20	5.0	0.0
(Bush's Best) 'Kraut' shredded	1/2 cup	20	5.0	0.0
(Claussen)	1/2 cup	17	3.2	0.2
(Del Monte)	1/2 cup	25	6.0	0.0
(Eden Foods) organic	1/2 cup	25	4.0	<1.0
(Finast)	1/2 cup	30	6.0	0.0
(Pathmark)	1/2 cup	20	4.0	0.0
(Snow Floss)	1/2 cup	28	4.0	0.0
(Stokely) 'Bavarian'	1/2 cup	30	7.0	0.0
(Stokely) w/liquid, shredded and chopped	1/2 cup	20	4.0	0.0
(Vlasic) 'Old Fashioned'	1 oz	4	1.0	0.0
SAUERKRAUT JUICE				
canned	1 cup	24	5.6	0.0
canned or bottled (Biotta)	6 oz	21	4.0	0.1
canned or bottled (S&W)	5 oz	14	3.0	0.0
SAUSAGE. See also individual listings.				
(Hickory Farms) 'Safari'	1 oz	98	1.0	9.0
(Hillshire Farm) 'Country Recipe'	2 oz	180	2.0	16.0
(Hormel)	3 oz	290	1.0	27.0
(JM) .5-oz patties, cooked	1 patty	70	1.0	6.0
(JM) raw	1 oz	130	1.0	14.0
(Jones Dairy Farm)	1 patty	155	tr	14.4
(Jones Dairy Farm) 'Golden Brown'	1 patty	155	tr	14.7
(Jones Dairy Farm) 'Golden Brown' mild	1 link	100	tr	9.8
(Jones Dairy Farm) 'Golden Brown' spicy	1 link	100	tr	9.5
Brown and serve				
(Eckrich) 'Lean Supreme Heat 'n Serve'	2 links	120	1.0	10.0
(Hormel)	2 links	140	0.0	13.0
(Hormel) uncooked	2 links	180	0.0	17.0
(Jones Dairy Farm) 'Light'	1 link	60	1.0	4.1
(Swift) 'Country Recipe'	1 link	130	1.0	12.0
(Swift) 'Country Recipe'	1 patty	130	1.0	12.0

Food Name	Serv. Size	Total Cal.	Carbs GMS	Fat GMS
(Swift) microwave	1 link	120	1.0	12.0
(Swift) 'Premium Original'	1 link	130	1.0	12.0
(Swift) 'Premium Original'	1 patty	120	1.0	12.0
(Swift) smoked flavor	1 link	120	1.0	11.0
Roll				
(Eckrich) minced	1-oz slice	80	1.0	7.0
(Jones Dairy Farm) 'Cello Roll'	1 slice	105	tr	9.6
BEEF				
(Eckrich)	1 oz	100	<1.0	9.0
(Eckrich) 'Lean Supreme'	1 oz	80	1.0	7.0
(Eckrich) 'Smok-Y-Links'	2 links	160	2.0	14.0
(Hillshire Farm) 'Bun Size'	2 oz	180	2.0	16.0
(Hillshire Farm) 'Flavorseal'	2 oz	180	2.0	16.0
(Jones Dairy Farm) 'Golden Brown'	1 link	75	tr	6.1
(Oscar Mayer) 'Smokies' 1.5-oz links	1 link	124	0.7	11.0
(Swift) 'Premium Brown 'N Serve'	1 link	120	1.0	12.0
BEEF AND CHEDDAR *(Hillshire Farms)* 'Flavorseal'	2 oz	190	1.0	15.0
CHEESE				
(Hormel) 'Smokie Cheezers'	2 links	168	1.0	15.0
(Oscar Mayer) 'Smokies'	1.5 oz	126	0.7	11.2
Hot				
(Eckrich) 'Smok-Y-Links'	2 links	150	1.0	14.0
(Hillshire Farm) 'Flavorseal'	2 oz	180	2.0	16.0
Maple-flavored *(Eckrich)* 'Smok-Y-Links'	2 links	160	2.0	14.0
W/ham *(Eckrich)* 'Smok-Y-Links'	2 links	160	2.0	15.0
HOT				
(JM) .5-oz patties, cooked	1 patty	70	1.0	6.0
(JM) patties, raw	1 oz	130	1.0	14.0
(OHSE) 'Hot Links'	1 oz	80	4.0	3.0
ITALIAN STYLE				
cooked	3 oz	268	1.3	21.3
cooked	2.4 oz	216	1.0	17.2
pork, cooked	1 oz	92	0.4	7.3
pork, raw	1 oz	98	0.2	8.9
raw	4 oz	391	0.7	35.4
raw	3.2 oz	315	0.6	28.5
Hot *(Hillshire Farm)* 'Links'	2 oz	180	1.0	17.0
Mild *(Hillshire Farm)* 'Links'	2 oz	190	1.0	17.0
Smoked *(Hillshire Farm)* 'Flavorseal'	2 oz	200	1.0	18.0
MAPLE-FLAVORED *(Swift)* brown and serve	1 link	120	1.0	12.0
NEW ENGLAND STYLE				
(Eckrich)	1 oz	35	1.0	1.0
(Light & Lean)	2 slices	90	0.0	6.0

Food Name	Serv. Size	Total Cal.	Carbs GMS	Fat GMS
(Oscar Mayer) .8-oz slices	1 slice	29	0.4	1.3
PICKLED				
(Penrose) beer, .5-oz links	1 link	40	1.0	3.0
(Penrose) firecracker, 1.5-oz links	1 link	120	1.0	10.0
(Penrose) firecracker, .5-oz links	1 link	40	1.0	3.0
(Penrose) firecracker, giant, 2.1-oz links	1 link	170	1.0	14.0
(Penrose) hot, .5-oz links	1 link	40	1.0	3.0
(Penrose) Polish, .5-oz links	1 link	40	1.0	3.0
(Penrose) red hot, .5-oz links	1 link	40	1.0	3.0
POLISH STYLE				
	1 oz	92	0.5	8.1
10-inch sausage	1 link	740	3.7	65.2
PORK				
4-inch links, cooked	1 link	48	0.1	4.1
4-inch links, raw	1 link	117	0.3	11.3
fresh, cooked	1 oz	105	0.3	8.8
fresh, raw	2 oz	238	0.6	23.0
patties, 1/4 inch x 3 7/8 inch diam, cooked	1 patty	100	0.3	8.4
patties, 1/4 inch x 3 7/8 inch diam, raw	1 patty	238	0.6	23.0
(Hormel) 'Little Sizzlers'	2 links	103	0.0	9.0
(Hormel) 'Little Sizzlers'	1 oz	130	2.0	13.0
(Hormel) 'Midget Links'	2 links	143	0.0	13.0
(Jimmy Dean) cooked	1 oz	120	<1.0	11.0
(Jimmy Dean) links	2 links	180	<1.0	17.0
(Jimmy Dean) 'Light'	1.2 oz	80	<1.0	7.0
(Jimmy Dean) patties	1 patty	140	<1.0	13.0
(JM) 'Tasty Link' cooked	1.4 oz	190	1.0	18.0
(JM) 'Tasty Link' raw	1.8 oz	260	1.0	26.0
(Jones Dairy Farm)	1 link	140	tr	13.7
(Jones Dairy Farm) 'Golden Brown Light'	1 link	55	0.5	4.2
(Jones Dairy Farm) 'Light'	1 link	70	1.0	5.0
(Oscar Mayer) 'Little Friers' cooked	8.9 oz	989	2.8	90.3
(Oscar Mayer) 'Little Friers' cooked	1 link	82	0.2	7.5
(Tyson) country, whole hog	3.5 oz	320	1.0	29.0
PORK AND BACON *(JM)* 'Tasty Link' raw	1.8 oz	220	1.0	21.0
PORK AND BEEF				
fresh, cooked	1 oz	112	0.8	10.3
fresh, 1/4 inch x 3 7/8-inch diam patties, cooked	1 patty	107	0.7	9.8
fresh, 2 inch x 3/4-inch diam links, cooked	1 link	51	0.4	4.7
smoked, 4 inch x 1 1/8-inch diam links	1 link	228	1.0	20.6
smoked, 2 inch x 3/4-inch diam links	1 link	54	0.2	4.8
smoked, w/flour and nonfat dry milk added, 4 inch x 1 1/8-inch diam links	1 link	182	2.7	14.6

Food Name	Serv. Size	Total Cal.	Carbs GMS	Fat GMS
smoked, w/flour and nonfat dry milk added, 2 inch x 3/4-inch diam links	1 link	43	0.6	3.4
smoked, w/nonfat dry milk added, 4 inch x 1 1/8-inch diam links	1 link	213	1.3	18.8
smoked, w/nonfat dry milk added, 2 inch x 3/4-inch diam links	1 link	50	0.3	4.4
SAGE *(Jimmy Dean)* cooked	1 oz	120	<1.0	11.0
SMOKED				
(Eckrich) 'Lean Supreme'	1 oz	70	1.0	6.0
(Eckrich) 'Skinless'	1 link	180	2.0	16.0
(Hillshire Farm) 'Bun Size'	2 oz	180	2.0	16.0
(Hillshire Farm) 'Flavorseal'	2 oz	190	1.0	17.0
(Hillshire Farm) 'Links'	2 oz	190	1.0	18.0
(Hillshire Farm) 'Lite'	2 oz	160	2.0	13.0
(Hormel) 'Smokies'	2 links	160	2.0	14.0
(OHSE)	1 oz	80	1.0	7.0
(Oscar Mayer) 'Big & Juicy Smokie Links' 2.7-oz links	1 link	227	1.2	20.5
(Oscar Mayer) 'Little Smokies' .3-oz links	1 link	27	0.1	2.5
(Oscar Mayer) 'Smokie Links' 1.5-oz links	1 link	126	0.6	11.3
(Pilgrim's Pride)	3 oz	144	2.5	9.1
SWEDISH STYLE *(Hickory Farms)*	1 oz	100	0.0	9.0
TURKEY				
(Butterball)	1 oz	50	<1.0	4.0
(Jimmy Dean) 'Light'	1.2 oz	80	<1.0	7.0
(Louis Rich) cooked	1 link	46	0.1	2.7
(Louis Rich) 85% fat-free, cooked	24 gm	45	<1.0	3.0
(Norbest) 'Tasti-Lean' chub or links	1 oz	53	0.3	2.8
Breakfast type				
(Hudson's) ground	1 oz	65	0.0	5.3
(Louis Rich) 85% fat-free	1 oz	55	<1.0	3.0
(Louis Rich) ground, cooked	1 oz	56	0.2	3.5
(Mr. Turkey)	1 oz	58	0.4	4.3
Smoked				
(Louis Rich)	1 oz	43	0.7	2.4
(Louis Rich) 90% fat-free	1 oz	40	<1.0	2.0
(Louis Rich) w/cheese	1 oz	47	0.7	2.8
(Louis Rich) w/cheddar, 90% fat-free	1 oz	45	<1.0	3.0
(Mr. Turkey)	1 oz	47	0.5	3.4
TURKEY AND PORK *(Jimmy Dean)* 'Light'	1.2 oz	80	<1.0	7.0
W/BACON *(Swift)* brown and serve	1 link	120	1.0	11.0
W/HAM *(Swift)* brown and serve	1 link	130	1.0	13.0
SAUSAGE, ALTERNATIVE				
(Heartline) 'Italian Sausage Style'	2 oz	176	9.0	7.0

Food Name	Serv. Size	Total Cal.	Carbs GMS	Fat GMS
(Heartline) 'Pepperoni Style' lite	.5 oz	22	1.0	0.0
Canned *(Worthington)* 'Saucettes'	2 links	140	5.0	9.0
Frozen				
(Morningstar Farms) links, 'Breakfast Links'	3 links	190	3.0	14.0
(Morningstar Farms) patties, 'Breakfast Patties'	2 patties	190	7.0	12.0
(Worthington) links, 'Prosage'	3 links	190	4.0	14.0
(Worthington) patties, 'Prosage'	2 patties	210	4.0	14.0
(Worthington) roll, 'Prosage' 3/8-inch slice	2 slices	180	4.0	12.0
SAUSAGE, CANNED				
(Hormel) hot	1 patty	150	0.0	13.0
(Hormel) mild	1 patty	150	0.0	13.0
SAUSAGE SEASONING, pork *(Tone's)*	1 tsp	12	2.7	0.3
SAUSAGE STICK				
(Hickory Farms) 'Sportsman Stick'	1 oz	138	4.0	10.0
BEEF				
(Pemmican) Pepperoni	1.1 oz	170	2.0	14.0
(Pemmican) Tabasco	1.1 oz	120	2.0	10.0
(Pemmican) Teriyaki	1.1 oz	150	5.0	11.0
SMOKED				
(Slim Jim) 'Big Slim'	.52 oz	80	1.0	7.0
(Slim Jim) 'Giant Slim'	1.1 oz	180	2.0	16.0
(Slim Jim) 'Jumbo Jim'	1 oz	150	2.0	12.0
(Slim Jim) 'Super Slim'	.7 oz	110	1.0	10.0
Mild *(Slim Jim)* 'Handi-Paks'	.31 oz	50	1.0	4.0
Nacho *(Slim Jim)* 'Super Slim'	.31 oz	40	1.0	3.0
Pepperoni *(Slim Jim)* 'Handi-Paks'	.31 oz	50	1.0	4.0
Spicy				
(Slim Jim) 'Handi-Paks'	.31 oz	50	1.0	4.0
(Pemmican)	.8 oz	110	1.0	10.0
Tabasco *(Slim Jim)* 'Handi-Paks'	.31 oz	50	1.0	4.0
SUMMER SAUSAGE				
Beef *(Hickory Farms)*	1 oz	100	1.0	8.0
Smoked *(Slim Jim)*	.5 oz	80	1.0	7.0
Teriyaki *(Pemmican)*	.8 oz	110	1.0	10.0
SAUSAGE TACO				
refrigerated *(Owens)* 'Border Breakfasts'	2.17 oz	190	11.0	12.0
SAVORY				
ground	1 oz	77	19.5	1.7
ground	1 tbsp	12	3.0	0.3
ground	1 tsp	4	1.0	0.1
ground *(Durkee)*	1 tsp	5	0.0	tr
ground *(Laurel Leaf)*	1 tsp	5	0.0	tr
ground *(Spice Islands)*	1 tsp	5	1.0	0.1

Food Name	Serv. Size	Total Cal.	Carbs GMS	Fat GMS
SAVOY CABBAGE. See CABBAGE, SAVOY.				
SCALLION. See ONION, GREEN.				
SCALLOP, ALTERNATIVE				
canned *(Worthington)* 'Vegetable Skallops'	1/2 cup	90	4.0	2.0
canned *(Worthington)* 'Vegetable Skallops' no salt	1/2 cup	80	4.0	1.0
mixed species, made from surimi	3 oz	84	9.0	0.4
SCALLOP, MIXED SPECIES				
breaded, fried	4 oz	244	11.5	12.4
fried, frozen *(Mrs. Paul's)*	3 oz	200	22.0	8.0
raw	1 lb	400	10.7	3.4
raw	3 oz	75	2.0	0.7
raw	1 oz	25	0.7	0.2
SCALLOP SQUASH. See SQUASH, SCALLOP.				
SCORZONERA. See SALSIFY, BLACK.				
SCRAPPLE				
	1 oz	60	4.1	3.8
(Jones Dairy Farm)	1 slice	65	4.2	3.7
SCOTCH. See ALCOHOLIC BEVERAGES.				
SCHAV. See SOUP.				
SCREWDRIVER. See ALCOHOLIC BEVERAGES.				
SCROD ENTRÉE, FROZEN				
baked 'Microwave Entrees' *(Gorton's)*	1 pkg	320	17.0	18.0
SCUP/sea bream				
dry-heat cooked	3 oz	115	0.0	3.0
raw	1 lb	477	0.0	12.4
raw	3 oz	89	0.0	2.3
raw	1 oz	30	0.0	0.8
SEA BASS. See BASS, SEA, MIXED SPECIES.				
SEA BREAM. See SCUP.				
SEA DEVIL. See MONKFISH.				
SEA PERCH. See OCEAN PERCH, ATLANTIC.				
SEA TROUT. See TROUT, SEA, MIXED SPECIES.				
SEAFOOD ENTRÉE, CANNED. See individual listings.				
SEAFOOD ENTRÉE, FROZEN. See also individual listings.				
(Armour) w/natural herbs 'Classics Lite'	10 oz	190	29.0	2.0
(Budget Gourmet) Newburg	10 oz	350	43.0	12.0
(Budget Gourmet) scallop and shrimp 'Mariner'	11.5 oz	320	43.0	9.0
(Cajun Cookin') gumbo	17 oz	330	51.0	7.0
(Gorton's) clam 'Crunchy Clam Strips' microwave, 5.8-oz pkg	2.9 oz	270	20.0	17.0
(Pillsbury) casserole 'Microwave Classic'	1 pkg	420	37.0	24.0
(Swanson) Creole, w/rice 'Homestyle Recipe'	9 oz	240	40.0	6.0

Food Name	Serv. Size	Total Cal.	Carbs GMS	Fat GMS
SEAFOOD FRYING MIX				
(Golden Dipt)	2/3 oz	60	14.0	0.0
(Golden Dipt) fish fry	2/3 oz	60	14.0	0.0
(Golden Dipt) fish fry, Cajun style	2/3 oz	60	14.0	0.0
SEAFOOD SALAD. See also individual listings.				
(Longacre) w/crabmeat 'Saladfest'	1 oz	45	3.0	3.0
SEAFOOD SEASONING MIX				
(Featherweight)	1/4 pkg	18	8.0	0.0
(Golden Dipt) all-purpose	1/4 tsp	2	0.0	0.0
(Golden Dipt) blackened redfish	1/4 tsp	2	0.0	0.0
(Golden Dipt) fish, broiled	1/4 tsp	2	0.0	0.0
(Golden Dipt) lemon pepper	1/4 tsp	8	1.0	0.0
(Golden Dipt) shrimp and crab, Cajun style	1/4 tsp	2	0.0	0.0
(Schilling) Chesapeake Bay	1/2 tsp	2	0.2	0.1
SEASONING AND COATING MIX. See also individual listings.				
(Golden Dipt) breading	1 oz	90	20.0	0.0
(Shake 'N Bake) country mild recipe	1/4 pkt	80	10.0	4.0
(Shake 'N Bake) Italian herb recipe	1/4 pkt	80	14.0	1.0
For chicken				
(Oven Fry) 'Extra Crispy'	1/4 pkt	120	21.0	2.0
(Oven Fry) 'Home Style Flour Recipe'	1/4 pkt	90	15.0	2.0
(Shake 'N Bake) hot and spicy	1/4 pkt	80	15.0	2.0
(Shake 'N Bake) 'Original Barbecue Recipe'	1/4 pkt	90	18.0	2.0
(Shake 'N Bake) 'Original Recipe'	1/4 pkt	80	14.0	2.0
For fish (Shake 'N Bake) 'Original Recipe'	1/4 pkt	70	14.0	1.0
For pork				
(Oven Fry) 'Extra Crispy'	1/8 pkt	60	10.0	1.0
(Shake 'N Bake) hot and spicy	1/8 pkt	45	8.0	1.0
(Shake 'N Bake) 'Original Barbecue Recipe'	1/8 pkt	35	8.0	0.0
(Shake 'N Bake) 'Original Recipe'	1/8 pkt	40	8.0	1.0
SEAWEED				
Dried				
agar	1 oz	87	22.9	0.1
nori	1 lb	158	23.2	1.3
nori	1 oz	10	1.4	0.1
spirulina	1 oz	82	6.8	2.2
Raw				
agar	1 lb	116	30.6	0.1
agar	1 oz	7	1.9	tr
Irish moss	1 lb	222	55.8	0.7
Irish moss	1 oz	14	3.5	<.1
kelp	1 lb	195	43.4	2.5
kelp	100 gm	43	9.6	0.6

Food Name	Serv. Size	Total Cal.	Carbs GMS	Fa GM
kelp	1 oz	12	2.7	0.2
laver	1 lb	158	23.2	1.3
laver	100 gm	35	5.1	0.3
laver	1 oz	10	1.4	0.1
spirulina	1 lb	120	11.0	1.8
spirulina	1 oz	8	0.7	0.1
wakame	1 lb	206	41.5	2.9
wakame	1 oz	13	2.6	0.2
SELTZER. See SOFT DRINKS AND MIXERS.				
SEMOLINA				
enriched	1/2 cup	311	68.6	0.5
unenriched	1/2 cup	109	23.7	0.2
whole grain	1 cup	602	121.6	1.8
whole grain	1 oz	102	20.6	0.3
SESAME BUTTER. See also TAHINI MIX.				
gourmet *(Roaster Fresh)*	1 oz	168	6.0	15.0
made from raw and stone ground kernels	1 oz	162	7.4	13.6
made from raw and stone ground kernels	1 tbsp	86	3.9	7.2
made from roasted kernels	1 oz	169	6.0	15.3
made from roasted kernels	1 tbsp	89	3.2	8.1
made from unroasted kernels	1 oz	172	5.1	16.0
made from unroasted kernels	1 tbsp	85	2.5	7.9
organic *(Arrowhead Mills)*	1 oz	170	4.0	17.0
organic, Mid-Eastern *(Westbrae)*	2 tbsp	220	3.0	20.0
organic 'Natural' *(Westbrae)*	2 tbsp	220	6.0	19.0
paste	1 oz	169	7.2	14.4
paste	1 tbsp	95	4.1	8.1
SESAME FLOUR				
high-fat	1 oz	149	7.6	10.5
low-fat	1 oz	95	10.1	0.5
partially defatted	1 oz	108	10.0	3.4
SESAME MEAL, partially defatted	1 oz	161	7.4	13.6
SESAME OIL				
	1/2 cup	964	0.0	109.0
	1 oz	251	0.0	28.4
	1 tbsp	120	0.0	13.6
(Eden Foods) hot pepper	1 tbsp	120	0.0	14.0
(Eden Foods) toasted	1 tbsp	120	0.0	14.0
(Eden Foods) unrefined	1 tbsp	120	0.0	14.0
(Hain)	1 tbsp	120	0.0	14.0
(Spectrum Naturals)	1 tbsp	120	0.0	14.0
(Spectrum Naturals) unrefined	1 tbsp	120	0.0	14.0

Food Name	Serv. Size	Total Cal.	Carbs GMS	Fat GMS
SESAME SEASONING				
(Schilling) all-purpose 'Parsley Patch'	1 tsp	15	1.0	1.0
SESAME SEED/sim sim				
Decorticated				
dried	1 tbsp	47	0.8	4.4
dried	1 tsp	16	.3	1.5
Kernels				
dried	1 cup	882	14.1	82.2
dried	1 oz	167	2.7	15.5
dried	1 tbsp	47	0.8	4.4
dried	1 tsp	16	0.3	1.5
dried (Arrowhead Mills)	1 oz	160	4.0	14.0
dried, toasted	1 oz	161	7.4	13.6
Whole				
dried	1 lb	2598	106.4	225.3
dried	1 cup	825	33.8	71.5
dried	1 oz	162	6.6	14.1
dried	1 tbsp	52	2.1	4.5
dried (Arrowhead Mills)	1 oz	160	6.0	14.0
dried (Durkee)	1 tsp	13	0.0	<0.1
dried (Laurel Leaf)	1 tsp	13	0.0	<0.1
roasted	1 oz	160	7.3	13.6
SESAME STICKS				
(Barbara's Bakery)	1 oz	130	20.0	4.0
(Flavor Tree)	1/4 cup	133	10.6	9.1
(Flavor Tree) 'No Salt'	1/4 cup	131	13.4	8.1
SESBANIA FLOWER. See KATURAY.				
SHAD, AMERICAN				
dry-heat cooked	3 oz	214	0.0	15.0
raw	1 lb	891	0.0	62.5
raw	3 oz	167	0.0	11.7
raw	1 oz	56	0.0	3.9
SHAKE 'N BAKE. See SEASONING AND COATING MIX.				
SHALLOT				
freeze-dried	1 oz	99	22.9	0.1
freeze-dried	1/4 cup	13	2.9	0.0
freeze-dried	1 tbsp	3	0.7	0.0
raw	100 gm	72	16.8	0.1
raw	1 tbsp	7	1.7	0.0
raw, trimmed	1 oz	20	4.8	<.1
raw, untrimmed	1 lb	287	67.1	0.4
SHARK				
Mako, boneless steak, raw (Peter Pan Seafoods)	3.5 oz	87	na	1.2

Food Name	Serv. Size	Total Cal.	Carbs GMS	Fat GMS
Mixed species				
batter-dipped, fried	3 oz	194	5.4	11.7
raw	1 lb	591	0.0	20.5
raw	3 oz	110	0.0	3.8
raw	1 oz	37	0.0	1.3
SHEANUT OIL				
	1/2 cup	964	0.0	109.0
	1 oz	251	0.0	28.4
	1 tbsp	120	0.0	13.6
SHEEPSHEAD/California sheepshead/fathead/redhead				
baked	6.6-oz fillet	234	0.0	3.0
baked	4 oz	143	0.0	1.8
baked	3 oz	107	0.0	1.4
broiled	6.6-oz fillet	234	0.0	3.0
broiled	4 oz	143	0.0	1.8
microwaved	6.6-oz fillet	234	0.0	3.0
microwaved	4 oz	143	0.0	1.8
raw	1 lb	490	0.0	10.9
raw	3 oz	92	0.0	2.0
raw	1 oz	31	0.0	0.7
roasted	4 oz	143	0.0	1.8
SHELLIE BEAN, CANNED				
w/liquid	1/2 cup	37	7.6	0.2
w/liquid	4 oz	34	7.0	0.2
(Stokely)	1/2 cup	35	7.0	0.0
SHERBET. See also FRUIT BAR, FROZEN; ICE BARS AND DESSERTS; SORBET.				
all flavors (Sealtest)	1/2 cup	130	28.0	1.0
orange	1/2 cup	132	29.2	1.9
orange	1 oz	40	8.6	0.6
orange (Borden)	1/2 cup	110	25.0	1.0
orange (Darigold)	1/2 cup	120	26.0	1.0
vanilla-orange 'Cubic Scoops' (Sealtest)	4 oz	130	22.0	4.0
vanilla-red raspberry 'Cubic Scoops' (Sealtest)	4 oz	130	22.0	4.0
SHERBET BAR				
all flavors 'Fat-Free' (Fudgsicle)	1 bar	70	14.0	0.0
all flavors 'Sugar-Free' (Fudgsicle)	1 bar	35	6.0	1.0
chocolate (Fudgsicle)	1 bar	70	12.0	1.0
chocolate, w/nuts 'Sugar-Free Fudge Nut Dip' (Fudgsicle)	1 bar	130	12.0	8.0
orange	2.75-oz bar	91	20.1	1.3
w/cream, all flavors 'Sugar-Free' (Creamsicle)	1 bar	25	5.0	1.0
SHORT RIBS ENTRÉE, FROZEN				
(Armour) boneless 'Classics'	9.75 oz	380	34.0	16.0
(Stouffer's) in gravy	9 oz	350	12.0	20.0

Food Name	Serv. Size	Total Cal.	Carbs GMS	Fat GMS
(Tyson) 'Gourmet Selection'	11 oz	470	38.0	24.0
SHORTENING				
COMMERCIAL				
hydrogenated soybean oil and cottonseed oil	1 cup	1812	0.0	205.0
hydrogenated soybean oil and cottonseed oil	1 tbsp	113	0.0	12.8
lard and vegetable oil	1 cup	1845	0.0	205.0
lard and vegetable oil	1 tbsp	115	0.0	12.8
(Wesson) 'Crystal'	1 tbsp	122	0.0	13.5
(Wesson) 'Lo-Melt'	1 tbsp	122	0.0	13.5
(Wesson) 'Super'	1 tbsp	122	0.0	13.5
(Wesson) 'Wesgold'	1 tbsp	122	0.0	13.5
(Wesson) 'Wespour'	1 tbsp	122	0.0	13.5
For baking				
hydrogenated soybean, palm, and cottonseed oils	1 cup	1812	0.0	205.0
hydrogenated soybean, palm, and cottonseed oils	1 tbsp	113	0.0	12.8
For bread				
hydrogenated soybean oil and cottonseed oil	1 cup	1812	0.0	205.0
hydrogenated soybean oil and cottonseed oil	1 tbsp	113	0.0	12.8
For cakes and frostings				
hydrogenated soybean and cottonseed oils	1 cup	1812	0.0	205.0
hydrogenated soybean and cottonseed oils	1 tbsp	113	0.0	12.8
hydrogenated soybean oil	1 cup	1812	0.0	205.0
hydrogenated soybean oil	1 tbsp	113	0.0	12.8
For confectionery				
fractionated palm oil	1 cup	1927	0.0	218.0
fractionated palm oil	1 tbsp	120	0.0	13.6
hydrogenated coconut and/or palm kernel oil	1 cup	1812	0.0	205.0
hydrogenated coconut and/or palm kernel oil	1 tbsp	113	0.0	12.8
Heavy duty, for frying				
beef tallow and cottonseed oil	1 cup	1845	0.0	205.0
beef tallow and cottonseed oil	1 tbsp	115	0.0	12.8
hydrogenated palm oil	1 cup	1812	0.0	205.0
hydrogenated palm oil	1 tbsp	113	0.0	12.8
hydrogenated soybean and cottonseed oils	1 cup	1812	0.0	205.0
hydrogenated soybean and cottonseed oils	1 tbsp	113	0.0	12.8
hydrogenated soybean oil, 30% linoleic	1 cup	1812	0.0	205.0
hydrogenated soybean oil, 30% linoleic	1 tbsp	113	0.0	12.8
hydrogenated soybean oil, under 1% linoleic	1 cup	1812	0.0	205.0
hydrogenated soybean oil, under 1% linoleic	1 tbsp	113	0.0	12.8
Multi-purpose				
hydrogenated soybean and palm oils	1 cup	1812	0.0	205.0
hydrogenated soybean and palm oils	1 tbsp	113	0.0	12.8

Food Name	Serv. Size	Total Cal.	Carbs GMS	Fat GMS
HOUSEHOLD				
hydrogenated soybean and cottonseed oils	1 cup	1812	0.0	205.0
hydrogenated soybean and cottonseed oils	1 tbsp	113	0.0	12.8
hydrogenated soybean oil and palm oil	1 cup	1812	0.0	205.0
hydrogenated soybean oil and palm oil	1 tbsp	113	0.0	12.8
lard and vegetable oil	1 cup	1845	0.0	205.0
lard and vegetable oil	1 tbsp	115	0.0	12.8
(Crisco) vegetable	1 tbsp	110	0.0	12.0
(Crisco) vegetable, butter flavor	1 tbsp	110	0.0	12.0
(Finast) vegetable	1 tbsp	110	0.0	13.0
(Finast) vegetable, butter flavor	1 tbsp	110	0.0	12.0
(Wesson)	1 tbsp	100	0.0	12.0
SHOYU. See SAUCE, SOY.				
SHRIMP, ALTERNATIVE				
made from surimi	1 lb	458	41.4	6.7
made from surimi	1 oz	29	2.6	0.4
made from surimi	3 oz	86	7.8	1.3
SHRIMP, MIXED SPECIES				
boiled	4 oz	112	(mq)	1.2
boiled, .8-oz size	4 shrimp	22	(mq)	0.2
breaded, fried	3 oz	206	9.8	10.4
breaded, fried	1.1 oz	73	3.4	3.7
breaded, fried, .8-oz size	4 shrimp	73	3.4	3.7
fried	4 oz	274	13.0	13.9
moist-heat cooked	3 oz	84	0.0	0.9
moist-heat cooked, .8-oz size	4 shrimp	22	0.0	0.2
poached	4 oz	112	(mq)	1.2
poached, .8-oz size	4 shrimp	22	(mq)	0.2
raw	1 lb	481	4.1	7.8
raw	3 oz	90	0.8	1.5
raw, .8-oz size	4 shrimp	30	0.3	0.5
steamed	4 oz	112	(mq)	1.2
steamed, .8-oz size	4 shrimp	22	(mq)	0.2
Canned				
drained	1 cup	154	1.3	2.5
drained	3 oz	102	0.9	1.7
drained	4 oz	136	1.2	2.2
drained *(Louisiana Brand)*	2 oz	58	0.0	1.0
large, drained *(ShopRite)*	2 oz	50	0.0	1.0
SHRIMP CHOW MEIN, canned				
(LaChoy)	3/4 cup	35	4.0	1.0
(LaChoy) 'Bi-Pack'	8.536 oz	60	10.2	1.0
(LaChoy) 'Bi-Pack'	3/4 cup	50	7.0	1.0

Food Name	Serv. Size	Total Cal.	Carbs GMS	Fat GMS
SHRIMP COCKTAIL				
(Booth) w/garlic butter sauce and vegetable rice	10 oz	400	40.0	25.0
(Budget Gourmet) w/fettuccine	9.5 oz	375	38.0	20.0
(LaChoy) w/lobster sauce 'Fresh & Lite'	10 oz	240	36.4	6.2
(Mrs. Paul's) w/clams and linguini 'Light'	10 oz	240	36.0	5.0
(Sau-Sea)	4 oz	113	19.0	1.0
(SeaPak) 'Super Valu' heat and serve	4 oz	210	30.0	4.0
SHRIMP ENTRÉE, FROZEN				
BAY, BABY (Armour) 'Classics Lite'	9.75 oz	220	31.0	6.0
BATTERED				
(SeaPak) 'Shrimp 'n Batter'	4 oz	260	20.0	15.0
(SeaPak) w/crabmeat stuffing	4 oz	260	27.0	13.0
BREADED				
(Gorton's) original seasoning	2.7 oz	200	15.0	12.0
(Gorton's) popcorn style	2.7 oz	220	16.0	14.0
(Gorton's) scampi seasoning	2.7 oz	210	16.0	12.0
(Mrs. Paul's) fried	3 oz	200	16.0	11.0
BUTTERFLY				
(Gorton's) 'Specialty'	4 oz	160	16.0	<1.0
(SeaPak) breaded 'Mikado'	4 oz	160	26.0	1.0
BUTTERFLY/ROUND (SeaPak) breaded	4 oz	150	20.0	1.0
CAJUN STYLE (Mrs. Paul's) 'Light'	9 oz	230	37.0	5.0
CREOLE				
(Armour) 'Classics Lite'	11.25 oz	260	53.0	2.0
(Cajun Cookin')	12 oz	390	55.0	11.0
(Healthy Choice)	11.25 oz	230	45.0	2.0
CRISP (Gorton's) 'Specialty'	4 oz	280	26.0	15.0
CRUNCHY				
(Gorton's) 'Crunchy Shrimp' microwave	2 oz	160	12.0	9.0
(Gorton's) whole 'Microwave Specialty'	5 oz	380	35.0	20.0
ETOUFFEE (Cajun Cookin')	17 oz	360	52.0	9.0
FETTUCCINE ALFREDO (Booth)	10 oz	260	28.0	8.0
JAMBALAYA (Cajun Cookin')	12 oz	450	43.0	20.0
MARINARA				
(Healthy Choice)	10.5 oz	260	51.0	1.0
(Smart Ones) w/linguini	8 oz	150	26.0	<1.0
NEW ORLEANS, w/wild rice (Booth)	10 oz	230	35.0	5.0
ORIENTAL, w/pineapple rice (Booth)	10 oz	190	30.0	3.0
PRIMAVERA				
(Booth) w/fettucini	10 oz	200	28.0	3.0
(Mrs. Paul's) 'Light'	9.5 oz	180	28.0	3.0
(Right Course)	9 5/8 oz	240	32.0	7.0
SCAMPI (Gorton's) 'Microwave Entrées'	1 pkg	390	21.0	30.0

Food Name	Serv. Size	Total Cal.	Carbs GMS	Fat GMS
STIR-FRY (Shanghai)	10.3 oz	170	19.0	2.0
SHRIMP ENTRÉE, PACKAGED				
(Ultra Slim Fast) creole	12 oz	240	45.0	4.0
(Ultra Slim Fast) marinara	12 oz	290	53.0	3.0
SHRIMP PASTE, canned	1 tsp	13	0.1	0.7
SHRIMP SALAD				
(Longacre) 'Saladfest'	1 oz	45	2.0	3.0
(Longacre) 'Saladfest' w/seafood	1 oz	42	2.0	3.0
SICAMA. See JICAMA.				
SILVER HAKE. See WHITING, MIXED SPECIES.				
SIM SIM. See SESAME SEED.				
SISYMBRIUM SEED				
whole, dried	1 cup	235	43.1	3.4
whole, dried	1 oz	90	16.5	1.3
SKIL. See SABLEFISH.				
SKUNK CABBAGE. See CABBAGE, SKUNK.				
SLIMEHEAD. See ORANGE ROUGHY.				
SLOPPY JOE SEASONING MIX				
(French's)	1/8 pkg	16	4.0	0.0
(Lawry's) 'Seasoning Blends'	1 pkg	126	27.7	0.4
(Schilling)	1/4 pkg	26	6.0	0.5
SMELT, RAINBOW				
broiled	4 oz	141	0.0	3.5
dry-heat cooked	4 oz	141	0.0	3.5
dry-heat cooked	3 oz	105	0.0	2.6
microwaved	4 oz	141	0.0	3.5
raw	1 lb	440	0.0	11.0
raw	3 oz	82	0.0	2.1
raw	1 oz	27	0.0	0.7
SNACK. See CORN CHIPS AND SNACKS; SNACK BAR; SNACK MIX.				
SNACK BAR. See also DIET BAR.				
(Barbara's Bakery)				
apple, real fruit, .5 oz	1 bar	50	11.0	0.0
apricot, real fruit, .5 oz	1 bar	50	11.0	0.0
cherry, real fruit, .5 oz	1 bar	50	11.0	0.0
grape, real fruit, .5 oz	1 bar	50	11.0	0.0
raspberry, real fruit, .5 oz	1 bar	50	11.0	0.0
(Bear Valley)				
carob-cocoa, food bar 'Pemmican'	3.75 oz	440	68.0	12.0
coconut almond, food bar 'Meal Pack'	3.75 oz	400	56.0	12.0
fruit 'n nut, food bar 'Pemmican'	3.75 oz	420	59.0	13.0
sesame lemon, food bar 'Meal Pack'	3.75 oz	410	57.0	13.0

Food Name	Serv. Size	Total Cal.	Carbs GMS	Fat GMS
(Carnation)				
chocolate chip, breakfast bar	1 bar	200	20.0	11.0
chocolate crunch, breakfast bar	1 bar	190	20.0	10.0
peanut butter chocolate chip, breakfast bar	1 bar	200	20.0	11.0
peanut butter crunch, breakfast bar	1 bar	190	20.0	10.0
(Earth Grains)				
banana apple walnut 'Bagel Power Bar'	1 bar	270	45.0	6.0
citrus almond w/mixed fruit 'Bagel Power Bar'	1 bar	260	45.0	4.0
fruit and nut 'Bagel Power Bar'	1 bar	240	48.0	3.0
(Glenny's)				
apple-cinnamon	1.25 oz	120	28.0	<1.0
caramel	1.25 oz	120	29.0	<1.0
chocolate	1.25 oz	120	28.0	<1.0
raspberry	1.25 oz	120	29.0	<1.0
(Health Valley)				
apple, fat-free	1 bar	140	33.0	0.0
'Apple Bakes'	1 bar	100	16.0	3.0
apricot, fat-free	1 bar	140	33.0	0.0
date, fat-free	1 bar	140	33.0	0.0
'Date Bakes'	1 bar	100	16.0	3.0
'Fruit & Fitness'	1 bar	200	39.0	3.0
'Oat Bran, Fig & Nut Bakes'	1 bar	110	19.0	3.0
oat bran, raisin, and cinnamon	1 bar	140	32.0	2.0
'Oat Bran Apricot Bakes'	1 bar	100	19.0	2.0
'Oat Bran Jumbo Fruit and Nut Bars'	1 bar	150	29.0	4.0
'Oat Bran Jumbo Fruit Bars'	1 bar	170	28.0	5.0
raisin, fat-free	1 bar	140	33.0	0.0
'Raisin Bakes'	1 bar	100	16.0	3.0
rice bran, almond, and date	1 bar	190	29.0	6.0
(Kudos)				
peaches and cream 'Pan Squares'	1 square	150	22.0	6.0
peanut butter and chocolate chip 'Pan Squares'	1 square	170	20.0	9.0
strawberry and cream cheese 'Pan Squares'	1 square	150	22.0	6.0
(Tiger's Milk) peanut butter and honey, carob coated	1 bar	160	23.0	5.0
(Weider)				
'Sportsfood Enerquench Bar'	1 bar	200	44.0	1.0
'Sportsfood Protein Bar'	1 bar	160	21.0	4.0
SNACK BAR MIX, PREPARED				
(Betty Crocker)				
caramel oatmeal 'Supreme Dessert'	1 bar	110	15.0	5.0
chocolate and toffee 'Supreme Dessert'	1 bar	110	17.0	4.0
chocolate peanut butter 'Supreme Dessert'	1 bar	110	14.0	5.0
date 'Classic'	1 bar	60	9.0	2.0

Food Name	Serv. Size	Total Cal.	Carbs GMS	Fat GMS
lemon-Sunkist 'Supreme Dessert' prepared w/4 eggs	1 bar	110	17.0	4.0
M&M cookie bars 'Supreme Dessert'	1 bar	110	16.0	5.0
raspberry 'Supreme Dessert'	1 bar	100	16.0	4.0
SNACK MIX				
(Doo Dads) original recipe, 1 oz	1/2 cup	129	18.2	5.2
(Flavor Tree)				
'Party Mix'	1/4 cup	163	12.3	11.0
'Party Mix No Salt'	1 1/2 cup	163	13.2	10.8
(Pepperidge Farm)				
cheese, super cheddar 'Goldfish Party Mix'	1 oz	140	15.0	7.0
'Classic'	1 oz	140	14.0	8.0
lightly smoked	1 oz	150	13.0	9.0
nutty deluxe, cashews and almonds 'Goldfish'	1/2 cup	180	20.0	9.0
original, honey roasted peanuts 'Goldfish'	1/2 cup	170	21.0	8.0
spicy	1 oz	140	14.0	8.0
(Ralston)				
barbecue 'Chex' 2/3 cup	1 oz	130	18.0	5.0
'Chex Traditional' 2/3 cup	1 oz	120	18.5	4.9
cool sour cream and onion 'Chex' 2/3 cup	1 oz	130	19.0	5.0
golden cheddar 'Chex' 2/3 cup	1 oz	130	19.0	5.0
nacho cheese 'Chex' 2/3 cup	1 oz	130	19.0	5.0
(Ritz) traditional, baked	1 oz	130	18.0	6.0
SNAPPER, RED, MIXED SPECIES				
broiled	4 oz	145	0.0	2.0
dry-heat cooked	4 oz	145	0.0	2.0
dry-heat cooked	3 oz	109	0.0	1.5
microwaved	4 oz	145	0.0	2.0
raw	1 lb	452	0.0	6.1
raw	3 oz	85	0.0	1.1
raw	1 oz	28	0.0	0.4
SNOW PEAS. See PEAS, SNOW.				
SOBA NOODLE. See NOODLE, JAPANESE.				
SODA. See SOFT DRINKS AND MIXERS.				
SODA, CLUB. See SOFT DRINKS AND MIXERS.				
SOFT DRINKS AND MIXERS. See also WATER, SPARKLING, FLAVORED.				
(A&W)				
cream soda	1 oz	14	3.6	tr
cream soda, 'Diet'	1 oz	<1	0.0	<.1
root beer	1 oz	15	3.5	<.1
root beer, 'Diet'	1 oz	<1	0.0	tr
(Canada Dry)				
collins mixer	8 oz	80	20.0	0.0
ginger ale	8 oz	90	21.0	0.0

Food Name	Serv. Size	Total Cal.	Carbs GMS	Fat GMS
ginger ale, 'Golden'	8 oz	100	24.0	0.0
grape, 'Concord'	8 oz	130	32.0	0.0
half and half	8 oz	110	26.0	0.0
tonic	8 oz	90	22.0	0.0
whiskey sour mixer	8 oz	90	22.0	0.0
(Coca Cola)				
cherry cola	6 oz	76	20.0	0.0
cherry cola, 'Diet'	6 oz	<1	0.2	0.0
cola, caffeine-free	6 oz	77	20.0	0.0
cola, 'Classic'	6 oz	72	19.0	0.0
cola, diet, caffeine-free	6 oz	<1	0.2	0.0
cola, diet, w/caffeine	6 oz	<1	0.2	0.0
cola, w/caffeine	6 oz	77	20.0	0.0
(Dr. Diablo) cola	12 oz	140	38.0	0.0
(Dr. Pepper)				
cola	12 oz	150	38.4	0.0
cola, caffeine-free	12 oz	150	38.4	0.0
diet	12 oz	3	0.2	0.0
diet, caffeine-free	12 oz	3	0.2	0.0
(Fanta)				
ginger ale	6 oz	63	16.0	0.0
grape	6 oz	86	22.0	0.0
orange	6 oz	88	23.0	0.0
root beer	6 oz	78	20.0	0.0
(Fresca) citrus	6 oz	2	0.2	0.0
(Health Valley)				
ginger ale	12 oz	153	35.0	1.0
root beer, 'Old Fashioned'	12 oz	120	26.0	1.0
root beer, sarsaparilla	12 oz	153	35.0	1.0
wild berry	12 oz	142	33.0	1.0
(Hires)				
cream soda, caffeine-free	6 oz	90	24.0	<1.0
cream soda, 'Diet' caffeine-free	6 oz	2	<1.0	<1.0
root beer, caffeine-free	6 oz	90	23.0	<1.0
root beer, 'Diet' caffeine-free, w/NutraSweet	6 oz	2	<1.0	<1.0
(Jolt) cola	6 oz	85	20.7	0.0
(Mello Yello)				
citrus	6 oz	87	22.0	0.0
citrus, diet	6 oz	3	0.2	0.0
(Mountain Dew)				
citrus	12 oz	179	44.4	0.0
citrus, diet	12 oz	4	0.7	0.0
(Mr. Pibb) cola	6 oz	71	19.0	0.0

Food Name	Serv. Size	Total Cal.	Carbs GMS	Fat GMS
(Mug)				
root beer	12 oz	168	42.0	0.0
root beer, 'Diet'	12 oz	4	1.2	0.0
(Natural 90 Diet) all flavors	6 oz	2	<1.0	0.0
(Pathmark) cola, 'No Frills Sugar-free'	8 oz	0	tr	0.0
(Pepsi)				
cherry cola, 'Diet Wild Cherry'	12 oz	1	na	0.0
cherry cola, 'Wild Cherry'	12 oz	163	43.2	0.0
cola, caffeine-free	12 oz	160	39.6	0.0
cola, clear 'Diet Crystal' w/NutraSweet	6 oz	0	0.0	0.0
cola, diet, caffeine-free	12 oz	<1	0.2	0.0
cola, diet, w/caffeine	12 oz	<1	0.2	0.0
cola, 'Light'	12 oz	<1	0.1	0.0
cola, w/caffeine	12 oz	160	39.6	0.0
(Santa Cruz Naturals) ginger ale, organic 'Sparkling'	8 oz	155	36.0	<1.0
(Schweppes)				
blackberry, 'Royal'	6 oz	35	8.0	0.0
citrus, tropical 'Royal'	6 oz	35	8.0	0.0
club soda	6 oz	0	0.0	0.0
collins mixer	6 oz	75	18.0	0.0
ginger ale	6 oz	65	16.0	0.0
ginger ale, raspberry	6 oz	65	16.0	0.0
ginger ale, raspberry 'Diet'	6 oz	2	<1.0	0.0
ginger ale, 'Sugar-free'	6 oz	2	<1.0	0.0
ginger beer	6 oz	70	17.0	0.0
grape	6 oz	95	23.0	0.0
grapefruit	6 oz	80	20.0	0.0
kiwi-passion fruit, 'Royal'	6 oz	35	8.0	0.0
lemon, bitter	6 oz	82	20.0	0.0
lemon, sour	6 oz	79	19.0	0.0
lemon-lime	6 oz	72	18.0	0.0
orange, sparkling	6 oz	88	22.0	0.0
peaches and cream, 'Royal'	6 oz	35	8.0	0.0
root beer	6 oz	76	19.0	0.0
seltzer, all flavors	6 oz	0	0.0	0.0
seltzer, 'Low Sodium'	6 oz	0	0.0	0.0
seltzer, 'Sodium-free'	6 oz	0	0.0	0.0
strawberry-banana, 'Royal'	6 oz	35	8.0	0.0
tonic	6 oz	64	16.0	0.0
tonic, 'Diet'	6 oz	2	<1.0	0.0
vanilla bean, 'Royal'	6 oz	35	8.0	0.0
Vichy water	6 oz	0	0.0	0.0
wild cherry, 'Royal'	6 oz	35	8.0	0.0

Food Name	Serv. Size	Total Cal.	Carbs GMS	Fat GMS
wild raspberry, 'Royal'	6 oz	35	8.0	0.0
(7•Up)				
cherry citrus	12 oz	148	38.7	0.0
cherry citrus, diet	12 oz	4	tr	0.0
lemon-lime	12 oz	144	36.2	0.0
lemon-lime, diet	12 oz	4	0.0	0.0
(Shasta)				
apple, 'Yoshi Apple'	8 oz	130	31.0	0.0
berry, 'Luigi Berry'	8 oz	130	32.0	0.0
black cherry	12 oz	162	44.0	0.0
cherry, 'Princess Toadstool Cherry'	8 oz	130	31.0	0.0
cherry cola	12 oz	140	38.0	0.0
citrus mist	12 oz	170	46.0	0.0
club soda	12 oz	0	0.0	0.0
cola	12 oz	147	40.0	0.0
cola, 'Free'	12 oz	151	41.0	0.0
collins mixer	12 oz	118	32.0	0.0
cream soda, 'Creme'	12 oz	154	42.0	0.0
ginger ale	12 oz	120	33.0	0.0
grape	12 oz	177	48.0	0.0
lemon-lime	12 oz	146	39.0	0.0
orange	12 oz	177	48.0	0.0
red berry	12 oz	158	43.0	0.0
root beer	12 oz	154	42.0	0.0
strawberry	12 oz	147	40.0	0.0
tonic	12 oz	121	33.0	0.0
(Slice)				
lemon-lime	12 oz	150	38.4	0.0
lemon-lime, 'Diet'	12 oz	16	2.4	0.0
orange, 'Diet'	12 oz	12	2.3	0.0
orange, Mandarin	12 oz	193	50.4	0.0
(Snapple)				
'Amazin' Grape'	8 oz	120	28.0	0.0
'Cherry Lime Rickey'	8 oz	110	27.0	0.0
'Creme D'Vanilla'	8 oz	130	33.0	0.0
'French Cherry'	8 oz	120	29.0	0.0
'Kiwi Peach'	8 oz	120	29.0	0.0
'Kiwi Strawberry'	8 oz	130	33.0	0.0
'Mango Madness'	8 oz	130	33.0	0.0
'Passion Supreme'	8 oz	120	29.0	0.0
'Peach Melba'	8 oz	120	31.0	0.0
'Raspberry'	8 oz	120	31.0	0.0
'Tru Root Beer'	8 oz	110	29.0	0.0

Food Name	Serv. Size	Total Cal.	Carbs GMS	Fat GMS
(Spree)				
cherry-lime	12 oz	158	43.0	0.0
cola	12 oz	147	40.0	0.0
ginger ale	12 oz	120	33.0	0.0
grapefruit	12 oz	154	42.0	0.0
lemon-lime	12 oz	154	42.0	0.0
lemon-tangerine	12 oz	165	45.0	0.0
lime, Mandarin	12 oz	154	42.0	0.0
root beer	12 oz	154	42.0	0.0
tropical blend	12 oz	146	41.0	0.0
(Sprite)				
lemon-lime	6 oz	71	18.0	0.0
lemon-lime, diet	6 oz	2	0.0	0.0
(Squirt)				
citrus	1 oz	13	3.2	tr
citrus, 'Diet'	1 oz	<1	0.1	tr
citrus berry, 'Ruby Red'	8 oz	120	30.0	0.0
(Tab)				
cola, caffeine-free	6 oz	<1	0.2	0.0
cola, w/caffeine	6 oz	<1	0.2	0.0
(Vernor's)				
ginger	3.5 oz	40	10.0	0.1
ginger, 'Diet'	3.5 oz	<1	0.1	0.1
(Wink) grapefruit	8 oz	120	30.0	0.0
(Yoo-Hoo) chocolate	9 oz	140	27.0	1.0
SOLE				
dry-heat cooked	3 oz	99	0.0	1.3
raw	3 oz	77	0.0	1.0
SOLE, FROZEN				
Dinner *(Healthy Choice)* au gratin	11 oz	270	40.0	5.0
Entrée				
(Gorton's) in lemon butter 'Microwave Entrees'	1 pkg	380	17.0	24.0
(Gorton's) seafood stuffed 'Select' approx 5 oz	1 fillet	160	18.0	3.0
(Healthy Choice) w/lemon butter sauce	8.25 oz	230	33.0	4.0
Fillet				
(Booth) Atlantic	4 oz	90	0.0	1.0
(Gorton's) 'Fishmarket Fresh'	5 oz	110	1.0	1.0
(Mrs. Paul's) breaded 'Light'	1 fillet	240	20.0	10.0
(SeaPak)	4 oz	90	0.0	1.0
(Van de Kamp's) breaded 'Light'	1 fillet	250	18.0	12.0
(Van de Kamp's) 'Natural'	4 oz	100	0.0	2.0

SOMEN NOODLE. See NOODLE, JAPANESE.

Food Name	Serv. Size	Total Cal.	Carbs GMS	Fat GMS
SORBET. See also FRUIT BARS, FROZEN; ICE BARS AND DESSERTS; SHERBET.				
(Baskin-Robbins)				
fruit whip	1 scoop	80	24.0	0.0
red raspberry	1 scoop	140	34.0	0.0
(Cascadian Farms)				
blackberry	1 oz	25	21.2	0.1
raspberry	1 oz	28	20.9	0.2
strawberry	1 oz	26	22.0	0.1
(Dole)				
Mandarin orange	4 oz	110	28.0	0.1
peach	4 oz	120	28.0	0.6
pineapple	4 oz	120	28.0	0.1
raspberry	4 oz	110	28.0	<.1
strawberry	4 oz	110	28.0	0.1
(Frusen Glädjé) raspberry	1/2 cup	140	36.0	0.0
(Häagen Dazs)				
blueberry, and vanilla ice cream	1/2 cup	190	25.0	8.0
Key lime, and vanilla ice cream	1/2 cup	200	29.0	7.0
lemon 'Ice Cream Shop'	4 oz	140	34.0	0.0
orange, and vanilla ice cream	1/2 cup	190	27.0	8.0
orange 'Ice Cream Shop'	4 oz	113	30.0	0.0
raspberry, and vanilla ice cream	1/2 cup	180	23.0	8.0
raspberry 'Ice Cream Shop'	4 oz	93	22.0	0.0
SORGHUM				
broomcorn, whole grain	100 gm	327	72.9	2.9
whole grain	1 cup	650	143.3	6.3
whole grain	1 oz	96	21.2	0.9
SORGHUM SYRUP				
	1/2 cup	424	112.2	0.0
	1 tbsp	53	4.0	0.0
SORREL				
boiled, drained	4 oz	23	3.3	0.7
raw, trimmed	1 oz	6	0.9	0.2
raw, trimmed, chopped	1/2 cup	15	2.1	0.5
raw, untrimmed	1 lb	70	10.2	2.2
SOUP, CANNED, CONDENSED				
(NOTE: Unless otherwise specified, PREPARED = prepared as directed w/water.)				
ASPARAGUS, CREAM OF				
prepared	1 cup	87	10.7	4.1
prepared w/whole milk	8 oz	161	16.4	8.2
unprepared	10.75 oz	210	26.0	9.9
(Campbell's) prepared	8 oz	80	10.0	4.0

Food Name	Serv. Size	Total Cal.	Carbs GMS	Fat GMS
BEAN				
(Campbell's) 'Homestyle' prepared	8 oz	130	25.0	1.0
W/bacon				
(Campbell's) 'Healthy Request'	4 oz	140	22.0	4.0
(Campbell's) 'Healthy Request' prepared	8 oz	140	21.0	4.0
(Campbell's) prepared	8 oz	140	21.0	4.0
W/frankfurters				
prepared	1 cup	188	22.0	7.0
unprepared	11.25 oz	455	53.4	16.9
W/pork				
prepared	1 cup	172	22.8	5.9
unprepared	11.5 oz	418	55.3	14.4
BEEF				
(Campbell's) prepared	8 oz	80	10.0	2.0
W/bouillon *(Campbell's)* prepared	8 oz	16	1.0	0.0
W/broth *(Campbell's)* prepared	8 oz	16	1.0	0.0
W/vegetables *(Campbell's)* 'Healthy Request'	4 oz	70	9.0	2.0
BEEF MUSHROOM				
prepared	1 cup	73	6.3	3.0
unprepared	10.75 oz	186	15.9	7.3
BEEF NOODLE				
prepared	1 cup	83	9.0	3.1
unprepared	10.75 oz	204	21.8	7.5
(Campbell's) prepared	8 oz	70	7.0	3.0
(Campbell's) 'Homestyle' prepared	8 oz	80	7.0	4.0
W/ground beef *(Campbell's)* prepared	8 oz	90	10.0	4.0
BLACK BEAN				
prepared	1 cup	116	19.8	1.5
unprepared	11 oz	282	48.1	3.7
BROCCOLI, CREAM OF				
(Campbell's) prepared	8 oz	80	8.0	5.0
(Campbell's) prepared w/whole milk	8 oz	140	14.0	7.0
CELERY, CREAM OF				
prepared	1 cup	90	8.8	5.6
prepared w/whole milk	1 cup	164	14.5	9.7
unprepared	10.75 oz	220	21.4	13.6
(Campbell's) prepared	8 oz	100	8.0	7.0
CHEESE				
prepared	1 cup	156	10.5	10.5
prepared w/whole milk	1 cup	231	16.2	14.6
unprepared	11 oz	378	25.6	25.4
Cheddar *(Campbell's)* prepared	8 oz	110	10.0	6.0

Food Name	Serv. Size	Total Cal.	Carbs GMS	Fat GMS
Nacho				
(Campbell's) prepared	8 oz	110	8.0	8.0
(Campbell's) prepared w/whole milk	8 oz	180	13.0	12.0
CHICKEN				
W/barley *(Campbell's)* prepared	8 oz	70	10.0	2.0
W/dumplings				
prepared	1 cup	96	6.1	5.5
unprepared	10.5 oz	235	14.7	13.4
(Campbell's) 'Chicken 'n Dumplings' prepared	8 oz	80	9.0	3.0
W/rice				
prepared	1 cup	60	7.2	1.9
unprepared	10.5 oz	146	17.4	4.7
(Campbell's) prepared	8 oz	60	7.0	3.0
(Campbell's) 'Healthy Request'	4 oz	60	7.0	2.0
(Campbell's) 'Healthy Request' prepared	8 oz	60	7.0	3.0
CHICKEN, CREAM OF				
prepared	1 cup	117	9.3	7.4
unprepared	10.75 oz	284	22.5	17.9
(Campbell's) prepared	8 oz	110	9.0	7.0
(Campbell's) 'Healthy Request'	4 oz	70	11.0	2.0
(Campbell's) 'Healthy Request' prepared	8 oz	70	11.0	2.0
W/broccoli				
(Campbell's)	4 oz	110	9.0	7.0
(Campbell's) prepared	8 oz	110	9.0	7.0
CHICKEN BROTH				
prepared	1 cup	39	0.9	1.4
unprepared	10.75 oz	95	2.3	3.2
(Campbell's) prepared	8 oz	30	2.0	2.0
CHICKEN GUMBO				
prepared	1 cup	56	8.4	1.4
unprepared	10.75 oz	137	20.3	3.5
CHICKEN MUSHROOM				
prepared	1 cup	132	9.3	9.1
unprepared	10.75 oz	332	23.2	22.3
Creamy *(Campbell's)* prepared	8 oz	120	8.0	8.0
CHICKEN NOODLE				
prepared	1 cup	75	9.4	2.5
unprepared	10.5 oz	182	22.7	5.5
(Campbell's) prepared	8 oz	60	8.0	2.0
(Campbell's) 'Healthy Request'	4 oz	60	8.0	2.0
(Campbell's) 'Healthy Request' prepared	8 oz	60	8.0	2.0
(Campbell's) 'Homestyle' prepared	8 oz	70	8.0	3.0
Broth and noodles *(Campbell's)* prepared	8 oz	45	8.0	1.0

Food Name	Serv. Size	Total Cal.	Carbs GMS	Fat GMS
Creamy				
(Campbell's)	4 oz	120	10.0	7.0
(Campbell's) prepared	8 oz	120	10.0	7.0
(Campbell's) prepared w/2% milk	8 oz	180	16.0	9.0
Curly noodle *(Campbell's)* prepared	8 oz	80	11.0	3.0
Double noodle in broth				
(Campbell's)	4 oz	90	13.0	2.0
(Campbell's) prepared	8 oz	90	13.0	2.0
Ring noodle *(Campbell's)* 'Noodle-O's' prepared	8 oz	70	9.0	2.0
CHICKEN VEGETABLE				
prepared	1 cup	75	8.6	2.8
unprepared	10.5 oz	182	20.9	6.9
(Campbell's) prepared	8 oz	70	8.0	3.0
CHILI BEEF				
prepared	1 cup	170	21.5	6.6
unprepared	11.25 oz	412	52.1	16.0
(Campbell's) prepared	8 oz	140	20.0	5.0
CLAM CHOWDER				
Manhattan style				
prepared	1 cup	78	12.2	2.2
unprepared	10.75 oz	186	29.7	5.4
(Campbell's) prepared	8 oz	70	10.0	2.0
(Campbell's) 'Seashore Soups'	4 oz	70	10.0	2.0
(Doxsee) prepared	7.5 oz	70	11.0	2.0
(Snow's)	3.75 oz	70	9.0	2.0
(Snow's) prepared	7.5 oz	70	11.0	2.0
New England style				
prepared	8 oz	95	12.4	2.9
prepared w/whole milk	8 oz	164	16.6	6.6
(Campbell's) prepared	8 oz	80	12.0	3.0
(Campbell's) prepared w/whole milk	8 oz	150	17.0	7.0
(Campbell's) 'Seashore Soups'	4 oz	80	12.0	3.0
(Gorton's) prepared w/whole milk	1/4 can	140	17.0	5.0
(Snow's)	3.75 oz	70	8.0	2.0
(Snow's) prepared w/whole milk	7.5 oz	140	13.0	6.0
CONSOMMÉ				
Beef	10.5 oz	72	4.3	0.0
Beef, w/gelatin				
prepared	1 cup	29	1.8	0.0
unprepared	10.5 oz	71	4.3	0.0
(Campbell's) prepared	8 oz	25	2.0	0.0
CORN, CREAM OF, GOLDEN				
(Campbell's)	4 oz	110	18.0	3.0

Food Name	Serv. Size	Total Cal.	Carbs GMS	Fat GMS
(Campbell's) prepared	8 oz	110	18.0	3.0
(Campbell's) prepared w/2% milk	8 oz	160	23.0	5.0
CORN CHOWDER, NEW ENGLAND				
(Snow's)	3.75 oz	80	13.0	2.0
(Snow's) prepared w/whole milk	7.5 oz	150	18.0	6.0
FISH CHOWDER, NEW ENGLAND				
(Snow's)	3.75 oz	60	6.0	2.0
(Snow's) prepared w/whole milk	7.5 oz	130	11.0	6.0
GREEN PEA				
prepared	1 cup	165	26.5	2.9
prepared w/whole milk	1 cup	239	32.2	7.0
unprepared	11.25 oz	399	64.4	7.1
(Campbell's) prepared	8 oz	160	25.0	3.0
MINESTRONE				
prepared	1 cup	82	11.2	2.5
unprepared	10.5 oz	203	27.3	6.1
(Campbell's) prepared	8 oz	80	13.0	2.0
MUSHROOM				
Beefy *(Campbell's)* prepared	8 oz	60	5.0	3.0
Golden *(Campbell's)* prepared	8 oz	70	9.0	3.0
W/beef stock				
prepared	1 cup	85	9.3	4.0
unprepared	10.75 oz	207	22.6	9.8
MUSHROOM, CREAM OF				
prepared	1 cup	129	9.3	9.0
prepared w/whole milk	1 cup	203	15.0	13.6
unprepared	10.75 oz	314	22.6	23.1
(Campbell's) prepared	8 oz	100	8.0	7.0
(Campbell's) 'Healthy Request'	4 oz	60	9.0	2.0
(Campbell's) 'Healthy Request' prepared	8 oz	60	9.0	2.0
MUSHROOM BARLEY				
prepared	1 cup	73	11.7	2.3
unprepared	10.75 oz	186	29.3	5.5
(Rokeach) prepared	1 cup	85	17.3	0.2
ONION				
prepared	1 cup	58	8.2	1.7
unprepared	10.5 oz	137	19.9	4.2
unprepared	8 oz	113	16.4	3.5
French *(Campbell's)* prepared	8 oz	60	9.0	2.0
ONION, CREAM OF				
prepared	1 cup	107	12.7	5.3
prepared w/whole milk	1 cup	186	18.4	9.4
unprepared	10.75 oz	268	31.7	12.8

Food Name	Serv. Size	Total Cal.	Carbs GMS	Fat GMS
(Campbell's) prepared	8 oz	100	12.0	5.0
(Campbell's) prepared w/half water, half milk	8 oz	140	15.0	7.0
OYSTER STEW				
prepared	1 cup	58	4.1	3.8
prepared w/whole milk	1 cup	135	9.8	7.9
unprepared	10.5 oz	143	9.9	9.3
(Campbell's) prepared	8 oz	70	5.0	5.0
(Campbell's) prepared w/whole milk	8 oz	140	10.0	9.0
PASTA				
Alphabet *(Campbell's)* prepared	8 oz	80	10.0	3.0
Chicken and stars *(Campbell's)* prepared	8 oz	60	7.0	2.0
Teddy bears in chicken broth				
(Campbell's)	4 oz	60	11.0	1.0
(Campbell's) prepared	8 oz	60	11.0	1.0
PEPPER POT				
prepared	1 cup	104	9.4	4.6
unprepared	10.5 oz	250	22.8	11.3
(Campbell's) prepared	8 oz	90	9.0	4.0
POTATO, CREAM OF				
prepared	1 cup	73	11.5	2.4
prepared w/whole milk	1 cup	149	17.2	6.4
unprepared	10.75 oz	180	27.9	5.7
(Campbell's) prepared	8 oz	80	12.0	3.0
(Campbell's) prepared w/tofu, 1 tbsp oil	8 oz	120	15.0	4.0
SCOTCH BROTH				
prepared	1 cup	80	9.5	2.6
unprepared	10.5 oz	197	23.0	6.4
(Campbell's) prepared	8 oz	80	9.0	3.0
SEAFOOD CHOWDER, NEW ENGLAND				
(Snow's)	3.75 oz	60	6.0	2.0
(Snow's) prepared w/whole milk	7.5 oz	140	14.0	6.0
SHRIMP, CREAM OF				
prepared	1 cup	90	8.2	5.2
prepared w/whole milk	1 cup	164	13.9	9.3
unprepared	10.75 oz	220	19.9	12.6
(Campbell's) prepared	8 oz	90	8.0	6.0
(Campbell's) prepared w/whole milk	8 oz	160	13.0	10.0
(Campbell's) 'Seashore Soups'	4 oz	90	8.0	6.0
(Campbell's) 'Seashore Soups' prepared w/2% milk	4 oz	140	13.0	10.0
SPLIT PEA				
W/egg barley *(Rokeach)* prepared	1 cup	132	23.6	0.5
W/ham				
prepared	1 cup	190	28.0	4.4

Food Name	Serv. Size	Total Cal.	Carbs GMS	Fat GMS
unprepared	11.5 oz	460	67.8	10.7
W/ham and bacon *(Campbell's)* prepared	8 oz	160	24.0	4.0
STOCKPOT				
prepared	1 cup	99	11.5	3.9
unprepared	11 oz	243	27.9	9.5
TOMATO				
prepared	1 cup	85	16.6	1.9
prepared w/whole milk	1 cup	161	22.3	6.0
unprepared	10.75 oz	207	40.3	4.7
(Campbell's) prepared	8 oz	90	17.0	2.0
(Campbell's) prepared w/whole milk	8 oz	150	22.0	4.0
(Campbell's) 'Healthy Request'	4 oz	90	17.0	2.0
(Campbell's) 'Healthy Request' prepared	8 oz	90	17.0	2.0
(Campbell's) 'Healthy Request' prepared w/half 2% milk, half water	8 oz	140	22.0	3.0
(Campbell's) 'Healthy Request' prepared w/skim milk	4 oz	130	22.0	2.0
(Campbell's) 'Healthy Request' prepared w/whole milk	8 oz	150	22.0	4.0
Italian, w/basil and oregano				
(Campbell's)	4 oz	90	21.0	0.0
(Campbell's) prepared	8 oz	90	21.0	0.0
Zesty *(Campbell's)* prepared	8 oz	100	20.0	2.0
TOMATO, CREAM OF				
(Campbell's) 'Homestyle' prepared	8 oz	110	20.0	3.0
(Campbell's) 'Homestyle' prepared w/whole milk	8 oz	180	25.0	7.0
TOMATO BEEF W/NOODLES				
prepared	1 cup	139	21.1	4.3
unprepared	10.75 oz	342	51.5	10.4
TOMATO BISQUE				
prepared w/milk	1 cup	198	29.4	6.6
unprepared	11 oz	300	57.6	6.1
(Campbell's) prepared	8 oz	120	22.0	3.0
TOMATO RICE				
prepared	1 cup	119	21.9	2.7
unprepared	11 oz	290	53.3	6.6
(Campbell's) 'Old Fashioned' prepared	8 oz	110	22.0	2.0
TURKEY NOODLE				
prepared	1 cup	68	8.6	2.0
unprepared	10.75 oz	168	21.0	4.8
(Campbell's) prepared	8 oz	70	9.0	2.0
TURKEY VEGETABLE				
prepared	1 cup	72	8.6	3.0
unprepared	10.5 oz	179	21.0	7.4
(Campbell's) prepared	8 oz	70	8.0	3.0

Food Name	Serv. Size	Total Cal.	Carbs GMS	Fat GMS
VEGETABLE				
(Campbell's) prepared	8 oz	90	14.0	2.0
(Campbell's) 'Homestyle' prepared	8 oz	60	9.0	2.0
(Campbell's) 'Old Fashioned' prepared	8 oz	60	9.0	2.0
Hearty, w/pasta				
(Campbell's)	4 oz	70	15.0	<1.0
(Campbell's) prepared	8 oz	70	15.0	<1.0
Vegetarian				
prepared	1 cup	72	12.0	1.9
unprepared	10.5 oz	176	29.1	4.7
(Campbell's) prepared	8 oz	80	13.0	2.0
W/beef broth				
prepared	1 cup	82	13.1	1.9
unprepared	10.5 oz	197	31.9	4.7
W/beef stock				
(Campbell's) 'Healthy Request'	4 oz	90	14.0	2.0
(Campbell's) 'Healthy Request' prepared	8 oz	90	14.0	2.0
VEGETABLE BEEF				
prepared	1 cup	78	10.2	1.9
unprepared	10.75 oz	192	24.7	4.6
(Campbell's) prepared	8 oz	70	10.0	2.0
(Campbell's) 'Healthy Request' prepared	8 oz	70	10.0	2.0
WON TON *(Campbell's)* prepared	8 oz	40	5.0	1.0
SOUP, CANNED, READY-TO-SERVE				
BEAN				
(Grandma Brown's)	1 cup	190	30.9	3.4
W/ham				
(Campbell's) 'Chunky Old Fashioned'	11 oz	290	38.0	9.0
(Campbell's) 'Chunky Old Fashioned'	9 5/8 oz	250	33.0	8.0
(Campbell's) 'Home Cookin''	9.5 oz	180	25.0	4.0
(Campbell's) 'Home Cookin''	10.75 oz	210	29.0	4.0
(Healthy Choice)	7.5 oz	220	35.0	4.0
(Hormel) 'Hearty Soup'	7.5 oz	190	29.0	4.0
BEEF				
(Progresso)	10.5 oz	180	17.0	6.0
(Progresso)	9.5 oz	160	15.0	5.0
Bouillon	8 oz	17	0.1	0.5
Broth *(College Inn)*	7 oz	16	1.0	0.0
Chunky				
(Campbell's) 'Chunky'	10.75 oz	200	24.0	5.0
(Campbell's) 'Chunky'	9.5 oz	170	21.0	4.0
Fat-free *(Health Valley)*	6.9 oz	10	2.0	0.0
Fat-free, no salt added *(Health Valley)*	6.9 oz	10	2.0	0.0

Food Name	Serv. Size	Total Cal.	Carbs GMS	Fat GMS
Hearty				
(Healthy Choice) 'Hearty Beef'	7.5 oz	120	17.0	2.0
(Progresso)	9.5 oz	160	15.0	4.0
Stroganoff style *(Campbell's)* 'Chunky'	10.75 oz	320	28.0	16.0
W/barley				
(Progresso)	10.5 oz	150	16.0	5.0
(Progresso)	9.5 oz	140	16.0	4.0
W/broth				
(College Inn)	1 cup	18	1.0	0.0
(Health Valley)	7.5 oz	17	2.0	1.0
(Health Valley) 'No Salt Added'	7.5 oz	17	2.0	1.0
(Progresso) seasoned	4 oz	10	<1.0	<1.0
(Swanson)	7.25 oz	18	0.0	1.0
W/minestrone				
(Progresso)	10.5 oz	180	18.0	6.0
(Progresso)	9.5 oz	170	16.0	5.0
W/noodles *(Progresso)*	9.5 oz	170	18.0	4.0
W/tomato juice	1 oz	11	2.6	0.0
W/vegetables				
(Lipton) 'Hearty Ones'	11 oz	229	40.0	3.0
(Progresso)	10.5 oz	170	18.0	3.0
(Progresso)	9.5 oz	150	16.0	3.0
W/vegetables and pasta				
(Campbell's) 'Home Cookin'	10.75 oz	140	18.0	2.0
(Campbell's) 'Home Cookin'	9.5 oz	120	16.0	2.0
BERRY				
Blueberry *(Great Impressions)*	6 oz	95	22.5	0.3
Three berry *(Great Impressions)*	6 oz	107	25.8	0.2
BLACK BEAN				
(Health Valley)	7.5 oz	160	24.0	3.0
(Health Valley) 'No Salt Added'	7.5 oz	160	24.0	3.0
(Health Valley) w/vegetables, fat-free	7.5 oz	70	9.0	0.0
BORSCHT				
(Gold's)	8 oz	100	21.0	0.0
(Rokeach)	1 cup	96	23.0	0.3
(Rokeach) 'Unsalted'	1 cup	103	23.0	0.3
Low-calorie				
(Gold's)	8 oz	20	5.0	<1.0
(Manischewitz)	1 cup	20	4.0	0.0
(Rokeach) 'Diet'	1 cup	29	5.8	0.2
W/beets *(Manischewitz)*	1 cup	80	20.0	0.0
BROCCOLI, CREAM OF *(Andersen's)*	7.5 oz	170	20.0	8.0
CHERRY *(Great Impressions)*	6 oz	123	29.6	0.2

Food Name	Serv. Size	Total Cal.	Carbs GMS	Fat GMS
CHICKEN				
(Progresso) 'Homestyle'	9.5 oz	110	12.0	3.0
Broth				
(Campbell's) 'Healthy Request'	8 oz	16	1.0	0.0
(Campbell's) 'Low Sodium'	10.5 oz	30	2.0	1.0
(College Inn)	1 cup	35	0.0	3.0
(College Inn)	7 oz	35	0.0	3.0
(College Inn) lower salt	7 oz	20	0.0	2.0
(Hain)	8.75 oz	70	0.0	6.0
(Health Valley) fat-free	6.9 oz	20	1.0	0.0
(Hain) 'No Salt Added'	8.75 oz	60	0.0	5.0
(Health Valley)	7.5 oz	35	1.0	2.0
(Health Valley) 'No Salt Added'	7.5 oz	35	1.0	2.0
(Pritikin) defatted	1 cup	18	1.0	1.0
(Progresso)	4 oz	8	0.0	0.0
(Swanson)	7.25 oz	30	2.0	2.0
(Swanson) 'Natural Goodness'	7.25 oz	20	1.0	1.0
Chunky				
(Campbell's) 'Chunky Old Fashioned'	10.75 oz	180	21.0	5.0
(Campbell's) 'Chunky Old Fashioned'	9.5 oz	150	18.0	4.0
(Healthy Choice) 'Hearty Chicken'	7.5 oz	150	17.0	5.0
Hearty				
(Progresso)	10.5 oz	130	9.0	4.0
(Progresso)	9.5 oz	130	11.0	4.0
Nuggets, w/vegetables and noodles				
(Campbell's) 'Chunky'	10.75 oz	190	24.0	6.0
(Campbell's) 'Chunky'	9.5 oz	170	21.0	6.0
W/meatballs (Progresso) 'Chickarina'	9.5 oz	130	13.0	5.0
W/noodles				
(Campbell's) 'Home Cookin'	10.75 oz	140	12.0	4.0
(Campbell's) 'Home Cookin'	9.5 oz	110	10.0	3.0
(Campbell's) 'Low Sodium'	10.75 oz	170	17.0	5.0
W/ribbon pasta (Pritikin)	1 cup	80	13.0	1.0
W/rice				
(Campbell's) 'Chunky'	9.5 oz	140	16.0	4.0
(Healthy Choice)	7.5 oz	140	18.0	4.0
(Hormel) 'Hearty Soup'	7.5 oz	110	17.0	2.0
W/wild rice (Progresso)	9.5 oz	120	17.0	3.0
CHICKEN, CREAM OF (Progresso)	9.5 oz	190	12.0	11.0
CHICKEN BARLEY (Progresso)	9.25 oz	100	12.0	2.0
CHICKEN GUMBO, w/sausage				
(Campbell's) 'Home Cookin'	10.75 oz	140	15.0	4.0
(Campbell's) 'Home Cookin'	9.5 oz	120	13.0	3.0

Food Name	Serv. Size	Total Cal.	Carbs GMS	Fat GMS
CHICKEN MINESTRONE				
(Campbell's) 'Home Cookin'	10.75 oz	180	17.0	6.0
(Campbell's) 'Home Cookin'	9.5 oz	160	15.0	5.0
(Progresso)	10.5 oz	140	14.0	4.0
(Progresso)	9.5 oz	130	12.0	3.0
CHICKEN MUSHROOM, CREAMY				
(Campbell's) 'Chunky'	10.5 oz	270	13.0	19.0
(Campbell's) 'Chunky'	9 3/8 oz	240	12.0	17.0
CHICKEN NOODLE				
(Hain)	9.5 oz	120	11.0	4.0
(Hain) 'No Salt Added'	9.5 oz	120	12.0	4.0
(Healthy Choice) 'Old Fashioned Chicken Noodle'	7.5 oz	90	9.0	3.0
(Hormel) 'Hearty Soup'	7.5 oz	110	14.0	3.0
(Lipton) 'Hearty Ones Homestyle'	11 oz	227	37.4	4.0
(Progresso)	10.5 oz	120	8.0	4.0
(Progresso)	9.5 oz	120	10.0	4.0
(Progresso) 'Healthy Classics'	8 oz	80	10.0	2.0
(Weight Watchers)	10.5 oz	80	9.0	2.0
Chunky				
(Campbell's) 'Chunky'	10.75 oz	200	20.0	7.0
(Campbell's) 'Chunky'	9.5 oz	180	18.0	7.0
Hearty (Campbell's) 'Healthy Request'	8 oz	80	7.0	2.0
CHICKEN RICE				
(Campbell's) 'Home Cookin'	10.75 oz	150	10.0	6.0
(Campbell's) 'Home Cookin'	9.5 oz	130	9.0	5.0
(Progresso)	10.5 oz	120	12.0	4.0
(Progresso)	9.5 oz	130	16.0	3.0
Chunky	8 oz	127	13.0	3.2
Hearty (Campbell's) 'Healthy Request'	8 oz	110	15.0	3.0
W/vegetables (Progresso) 'Healthy Classics'	8 oz	80	11.0	2.0
CHICKEN VEGETABLE				
(Hain)	9.5 oz	120	14.0	4.0
(Hain) 'No Salt Added'	9.5 oz	130	14.0	4.0
(Campbell's) 'Chunky'	9.5 oz	170	19.0	6.0
(Campbell's) 'Chunky Low Sodium'	10.75 oz	240	21.0	11.0
(Campbell's) 'Home Cookin'	10.75 oz	180	25.0	4.0
(Pritikin)	1 cup	70	12.0	1.0
(Progresso)	9.5 oz	140	17.0	4.0
Chunky				
(Health Valley)	7.5 oz	125	20.0	2.0
(Health Valley) 'No Salt Added'	7.5 oz	125	20.0	2.0
Hearty (Campbell's) 'Healthy Request'	8 oz	120	16.0	3.0

Food Name	Serv. Size	Total Cal.	Carbs GMS	Fat GMS
CHILI BEEF				
(Campbell's) 'Chunky'	11 oz	290	37.0	7.0
(Campbell's) 'Chunky'	9.75 oz	260	33.0	6.0
(Healthy Choice) thick and hearty	7.5 oz	150	22.0	1.0
CLAM CHOWDER				
Manhattan style				
(Campbell's) 'Chunky'	10.75 oz	160	24.0	4.0
(Campbell's) 'Chunky'	9.5 oz	150	21.0	4.0
(Health Valley)	7.5 oz	110	15.0	2.0
(Health Valley) 'No Salt Added'	7.5 oz	110	15.0	2.0
(Progresso)	9.5 oz	120	13.0	2.0
New England style				
(Campbell's) 'Chunky'	10.75 oz	290	26.0	17.0
(Campbell's) 'Chunky'	9.5 oz	260	23.0	15.0
(Campbell's) 'Healthy Request'	8 oz	100	14.0	3.0
(Campbell's) 'Home Cookin'	10.75 oz	260	15.0	18.0
(Gorton's) 'New England Style'	7.5 oz	140	17.0	5.0
(Hain)	9.25 oz	180	26.0	4.0
(Hormel) 'Hearty Soup'	7.5 oz	130	16.0	5.0
(Progresso)	10.5 oz	220	21.0	12.0
(Progresso)	9.25 oz	220	20.0	12.0
(Weight Watchers)	7.5 oz	90	16.0	0.0
CORN AND VEGETABLE, fat-free (Health Valley)	7.5 oz	70	13.0	0.0
CORN CHOWDER				
(Campbell's) 'Chunky'	10.75 oz	340	23.0	21.0
(Campbell's) 'Chunky'	9.5 oz	300	21.0	19.0
(Progresso)	9.25 oz	200	22.0	10.0
CRAB	8 oz	76	10.3	1.5
CREOLE				
(Campbell's) 'Chunky'	10.75 oz	240	31.0	8.0
(Campbell's) 'Chunky'	9.5 oz	220	28.0	7.0
ESCAROLE, in chicken broth (Progresso)	9.25 oz	30	2.0	1.0
GAZPACHO	8 oz	56	0.8	2.2
HAM AND BEAN				
(Campbell's) w/butterbeans 'Chunky'	10.75 oz	280	34.0	10.0
(Progresso)	9.5 oz	140	28.0	2.0
LEMON (Great Impressions)	6 oz	90	22.1	<1.0
LENTIL				
(Health Valley)	7.5 oz	170	28.0	2.0
(Health Valley) 'No Salt Added'	7.5 oz	170	28.0	2.0
(Progresso)	10.5 oz	140	24.0	4.0
(Progresso)	9.5 oz	140	25.0	4.0
(Progresso) 'Healthy Classics'	8 oz	120	19.0	1.0

Food Name	Serv. Size	Total Cal.	Carbs GMS	Fat GMS
Hearty				
(Campbell's) 'Home Cookin'	10.75 oz	170	28.0	2.0
(Campbell's) 'Home Cookin'	9.5 oz	140	24.0	1.0
Vegetarian				
(Hain)	9.5 oz	160	25.0	3.0
(Hain) 'No Salt Added'	9.5 oz	160	24.0	3.0
W/carrots, fat-free (Health Valley)	7.5 oz	70	10.0	0.0
W/ham	8 oz	139	20.2	2.8
W/sausage (Progresso)	9.5 oz	170	21.0	8.0
MACARONI AND BEAN				
(Progresso)	10.5 oz	150	27.0	4.0
(Progresso)	9.5 oz	140	25.0	5.0
MENUDO (Old El Paso)	1/2 can	476	14.0	52.0
MINESTRONE				
(Campbell's) 'Chunky'	9.5 oz	160	24.0	4.0
(Campbell's) 'Healthy Request'	8 oz	90	13.0	2.0
(Campbell's) 'Home Cookin'	10.75 oz	140	22.0	3.0
(Campbell's) 'Home Cookin'	9.5 oz	120	20.0	3.0
(Hain)	9.5 oz	170	27.0	2.0
(Hain) 'No Salt Added'	9.5 oz	160	28.0	4.0
(Health Valley)	7.5 oz	130	19.0	3.0
(Health Valley) 'No Salt Added'	7.5 oz	130	19.0	3.0
(Health Valley) 'Real Italian Fat-Free'	7.5 oz	80	12.0	0.0
(Healthy Choice)	7.5 oz	160	30.0	2.0
(Hormel) 'Hearty Soup'	7.5 oz	100	17.0	1.0
(Lipton) 'Hearty Ones'	11 oz	189	36.1	3.2
(Progresso)	10.5 oz	120	25.0	3.0
(Progresso)	9.5 oz	130	22.0	4.0
(Progresso) chunky, hearty	9.25 oz	110	16.0	2.0
(Progresso) chunky, zesty	9.5 oz	150	19.0	8.0
(Progresso) 'Healthy Classics'	8 oz	120	19.0	2.0
MUSHROOM, CREAM OF				
(Campbell's) 'Low Sodium'	10.5 oz	210	18.0	14.0
(Hain)	9.25 oz	110	16.0	4.0
(Progresso)	9.25 oz	160	14.0	10.0
(Weight Watchers)	10.5 oz	90	14.0	2.0
MUSHROOM BARLEY				
(Hain)	9.5 oz	100	17.0	2.0
(Health Valley)	7.5 oz	100	16.0	2.0
(Health Valley) 'No Salt Added'	7.5 oz	100	16.0	2.0
PEPPER STEAK				
(Campbell's) 'Chunky'	9.5 oz	160	21.0	3.0
(Campbell's) 'Chunky'	10.75 oz	180	24.0	3.0

Food Name	Serv. Size	Total Cal.	Carbs GMS	Fat GMS
POTATO, CREAM OF *(Andersen's)*	7.5 oz	200	25.0	10.0
POTATO LEEK				
(Health Valley)	7.5 oz	130	23.0	2.0
(Health Valley) 'No Salt Added'	7.5 oz	130	23.0	2.0
SCHAV *(Gold's)*	8 oz	25	4.0	0.0
SIRLOIN BURGER				
(Campbell's) 'Chunky'	10.75 oz	220	23.0	9.0
(Campbell's) 'Chunky'	9.5 oz	200	20.0	8.0
SPLIT PEA				
(Andersen's)	7.5 oz	130	24.0	0.0
(Campbell's) 'Low Sodium'	10.75 oz	230	37.0	4.0
(Grandma Brown's)	1 cup	208	31.0	4.1
(Hain)	9.5 oz	170	28.0	1.0
(Hain) 'No Salt Added'	9.5 oz	170	29.0	1.0
(Progresso)	9.5 oz	160	27.0	3.0
Green				
(Health Valley)	7.5 oz	190	34.0	0.3
(Health Valley) 'No Salt Added'	7.5 oz	190	34.0	0.3
(Hain) vegetarian	9.5 oz	170	28.0	1.0
(Hain) vegetarian 'No Salt Added'	9.5 oz	170	27.0	1.0
(Progresso)	10.5 oz	201	31.0	3.0
W/ham				
(Campbell's) 'Chunky'	10.5 oz	230	33.0	6.0
(Campbell's) 'Chunky'	9.5 oz	210	30.0	5.0
(Campbell's) 'Home Cookin'	10.75 oz	230	38.0	1.0
(Campbell's) 'Home Cookin'	9.5 oz	200	34.0	1.0
(Healthy Choice)	7.5 oz	170	25.0	3.0
(Progresso)	10.5 oz	160	24.0	5.0
(Progresso)	9.5 oz	150	23.0	5.0
STEAK AND POTATO				
(Campbell's) 'Chunky'	10.75 oz	200	24.0	5.0
(Campbell's) 'Chunky'	9.5 oz	170	21.0	4.0
TOMATO				
(Health Valley)	7.5 oz	100	17.0	3.0
(Health Valley) 'No Salt Added'	7.5 oz	100	17.0	3.0
(Healthy Choice) 'Tomato Garden'	7.5 oz	130	22.0	3.0
(Progresso)	9.5 oz	120	20.0	3.0
Beef, w/rotini *(Progresso)*	9.5 oz	170	18.0	6.0
Garden				
(Campbell's) 'Home Cookin'	10.75 oz	150	29.0	3.0
(Campbell's) 'Home Cookin'	9.5 oz	130	25.0	2.0
W/tomato pieces *(Campbell's)* 'Low Sodium'	10.5 oz	190	30.0	6.0
W/tortellini *(Progresso)*	9.25 oz	130	16.0	5.0

Food Name	Serv. Size	Total Cal.	Carbs GMS	Fat GMS
TOMATO VEGETABLE, fat-free *(Health Valley)*	7.5 oz	50	8.0	0.0
TORTELLINI				
(Progresso)	9.5 oz	90	11.0	3.0
(Progresso) Creamy	9.25 oz	240	17.0	16.0
TURKEY	8 oz	135	14.1	4.4
TURKEY RICE				
(Hain)	9.5 oz	100	10.0	3.0
(Hain) 'No Salt Added'	9.5 oz	120	13.0	4.0
TURKEY VEGETABLE				
(Campbell's) 'Chunky'	9 3/8 oz	150	16.0	6.0
(Weight Watchers)	10.5 oz	70	10.0	2.0
VEGETABLE				
(Campbell's) 'Chunky'	10.75 oz	160	28.0	4.0
(Campbell's) 'Chunky'	9.5 oz	150	25.0	4.0
(Health Valley)	7.5 oz	110	20.0	1.0
(Health Valley) 'No Salt Added'	7.5 oz	110	20.0	1.0
(Healthy Choice) 'Country Vegetable'	7.5 oz	120	23.0	1.0
(Progresso)	9.5 oz	80	15.0	2.0
(Progresso) 'Healthy Classics'	8 oz	80	13.0	1.0
Country				
(Campbell's) 'Home Cookin'	10.75 oz	120	20.0	2.0
(Campbell's) 'Home Cookin'	9.5 oz	100	18.0	2.0
(Hormel) 'Hearty Soup'	7.5 oz	90	14.0	2.0
Five bean, chunky				
(Health Valley)	7.5 oz	110	21.0	2.0
(Health Valley) 'No Salt Added'	7.5 oz	110	21.0	2.0
Fourteen garden vegetables, fat-free *(Health Valley)*	7.5 oz	50	9.0	0.0
Hearty *(Campbell's)* 'Healthy Request'	8 oz	90	17.0	1.0
Italian, w/pasta				
(Hain)	9.5 oz	160	25.0	5.0
(Hain) 'Low Sodium'	9.5 oz	140	22.0	6.0
Mediterranean *(Campbell's)* 'Chunky'	9.5 oz	170	24.0	6.0
Vegetarian				
chunky *(Weight Watchers)*	10.5 oz	100	18.0	2.0
(Hain)	9.5 oz	140	22.0	4.0
(Hain) 'No Salt Added'	9.5 oz	150	23.0	5.0
W/barley, fat-free *(Health Valley)*	7.5 oz	60	11.0	0.0
W/beef stock *(Weight Watchers)*	10.5 oz	90	13.0	2.0
VEGETABLE BEEF				
(Campbell's) 'Chunky Low Sodium'	10.75 oz	180	19.0	5.0
(Campbell's) 'Chunky Old Fashioned'	10.75 oz	190	20.0	6.0
(Campbell's) 'Chunky Old Fashioned'	9.5 oz	160	17.0	5.0
(Campbell's) hearty	8 oz	120	17.0	2.0

Food Name	Serv. Size	Total Cal.	Carbs GMS	Fat GMS
(Campbell's) 'Home Cookin'	10.75 oz	140	17.0	3.0
(Campbell's) 'Home Cookin'	9.5 oz	120	15.0	2.0
(Hormel) 'Hearty Soup'	7.5 oz	90	15.0	1.0
(Healthy Choice) 'Vegetable Beef'	7.5 oz	130	21.0	1.0
VEGETABLE BROTH				
(Hain)	9.5 oz	45	10.0	0.0
(Hain) 'Low Sodium'	9.5 oz	40	8.0	<1.0
SOUP, FROZEN				
ASPARAGUS, CREAM OF				
(Kettle Ready)	6 oz	62	5.1	4.3
(Myers)	9.75 oz	152	10.0	8.0
BARLEY BEAN *(Tabatchnick)*	7.5 oz	130	22.0	2.0
BEAN				
Northern bean *(Tabatchnick)*	7.5 oz	164	29.0	2.0
Savory, w/ham *(Kettle Ready)*	6 oz	113	20.2	3.6
W/beef and vegetables, hearty *(Kettle Ready)*	6 oz	85	10.7	3.0
BLACK BEAN, w/ham *(Kettle Ready)*	6 oz	154	23.0	6.2
BROCCOLI, CREAM OF				
(Kettle Ready)	6 oz	94	6.4	7.2
(Myers)	9.75 oz	174	11.0	11.0
(Tabatchnick)	7.5 oz	90	10.0	4.0
CABBAGE *(Tabatchnick)*	7.5 oz	110	21.0	2.0
CAULIFLOWER, CREAM OF *(Kettle Ready)*	6 oz	93	5.5	7.0
CHEDDAR CHEESE, CREAM OF				
(Kettle Ready)	6 oz	158	7.3	12.5
(Kettle Ready) w/broccoli	6 oz	137	4.7	11.3
CHEESE, w/broccoli *(Myers)*	9.75 oz	325	19.0	23.0
CHICKEN *(Tabatchnick)*	7.5 oz	65	10.0	2.0
CHICKEN, CREAM OF *(Kettle Ready)*	6 oz	98	5.0	6.2
CHICKEN GUMBO *(Kettle Ready)*	6 oz	94	12.1	3.5
CHICKEN NOODLE				
(Kettle Ready)	6 oz	94	12.0	3.0
(Myers)	9.75 oz	87	5.0	5.0
CHILI				
(Kettle Ready)	6 oz	161	14.0	6.5
(Kettle Ready) jalapeño	6 oz	173	14.7	8.0
CLAM CHOWDER				
Boston *(Kettle Ready)*	6 oz	131	13.0	7.3
Manhattan style *(Kettle Ready)*	6 oz	69	8.0	2.6
New England style				
(Kettle Ready)	6 oz	116	11.4	6.5
(Myers)	9.75 oz	152	21.0	5.0
(Stouffer's)	8 oz	180	16.0	9.0

Food Name	Serv. Size	Total Cal.	Carbs GMS	Fat GMS
(Tabatchnick)	7.5 oz	98	14.0	2.0
CORN CHOWDER w/broccoli *(Kettle Ready)*	6 oz	102	13.0	5.0
LENTIL *(Tabatchnick)*	7.5 oz	170	27.0	2.0
MINESTRONE				
(Kettle Ready) hearty	6 oz	104	15.2	4.4
(Tabatchnick)	7.5 oz	137	24.0	2.0
MUSHROOM, CREAM OF				
(Kettle Ready)	6 oz	85	6.2	6.4
(Tabatchnick)	6 oz	75	11.0	2.0
MUSHROOM BARLEY				
(Tabatchnick)	7.5 oz	92	16.0	2.0
(Tabatchnick) 'No Salt'	7.5 oz	97	18.0	1.0
ONION, French *(Kettle Ready)*	6 oz	42	5.0	2.2
PEA				
(Tabatchnick)	7.5 oz	175	31.0	1.0
(Tabatchnick) 'No Salt'	7.5 oz	175	31.0	1.0
SEAFOOD BISQUE *(Myers)*	9.75 oz	163	13.0	8.0
SPINACH, CREAM OF				
(Myers)	9.75 oz	174	10.0	11.0
(Stouffer's)	8 oz	210	12.0	15.0
(Tabatchnick)	7.5 oz	85	12.0	2.0
SPLIT PEA W/HAM *(Kettle Ready)*	6 oz	155	25.3	4.4
TOMATO RICE *(Tabatchnick)*	6 oz	73	14.0	1.0
TOMATO TORTELLINI *(Kettle Ready)*	6 oz	122	15.0	5.4
VEGETABLE				
(Kettle Ready) garden	6 oz	85	12.3	3.0
(Tabatchnick)	7.5 oz	97	18.0	1.0
(Tabatchnick) 'No Salt'	7.5 oz	92	16.0	2.0
VEGETABLE BEEF *(Myers)*	9.75 oz	120	8.0	6.0
ZUCCHINI *(Tabatchnick)*	6 oz	80	12.0	2.0
SOUP, MICROWAVE				
BEAN				
W/bacon and ham *(Campbell's)*	7.5 oz	230	38.0	5.0
W/ham, chowder *(Hormel)* 'Micro-Cup Hearty Soups'	1 pkg	191	31.0	3.0
BEEF, w/vegetable *(Hormel)* 'Micro-Cup Hearty Soups'	1 pkg	71	12.0	1.0
CHICKEN				
W/rice *(Campbell's)* 'Microwave'	7.5 oz	100	14.0	4.0
W/vegetables and rice *(Hormel)* 'Micro-Cup Hearty Soups'	1 pkg	114	16.0	3.0
CHICKEN NOODLE				
(Campbell's) 'Microwave'	7.5 oz	100	11.0	4.0
(Hormel) 'Micro-Cup Hearty Soups'	1 pkg	108	14.0	3.0
(Lunch Bucket) microwave cup	7.25 oz	90	13.0	2.0
(Weight Watchers) microwave cup	7.5 oz	90	13.0	1.0

Food Name	Serv. Size	Total Cal.	Carbs GMS	Fat GMS
CHILI BEEF *(Campbell's)* 'Microwave'	7.5 oz	190	32.0	4.0
CLAM CHOWDER				
New England *(Hormel)* 'Micro-Cup Hearty Soups'	1 pkg	118	15.0	5.0
MINESTRONE *(Hormel)* 'Micro-Cup Hearty Soups'	1 pkg	104	15.0	2.0
NOODLE				
Beef flavor *(Campbell's)* 'Cup Microwave'	1.35 oz	130	23.0	2.0
Chicken flavor *(Campbell's)* 'Cup Microwave'	1.35 oz	140	22.0	3.0
Pork flavor, w/vegetables *(Campbell's)* 'Hearty Microwave'	1.7 oz	180	32.0	2.0
W/chicken broth *(Campbell's)* 'Cup Microwave'	1.35 oz	130	23.0	2.0
VEGETABLE, country				
(Hormel) 'Micro-Cup Hearty Soups'	1 pkg	89	13.0	2.0
(Lunch Bucket) microwave cup	7.25 oz	70	15.0	1.0
VEGETABLE BEEF				
(Campbell's) 'Microwave'	7.5 oz	100	16.0	2.0
(Weight Watchers) microwave cup	7.5 oz	90	13.0	1.0
SOUP MIX				
(NOTE: Unless otherwise specified, PREPARED = prepared as directed w/water.)				
ASPARAGUS, prepared	8 oz	52	7.9	1.5
ASPARAGUS, CREAM OF, prepared	8 oz	58	8.9	1.7
BEAN W/BACON, prepared	1 cup	106	16.4	2.2
BEEF				
Beef flavor, w/noodles				
(Campbell's) 'Ramen Noodle' prepared	6 oz	160	32.0	1.0
(Estee) prepared	6 oz	20	3.0	<1.0
(Lipton) 'Cup-A-Soup' prepared	6 oz	44	7.6	0.7
(Lipton) 'Hearty' prepared	6 oz	107	20.2	1.4
Beef flavor, w/noodles and vegetables				
(Campbell's) prepared	6 oz	220	44.0	2.0
Broth				
cubed	1 cube	6	0.6	0.1
cubed, prepared	6 oz	5	0.6	0.1
powder, prepared	8 oz	20	1.9	0.7
Hearty *(Soup Starter)* 'Homestyle'	.945 oz	90	20.0	<1.0
Vegetable *(Soup Starter)* 'Homestyle'	.91 oz	90	18.0	<1.0
W/noodles *(Ultra Slim Fast)* 1 envelope, prepared	6 oz	45	7.0	<1.0
BEEF NOODLE, prepared	8 oz	40	6.0	0.8
BLACK BEAN				
(Fantastic Foods) 'Jumpin' black beans, prepared	10 oz	170	40.0	1.0
BROCCOLI				
Creamy				
(Lipton) 'Cup-A-Soup' prepared	6 oz	62	9.1	2.4
(Lipton) 'Cup-A-Soup Food Service' prepared	6 oz	62	8.9	2.3
(Ultra Slim Fast) 1 envelope, prepared	6 oz	75	14.0	<1.0

Food Name	Serv. Size	Total Cal.	Carbs GMS	Fat GMS
Golden *(Lipton)* 'Cup-A-Soup Lite' prepared	6 oz	42	16.3	1.2
W/cheese *(Lipton)* 'Cup-A-Soup' prepared	6 oz	70	9.8	3.4
BOUILLON				
Beef flavor				
cubed	1 cube	6	0.6	0.1
cubed *(Steero)*	1 cube	6	1.0	<1.0
cubed *(Wyler's)*	1 cube	6	1.0	<1.0
instant *(Featherweight)*	1 tsp	18	2.0	1.0
instant *(Lite-Line)* 'Low Sodium'	1 tsp	12	2.0	<1.0
instant *(Steero)*	1 tsp	6	1.0	<1.0
instant *(Weight Watchers)* 'Broth Mix'	1 pkt	8	1.0	0.0
instant *(Wyler's)*	1 tsp	6	1.0	<1.0
powder	1 pkt	14	1.4	0.5
powder, prepared	8 oz	19	1.9	0.7
Brown				
(G. Washington's) 'Seasoning & Broth'	.14 oz	6	1.0	0.0
(G. Washington's) 'Seasoning & Broth' kosher	.14 oz	6	1.0	0.0
Chicken flavor				
cubed	1 cube	9	1.1	0.2
cubed *(Steero)*	1 cube	8	1.0	<1.0
cubed *(Wyler's)*	1 cube	8	1.0	<1.0
instant *(Featherweight)*	1 tsp	18	2.0	1.0
instant *(Lite-Line)* 'Low Sodium'	1 tsp	12	2.0	<1.0
instant *(Steero)*	1 tsp	8	1.0	<1.0
instant *(Weight Watchers)* 'Broth Mix'	1 pkt	8	1.0	0.0
instant *(Wyler's)*	1 tsp	8	1.0	<1.0
Golden				
(G. Washington's') 'Seasoning & Broth'	.13 oz	6	1.0	0.0
(G. Washington's) 'Seasoning & Broth' kosher	.13 oz	6	1.0	0.0
Onion flavor				
(G. Washington's) 'Seasoning and Broth'	.18 oz	12	2.0	0.0
(Wyler's) instant	1 tsp	10	1.0	<1.0
Vegetable flavor				
(G. Washington's) 'Seasoning & Broth'	.18 oz	12	2.0	0.0
(Wyler's) instant	1 tsp	6	1.0	<1.0
CAULIFLOWER, prepared	8 oz	69	10.7	1.7
CELERY, prepared	8 oz	63	9.8	1.6
CHEESE				
(Fantastic Noodles) creamy cheddar w/noodles, prepared	7 oz	178	21.0	8.0
(Hain) cheese and broccoli, prepared	6 oz	310	19.0	22.0
(Hain) 'Savory Soup & Sauce Mix' prepared	6 oz	250	20.0	16.0
CHICKEN				
prepared	8 oz	107	13.3	5.3

Food Name	Serv. Size	Total Cal.	Carbs GMS	Fat GMS
(Soup Starter) 'Homestyle'	.735 oz	70	15.0	<1.0
Broth				
cubed	1 cube	10	1.1	0.2
cubed, prepared	6 oz	9	1.1	0.2
(Lipton) 'Cup-A-Soup' prepared	6 oz	20	3.3	0.6
Creamy, w/vegetables (Lipton) prepared	6 oz	93	14.4	3.1
Creamy, w/white meat (Campbell's) prepared	6 oz	90	12.0	4.0
Florentine (Lipton) 'Lite'	6 oz	42	7.6	0.5
Hearty				
(Lipton) 'Country Style'	6 oz	69	11.1	1.1
(Lipton) 'Supreme' prepared	6 oz	107	11.4	5.9
Lemon (Lipton) 'Cup-A-Soup Lite' prepared	6 oz	48	9.1	0.4
W/corn (Lipton) 'Country' prepared	6 oz	133	17.5	5.5
W/noodles (Ultra Slim Fast) 1 envelope, prepared	6 oz	45	6.0	<1.0
CHICKEN, CREAM OF				
(Lipton) 'Cup-A-Soup' prepared	6 oz	84	9.7	4.4
(Lipton) 'Food Service' prepared	6 oz	84	9.4	4.4
CHICKEN LEEK				
creamy (Ultra Slim Fast) 1 envelope, prepared	6 oz	50	7.0	<1.0
CHICKEN NOODLE				
prepared	1 cup	53	7.4	1.2
(Campbell's) 'Lowfat Block' prepared	1 cup	160	32.0	1.0
(Campbell's) 'Quality Recipe' prepared	1 cup	100	16.0	2.0
(Campbell's) 'Ramen Noodle' prepared	1 cup	190	26.0	8.0
(Estee) 'Instant' prepared	6 oz	25	4.0	<1.0
(Lipton) 'Cup-A-Soup' prepared	6 oz	48	6.6	1.1
(Lipton) 'Supreme' prepared	6 oz	107	11.8	5.9
(Mrs. Grass) 'Chickeny Rich'	1/4 pkg	70	10.0	2.0
Creamy, hearty (Lipton) prepared	7 oz	179	21.4	8.2
Hearty				
(Lipton) prepared	1 cup	83	13.3	1.3
(Lipton) prepared	7 oz	118	21.2	1.5
W/meat				
(Campbell's) white meat	6 oz	90	12.0	2.0
(Lipton) 'Cup' prepared	6 oz	46	6.6	1.0
(Lipton) 'Value Pack' prepared	6 oz	46	6.6	1.0
(Lipton) white meat, diced, prepared	1 cup	81	12.1	1.8
W/rice (Lipton) prepared	6 oz	47	7.7	0.8
W/vegetables				
(Campbell's) prepared	1 cup	270	38.0	10.0
(Campbell's) lowfat, prepared	1 cup	220	44.0	2.0
(Lipton) 'Cup' prepared	6 oz	47	7.8	0.6
(Lipton) hearty, prepared	1 cup	75	12.3	1.6

Food Name	Serv. Size	Total Cal.	Carbs GMS	Fat GMS
CHICKEN RICE, prepared	8 oz	61	9.3	1.4
CHICKEN VEGETABLE, prepared	8 oz	50	7.8	0.8
CHILI PEPPER (A Taste of Thai) hot and sour, prepared	1 cup	40	5.0	2.0
CLAM CHOWDER				
Manhattan style (Golden Dipt)	1/4 pkg	80	13.0	2.0
New England style (Golden Dipt)	1/4 pkg	70	12.0	2.0
CONSOMMÉ, w/gelatin, prepared	1 cup	17	2.1	0.0
GINGER (A Taste of Thai) tangy coconut, prepared	1 cup	250	3.0	1.5
GREEN PEA				
(Lipton) 'Cup-A-Soup' prepared	6 oz	113	14.4	4.2
(Lipton) 'Cup-A-Soup Food Service' prepared	6 oz	115	15.1	4.5
HERB (Lipton) savory, w/garlic 'Recipe Secrets' prepared	8 oz	35	7.0	<1.0
LEEK				
Creamy (Ultra Slim Fast) 1 envelope prepared	6 oz	80	15.0	<1.0
LENTIL (Hain) 'Savory Soup Mix' prepared	6 oz	130	20.0	2.0
LOBSTER BISQUE (Golden Dipt) prepared	1/4 pkg	30	5.0	1.0
MINESTRONE				
(Hain) 'Savory Soup Mix' prepared	6 oz	110	20.0	1.0
(Manischewitz) prepared	6 oz	50	9.0	<1.0
MUSHROOM				
(Estee) 'Instant' prepared	6 oz	40	3.0	2.0
(Hain) 'Savory Soup & Recipe Mix' prepared	6 oz	210	11.0	15.0
(Hain) 'Savory Soup & Recipe Mix No Salt Added' prepared	6 oz	250	15.0	20.0
Beef flavor (Lipton) prepared	1 cup	38	6.7	0.5
MUSHROOM, CREAM OF (Lipton) 'Cup-A-Soup' prepared	6 oz	71	9.1	3.2
NOODLE				
(Campbell's) 'Quality Soup & Recipe' prepared	1 cup	110	19.0	2.0
(Lipton) 'Cup-A-Soup Ring Noodle' prepared	6 oz	47	7.6	0.7
(Lipton) 'Giggle Noodle' prepared	1 cup	77	11.4	2.1
(Lipton) 'Ring-O-Noodle' prepared	1 cup	71	10.4	2.0
Beef flavor				
(Cup O'Noodles) prepared	1 cup	290	33.0	14.0
(Oodles of Noodles) prepared	1 cup	390	49.0	18.0
(Top Ramen) prepared	1 cup	390	49.0	18.0
Beefy, w/vegetables (Lipton) prepared	1 cup	85	16.7	0.9
Chicken flavor				
(Cup O'Noodles) prepared	1 cup	300	32.0	16.0
(Cup O'Noodles) 'Hearty' prepared	1 cup	300	35.0	14.0
(Oodles of Noodles) prepared	1 cup	400	48.0	18.0
(Top Ramen) prepared	1 cup	400	48.0	18.0
Hearty (Campbell's) 'Quality Soup & Recipe' prepared	1 cup	90	15.0	1.0
Hearty, w/vegetables (Lipton) prepared	1 cup	75	12.3	1.6

Food Name	Serv. Size	Total Cal.	Carbs GMS	Fat GMS
Oriental				
(Campbell's) 'Ramen Noodle' prepared	1 cup	190	26.0	8.0
(Campbell's) 'Ramen Noodle Lowfat Block' prepared	1 cup	150	31.0	1.0
(Oodles of Noodles) prepared	1 cup	390	49.0	18.0
(Top Ramen) prepared	1 cup	390	49.0	18.0
Oriental, w/vegetables				
(Campbell's) 'Cup-A-Ramen' prepared	1 cup	270	38.0	10.0
(Campbell's) 'Cup-A-Ramen Lowfat' prepared	1 cup	220	44.0	2.0
Pork flavor				
(Campbell's) 'Ramen Noodle' prepared	1 cup	200	26.0	8.0
(Campbell's) 'Ramen Noodle Lowfat Block' prepared	1 cup	150	31.0	1.0
(Oodles of Noodles) prepared	1 cup	390	51.0	20.0
(Top Ramen) prepared	1 cup	390	51.0	20.0
Pork flavor, w/old-fashioned vegetables				
(Cup O'Noodles) 'Hearty' prepared	6 oz	290	34.0	15.0
Pork flavor, w/seafood (Cup O'Noodles) 'Hearty' prepared	1 cup	300	34.0	15.0
Pork flavor, w/shrimp (Cup O'Noodles) prepared	1 cup	300	32.0	14.0
W/chicken broth				
(Campbell's) 'Cup 2 Minute Soup' prepared	6 oz	90	15.0	2.0
(Campbell's) 'Double Noodle'	1.78 oz	200	36.0	2.0
(Campbell's) 'Double Noodle' prepared	8 oz	200	36.0	2.0
ONION				
(Campbell's) 'Quality Soup & Recipe' prepared	1 cup	30	7.0	0.0
(Estee) prepared	6 oz	25	4.0	<1.0
(Hain) 'Savory Soup, Dip & Recipe Mix' prepared	6 oz	50	6.0	2.0
(Hain) 'Savory Soup, Dip & Recipe Mix' no salt, prepared	6 oz	50	9.0	1.0
(Lipton) prepared	1 cup	20	4.3	0.2
(Lipton) 'Cup-A-Soup' prepared	6 oz	27	4.7	0.5
(Mrs. Grass) 'Soup & Dip Mix' prepared	1/4 pkg	35	6.0	<1.0
Beefy (Lipton) prepared	1 cup	29	4.2	1.0
Creamy				
(Lipton) 'Cup-A-Soup' prepared	6 oz	70	9.5	3.2
(Ultra Slim Fast) 1 envelope, prepared	6 oz	45	7.0	<1.0
Golden, w/chicken broth (Lipton) prepared	1 cup	62	11.0	1.5
Mushroom (Lipton) prepared	1 cup	41	6.8	0.9
ORIENTAL (Lipton) 'Cup-A-Soup Lite' prepared	6 oz	45	5.8	1.7
OXTAIL prepared	8 oz	71	9.0	2.6
POTATO LEEK (Hain) 'Savory Soup Mix' prepared	6 oz	260	20.0	18.0
SPLIT PEA				
Green				
(Hain) 'Savory Soup Mix' prepared	6 oz	310	16.0	10.0
(Manischewitz) prepared	6 oz	45	9.0	<1.0
Fat-free, thick and creamy (Fantastic Foods) 'Splittin Pea'	10 oz	145	31.0	1.0

Food Name	Serv. Size	Total Cal.	Carbs GMS	Fat GMS
W/carrots (Health Valley)	7.5 oz	80	17.0	0.0
SEAFOOD CHOWDER (Golden Dipt)	1/4 pkg	70	12.0	2.0
SHRIMP				
Bisque (Golden Dipt) dry mix	1/4 pkg	30	5.0	1.0
W/vegetables				
(Campbell's) 'Cup-A-Ramen' prepared	1 cup	280	40.0	10.0
(Campbell's) 'Lowfat' prepared	1 cup	230	45.0	2.0
TOMATO				
(Estee) 'Instant' prepared	6 oz	40	5.0	<1.0
(Hain) 'Savory Soup & Recipe Mix' prepared	6 oz	220	19.0	14.0
(Lipton) 'Cup-A-Soup' prepared	6 oz	103	21.2	0.9
(Lipton) 'Cup-A-Soup Food Service' prepared	6 oz	100	20.1	0.9
Creamy (Ultra Slim Fast) 1 envelope, prepared	6 oz	60	10.0	<1.0
Creamy, w/herb (Lipton) 'Cup-A-Soup Lite' prepared	6 oz	66	14.1	0.3
Minestrone (Cous•cous)	10 oz	200	41.0	0.0
TOMATO VEGETABLE				
prepared	8 oz	56	10.2	0.9
W/noodles (Fantastic Noodles) prepared	7 oz	158	20.0	8.0
VEGETABLE				
(Campbell's) 'Quality Soup & Recipe' prepared	1 cup	40	8.0	0.0
(Hain) 'Savory Soup Mix' prepared	6 oz	80	13.0	1.0
(Hain) 'Savory Soup Mix No Salt Added' prepared	6 oz	80	13.0	1.0
(Lipton) prepared	1 cup	39	6.9	0.5
(Manischewitz) prepared	6 oz	50	9.0	<1.0
Country (Lipton) prepared	1 cup	80	15.7	0.7
Curry, w/noodles (Fantastic Noodles) prepared	7 oz	150	18.0	7.0
Garden (Lipton) 'Lots-A-Noodles Cup-A-Soup' prepared	7 oz	123	23.1	1.5
Harvest				
(Lipton) 'Country Style' prepared	6 oz	95	18.9	1.2
(Lipton) 'Cup-A-Soup Country Style' prepared	6 oz	91	18.8	1.2
Hearty (Ultra Slim Fast) 1 envelope, prepared	6 oz	45	5.0	<1.0
Miso, w/noodles (Fantastic Noodles) prepared	7 oz	152	19.0	7.0
Noodle, w/meatballs (Lipton) 'Country Style' prepared	6 oz	95	15.4	1.6
Parmesan (Cous•cous)	10 oz	200	35.0	3.0
Spring (Lipton) 'Cup-A-Soup' prepared	6 oz	33	5.9	0.8
VEGETABLE BEEF, prepared	8 oz	53	8.0	1.1
VIRGINIA PEA				
(Lipton) prepared	6 oz	113	14.6	4.1
(Lipton) 'Country Style' prepared	6 oz	148	17.3	6.4
SOUR CREAM				
	1 cup	493	9.8	48.2
	1 oz	61	1.2	5.9
	1 tbsp	26	0.5	2.5

Food Name	Serv. Size	Total Cal.	Carbs GMS	Fat GMS
(Bison)	1 oz	50	1.0	5.0
(Breakstone's)	1 tbsp	30	1.0	3.0
(Crowley)	1 oz	50	1.0	5.0
(Darigold)	1 tbsp	23	1.1	2.8
(Friendship)	2 tbsp	55	1.0	5.0
(Knudsen) 'Hampshire'	1 oz	60	1.0	6.0
(Sealtest)	1 tbsp	30	1.0	3.0
French onion *(Crowley)*	1 oz	50	1.0	5.0
Pasteurized, 100% natural *(Alta•Dena)*	1 oz	60	1.0	6.0
W/acidophilus, cultured *(Alta•Dena)* 'Kefir'	1 oz	70	1.0	6.0
W/chives *(Land O'Lakes)* 'Light'	2 tbsp	40	4.0	2.0
HALF AND HALF				
(Breakstone's) 'Light Choice'	1 tbsp	25	1.0	2.0
(Sealtest) 'Light'	1 tbsp	25	1.0	2.0
Cultured	1 tbsp	20	0.6	1.8
LIGHT/LOW-FAT				
(Crowley)	1 oz	30	2.0	2.0
(Friendship) 'Lite Delite'	2 tbsp	35	2.0	2.0
(Knudsen)	1 oz	40	2.0	3.0
(Land O'Lakes) 'Light'	2 tbsp	40	4.0	2.0
(Naturally Yours) 'Real•Dairy' no fat	2 tbsp	15	1.0	0.0
(Weight Watchers)	2 tbsp	35	2.0	2.0
SOUR CREAM, ALTERNATIVE/NONDAIRY				
	1 cup	479	15.3	44.9
	1 oz	59	1.9	5.5
(Crowley) dressing	1 oz	40	1.0	4.0
(Pet)	1 tbsp	25	<1.0	2.0
Cultured				
	1 cup	479	15.2	44.9
	1 oz	58	1.9	5.5
(Light n' Lively) nonfat	1 tbsp	10	1.0	0.0
SOURSOP. See GUANABANA.				
SOY BEVERAGE				
(Edensoy) 'Extra' original	8.45 oz	140	14.0	4.0
(Edensoy) original	8.45 oz	140	14.0	4.0
(Health Valley) fat-free 'Soy Moo'	1 cup	110	19.0	0.0
(Soyamel) powdered mix, prepared	8 oz	130	10.0	7.0
(WestSoy) 'Lite' plain	8 oz	100	16.0	2.0
(WestSoy) 'Natural' original	8 oz	150	18.0	5.0
(WestSoy) 'Natural' unsweetened	8 oz	100	5.0	5.0
(WestSoy) 'Plus' plain	8 oz	150	18.0	5.0
ALMOND FLAVOR				
(WestSoy) 'Lite'	6 oz	160	26.0	4.0

Food Name	Serv. Size	Total Cal.	Carbs GMS	Fat GMS
(WestSoy) 'Natural'	6 oz	250	31.0	11.0
BANANA FLAVOR *(WestSoy)* 'Lite' creamy banana	6 oz	160	26.0	3.0
CAROB FLAVOR				
(Ah Soy)	6 oz	160	30.0	3.0
(Edensoy)	8.45 oz	160	30.0	5.0
(WestSoy) 'Plus'	8 oz	160	21.0	5.0
Malted				
(WestSoy) 'Lite'	6 oz	160	27.0	3.0
(WestSoy) 'Natural'	6 oz	270	37.0	11.0
CHOCOLATE FLAVOR *(Ah Soy)*	6 oz	160	29.0	3.0
COCOA FLAVOR				
(WestSoy) 'Lite'	8 oz	140	27.0	2.0
(WestSoy) 'Lite' w/mint	6 oz	160	26.0	3.0
COFFEE FLAVOR *(WestSoy)* 'Natural' java malted	6 oz	270	37.0	11.0
VANILLA FLAVOR				
(Ah Soy)	6 oz	160	23.0	5.0
(Edensoy) 'Extra'	8.45 oz	150	25.0	3.0
(Edensoy) 'Natural Vanilla'	8.45 oz	150	25.0	3.0
(WestSoy) 'Lite'	8 oz	110	20.0	2.0
(WestSoy) 'Lite' vanilla royale	6 oz	160	26.0	3.0
(WestSoy) 'Plus'	8 oz	150	20.0	5.0
All natural *(WestSoy)*	8 oz	120	22.0	2.5
Malted *(WestSoy)* 'Natural'	6 oz	250	31.0	11.0
SOY FLOUR				
defatted	1 oz	93	10.9	0.3
defatted, stirred	1/2 cup	165	19.2	0.6
full-fat	1 oz	124	10.0	5.9
full-fat *(Arrowhead Mills)*	2 oz	250	18.0	11.0
full-fat, roasted	1 oz	125	9.5	6.2
full-fat, roasted, stirred	1/2 cup	185	14.1	9.2
full-fat, stirred	1/2 cup	183	14.8	8.7
low-fat	1 oz	92	10.8	1.9
low-fat, stirred	1/2 cup	143	16.7	3.0
SOY MEAL				
defatted, raw	1/2 cup	207	24.5	1.5
defatted, raw	1 oz	96	11.4	0.7
SOY MILK. See SOY BEVERAGE.				
SOY PROTEIN CONCENTRATE				
acid wash extracted	1 oz	93	8.7	0.1
acid/water wash extracted	1 oz	94	8.8	0.1
alcohol extracted	1 oz	93	8.7	0.1
SOY PROTEIN ISOLATE				
	1 oz	95	2.1	1.0

Food Name	Serv. Size	Total Cal.	Carbs GMS	Fat GMS
potassium type	1 oz	91	2.9	0.2
w/potassium	1 oz	96	0.2	1.0
w/sodium	1 oz	96	0.2	1.0
SOYBEAN				
Dried				
boiled	4 oz	196	11.2	10.2
boiled	1/2 cup	149	8.5	7.7
dry-roasted	1/2 cup	387	28.1	18.6
dry-roasted	1 oz	128	9.3	6.1
raw	1/2 cup	387	28.1	18.5
raw	1 oz	118	8.6	5.7
raw (Arrowhead Mills)	2 oz	230	19.0	10.0
roasted	1/2 cup	405	28.9	21.8
roasted	1 oz	134	9.5	7.2
Green				
boiled, drained	4 oz	160	12.5	7.3
boiled, drained	1/2 cup	127	9.9	5.8
raw	1/2 cup	188	14.1	8.7
raw, in pods	1 lb	353	26.6	16.4
raw, shelled	1 oz	42	3.1	1.9
Kernels, roasted/toasted				
whole	1 cup	489	33.0	25.9
whole	1 oz	129	8.7	6.8
Mature				
boiled	1/2 cup	149	8.5	7.7
dry-roasted	1/2 cup	387	28.1	18.6
raw	1/2 cup	387	28.1	18.5
roasted	1/2 cup	405	28.9	21.8
Mature, sprouted				
boiled, drained	1 cup	48	4.6	1.8
raw	1 lb	580	50.7	30.4
raw	1/2 cup	43	3.3	2.3
steamed	1/2 cup	38	3.1	2.1
stir-fried	3.5 oz	125	9.4	7.1
SOYBEAN, FERMENTED. See also MISO.				
natto	1/2 cup	187	12.6	9.7
natto	1 oz	60	4.1	3.1
SOYBEAN CURD CAKE. See TOFU.				
SOYBEAN FLAKES (Arrowhead Mills)	2 oz	250	18.0	11.0
SOYBEAN LECITHIN OIL				
	1/2 cup	964	0.0	109.0
	1 oz	251	0.0	28.4
	1 tbsp	120	0.0	13.6

Food Name	Serv. Size	Total Cal.	Carbs GMS	Fat GMS
SOYBEAN OIL				
. . . .	1 cup	1927	0.0	218.0
hydrogenated	1 cup	1927	0.0	218.0
hydrogenated	1 oz	251	0.0	28.4
hydrogenated	1 tbsp	120	0.0	13.6
(Hain)	1 tbsp	120	0.0	14.0
(IGA)	1 tbsp	120	0.0	14.0
SOYBEAN-COTTONSEED OIL				
hydrogenated	1/2 cup	964	0.0	109.0
hydrogenated	1 oz	251	0.0	28.4
hydrogenated	1 tbsp	120	0.0	13.6
SPAGHETTI. See PASTA.				
SPAGHETTI ENTRÉE, CANNED				
W/beef (Chef Boyardee) 'Beef-O-Getti'	7.5 oz	220	27.0	9.0
W/beef, in tomato sauce (Chef Boyardee)	7.5 oz	240	30.0	9.0
W/frankfurters (Van Camp's) 'Spaghettee Weenie'	1 cup	243	34.7	7.4
W/frankfurters, in tomato sauce (Franco-American)				
'SpaghettiOs'	7.5 oz	220	26.0	9.0
W/meatballs				
(Estee)	7.5 oz	240	19.0	14.0
(Featherweight)	7.5 oz	160	23.0	3.0
(Nalley's)	7.5 oz	190	29.0	4.0
W/meatballs, in sauce (Buitoni)	7.5 oz	190	21.0	8.0
W/meatballs, in tomato sauce				
(Chef Boyardee)	7.5 oz	230	30.0	9.0
(Franco-American)	7 3/8 oz	220	28.0	8.0
(Franco-American) 'SpaghettiOs'	7 3/8 oz	220	25.0	9.0
(Pathmark) 'No Frills'	7.5 oz	200	22.0	8.0
W/tomato and cheese sauce (Franco-American)				
'SpaghettiOs'	7.5 oz	170	33.0	2.0
W/tomato sauce, rings (Finast)	7.5 oz	150	31.0	1.0
SPAGHETTI ENTRÉE, FREEZE-DRIED				
(Mountain House) w/meat and sauce, prepared	1 cup	260	41.0	5.0
SPAGHETTI ENTRÉE, FROZEN				
Parmesan, w/Italian-style green beans (Stouffer's)	10.25 oz	240	30.0	9.0
W/beef (Dining Lite)	9 oz	220	25.0	8.0
W/beef sauce and mushrooms (Le Menu) 'LightStyle' . . .	9 oz	280	45.0	6.0
W/Italian-style meatballs (Swanson) 'Homestyle Recipe' . . .	13 oz	490	60.0	18.0
W/meat sauce				
(Banquet) 'Casserole'	8 oz	270	35.0	8.0
(Freezer Queen) 'Single Serve'	10 oz	350	47.0	12.0
(Kid Cuisine)	9.25 oz	310	43.0	12.0
(Lean Cuisine)	11.5 oz	290	45.0	6.0

Food Name	Serv. Size	Total Cal.	Carbs GMS	Fat GMS
(Stouffer's)	12 7/8 oz	320	38.0	12.0
(Weight Watchers)	10 oz	240	28.0	7.0
W/meatballs				
(Banquet)	10 oz	290	44.0	10.0
(Morton)	10 oz	200	39.0	3.0
(Stouffer's) 19.5-oz pkg	1/2 pkg	290	37.0	9.0
(Stouffer's) 12 5/8-oz pkg	1 pkg	440	53.0	16.0
(Swanson)	12.5 oz	390	46.0	17.0
W/meatballs and sauce *(Lean Cuisine)*	9.5 oz	290	36.0	7.0
SPAGHETTI ENTRÉE, MICROWAVE				
(Lunch Bucket) 'Spaghetti 'n Meatsauce' microwave cup	7.5 oz	240	39.0	5.0
Rings *(Kid's Kitchen)* microwave cup	7.5 oz	180	35.0	1.0
Rings and franks in tomato sauce *(Kid's Kitchen)* microwave cup	7.5 oz	290	33.0	12.0
W/meatballs				
(Chef Boyardee) 'Microwave'	7.5 oz	230	29.0	10.0
(Hormel) micro cup	7.5 oz	210	27.0	7.0
(Kid's Kitchen) microwave cup	7.5 oz	220	26.0	8.0
W/meatballs, in sauce *(Libby's)* 'Diner'	7.75 oz	190	31.0	3.0
SPAGHETTI ENTRÉE, PACKAGED				
Spaghettini *(Top Shelf)*	1 serving	240	35.0	5.0
W/beef and mushroom sauce *(Ultra Slim Fast)*	12 oz	370	49.0	10.0
W/meat sauce *(Top Shelf)*	10 oz	260	37.0	6.0
SPAGHETTI ENTRÉE MIX				
(Kraft) 'Mild American Dinner' prepared	1 cup	300	50.0	7.0
(Kraft) 'Tangy Italian Style Dinner' prepared	1 cup	310	49.0	8.0
Low-fat, w/whole wheat noodles *(Fantastic Foods)* 'All-O-Round'	10 oz	211	45.0	2.0
W/condensed meat sauce *(Chef Boyardee)* 'Dinner' prepared	3.25 oz	250	37.0	6.0
W/meat sauce				
(Chef Boyardee) 'Dinner' prepared	7.9 oz	240	42.0	3.0
(Kraft) 'Dinner' prepared	1 cup	360	47.0	14.0
W/mushroom sauce *(Chef Boyardee)* 'Dinner' prepared	7.9 oz	210	41.0	1.0
SPAGHETTI SEASONING *(Tone's)*	1 tsp	11	2.5	<.1
SPAGHETTI SQUASH. See SQUASH, SPAGHETTI.				
SPAM. See LUNCHEON MEAT, CANNED.				
SPARE RIB SEASONING MIX, 'Bag 'n Season' *(Schilling)*	1 pkg	185	42.0	1.5
SPINACH				
boiled, drained	4 oz	26	4.3	0.3
boiled, drained	1/2 cup	21	3.4	0.2
raw	10-oz pkg	62	9.9	1.0
raw *(Dole)*	3 oz	9	0.1	0.3

Food Name	Serv. Size	Total Cal.	Carbs GMS	Fat GMS
raw, chopped	1/2 cup	6	1.0	0.1
raw, chopped	1 oz	6	1.0	0.1
raw, untrimmed	1 lb	73	11.4	1.1
SPINACH, CANNED				
drained solids	1/2 cup	25	3.6	0.5
drained solids, no salt added	4 oz	26	3.9	0.6
w/liquid	4 oz	22	3.3	0.4
w/liquid, low-sodium	4 oz	22	3.3	0.4
(Allens)	1/2 cup	28	3.0	<1.0
(Allens) chopped	1/2 cup	28	3.0	<1.0
(Allens) sliced	1/2 cup	28	3.0	<1.0
(Allens) whole	1/2 cup	28	3.0	<1.0
(Bush's Best) chopped	1/2 cup	25	4.0	0.0
(Del Monte) chopped, w/liquid	1/2 cup	25	4.0	0.0
(Del Monte) whole, w/liquid	1/2 cup	25	4.0	0.0
(Del Monte) whole, w/liquid, 'No Salt Added'	1/2 cup	25	4.0	0.0
(Featherweight)	1/2 cup	35	4.0	1.0
(Finast)	1/2 cup	25	4.0	0.0
(Finast) 'No Salt Added'	1/2 cup	25	4.0	0.0
(Freshlike) cut	1/2 cup	20	4.0	0.0
(Freshlike) cut, water-packed, w/o salt	1/2 cup	20	4.0	0.0
(Freshlike) cut, water packed, w/o sugar or salt	1/2 cup	20	4.0	0.0
(Pathmark) 'No Frills'	1 cup	45	8.0	1.0
(Pathmark) 'No Salt Added'	1/2 cup	30	4.0	1.0
(Pathmark) whole	1/2 cup	30	4.0	1.0
(S&W) 'Premium Northwest'	1/2 cup	25	3.0	0.0
(Stokely)	1/2 cup	30	3.0	0.0
(Veg•All) cut	1/2 cup	20	4.0	0.0
SPINACH, FROZEN				
Chopped				
boiled, drained	10-oz pkg	62	11.7	0.5
boiled, drained	1/2 cup	27	5.1	0.2
unprepared	10-oz pkg	68	11.4	0.9
unprepared	1 cup	37	6.2	0.5
(A&P)	3.3 oz	20	4.0	<1.0
(Birds Eye)	3.3 oz	20	3.0	0.0
(Finast)	3.3 oz	20	3.0	0.0
(Frosty Acres)	3.3 oz	20	3.0	0.0
(Seabrook)	3.3 oz	20	3.0	0.0
(Southern)	3.5 oz	25	3.5	0.3
Creamed				
(Birds Eye) 'Combination Vegetables'	3 oz	60	5.0	4.0
(Green Giant)	1/2 cup	70	10.0	3.0

Food Name	Serv. Size	Total Cal.	Carbs GMS	Fat GMS
(Stouffer's)	4.5 oz	170	7.0	14.0
Leaf				
boiled, drained	10-oz pkg	62	11.7	0.5
boiled, drained	4 oz	32	6.1	0.2
unprepared	10-oz pkg	68	11.4	0.9
unprepared	1 cup	37	6.2	0.5
(A&P)	3.3 oz	25	4.0	<1.0
(Birds Eye) 'Portion Pack'	3.2 oz	20	3.0	0.0
(Birds Eye) whole leaf	3.3 oz	20	4.0	0.0
(Finast)	3.3 oz	20	4.0	0.0
(Freshlike) cut	3.3 oz	20	4.0	0.0
(Frosty Acres)	3.3 oz	20	4.0	0.0
(Green Giant) cut, in butter sauce	1/2 cup	40	6.0	2.0
(Green Giant) 'Harvest Fresh'	1/2 cup	25	5.0	0.0
(Green Giant) 'Plain Polybag'	1/2 cup	25	6.0	0.0
(Seabrook) cut	3.3 oz	20	4.0	0.0
(Southern) whole	3.5 oz	25	3.6	0.3
(Veg•All) cut	3.3 oz	20	4.0	0.0
SPINACH, NEW ZEALAND				
boiled, drained	4 oz	14	2.5	0.2
boiled, drained, chopped	1/2 cup	11	2.0	0.2
raw, chopped	1/2 cup	4	0.7	0.1
raw, untrimmed	1 lb	47	8.2	0.7
SPINACH ENTRÉE, FROZEN				
au gratin (Budget Gourmet)	6 oz	120	14.0	5.0
creamed (Stouffer's)	4.5 oz	190	8.0	16.0
soufflé (Stouffer's)	6 oz	220	11.0	15.0
SPINACH SALAD, 'Sassy Spinach Kit' (Saco)	1/2 cup	157	14.0	11.0
SPIRULINA				
dried	100 gm	290	23.9	7.7
dried	1 oz	82	6.8	2.2
raw	100 gm	26	2.4	0.4
SPLIT PEAS				
boiled	4 oz	134	23.9	0.4
boiled (A&P)	1 cup	220	40.0	<1.0
boiled, mature seeds	1/2 cup	116	20.7	0.4
raw	1 oz	97	17.1	0.3
raw, green (Arrowhead Mills)	2 oz	200	35.0	1.0
raw, mature seeds	1/2 cup	334	59.2	1.1
SPONGE GOURD. See GOURD, DISHCLOTH.				
SPORTS DRINK				
CHOCOLATE				
(Weider) 'Dynamic Muscle Builder'	11 oz	220	36.0	<1.0

Food Name	Serv. Size	Total Cal.	Carbs GMS	Fat GMS
(Weider) 'Dynamic Weight Gainer'	11 oz	280	48.0	2.0
(Weider) high-energy 'Protein Blast'	11.5 oz	270	44.0	<1.0
(Weider) 'Sports Line Power Shake' Dutch chocolate	11 oz	220	37.0	<1.0
FRUIT PUNCH *(Pro-formance)*	8 oz	99	26.0	0.0
GRAPE				
(Opti-Carb 140)	16 oz	140	35.0	0.0
(Pro-formance)	8 oz	99	26.0	0.0
LEMON				
(Knudsen & Sons) 'Isotonic Sports Beverage'	8 oz	60	21.0	0.0
(Pro-formance)	8 oz	99	26.0	0.0
LEMONADE				
(Power Burst) advanced performance beverage	8 oz	50	14.0	0.0
LEMON-LIME *(Shasta)* caffeine-free, 'Body Works'	8 oz	60	15.0	0.0
ORANGE				
(All Sport) caffeine-free	8 oz	70	19.0	0.0
(Gatorade)	8 oz	50	14.0	0.0
(Opti-Carb 140)	16 oz	140	35.0	0.0
(PowerAde)	8 oz	70	19.0	0.0
(Pro-formance)	8 oz	99	26.0	0.0
(Shasta) caffeine-free, 'Body Works'	8 oz	60	15.0	0.0
(10-K)	8 oz	60	15.0	0.0
SPORTS DRINK MIX				
(Tiger's Milk)				
'Breakfast Booster' dry	2 level tbsp	70	14.0	<1.0
'Energy Booster' dry	3 heap tbsp	120	28.0	<1.0
'Protein Booster' Dutch chocolate, dry	3 heap tbsp	90	12.0	<1.0
'Protein Booster' vanilla-orange creme, dry	3 heap tbsp	90	12.0	<1.0
(Weider)				
'Big' chocolate malt, sugar-free, dry	4 scoops	320	58.0	2.0
'Carbo Energizer' orange, dry	4 scoops	230	58.0	0.0
'Crash Weight Gain No. 7' vanilla, dry	4 heap tbsp	300	61.0	3.0
'Dynamic Body Shaper' Dutch chocolate, dry	2 scoops	110	12.0	<1.0
'Dynamic Muscle Builder' dry	3 heap tbsp	100	6.0	0.0
'Dynamic Muscle Builder' natural chocolate, dry	2 scoops	120	9.0	1.0
'Dynamic Muscle Builder' natural vanilla, dry	2 scoops	120	9.0	<1.0
'Dynamic Weight Gainer' Dutch chocolate, dry	4 scoops	320	61.0	<1.0
'Dynamic Weight Gainer' peanut butter, dry	4 scoops	330	61.0	2.0
'90 Plus' vanilla, sugar-free, dry	2 scoops	100	1.0	0.0
'N2itro-Fire' protein blend, dry	2 tbsp	110	17.0	1.0
'Victory Explosive Workout' citrus, dry	4 tbsp	190	48.0	0.0
SPOT				
dry-heat cooked	3 oz	134	0.0	5.3
raw	1 lb	559	0.0	22.2

Food Name	Serv. Size	Total Cal.	Carbs GMS	Fat GMS
raw	1 oz	35	0.0	1.4
SPREAD, VEGETARIAN				
	1 cup	953	54.9	83.2
	1 oz	110	6.4	9.6
	1 tbsp	60	3.4	5.2
(Best Foods)	1 tbsp	50	2.0	5.0
(Hellmann's)	1 tbsp	50	2.0	5.0
(Kraft)	1 tbsp	50	3.0	5.0
SPREADS. See CHEESE SPREAD; SPREAD, VEGETARIAN; and individual listings.				
SPRING ONION. See ONION, GREEN.				
SPRINKLES				
milk chocolate (Snack Pack)	3.88 oz	178	28.4	6.3
vanilla chocolate (Snack Pack)	3.88 oz	166	26.3	6.1
SQUAB/pigeon				
Raw				
breast meat only	1 oz	38	0.0	1.3
giblets	100 gm	154	1.2	7.2
light meat w/o skin	1 lb	202	0.0	6.8
meat and skin	1 oz	83	0.0	6.7
meat and skin, approx 7 oz	1 squab	584	0.0	47.4
meat only	1 oz	40	0.0	2.1
SQUASH SEED. See PUMPKIN SEED.				
SQUASH, ACORN/table queen squash				
boiled, mashed	1/2 cup	41	10.7	0.1
boiled, mashed	4 oz	39	10.0	0.1
raw (Frieda's)	1 lb	249	63.5	0.5
raw (Frieda's)	1 oz	16	4.0	<.1
raw, approx 4-inch diam	1 squash	172	44.9	0.4
raw, cubes	1/2 cup	28	7.3	0.1
raw, trimmed	1 oz	11	3.0	<.1
raw, untrimmed	1 lb	138	35.9	0.3
SQUASH, BANANA				
baked (Frieda's)	1 lb	286	69.9	1.8
baked (Frieda's)	1 oz	18	4.4	0.1
SQUASH, BUTTERNUT				
baked	4 oz	45	11.9	0.1
baked, cubes	1/2 cup	41	10.7	0.1
boiled, mashed	1/2 cup	47	12.1	0.1
raw, cubes	1/2 cup	32	8.2	0.1
raw, trimmed	1 oz	13	3.3	<.1
raw, untrimmed	1 lb	172	44.6	0.4
SQUASH, CROOKNECK				
boiled, drained	4 oz	23	4.9	0.4

Food Name	Serv. Size	Total Cal.	Carbs GMS	Fat GMS
boiled, drained, slices	1/2 cup	18	3.9	0.3
canned, drained, no salt added	4 oz	15	3.4	0.1
canned, yellow, cut (Allens)	1/2 cup	16	3.0	<1.0
frozen, boiled, drained	4 oz	28	6.3	0.2
frozen, cooked (Kohl's)	4 oz	45	11.0	<1.0
frozen, yellow (Seabrook)	3.3 oz	18	4.0	0.0
frozen, yellow (Southern)	3.5 oz	21	4.1	0.1
raw, ends trimmed	1 oz	5	1.1	0.1
raw, slices	1/2 cup	12	2.6	0.2
raw, untrimmed	1 lb	84	18.2	1.1
SQUASH, HUBBARD				
baked	4 oz	57	12.3	0.7
baked, cubes	1/2 cup	51	11.0	0.6
boiled, mashed	1/2 cup	35	7.6	0.4
boiled, mashed	4 oz	34	7.3	0.4
raw, cubes	1/2 cup	23	5.1	0.3
raw, trimmed	1 oz	11	2.5	0.1
raw, untrimmed	1 lb	116	25.3	1.5
SQUASH, MARROW/vegetable marrow squash				
raw, trimmed	1 oz	4	1.0	<.1
SQUASH, SCALLOP/cymling/pattypan squash				
boiled, drained	4 oz	18	3.7	0.2
boiled, drained, mashed	1/2 cup	19	4.0	0.2
boiled, drained, slices	1/2 cup	14	3.0	0.2
raw, slices	1/2 cup	12	2.5	0.1
raw, trimmed	1 oz	5	1.1	0.1
raw, untrimmed	1 lb	81	17.1	0.9
SQUASH, SPAGHETTI				
baked or boiled, drained	4 oz	33	7.3	0.3
baked or boiled, drained	1/2 cup	23	5.0	0.2
raw, cubes	1/2 cup	16	3.5	0.3
raw, trimmed	1 oz	9	2.0	0.2
raw, untrimmed	1 lb	106	22.3	1.8
SQUASH, STRAIGHTNECK, raw, slices	1/2 cup	12	2.6	0.2
SQUASH, SUMMER, all varieties				
boiled, drained	4 oz	23	4.9	0.4
boiled, drained, slices	1/2 cup	18	3.9	0.3
raw, slices	1/2 cup	13	2.8	0.1
raw, trimmed	1 oz	6	1.2	0.1
raw, untrimmed	1 lb	87	18.7	0.9
SQUASH, WINTER, all varieties				
baked	4 oz	44	9.9	0.7
baked, cubes	1/2 cup	40	8.9	0.6

Food Name	Serv. Size	Total Cal.	Carbs GMS	Fat GMS
frozen, cooked *(Birds Eye)*	4 oz	45	11.0	0.0
frozen, cooked *(Seabrook)*	4 oz	45	11.0	0.0
raw, cubes	1/2 cup	21	5.1	0.1
raw, trimmed	1 oz	11	2.5	0.1
raw, untrimmed	1 lb	119	28.4	0.7
SQUID, MIXED SPECIES/calamari				
fried	3 oz	149	6.6	6.4
raw	1 lb	416	14.0	6.3
raw	3 oz	78	2.6	1.2
raw	1 oz	26	0.9	0.4
SQUIRREL				
raw	1 oz	34	0.0	0.9
roasted	4 oz	154	0.0	4.1
roasted, diced	1 cup	190	0.0	5.1
STAR APPLE. See CAIMIT.				
STAR FRUIT/carambola				
cubed	1 cup	45	10.7	0.5
trimmed	1 oz	9	2.2	0.1
untrimmed	1 lb	142	33.7	1.5
STEAK SEASONING 'Spice Blends' *(Schilling)*	1/4 tsp	1	0.1	(tr)
STIR-FRY ENTRÉE KIT				
(Tyson)	9 oz	230	15.0	9.0
(Tyson) 'Yoshida Oriental Sauce'	1.6 oz	100	22.0	1.0
STIR-FRY SEASONING *(Gilroy)*	1 tsp	6	1.0	0.0
STRAIGHTNECK SQUASH. See SQUASH, STRAIGHTNECK.				
STRAWBERRY				
trimmed	1 pint	96	22.5	1.2
trimmed	1 cup	45	10.5	0.6
trimmed	1 oz	9	2.0	0.1
untrimmed	1 lb	130	30.0	1.6
Canned, in heavy syrup	4 oz	104	26.7	0.3
Freeze-dried *(Mountain House)* prepared	1/4 cup	45	12.0	0.0
Frozen				
in light syrup, halves 'Quick Thaw Pouch' *(Birds Eye)*	5 oz	90	22.0	0.0
in light syrup, whole *(Birds Eye)*	4 oz	80	20.0	0.0
sweetened, sliced	10-oz pkg	273	73.6	0.4
sweetened, sliced	1 cup	245	66.1	0.3
sweetened, sliced	4 oz	109	29.4	0.1
sweetened, sliced *(Finast)*	3.3 oz	125	30.0	0.0
sweetened, whole	10-oz pkg	222	59.6	0.4
sweetened, whole	1 cup	199	53.5	0.4
sweetened, whole	4 oz	88	23.8	0.2
unsweetened	20-oz pkg	198	51.8	0.6

Food Name	Serv. Size	Total Cal.	Carbs GMS	Fat GMS
unsweetened	1 cup	52	13.6	0.2
unsweetened	4 oz	40	10.4	0.1
STRAWBERRY BANANA NECTAR *(Kern's)*	6 oz	110	28.0	0.0
STRAWBERRY COLADA. See ALCOHOLIC BEVERAGES.				
STRAWBERRY DAIQUIRI. See ALCOHOLIC BEVERAGES.				
STRAWBERRY DRINK				
(Snapple) 'Strawberry Passion Awareness' real fruit	8 oz	120	31.0	0.0
STRAWBERRY FLAVOR DRINK				
(Ensure) liquid nutrition	8 oz	250	34.3	8.8
(Ensure) liquid nutrition 'Plus'	8 oz	355	47.3	12.6
(Frostee)	8 oz	180	27.0	7.0
(Sego) 'Lite'	10 oz	150	17.0	4.0
(Sego) 'Very Strawberry'	10 oz	225	34.0	5.0
(Squeezit) 'Silly Billy Strawberry'	6.75 oz	90	23.0	0.0
(Tang)	8.45 oz	120	32.0	0.0
(10-K)	8 oz	60	15.0	0.0
STRAWBERRY FLAVOR DRINK MIX, PREPARED				
(Kool-Aid) presweetened	8 oz	80	20.0	0.0
(Nestlé) 'Quik' 2 1/2 heap tsp w/whole milk	8 oz	220	32.0	8.0
(Nestlé) 'Quik' 2 1/2 heap tsp w/2% milk	8 oz	200	32.0	5.0
(Nestlé) 'Quik' 2 1/2 heap tsp w/skim milk	8 oz	160	32.0	0.0
(Turbo Nutrition) weight gain protein powder, 2 oz w/whole milk	8 oz	360	33.0	9.0
(Wylers) 'Crystals'	8 oz	85	20.7	0.3
STRAWBERRY GUAVA JUICE *(Knudsen & Sons)*	8 oz	105	26.0	0.0
STRAWBERRY GUAVA NECTAR				
(Santa Cruz Natural) organic	8 oz	90	24.0	<1.0
STRAWBERRY JUICE DRINK				
(Knudsen & Sons) float	8 oz	130	32.0	0.0
(Tang) 'Fruit Box'	8.45 oz	120	32.0	0.0
(Wyler's) 'Fruit Slush'	4 oz	157	39.3	0.0
STRAWBERRY LEMONADE				
(Kern's)	6 oz	110	28.0	0.0
(Knudsen & Sons)	8 oz	90	21.0	0.0
(Santa Cruz Natural) organic	8 oz	60	20.0	<1.0
(Snapple)	8 oz	110	26.0	0.0
STRAWBERRY NECTAR				
(Knudsen & Sons)	8 oz	105	29.0	0.0
(Libby's)	6 oz	110	27.0	0.0
STRAWBERRY PUNCH DRINK				
(Arizona) 'Cowboy Cocktail'	8 oz	120	30.0	0.0
STRAWBERRY PUNCH MIX				
(Kool-Aid) sugar-sweetened, prepared	8 oz	80	20.0	0.0

Food Name	Serv. Size	Total Cal.	Carbs GMS	Fat GMS
(Kool-Aid) unsweetened, prepared w/sugar	8 oz	100	25.0	0.0
(Kool-Aid) unsweetened, prepared w/o sugar	8 oz	2	0.0	0.0
STRAWBERRY SYRUP				
(Knott's Berry Farm)	1 oz	120	30.0	0.0
(Knudsen & Sons)	1 oz	75	18.0	<1.0
(S&W) w/saccharin	1 tsp	4	1.0	0.0
STRAWBERRY TOPPING				
(Kraft)	1 tbsp	50	14.0	0.0
(Smucker's)	2 tbsp	120	30.0	0.0
(Smucker's) fat-free 'Light'	2 tbsp	55	14.0	0.0
STRING BEAN. See GREEN BEAN.				
STROGANOFF DINNER. See BEEF ENTRÉE.				
STRUDEL. See individual listings.				
STUFFED PEPPER				
(Celentano) sweet red, frozen	13 oz	350	28.0	20.0
(Stouffer's) green, w/beef in tomato sauce, frozen	7.75 oz	200	22.0	8.0
(Stouffer's) single serving	10 oz	220	28.0	8.0
STUFFING				
(Betty Crocker)				
chicken, dry	1/6 pkg	110	21.0	1.0
traditional herb, dry	1/6 pkg	110	22.0	1.0
traditional herb, prepared w/salted butter	1/2 cup	190	22.0	9.0
(Brownberry)				
corn, dry	1 oz	103	20.6	1.6
herb, dry	1 oz	100	20.7	1.3
(Croutettes) dry	.7 oz	70	14.0	0.0
(General Mills)				
chicken, dry	1/6 pkg	110	21.0	1.0
chicken, prepared w/margarine	1/2 cup	180	21.0	9.0
traditional herb, dry	1/6 pkg	110	22.0	<1.0
traditional herb, prepared w/margarine	1/2 cup	180	22.0	8.0
(Golden Dipt)				
Cajun style, dry	1/4 cup	40	9.0	0.0
cheddar and French, dry	1/2 cup	80	9.0	3.0
garden herb, dry	1/4 cup	40	9.0	0.0
(Golden Grain)				
chicken, dry	1 oz	106	20.0	1.2
cornbread, dry	1 oz	105	20.9	1.0
herb and butter, dry	1 oz	104	19.7	1.1
w/wild rice, dry	1 oz	108	20.9	1.1
(Pepperidge Farm)				
apple and raisin 'Distinctive Stuffing' dry	1 oz	110	21.0	1.0
classic chicken 'Distinctive Stuffing' dry	1 oz	110	20.0	1.0

Food Name	Serv. Size	Total Cal.	Carbs GMS	Fat GMS
cornbread, dry	1 oz	110	22.0	1.0
country style, dry	1 oz	100	21.0	1.0
cube, dry	1 oz	110	22.0	1.0
herb, country garden 'Distinctive Stuffing' dry	1 oz	120	18.0	4.0
herb, dry	1 oz	110	22.0	1.0
vegetable, harvest, w/almonds 'Distinctive' dry	1 oz	110	19.0	3.0
wild rice and mushroom 'Distinctive Stuffing' dry	1 oz	130	17.0	5.0
(Stove Top)				
Americana San Francisco, prepared w/salted butter	1/2 cup	170	20.0	9.0
beef, prepared w/salted butter	1/2 cup	180	21.0	9.0
chicken flavor, prepared w/salted butter	1/2 cup	180	20.0	9.0
cornbread 'Flexible Serving' prepared w/salted butter	1/2 cup	170	20.0	9.0
cornbread, prepared w/salted butter	1/2 cup	170	21.0	9.0
cornbread, prepared w/salted margarine	1/2 cup	180	22.0	9.0
homestyle herb 'Flexible Serving' prepared w/salted butter	1/2 cup	170	20.0	9.0
long grain and wild rice, prepared w/salted butter	1/2 cup	180	22.0	9.0
mushroom and onion, prepared w/salted butter	1/2 cup	180	20.0	9.0
pork 'Flexible Serving' prepared w/salted butter	1/2 cup	170	20.0	9.0
pork, prepared w/salted butter	1/2 cup	170	20.0	9.0
savory herbs, prepared w/salted butter	1/2 cup	170	20.0	9.0
turkey, prepared w/salted butter	1/2 cup	170	20.0	9.0
turkey, prepared w/salted margarine	1/2 cup	180	20.0	9.0
STUFFING, FROZEN				
chicken 'Stuffing Originals' *(Green Giant)*	1/2 cup	170	21.0	7.0
cornbread 'Stuffing Originals' *(Green Giant)*	1/2 cup	170	25.0	6.0
mushroom 'Stuffing Originals' *(Green Giant)*	1/2 cup	150	19.0	7.0
wild rice 'Stuffing Originals' *(Green Giant)*	1/2 cup	160	21.0	7.0
STUFFING MIX, MICROWAVE				
broccoli and cheese, prepared w/salted butter *(Stove Top)*	1/2 cup	170	20.0	8.0
cornbread, homestyle, prepared w/salted butter *(Stove Top)*	1/2 cup	160	20.0	7.0
mushroom and onion, prepared w/salted butter *(Stove Top)*	1/2 cup	170	21.0	7.0
STURGEON, MIXED SPECIES				
baked	4 oz	153	0.0	5.9
broiled	4 oz	153	0.0	5.9
dry-heat cooked	3 oz	115	0.0	4.4
microwaved	4 oz	153	0.0	5.9
raw	1 lb	478	0.0	18.3
raw	3 oz	89	0.0	3.4
raw	1 oz	30	0.0	1.1
smoked	4 oz	196	0.0	5.0

Food Name	Serv. Size	Total Cal.	Carbs GMS	Fc GM
SUCCOTASH				
boiled, drained	4 oz	130	27.6	0.
boiled, drained	1/2 cup	110	23.4	0.
raw	1 lb	451	88.9	4.
raw	1 oz	28	5.6	0.
Canned				
(S&W) 'Country Style'	1/2 cup	80	16.0	1.
(Stokely)	1/2 cup	90	20.0	0.
Frozen				
boiled, drained	4 oz	105	22.6	1.
boiled, drained	1/2 cup	79	17.0	0.
unprepared	1/2 cup	73	15.6	0.
(Frosty Acres)	3.3 oz	100	19.0	0.
(Seabrook)	3.3 oz	100	19.0	0.
SUCKER				
dry-heat cooked	3 oz	101	0.0	2.
raw	1 lb	419	0.0	10.5
SUGAR, ALTERNATIVE				
(Equal) aspartame	1 pkg	4	<1.0	0.
(Featherweight) saccharin	1 tablet	0	0.0	0.
(Featherweight) saccharin, liquid	3 drops	0	0.0	0.0
(Nutra Taste) saccharin	1 pkt	4	1.0	0.
(NutraSweet) aspartame 'Spoonful'	1 tsp	2	<1.0	0.
(S&W Nutradiet) saccharin, liquid	1/8 tsp	0	0.0	0.
(Sprinkle Sweet)	1 tsp	2	0.5	0.0
(Sugar Twin) saccharin	1 pkt	4	<1.0	0.0
(Sugar Twin) saccharin 'Plus'	1 pkt	3	<1.0	0.
(Sweet 'n Low)	1 pkt	4	1.0	0.0
(Sweet One)	1 pkt	4	1.0	0.0
(Sweet Plus)	1 pkt	4	1.0	0.0
(Sweet•10)	1/8 tsp	0	0.0	0.0
(Weight Watchers) 'Sweet'ner'	1 pkt	4	1.0	0.0
SUGAR, BEET OR CANE. See also SUGAR, ALTERNATIVE; SUGAR, DEXTROSE; SUGAR, MAPLE; SUGAR, TURBINADO; SUGAR CANE BATON.				
BROWN				
dark 'Old Fashioned' (Domino)	1 tsp	16	4.0	0.0
golden, fresh from Hawaii (C&H)	1 tsp	16	4.0	0.0
light 'Brownulated' (Domino)	1 tsp	12	3.0	0.0
light, golden, packed (Domino)	1 tsp	16	4.0	0.0
packed	1 cup	827	214.1	0.0
packed	1 oz	106	27.3	0.0
unpacked	1 cup	545	141.1	0.0

Food Name	Serv. Size	Total Cal.	Carbs GMS	Fat GMS
CONFECTIONER'S/powdered				
sifted	1 cup	385	99.5	0.0
sifted	1 oz	109	28.2	0.0
sifted, 10-X *(Domino)*	1/2 cup	240	60.0	0.0
unsifted	1 cup	462	119.4	0.0
unsifted	1 tbsp	31	8.0	0.0
GRANULATED				
	1 cup	774	199.8	0.0
	1 oz	109	28.2	0.0
	1 tsp	15	4.0	0.0
cubes 'Dots' *(Domino)*	1 cube	8	2.0	0.0
cubes, 1/2 inch	2 cubes	19	5.0	0.0
juice, organic *(Sucanat)*	1 tsp	12	3.0	0.0
lumps, 1 1/8 x 3/4 x 5/16 inches	1 lump	19	5.0	0.0
packet, approx .2 oz	1 pkt	23	6.0	0.0
'Packets' *(Domino)*	1 pkt	16	4.0	0.0
SUPERFINE, instant dissolving *(Domino)*	1 tsp	16	4.0	0.0
SUGAR, DEXTROSE				
anhydrous	100 gm	366	99.5	0.0
anhydrous	1 oz	104	28.2	0.0
crystallized	100 gm	335	91.0	0.0
crystallized	1 oz	95	25.8	0.0
SUGAR, MAPLE				
	100 gm	354	90.9	0.2
	1-oz piece	100	25.8	0.1
SUGAR, TURBINADO *(Hain)*	1 tbsp	50	12.0	0.0
SUGAR APPLE/sweetsop				
raw, approx 2 7/8-inch diam	1 med	146	36.6	0.5
raw, pulp	1 cup	235	59.1	0.7
trimmed	1/2 cup	118	29.6	0.4
trimmed	1 oz	27	6.7	0.1
untrimmed	1 lb	236	59.0	0.7
SUGAR CANE BATON *(Frieda's)*	1 oz	21	49.9	0.1
SUGAR CANE JUICE	1 oz	21	5.1	tr
SUMMER SAUSAGE				
(Eckrich)	1-oz slice	80	1.0	7.0
(Hillshire Farm)	2 oz	180	1.0	16.0
(Hormel) 'Perma-Fresh'	2 slices	140	0.0	11.0
(Hormel) 'Tangy Chub'	1 oz	90	0.0	7.0
(Hormel) 'Thuringer'	1 oz	90	0.0	9.0
BEEF				
(Hillshire Farm)	2 oz	190	1.0	17.0
(Hormel) 'Beefy'	1 oz	100	0.0	9.0

Food Name	Serv. Size	Total Cal.	Carbs GMS	Fe GMS
(Lean & Lite)	1 oz	43	1.0	2
(Light & Lean)	2 slices	100	0.0	8
(OHSE)	1 oz	75	2.0	5.
(Oscar Mayer)	.8-oz slice	69	0.2	6.
TURKEY (Louis Rich)	1-oz slice	55	0.4	3.
W/CHEESE (Hillshire Farm)	2 oz	200	1.0	18.
SUNCHOKE. See ARTICHOKE, JERUSALEM.				
SUN-DRIED TOMATOES, in oil and herbs (Bella Sun Luci)	2/3 oz	60	6.0	3.
SUNFISH/calico bass/crappie/pumpkinseed				
dry-heat cooked	3 oz	97	0.0	0.
raw	1 lb	404	0.0	3.
raw	3 oz	76	0.0	0.
raw	1 oz	25	0.0	0.
SUNFLOWER BUTTER				
	1 oz	165	7.8	13.
	1 tbsp	93	4.4	7.
gourmet (Roaster Fresh)	1 oz	160	5.0	13.
roasted (Maranatha Natural)	2 tbsp	170	8.0	14.
SUNFLOWER OIL				
hydrogenated	1/2 cup	964	0.0	109.
hydrogenated	1 oz	251	0.0	28.
linoleic	1/2 cup	964	0.0	109.
linoleic	1 oz	251	0.0	28.
(Hain)	1 tbsp	120	0.0	14.
(IGA)	1 tbsp	120	0.0	14.
(Kroger)	1 tbsp	122	0.0	13.
(Pathmark)	1 tbsp	130	0.0	14.
(Spectrum Naturals)	1 tbsp	120	0.0	14.
(Wesson)	1 tbsp	122	0.0	13.
SUNFLOWER SEED KERNELS				
Dried				
	1 cup	821	27.0	71.
	1 oz	162	5.3	14.
in shell	1 lb	1397	46.0	121.
(Arrowhead Mills)	1 oz	160	6.0	13.
(Frito-Lay's)	1 oz	160	6.0	14.0
Dry-roasted				
	1 cup	745	30.8	63.7
	1 oz	165	6.8	14.1
salted	1 cup	745	30.8	63.7
salted	1 oz	165	6.8	14.1
(Fisher)	1 oz	170	6.0	15.
(Fisher) in shell	1 oz	170	6.0	15.0

Food Name	Serv. Size	Total Cal.	Carbs GMS	Fat GMS
(Fisher) in shell, salted	1 oz	170	6.0	14.0
(Flavor House)	1 oz	180	4.0	15.0
(Pathmark)	1 oz	180	7.0	14.0
(Planters)	1 oz	160	6.0	14.0
Oil-roasted				
	1 cup	830	19.9	77.6
	1 oz	175	4.2	16.3
salted	1 cup	830	19.9	77.6
salted	1 oz	175	4.2	16.3
(Fisher)	1 oz	170	4.0	16.0
(Planters)	1 oz	170	5.0	15.0
Toasted				
	1 cup	829	27.6	76.1
	1 oz	176	5.9	16.1
salted	1 cup	829	27.6	76.1
salted	1 oz	176	5.9	16.1
(Fisher)	1 oz	170	6.0	14.0
SUNFLOWER SEED FLOUR				
partially defatted	1 cup	261	28.7	1.3
partially defatted	1 oz	92	10.2	0.5
partially defatted	1 tbsp	16	1.8	0.1
SUNSHINE JUICE, organic *(Santa Cruz Natural)*	8 oz	100	23.0	1.0
SURIMI				
	3 oz	84	5.8	0.8
leg style 'Classic Seablends' 10% crab *(Peter Pan Seafoods)*	3.5 oz	85	na	0.4
leg style 'Standard Seablends' *(Peter Pan Seafoods)*	3.5 oz	88	na	0.4
salad style 'Classic Seablends Combo' 10% crab				
(Peter Pan Seafoods)	3.5 oz	85	na	0.4
salad style 'Standard Seablends Combo'				
(Peter Pan Seafoods)	3.5 oz	88	na	0.4
SURINAM CHERRY. See PITANGA.				
SWAMP CABBAGE. See CABBAGE, SKUNK.				
SWEDISH MEATBALL DINNER/ENTRÉE				
frozen dinner, 'Classics' *(Armour)*	11.25 oz	330	23.0	18.0
frozen entrée, w/parsley noodles, gravy				
'Lean Cuisine' *(Stouffer's)*	9.25 oz	420	32.0	21.0
frozen entrée, w/pasta, gravy 'Lean Cuisine' *(Stouffer's)*	9 1/8 oz	290	31.0	8.0
SWEDISH TURNIP				
boiled, drained	4 oz	39	8.8	0.2
boiled, drained, cubed	1/2 cup	29	6.6	0.2
boiled, drained, mashed	1/2 cup	41	9.3	0.2
raw, cubed	1/2 cup	25	5.7	0.1
raw, trimmed	1 oz	10	2.3	0.1

Food Name	Serv. Size	Total Cal.	Carbs GMS	Fat GMS
raw, untrimmed	1 lb	140	31.4	0.8
SWEET AND SOUR DINNER (LaChoy)	4.48 oz	89	21.7	0.2
SWEET POTATO. See also YAM.				
baked in skin, pulp only	4 oz	117	27.5	0.1
baked in skin, pulp only, 5 inches long, 2 inches diam	1 potato	118	27.7	0.1
baked in skin, pulp only, mashed	1/2 cup	103	24.3	0.1
boiled, w/o skin	4 oz	119	27.5	0.3
boiled, w/o skin, mashed	1/2 cup	172	39.8	0.5
dehydrated flakes, dry	1 cup	455	108.0	0.7
dehydrated flakes, prepared w/water	1 lb	431	102.6	0.5
dehydrated flakes, prepared w/water	1 cup	242	57.6	0.3
raw, cubes	1 cup	140	32.3	0.4
raw, 5 inches long, 2 inches diam	1 potato	136	31.6	0.4
raw, trimmed	1 oz	30	6.9	0.1
raw, untrimmed	1 lb	343	79.3	1.0
SWEET POTATO, CANNED				
Candied				
(Joan of Arc)	1/2 cup	240	60.0	0.0
(Princella)	1/2 cup	240	60.0	0.0
(Royal Prince)	1/2 cup	240	60.0	0.0
(S&W)	1/2 cup	180	44.0	0.0
In extra heavy syrup (S&W) 'Southern'	1/2 cup	139	31.0	1.0
In heavy syrup				
(Joan of Arc)	1/2 cup	130	34.0	0.0
(Princella)	1/2 cup	130	34.0	0.0
(Royal Prince)	1/2 cup	130	34.0	0.0
In light syrup				
(Finast)	1/2 cup	110	25.0	<1.0
(Joan of Arc)	1/2 cup	110	28.0	0.0
(Princella)	1/2 cup	110	28.0	0.0
(Royal Prince)	1/2 cup	110	28.0	0.0
In pineapple-orange sauce				
(Joan of Arc)	1/2 cup	210	54.0	0.0
(Princella)	1/2 cup	210	54.0	0.0
(Royal Prince)	1/2 cup	210	54.0	0.0
In syrup				
(Allens) cut	1/2 cup	90	20.0	<1.0
(Allens) whole	1/2 cup	90	20.0	<1.0
(Joan of Arc)	1/2 cup	90	24.0	0.0
(Kohl's) cut	1/2 cup	110	31.0	<1.0
(Pathmark) 'No Frills'	1/2 cup	105	25.0	0.0
(Pathmark) 'Southern'	1 cup	230	55.0	0.0
(Princella)	1/2 cup	90	24.0	0.0

Food Name	Serv. Size	Total Cal.	Carbs GMS	Fat GMS
(Royal Prince)	1/2 cup	90	24.0	0.0
(Taylor's Brand) whole and cut	1 cup	240	58.0	0.0
In water (Allens) cut	1/2 cup	70	16.0	<1.0
SWEET POTATO, FROZEN				
unprepared, cubes	1/2 cup	84	19.5	0.2
(Mrs. Paul's) candied	4 oz	170	42.0	0.0
(Mrs. Paul's) candied, w/apples 'Sweets 'n Apples'	4 oz	160	38.0	0.0
SWEET POTATO LEAF				
raw, approx 12 1/4 inches long	1 leaf	6	1.0	0.1
raw, chopped	1 cup	12	2.2	0.1
raw, trimmed	1 oz	10	1.8	0.1
raw, untrimmed	1 lb	149	27.2	1.3
steamed	4 oz	39	8.3	0.3
steamed	1/2 cup	11	2.3	0.1
SWEETBREAD. See BEEF, PANCREAS; BEEF, THYMUS; LAMB, PANCREAS; VEAL, PANCREAS; VEAL, THYMUS.				
SWEETENERS. See SUGAR, ALTERNATIVE; SUGAR, BEET OR CANE; SUGAR, MAPLE; SUGAR, TURBINADO.				
SWEETSOP. See SUGAR APPLE.				
SWISS CHARD/chard				
boiled, drained	4 oz	23	4.7	0.1
boiled, drained, chopped	1/2 cup	18	3.6	0.1
raw, chopped	1/2 cup	3	0.7	0.0
raw, trimmed	1 oz	5	1.1	0.1
raw, untrimmed	1 lb	81	15.6	0.8
SWISS STEAK DINNER				
frozen (Budget Gourmet)	11.2 oz	450	40.0	22.0
frozen (Swanson)	10 oz	350	37.0	11.0
SWISS STEAK SEASONING MIX				
'Bag 'n Season' (Schilling)	1 pkg	81	17.0	0.4
SWORDFISH				
baked	4 oz	176	0.0	5.8
broiled	4 oz	176	0.0	5.8
dry-heat cooked	3 oz	132	0.0	4.4
frozen, steaks, w/o seasoning mix (SeaPak)	6-oz pkg	210	0.0	7.0
microwaved	4 oz	176	0.0	5.8
raw	1 lb	548	0.0	18.2
raw	3 oz	103	0.0	3.4
raw	1 oz	34	0.0	1.1
raw (Peter Pan Seafoods)	3.5 oz	118	na	4.0

T

Food Name	Serv. Size	Total Cal.	Carbs GMS	Fat GMS
TABBOULEH MIX				
(Casbah) dry	1 oz	126	28.0	1.
(Fantastic Foods) prepared w/oil and tomatoes	1/2 cup	161	17.0	10.
(Fantastic Foods) prepared w/o oil	1/2 cup	85	17.0	0.
(Near East) prepared	1/2 cup	170	20.0	9.
TABLE QUEEN SQUASH. See SQUASH, ACORN.				
TACO DIP. See DIP, TACO.				
TACO KIT				
(Natural Touch) vegetarian	2 tbsp	90	6.0	2.
(Old El Paso) prepared	1 taco	67	8.0	3.0
(Tio Sancho) 'Dinner Kit' prepared	1 taco	64	8.1	3.1
TACO SEASONING MIX				
(Hain)	1/10 pkg	10	2.0	0.0
(Lawry's) 'Seasoning Blends'	1 pkg	118	23.6	1.1
(Old El Paso)	1 pkg	100	21.0	1.0
(Old El Paso)	1/12 pkg	8	2.0	<1.0
(Schilling)	1/4 pkg	31	6.0	0.5
(Tio Sancho)	1.51 oz	132	26.0	1.7
(Tio Sancho) 'Dinner Kit' taco seasoning	1.25 oz	104	20.9	1.4
TACO SHELL				
(Azteca) corn	1 shell	60	7.0	3.0
(Azteca) flour	1 shell	200	18.0	12.0
(Chi-Chi's)	1 shell	140	17.0	7.0
(Gebhardt)	1 shell	50	7.0	2.0
(Lawry's)	1 shell	50	8.0	2.1
(Lawry's) 'Super'	1 shell	86	13.0	3.6
(Old El Paso)	1 shell	50	6.0	3.0
(Old El Paso) 'Mini'	3 shells	70	7.0	4.0
(Old El Paso) 'Super Size'	1 shell	100	11.0	6.0
(Ortega)	1 shell	50	8.0	2.0
(Rosarita)	1 shell	50	7.0	2.0
(Tio Sancho)	1 shell	64	8.1	3.1
(Tio Sancho) 'Super'	1 shell	94	11.3	4.7
TAFFY. See CANDY.				
TAHINI MIX				
(Arrowhead Mills) organic	1 oz	170	4.0	17.0
(Casbah) dry	1 oz	25	2.0	5.0
(Erewhon) 'Sesame Tahini'	2 tbsp	200	3.0	18.0
(Maranatha Natural) 'Sesame Tahini'	2 tbsp	210	3.0	19.0
(Westbrae) raw, organic	2 tbsp	210	1.0	19.0
(Westbrae) toasted, organic	2 tbsp	220	3.0	19.0

Food Name	Serv. Size	Total Cal.	Carbs GMS	Fat GMS
TAMALE				
(Derby) beef	2 tamales	160	15.0	7.0
(Gebhardt)	2 tamales	290	19.0	22.0
(Gebhardt) jumbo	2 tamales	400	26.0	30.0
Canned				
(Derby) beef	6.561 oz	253	20.8	17.4
(Gebhardt)	5.75 oz	269	18.6	20.7
(Gebhardt) beef	4 oz	230	15.0	17.0
(Gebhardt) jumbo	6.949 oz	332	24.0	25.2
(Hormel)	7.5 oz	280	19.0	20.0
(Hormel) beef	2 tamales	140	8.0	10.0
(Hormel) hot 'n spicy	7.5 oz	280	19.0	20.0
(Libby's) beef, w/sauce	7.5 oz	408	26.4	30.2
(Old El Paso)	2 tamales	190	16.0	12.0
(Van Camp's) w/sauce	1 cup	293	28.6	16.2
(Wolf Brand)	7.75 oz	328	24.9	24.5
Frozen				
(Amy's Kitchen) 'Mexican' organic	8 oz	170	36.0	3.0
(Hormel) beef	1 tamale	140	13.0	7.0
(Patio) dinner	13 oz	470	58.0	21.0
TAMALITO (Dennison's) in chili gravy, canned	7.5 oz	310	37.0	16.0
TAMARIND/Indian date				
pulp	1 cup	287	75.0	0.7
'Tamarindos' (Frieda's)	3.5 oz	239	62.5	0.6
trimmed	1 oz	68	17.7	0.2
untrimmed	1 lb	369	96.4	0.9
TANGELO JUICE, fresh	100 gm	41	9.7	0.1
TANGERINE				
peeled, seeded	1 oz	12	3.2	0.1
sections, w/o membrane	1/2 cup	43	10.9	0.2
untrimmed	1 lb	144	36.6	0.6
TANGERINE, CANNED				
in heavy syrup (S&W)	1/2 cup	76	20.0	0.0
in juice	4 oz	42	10.9	<.1
in light syrup	4 oz	69	18.4	0.1
in light syrup (A&P)	1/2 cup	80	20.0	<1.0
in light syrup (Dole)	1/2 cup	76	20.0	0.1
in light syrup (Empress)	5.5 oz	100	25.0	0.0
in light syrup (Finast)	5.5 oz	100	25.0	0.0
'Natural Style' (S&W)	1/2 cup	60	15.0	0.0
sections, in water (Featherweight)	1/2 cup	35	8.0	0.0
unsweetened (S&W Nutradiet)	1/2 cup	28	7.0	0.0

Food Name	Serv. Size	Total Cal.	Carbs GMS	Fat GMS
TANGERINE JUICE				
canned, sweetened	1 cup	125	29.9	0.5
canned, sweetened	1 oz	16	3.7	0.1
chilled 'Pure & Light Mandarin Tangerine' (Dole)	6 oz	97	25.0	0.1
fresh	1 cup	106	25.0	0.5
fresh	1 oz	13	3.1	0.1
frozen concentrate, sweetened, diluted w/3 vol water	1 cup	111	26.7	0.3
frozen concentrate, sweetened, diluted w/3 vol water	1 oz	14	3.3	0.0
frozen concentrate, sweetened, undiluted	6 oz	345	83.1	0.8
frozen or chilled (Minute Maid)	6 oz	90	23.0	0.0
TANGERINE ORANGE DRINK				
'Thirst Quencher Light' (Gatorade)	8 oz	25	7.0	0.0
TAPIOCA, PEARL				
dry	1 cup	518	134.8	0.0
dry	1 oz	97	25.1	tr
TARO				
cooked	4 oz	161	39.2	0.1
cooked, slices	1/2 cup	94	22.8	0.1
raw, slices	1/2 cup	56	13.8	0.1
raw, trimmed	1 oz	30	7.5	0.1
raw, untrimmed	1 lb	419	103.2	0.8
TARO, TAHITIAN				
cooked	4 oz	50	7.8	0.8
cooked, slices	1/2 cup	30	4.7	0.5
raw, slices	1/2 cup	25	4.3	0.6
raw, trimmed	1 lb	181	31.3	4.4
raw, trimmed	1 oz	11	2.0	0.3
TARO LEAF				
raw	1 cup	12	1.9	0.2
raw, 11 x 6 1/2 inches	1 leaf	4	0.7	0.1
raw, trimmed	1 oz	12	1.9	0.2
raw, untrimmed	1 lb	115	18.3	2.0
steamed	4 oz	27	4.6	0.5
steamed	1/2 cup	18	3.0	0.3
TARO SHOOTS				
cooked	4 oz	16	3.6	0.1
cooked, slices	1/2 cup	10	2.2	0.1
raw, 15 x 5 inches	1 shoot	9	1.9	0.1
raw, slices	1/2 cup	5	1.0	0.0
raw, trimmed	1 oz	3	0.7	<.1
raw, untrimmed	1 lb	45	9.3	0.4
TARPON, ATLANTIC				
raw	1 lb	422	0.0	1.8

Food Name	Serv. Size	Total Cal.	Carbs GMS	Fat GMS
raw	1 oz	26	0.0	0.1
TARRAGON				
ground	1 oz	84	14.2	2.1
ground	1 tbsp	14	2.4	0.4
ground	1 tsp	5	0.8	0.1
ground *(Durkee)*	1 tsp	10	0.0	<0.1
ground *(Laurel Leaf)*	1 tsp	10	0.0	<0.1
ground *(Spice Islands)*	1 tsp	5	0.7	0.1
TEA				
Brewed				
prepared w/distilled water	6 oz	2	0.5	0.0
prepared w/tap water	6 oz	2	0.5	0.0
(Celestial Seasonings) caffeine-free	8 oz	4	0.8	tr
(Nestea)	6 oz	0	0.0	0.0
Instant				
decaffeinated *(Lipton)*	6 oz	0	0.0	0.0
lemon flavor *(Lipton)*	6 oz	3	0.6	0.0
regular *(Lipton)*	6 oz	0	0.0	0.0
TEA, FLAVORED				
(Bigelow)				
'Chinese Fortune'	5.25 oz	1	0.1	tr
'Cinnamon Stick'	5.25 oz	1	0.1	tr
'Constant Comment'	5.25 oz	1	0.1	tr
'Darjeeling'	5.25 oz	1	0.1	tr
'Earl Grey'	5.25 oz	1	0.1	tr
'English Teatime'	5.25 oz	1	0.1	tr
'Lemon Lift'	5.25 oz	1	0.2	tr
'Plantation Mint'	5.25 oz	1	0.1	tr
'Raspberry Royale'	5.25 oz	1	0.1	tr
(Celestial Seasonings)				
'Amaretto Nights'	8 oz	3	0.6	tr
apple spice 'Fruit & Tea'	8 oz	3	0.2	tr
'Bavarian Chocolate Orange'	8 oz	7	1.6	tr
'Cinnamon Vienna'	8 oz	2	0.4	tr
'Classic English Breakfast'	8 oz	3	0.4	tr
'Darjeeling Gardens'	8 oz	3	0.5	tr
'Extraordinary Earl Grey'	8 oz	3	0.5	tr
'Irish Cream Mist'	8 oz	3	0.6	tr
lemon 'Fruit & Tea'	8 oz	3	0.5	tr
mint, Swiss	8 oz	3	0.4	tr
'Morning Thunder'	8 oz	3	0.4	tr
orange spice 'Fruit & Tea'	8 oz	3	0.4	tr
raspberry 'Fruit & Tea'	8 oz	2	0.5	tr

Food Name	Serv. Size	Total Cal.	Carbs GMS	Fat GMS
(Nestea)				
apple spice	16 oz	180	44.0	0.0
apple spice	6 oz	66	16.5	0.0
lemon, natural	16 oz	180	44.0	0.0
lemon, natural	6 oz	66	16.5	0.0
lemon, natural, diet	16 oz	180	44.0	0.0
lemon, natural, diet	6 oz	66	16.5	0.0
peach	16 oz	180	44.0	0.0
peach	6 oz	66	16.5	0.0
raspberry	16 oz	180	44.0	0.0
raspberry	6 oz	66	16.5	0.0
tropical	16 oz	180	44.0	0.0
tropical	6 oz	66	16.5	0.0
(Tetley)				
'Apple Freeze'	8 oz	79	20.0	0.0
'Classic'	8 oz	69	17.0	0.0
'Classic Lemon'	8 oz	108	27.0	0.0
'Diet Lemon Frost'	8 oz	10	2.3	0.0
'Diet Raspberry Blizzard'	8 oz	10	2.4	0.0
'Lemon Frost'	8 oz	89	22.0	0.0
'Orange Glazier'	8 oz	79	20.0	0.0
'Peach Chiller'	8 oz	79	20.0	0.0
'Raspberry Blizzard'	8 oz	95	24.0	0.0
(Wyler's) 'Fruit Tea Punch'	12 oz	118	29.6	0.0
TEA, HERBAL				
(Bigelow)				
almond orange	5 oz	<1	<.1	tr
'Apple Orchard'	5.25 oz	5	1.2	tr
apple spice	5 oz	<1	<.1	tr
chamomile	5 oz	<1	tr	tr
chamomile mint	5 oz	<1	tr	tr
cinnamon orange	5 oz	<1	0.1	tr
cranberry apple	5 oz	1	0.3	tr
'Fruit & Almond'	5.25 oz	1	<.1	tr
grains, roasted, w/carob	5 oz	3	0.6	tr
hibiscus and rose hips	5 oz	1	0.2	tr
'I Love Lemon'	5.25 oz	1	<.1	tr
'Lemon & C'	5 oz	<1	<.1	tr
'Mint Blend'	5 oz	<1	0.2	tr
'Mint Medley'	5.25 oz	1	0.2	tr
'Orange & C'	5 oz	<1	<.1	tr
'Orange & Spice'	5.25 oz	1	<.1	tr
peppermint	5 oz	<1	<.1	<.1

Food Name	Serv. Size	Total Cal.	Carbs GMS	Fat GMS
red raspberry	5 oz	1	0.2	tr
spearmint	5 oz	<1	<.1	tr
'Specially Strawberry'	5 oz	1	0.2	tr
'Sweet Dreams'	5.25 oz	1	0.1	tr
'Take-A-Break'	5.25 oz	1	0.6	tr
(Celestial Seasonings)				
'Almond Sunset'	8 oz	3	1.1	tr
chamomile	8 oz	2	0.5	tr
'Cinnamon Apple Spice'	8 oz	3	0.4	tr
'Cinnamon Rose'	8 oz	2	1.1	tr
'Country Peach Spice'	8 oz	3	0.7	tr
'Cranberry Cove'	8 oz	3	0.7	tr
'Emperor's Choice'	8 oz	4	0.9	<.1
'Ginseng Plus'	8 oz	3	<.5	tr
'Grandma's Tummy Mint'	8 oz	2	<.3	tr
'Lemon Mist'	8 oz	2	<.5	tr
'Lemon Zinger'	8 oz	4	0.7	tr
'Mandarin Orange Spice'	8 oz	5	1.1	tr
'Mellow Mint'	8 oz	2	0.4	tr
'Mint Magic'	8 oz	1	0.4	tr
'Mo's 24'	8 oz	2	0.2	tr
'Orange Zinger'	8 oz	5	1.2	tr
peppermint	8 oz	2	1.1	tr
'Raspberry Patch'	8 oz	4	1.1	tr
'Red Zinger'	8 oz	4	1.1	tr
'Roastaroma'	8 oz	11	2.0	<.1
'Sleepytime'	8 oz	5	1.1	tr
spearmint	8 oz	5	0.2	<.1
'Strawberry Fields'	8 oz	4	0.8	tr
'Sunburst C'	8 oz	3	1.1	tr
'Wild Forest Blackberry'	8 oz	2	1.8	tr
(Lipton)				
'Almond Pleasure'	8 oz	4	1.0	0.0
chamomile	8 oz	4	1.0	0.0
cinnamon apple	8 oz	2	<1.0	0.0
'Citrus Sunset'	8 oz	4	1.0	0.0
'Gentle/Tangy Orange'	8 oz	4	1.0	0.0
'Lemon Soother'	8 oz	4	1.0	0.0
'Toasty Spice'	8 oz	6	1.0	0.0

TEA, ICED

Can, bottle, or box

(Arizona)

'Diet'	8 oz	4	0.0	0.0

Food Name	Serv. Size	Total Cal.	Carbs GMS	Fa GM.
'Diet' with lemon	8 oz	4	0.0	0.0
raspberry flavor, sun-brewed style	8 oz	95	25.0	0.0
(Lipton) w/lemon, aseptic box	8.45 oz	96	24.0	0.3
(Nestea)				
	8 oz	90	22.0	0.0
diet	8 oz	4	1.0	0.0
(Shasta)	12 oz	124	34.0	0.0
(Snapple)				
cranberry	8 oz	110	27.0	0.0
'Diet'	8 oz	0	1.0	0.0
lemon	8 oz	110	27.0	0.0
mango	8 oz	110	27.0	0.0
mint	8 oz	120	29.0	0.0
old fashioned	8 oz	80	20.0	0.0
orange	8 oz	110	27.0	0.0
peach	8 oz	110	27.0	0.0
peach 'Diet'	8 oz	0	1.0	0.0
raspberry	8 oz	120	29.0	0.0
raspberry 'Diet'	8 oz	0	1.0	0.0
strawberry	8 oz	100	26.0	0.0
w/lemon, 'Diet'	8 oz	4	<1.0	<1.0
(Tetley)				
brewed	8 oz	74	19.0	0.0
brewed, w/lemon	8 oz	74	19.0	0.0
sweetened	8 oz	74	19.0	0.0
(Veryfine)				
peach kiwi flavored, brewed, 'Chillers'	8 oz	80	18.0	0.0
w/lemon	8 oz	80	16.0	0.0
Prepared from mix				
(Crystal Light)				
w/NutraSweet	8 oz	4	0.0	0.0
w/Nutrasweet, decaffeinated	8 oz	4	0.0	0.0
(Lipton)				
lemon flavor	6 oz	55	14.3	0.0
lemon flavor, decaffeinated	6 oz	55	14.2	0.0
lemon flavor, w/NutraSweet	8 oz	5	1.2	0.0
'Sugar-free'	8 oz	1	0.3	0.0
'Sugar-free' decaffeinated	8 oz	1	0.3	0.0
(Nestea)				
'Ice Teasers' all flavors	8 oz	6	1.0	0.0
lemon flavor	8 oz	6	1.0	0.0
lemon flavor, sugar-free	8 oz	4	1.0	0.0
lemon flavor, sugar-free, decaffeinated	2 tsp	6	1.0	0.0

Food Name	Serv. Size	Total Cal.	Carbs GMS	Fat GMS
'100%'	8 oz	2	0.0	0.0
'100%' decaffeinated	8 oz	0	0.0	0.0
sugar-free	8 oz	6	1.0	0.0
w/sugar and lemon	8 oz	70	19.0	0.0
(Pathmark)				
lemon flavor, low-calorie	8 oz	4	1.0	0.0
lemon flavor, low-calorie, decaffeinated	8 oz	4	1.0	0.0
lemon flavor, sugar-sweetened, decaffeinated	2 tbsp	80	20.0	0.0
TEA FLAVORED DRINK *(10-K)*	8 oz	60	15.0	0.0
TEASEED OIL				
	1 cup	1927	0.0	218.0
	1 oz	251	0.0	28.4
	1 tbsp	120	0.0	13.6
TEFF FLOUR, whole-grain *(Arrowhead Mills)*	2 oz	200	41.0	1.0
TEFF SEED *(Arrowhead Mills)*	1/2 cup	165	14.1	6.4
TEMPEH	1 oz	56	4.8	2.2
TENDERGREEN. See MUSTARD SPINACH.				
TEQUILA. See ALCOHOLIC BEVERAGES.				
TEQUILA SUNRISE. See ALCOHOLIC BEVERAGES.				
TERIYAKI MARINADE				
(Lawry's)	2 tbsp	72	11.0	0.4
(Lawry's) barbecue	1/4 cup	164	27.4	2.3
TERRAPIN, diamond back, raw	100 gm	111	0.0	3.5
THURINGER CERVELAT				
(Hillshire Farm)	2 oz	180	1.0	15.0
(Hormel) 'Old Smokehouse'	1 oz	90	1.0	8.0
(Hormel) 'Old Smokehouse Chub'	1 oz	100	0.0	9.0
(Hormel) 'Old Smokehouse Sliced'	1 oz	100	0.0	9.0
(Hormel) 'Viking Club Cervelat'	1 oz	90	0.0	8.0
(JM) beef	1-oz slice	80	1.0	7.0
(JM) 'Cervelat'	1-oz slice	70	1.0	6.0
THYME				
ground	1 oz	78	18.1	2.1
ground	1 tbsp	12	2.8	0.3
ground	1 tsp	4	0.9	0.1
ground *(Durkee)*	1 tsp	5	0.0	tr
ground *(Laurel Leaf)*	1 tsp	5	0.0	tr
ground *(Spice Islands)*	1 tsp	5	1.0	0.1
TILEFISH				
broiled	4 oz	167	0.0	5.3
dry-heat cooked	4 oz	167	0.0	5.3
dry-heat cooked	3 oz	125	0.0	4.0
microwaved	4 oz	167	0.0	5.3

Food Name	Serv. Size	Total Cal.	Carbs GMS	Fat GMS
raw	1 lb	433	0.0	10.5
raw	3 oz	82	0.0	2.0
raw	1 oz	27	0.0	0.7

TOASTED SESAME OIL. See SESAME OIL.

TOASTER BISCUIT. See BISCUIT, TOASTER.

TOASTER MUFFIN/PASTRY. See MUFFIN/PASTRY, TOASTER.

TOFFEE. See CANDY.

TOFU/soybean curd cake

raw	1 oz	22	0.5	1.4
raw	1/2 cup	94	2.3	5.9
Flavored				
Chinese five-spice (Nasoya)	5 oz	150	2.0	8.0
French, country herb (Nasoya)	5 oz	150	2.0	8.0
pasteurized (Frieda's)	4.2 oz	86	2.9	(mq)
Freeze-dried/koyadofu	1 oz	136	4.1	8.6
Fried	1 oz	77	3.0	5.7
Grilled/yakidofu	1 oz	25	0.3	1.7
Okara	1 oz	22	3.6	0.5
Salted and fermented/fuyu	1 oz	33	1.5	2.3
Silken (Mori-Nu)	1/2 pkg	90	4.0	4.0

TOFU PATTY, FROZEN

garden (Natural Touch)	2.5-oz patty	90	3.0	4.0
okara (Natural Touch)	2.25-oz patty	160	7.0	10.0

TOFU SPREAD

green chili 'Tofu Topper' canned (Natural Touch)	2 tbsp	50	2.0	4.0
herb and spice 'Tofu Topper' canned (Natural Touch)	2 tbsp	50	2.0	4.0
Mexican 'Tofu Topper' canned (Natural Touch)	2 tbsp	60	2.0	5.0

TOM COLLINS. See ALCOHOLIC BEVERAGES.

TOMATILLO/ground husk tomato

fresh (Frieda's)	3.5 oz	25	4.2	0.5
raw	1 med	11	2.0	0.4
raw, chopped	1/2 cup	21	3.8	0.7

TOMATO. See also TOMATO, SUN-DRIED.

Green

raw, 2 3/5-inch diam	1 tomato	30	6.3	0.3
trimmed	1 oz	7	1.4	0.1
untrimmed	1 lb	99	21.1	0.8
Red				
boiled	1/2 cup	32	7.0	0.5
boiled	4 oz	31	6.6	0.5
raw, chopped	1/2 cup	19	4.2	0.3
raw, 2 3/5-inch diam, 4.75 oz	1 tomato	26	5.7	0.4
raw, trimmed	1 oz	6	1.3	0.1

Food Name	Serv. Size	Total Cal.	Carbs GMS	Fat GMS
raw, untrimmed	1 lb	88	19.2	1.4
stewed	1 cup	80	13.2	2.7
stewed	4 oz	90	14.8	3.0
TOMATO, CANNED				
(A&P)				
sliced	1/2 cup	35	8.0	<1.0
whole	1/2 cup	25	6.0	<1.0
(Angela Mia)				
chopped 'Premium Choice'	4 oz	24	4.1	0.4
crushed	4 oz	25	5.1	0.2
crushed, chunky	4 oz	26	5.1	0.3
crushed 'Premium Choice'	2.222 oz	29	5.6	0.4
(Contadina)				
crushed, in purée	1/2 cup	30	6.0	<1.0
Italian style	1/2 cup	35	8.0	<1.0
Italian style, pear	1/2 cup	25	5.0	<1.0
'Recipe Ready'	1/2 cup	25	5.0	0.2
stewed	1/2 cup	35	8.0	<1.0
stewed, Mexican style	1/2 cup	35	8.0	0.3
whole, peeled	1/2 cup	25	5.0	<1.0
w/jalapeños	1/2 cup	35	8.0	<1.0
(Del Monte)				
stewed	1/2 cup	35	8.0	0.0
stewed 'No Salt Added'	1/2 cup	35	8.0	0.0
wedges, w/liquid	1/2 cup	30	8.0	0.0
whole, peeled, w/liquid	1/2 cup	25	5.0	0.0
(Eden Foods) crushed, organic, no salt added	4 oz	35	6.0	0.0
(Featherweight)	1/2 cup	20	4.0	0.0
(Finast)				
sliced	1/2 cup	35	9.0	0.0
whole, peeled	1/2 cup	25	6.0	0.0
(Hunt's)				
choice cut	4 oz	19	4.0	0.0
crushed	4 oz	31	7.2	0.4
crushed 'Angela Mia'	4 oz	35	7.0	<1.0
crushed, Italian flavored	4 oz	40	9.0	<1.0
diced, in juice	4 oz	19	4.0	0.1
diced, in juice 'No Salt Added'	4 oz	20	4.1	0.1
diced, in purée	4 oz	23	4.7	0.2
diced, w/green chilies	.3527 oz	2	0.2	0.1
pear shaped	4.868 oz	21	4.1	0.1
pear shaped	4.832 oz	21	4.1	0.1
pear shaped	4.656 oz	20	3.9	0.1

Food Name	Serv. Size	Total Cal.	Carbs GMS	Fat GMS
pear shaped, Italian flavored	4 oz	20	5.0	<1.0
peeled, choice cut	4 oz	20	5.0	<1.0
stewed	4 oz	33	6.7	0.1
stewed 'Food Service'	4 oz	29	6.7	0.1
stewed, Italian flavored	4 oz	35	8.0	<1.0
stewed 'No Salt Added'	1/2 cup	35	8.0	0.0
whole	4 oz	20	5.0	0.0
whole, Italian flavored	4 oz	25	6.0	<1.0
whole 'No Salt Added'	4 oz	20	5.0	0.0
whole, peeled	5.608 oz	24	4.7	0.3
whole, peeled	5.22 oz	22	4.4	0.1
whole, peeled	5.009 oz	22	4.2	0.1
whole, peeled	4.832 oz	21	4.1	0.1
whole, peeled 'No Salt Added'	4.832 oz	21	4.1	0.1
(Old El Paso) w/green chilies	1/4 cup	14	3.0	0.0
(Ortega) w/jalapeños	1 oz	8	1.0	0.0
(Pathmark)				
crushed	1/2 cup	40	9.0	0.0
crushed 'No Frills'	1 cup	90	20.0	0.0
'No Frills'	1 cup	50	11.0	0.0
sliced	1/2 cup	35	9.0	0.0
whole, peeled 'No Salt Added'	1/2 cup	25	6.0	0.0
whole, peeled, w/tomato juice	1/2 cup	25	6.0	0.0
(S&W)				
aspic, supreme	1/2 cup	60	16.0	0.0
cut, peeled 'Ready-Cut'	1/2 cup	25	6.0	0.0
diced, in rich purée	1/2 cup	35	8.0	0.0
Italian, sliced	1/2 cup	35	9.0	0.0
Mexican style	1/2 cup	40	8.0	0.0
sliced	1/2 cup	35	9.0	0.0
stewed '50% Salt Reduced'	1/2 cup	35	9.0	0.0
whole, peeled	1/2 cup	25	6.0	0.0
whole, peeled, Italian-style pear, w/basil	1/2 cup	25	5.0	0.0
(S&W Nutradiet) whole	1/2 cup	25	5.0	0.0
(Stokely)				
stewed	1/2 cup	35	8.0	0.0
whole	1/2 cup	25	5.0	0.0
TOMATO, PICKLED, kosher (Claussen)	1 oz	5	1.0	0.0
TOMATO-BEEF COCKTAIL (Beefamato)	6 oz	80	19.0	0.0
TOMATO-CHILE COCKTAIL (Snap-E-Tom)	6 oz	40	7.0	0.0
TOMATO-CLAM COCKTAIL (Clamato)	6 oz	96	23.0	0.0
TOMATO JUICE				
(A&P)	6 oz	30	7.0	0.0

Food Name	Serv. Size	Total Cal.	Carbs GMS	Fat GMS
(Biotta)	6 oz	28	5.8	0.1
(Campbell's)	6 oz	40	8.0	0.0
(Featherweight)	6 oz	35	8.0	0.0
(Hunt's)	9.03 oz	33	6.5	0.2
(Hunt's)	7.16 oz	28	5.5	0.2
(Hunt's)	6 oz	30	7.0	0.0
(Hunt's)	5.467 oz	22	4.2	0.1
(Hunt's) 'No Salt Added'	6 oz	45	11.0	0.0
(Knudsen & Sons) organic	8 oz	50	10.0	0.0
(Libby's)	6 oz	35	7.0	0.0
(Pathmark)	6 oz	30	6.0	0.0
(Pathmark) frozen, diluted	6 oz	35	8.0	0.0
(S&W) 'California'	6 oz	35	8.0	0.0
(S&W Nutradiet)	6 oz	35	8.0	0.0
(Stokely)	4 oz	20	4.0	0.0
(Welch's)	6 oz	35	7.0	0.0
TOMATO PASTE				
(Contadina)	2 oz	50	11.0	<1.0
(Contadina) Italian style	2 oz	65	12.0	1.0
(Hunt's)	1.164 oz	24	4.9	0.2
(Hunt's) 'Food Service'	1.164 oz	24	4.9	0.2
(Hunt's) Italian style	1.164 oz	25	4.7	0.4
(Hunt's) 'No Salt Added"	1.164 oz	24	4.9	0.2
(Hunt's) w/garlic	2 oz	50	11.0	<1.0
(Hunt's) w/garlic	1.164 oz	26	5.1	0.3
TOMATO POWDER				
ground	1 oz	86	21.2	0.1
ground	100 gm	302	74.7	0.4
TOMATO PURÉE				
(Angela Mia)	2.187 oz	16	2.9	0.3
(Contadina)	1/2 cup	40	8.0	<1.0
(Contadina) w/crushed tomatoes	1/2 cup	30	6.0	<1.0
(Hunt's)	2.187 oz	23	4.3	0.3
(Hunt's) 'Food Service'	2.222 oz	26	5.0	0.4
TOMATO SAUCE				
CANNED				
(A&P)	1/2 cup	45	9.0	<1.0
(Contadina)	1/2 cup	30	7.0	<1.0
(Del Monte)	1 cup	70	16.0	1.0
(Finast)	1/2 cup	45	9.0	0.0
(Health Valley)	1 cup	70	13.0	0.5
(Hunt's)	4 oz	30	7.0	0.0
(Hunt's)	2.187 oz	16	2.6	0.2

Food Name	Serv. Size	Total Cal.	Carbs GMS	Fat GMS
(Pathmark)	1/2 cup	40	9.0	0.0
(S&W)	1/2 cup	40	9.0	0.0
(Stokely)	1/2 cup	30	7.0	0.0
Casera (Hunt's)	2.187 oz	22	5.2	0.1
Chunky				
(Hunt's) chili	2.222 oz	21	4.1	0.4
(Hunt's) 'Food Service'	2.187 oz	15	2.8	0.2
(Hunt's) Italian	2.222 oz	29	4.5	1.1
(Hunt's) Mexican	2.222 oz	19	3.8	0.4
(Hunt's) tomato	2.187 oz	13	2.9	0.1
Garden vegetable (Contadina)	5 oz	80	9.0	3.0
Herb flavored (Hunt's)	4 oz	70	12.0	2.0
Hot, Maya (Hunt's)	1.058 oz	6	1.1	0.2
Italian style				
(Contadina)	1/2 cup	30	7.0	<1.0
(Contadina) sausage	5 oz	110	8.0	6.0
(Hunt's)	4 oz	60	11.0	2.0
(Hunt's)	2.222 oz	26	5.2	0.5
(Rokeach)	3 oz	60	8.0	2.0
Low sodium (Rokeach)	3 oz	50	8.0	2.0
Marinara				
(Buitoni)	1/2 cup	70	11.0	3.0
(Contadina)	4 oz	80	8.0	4.0
(Pathmark) 'No Frills'	1/2 cup	80	12.0	3.0
(Rokeach)	3 oz	60	9.0	2.0
'Meatloaf Fixin's' (Hunt's)	2 oz	20	5.0	<1.0
No salt added				
(Del Monte)	1 cup	70	16.0	1.0
(Finast)	8 oz	90	18.0	0.0
(Health Valley)	1 cup	70	13.0	0.5
(Hunt's)	4 oz	35	8.0	0.0
(Hunt's)	2.187 oz	16	2.6	0.2
(Pathmark)	1/2 cup	45	9.0	0.0
Pesto (Contadina)	2.33 oz	350	5.0	34.0
Plum (Contadina)	5 oz	80	8.0	4.0
'Special'				
(Hunt's)	4 oz	35	8.0	0.0
(Hunt's)	2.187 oz	21	3.8	0.6
'Thick and Zesty' (Contadina)	1/2 cup	40	8.0	<1.0
W/bits (Hunt's)	4 oz	30	7.0	<1.0
W/garlic				
(Hunt's)	4 oz	70	10.0	2.0
(Hunt's)	2.258 oz	29	4.9	1.0

Food Name	Serv. Size	Total Cal.	Carbs GMS	Fat GMS
W/green chilies *(Old El Paso)*	1/4 cup	14	3.0	<1.0
W/herbs *(Hunt's)*	2.187 oz	33	4.9	1.3
W/jalapeños *(Old El Paso)*	1/4 cup	11	2.0	1.0
W/mushrooms *(Hunt's)*	4 oz	25	6.0	<1.0
W/onions				
(Del Monte)	1 cup	100	23.0	1.0
(Hunt's)	4 oz	40	9.0	<1.0
REFRIGERATED				
(Contadina) 'Light'	.5 oz	50	9.0	0.0
(Contadina) marinara 'Fresh'	7.5 oz	100	12.0	4.0
(Contadina) plum w/basil 'Fresh'	7.5 oz	100	14.0	4.0
TOMATOES, SUN-DRIED. See SUN-DRIED TOMATOES.				
TOMATOSEED OIL				
	1/2 cup	964	0.0	109.0
	1 oz	251	0.0	28.4
	1 tbsp	120	0.0	13.6
TONIC. See SOFT DRINKS AND MIXERS.				
TORSK. See CUSK.				
TORTELLINI PASTA, NONDAIRY				
regular *(Tofutti)* frozen	2 oz	210	32.0	4.0
spinach *(Tofutti)* frozen	2 oz	210	32.0	4.0
TORTELLINI PASTA, REFRIGERATED				
CHEESE *(DiGiorno)* approx 1 cup cooked	1/3 pkg	270	41.0	6.0
CHICKEN AND HERB *(DiGiorno)* approx 1 cup cooked	1/3 pkg	240	37.0	5.0
EGG				
w/cheese 'Fresh' *(Contadina)*	4.5 oz	380	60.0	6.0
w/cheese 'Fresh' *(Contadina)*	3 oz	260	39.0	6.0
w/chicken and prosciutto 'Fresh' *(Contadina)*	4.5 oz	370	53.0	7.0
w/meat 'Fresh' *(Contadina)*	4.5 oz	380	60.0	6.0
MOZZARELLA GARLIC *(DiGiorno)* approx 1 cup cooked	1/3 pkg	260	35.0	8.0
SAUSAGE, Italian 'Fresh' *(Contadina)*	3 oz	260	37.0	7.0
SPINACH				
w/cheese 'Fresh' *(Contadina)*	4.5 oz	380	60.0	6.0
w/cheese 'Fresh' *(Contadina)*	3 oz	260	38.0	6.0
w/chicken and prosciutto 'Fresh' *(Contadina)*	4.5 oz	340	53.0	7.0
w/meat 'Fresh' *(Contadina)*	4.5 oz	380	60.0	6.0
W/CHICKEN AND PROSCIUTTO *(Contadina)*	3 oz	250	34.0	6.0
W/MEAT				
(Contadina) 'Fresh'	3 oz	260	39.0	6.0
(DiGiorno) approx 1 cup cooked	1/3 pkg	280	38.0	9.0
TORTELLINI DISH/ENTRÉE, FROZEN				
(Birds Eye) in tomato sauce 'For One'	5.5 oz	210	31.0	5.0
(Budget Gourmet) 'Side Dish'	5.5 oz	180	25.0	9.0

Food Name	Serv. Size	Total Cal.	Carbs GMS	Fat GMS
(Green Giant) marinara 'One Serving'	5.5 oz	260	37.0	9.0
(Green Giant) Provençal 'Microwave Garden Gourmet'	1 pkg	260	44.0	6.0
(Le Menu) and meat sauce 'LightStyle'	8 oz	250	34.0	8.0
(Stouffer's) in Alfredo sauce	8 7/8 oz	580	35.0	37.0
(Stouffer's) w/tomato sauce	9.25 oz	360	39.0	15.0
(Top Shelf) in marinara sauce	10 oz	211	37.0	3.0
(Top Shelf) w/shrimp and seafood	10 oz	278	36.0	8.0
(Weight Watchers)	9 oz	310	50.0	6.0
TORTILLA, CORN				
(Azteca)	1 tortilla	45	9.0	0.0
(Old El Paso)	1 tortilla	60	10.0	1.0
TORTILLA, FLOUR				
(Azteca) 9-inch diam	1 tortilla	130	23.0	3.0
(Azteca) 7-inch diam	1 tortilla	80	14.0	2.0
(Mission) 'Light'	1 tortilla	70	16.0	1.0
(Old El Paso)	1 tortilla	150	27.0	3.0
Burrito style				
(Garcia's)	1 tortilla	220	37.0	5.0
(Mission) 'Premium'	1 tortilla	230	40.0	6.0
(Tyson)	1 tortilla	173	29.0	4.0
(Tyson) large, heat-pressed	1 tortilla	182	33.0	4.0
(Tyson) small, hand-stretched	1 tortilla	106	19.0	2.0
Fajita style				
(Fry's) extra soft	1 tortilla	100	17.0	2.0
(Garcia's)	1 tortilla	100	17.0	2.5
(Tyson)	1 tortilla	84	18.0	2.0
Taco size				
(Mission) soft	1 tortilla	150	25.0	4.0
(Tyson) soft	1 tortilla	121	20.0	3.0
TORTILLA CHIPS. See also CORN CHIPS AND SNACKS.				
(Bachman)				
nacho	1 oz	140	18.0	6.0
'No Salt'	1 oz	140	19.0	6.0
(Barbara's Bakery)				
yellow corn, organic	1 oz	140	18.0	7.0
yellow corn, organic, no salt added	1 oz	140	18.0	7.0
(Bearitos)				
blue corn 'Organic'	1 oz	146	17.4	7.0
blue corn 'Organic No Salt'	1 oz	137	17.1	6.5
yellow corn 'Organic'	1 oz	143	18.1	6.4
yellow corn 'Organic No Salt'	1 oz	148	17.2	7.2
(Bravos)				
nacho cheese flavored, jalapeño	1 oz	150	19.0	7.0

Food Name	Serv. Size	Total Cal.	Carbs GMS	Fat GMS
nacho cheese flavored, round, crispy	1 oz	150	18.0	8.0
nacho cheese flavored, strips	1 oz	140	18.0	7.0
(Buenitos)				
'Tortilla Chips'	1 oz	150	18.0	8.0
'Tortilla Chips, No Salt Added'	1 oz	150	18.0	8.0
(Doritos)				
'Cool Ranch'	1 oz	140	18.0	7.0
'Cool Ranch Light'	1 oz	120	21.0	4.0
'Jumpin' Jack'	1 oz	140	18.0	7.0
nacho cheese	1 oz	140	18.0	7.0
nacho cheese 'Light'	1 oz	120	21.0	4.0
salsa and cheese 'Thins'	1 oz	150	17.0	8.0
'Salsa Rio'	1 oz	140	18.0	7.0
taco	1 oz	140	18.0	7.0
toasted corn	1 oz	140	19.0	7.0
white corn, lightly salted 'Thins'	1 oz	140	19.0	7.0
(Eagle) ranch	1 oz	140	17.0	8.0
(Featherweight)				
'Low Salt'	1 oz	150	18.0	8.0
nacho	1 oz	150	18.0	8.0
(Guiltless Gourmet)				
white corn, baked, salted	1 oz	110	22.0	1.5
yellow corn, baked, salted	1 oz	110	22.0	1.5
yellow corn, baked, unsalted	1 oz	110	22.0	1.5
(Hain)				
sesame	1 oz	140	19.0	7.0
sesame, cheese	1 oz	160	20.0	8.0
sesame 'No Salt Added'	1 oz	140	19.0	7.0
taco	1 oz	160	15.0	11.0
(Keebler)				
cinnamon crispaña, flour 'Chacho's'	1 oz	140	19.0	7.0
original, restaurant style 'Chacho's'	1 oz	140	18.0	7.0
(Kettle Ties)				
blue corn, lightly salted	1 oz	140	18.0	6.0
blue corn, no salt	1 oz	140	18.0	6.0
yellow corn, lightly salted	1 oz	140	19.0	7.0
yellow corn, no salt	1 oz	140	19.0	7.0
(La Famous)				
'No Salt Added'	1 oz	140	18.0	7.0
plain	1 oz	140	18.0	7.0
(Laura Scudder's)				
lightly salted 'Restaurant Style'	1 oz	140	18.0	7.0
nacho, jalapeño 'Strips'	1 oz	150	19.0	7.0

Food Name	Serv. Size	Total Cal.	Carbs GMS	Fat GMS
nacho 'Triangles'	1 oz	140	18.0	7.0
picante 'Restaurant Style Strips'	1 oz	150	19.0	7.0
(Old El Paso)				
crispy	1 oz	150	17.0	8.0
white, round 'NaChips' low sodium	1 oz	160	17.0	9.0
(Planters)				
nacho cheese	1 oz	150	18.0	8.0
traditional	1 oz	150	18.0	8.0
(Slimchips) fat-free	.4 oz	44	10.0	<.5
(Tio Sancho)				
'Microwave Snacks'	4 oz	567	74.4	26.1
nacho	.5 oz	70	0.7	5.7
(Tostitos)				
nacho, sharp	1 oz	150	17.0	8.0
white corn, baked 'Cool Ranch'	1 oz	130	21.0	3.0
white corn, baked, no salt	1 oz	110	24.0	1.0
white corn, baked 'Original'	1 oz	110	24.0	1.0
(Wise) nacho cheese flavored, crispy, round	1 oz	150	18.0	8.0
TORULA YEAST. See YEAST, TORULA.				
TOSTACO SHELL (Old El Paso)	1 shell	100	11.0	5.0
TOSTADA SHELL				
(Lawry's)	1 shell	73	9.5	3.5
(Old El Paso)	1 shell	55	6.0	3.0
(Ortega)	1 shell	50	8.0	2.0
(Pancho Villa)	1 shell	55	6.0	3.0
(Rosarita)	1 shell	60	8.0	3.0
(Tio Sancho)	1 shell	67	8.4	3.2
TOWEL GOURD. See GOURD, DISHCLOTH.				
TRAIL MIX				
(Harmony) 'Delux Super'	1/4 cup	150	23.0	7.0
(Harmony) nut and berry mix	1/4 cup	160	21.0	8.0
TREE FERN				
cooked	4 oz	45	12.5	0.1
cooked, chopped	1/2 cup	28	7.8	0.1
TRITICALE				
whole grain	1/2 cup	323	69.2	2.0
whole grain	1 oz	95	20.4	0.6
TRITICALE FLOUR				
whole grain	1/2 cup	220	47.5	1.2
whole grain	1 oz	96	20.7	0.5
TROPICAL CITRUS DRINK				
chilled (Five Alive)	6 oz	90	21.0	0.0
frozen, prepared (Five Alive)	6 oz	90	21.0	0.0

Food Name	Serv. Size	Total Cal.	Carbs GMS	Fat GMS
TROPICAL FRUIT DRINK				
bottled 'Thirst Quencher' (Gatorade)	8 oz	50	14.0	0.0
mix 'Thirst Quencher' prepared (Gatorade)	8 oz	60	15.0	0.0
TROPICAL FRUIT JUICE				
bottled (Juicy Juice)	6 oz	110	26.0	0.0
boxed (Juicy Juice)	8.45 oz	150	36.0	0.0
TROPICAL LIME COOLER (Knudsen & Sons)	8 oz	130	32.0	0.0
TROPICAL NECTAR, can or bottle (Kern's)	6 oz	110	27.0	0.0
TROPICAL ORANGE DRINK, 'Fruit Box' (Tang)	8.45 oz	150	37.0	0.0
TROPICAL PASSION JUICE (Knudsen & Sons)	8 oz	80	20.0	0.0
TROPICAL PUNCH				
Can, bottle, or box				
(Knudsen & Sons)	8 oz	105	33.0	0.0
(Kool-Aid) 'Koolers'	8.45 oz	130	35.0	0.0
(Minute Maid)	6 oz	90	22.0	0.0
(Santa Cruz Natural) organic	8 oz	110	26.0	<1.0
Mix				
(Kool-Aid) sugar-free, w/NutraSweet, prepared	8 oz	4	0.0	0.0
(Kool-Aid) sugar-sweetened, prepared	8 oz	80	21.0	0.0
(Kool-Aid) unsweetened, prepared w/sugar	8 oz	100	25.0	0.0
(Kool-Aid) unsweetened, prepared w/o sugar	8 oz	2	0.0	0.0
TROPICAL SALAD (Sun Fresh) chilled, packed in light syrup	3.5 oz	88	18.7	0.9
TROUT, MIXED SPECIES				
dry-heat cooked	3 oz	161	0.0	7.2
raw	1 lb	673	0.0	30.0
raw	3 oz	126	0.0	5.6
raw	1 oz	42	0.0	1.9
raw, approx 2.8 oz	1 fillet	117	0.0	5.2
TROUT, RAINBOW				
farmed, dry-heat cooked	3 oz	144	0.0	6.1
farmed, raw	3 oz	117	0.0	4.6
wild, dry-heat cooked	3 oz	127	0.0	4.9
wild, raw	3 oz	101	0.0	2.9
wild, raw, approx 2.8 oz	1 fillet	189	0.0	5.5
TROUT, SEA, MIXED SPECIES				
raw	1 lb	472	0.0	16.4
raw	3 oz	88	0.0	3.1
raw	1 oz	29	0.0	1.0
TUMERIC. See TURMERIC.				
TUNA, ALBACORE. See TUNA, CANNED; TUNA, FROZEN.				
TUNA, ALTERNATIVE, frozen 'Tuno' (Worthington)	2 oz	100	3.0	7.0
TUNA, BLUEFIN				
dry-heat cooked	4 oz	209	0.0	7.1

Food Name	Serv. Size	Total Cal.	Carbs GMS	Fat GMS
dry-heat cooked	3 oz	156	0.0	5.3
raw	1 lb	652	0.0	22.2
raw	3 oz	122	0.0	4.2
raw	1 oz	41	0.0	1.4
TUNA, CANNED				
LIGHT				
In canola oil, chunk (Chicken of the Sea)	2 oz	160	<1.0	12.0
In oil				
drained	3 oz	168	0.0	7.0
drained, approx 6 oz	1 can	339	0.0	14.0
w/o salt, drained	3 oz	168	0.0	7.0
w/o salt, drained, approx 6 oz	1 can	339	0.0	14.0
In pure vegetable oil, chunk, w/liquid (Chicken of the Sea)	2 oz	160	<1.0	12.0
In soybean oil				
chunk, drained	1 oz	56	0.0	2.3
chunk, drained (A&P)	2 oz	150	<1.0	13.0
chunk, drained (Bumble Bee)	2 oz	110	0.0	12.0
chunk, drained (Finast)	2 oz	150	<1.0	13.0
chunk, drained (Star-Kist)	2 oz	150	<1.0	13.0
chunk 'Fancy' drained (S&W)	2 oz	140	0.0	10.0
solid, drained (Progresso)	1/3 cup	150	<1.0	13.0
solid, drained (Star-Kist)	2 oz	150	<1.0	13.0
w/o salt, drained	1 oz	56	0.0	2.3
In spring water, chunk, w/liquid (Chicken of the Sea)	2 oz	60	<1.0	1.0
In water				
chunk, drained (Bumble Bee)	2 oz	50	0.0	1.0
chunk, drained (Finast)	2 oz	60	<1.0	<1.0
chunk, drained (Pathmark)	2 oz	70	0.0	2.0
chunk, drained (Star-Kist)	2 oz	60	<1.0	<1.0
chunk, diet, drained (Star-Kist)	2 oz	65	<1.0	<1.0
chunk 'Fancy' drained (S&W)	2 oz	60	0.0	1.0
chunk 'No Salt Added' drained (Weight Watchers)	2 oz	60	<1.0	<1.0
chunk '60% Less Salt' drained (Star-Kist)	2 oz	65	<1.0	1.0
drained	3 oz	111	0.0	0.4
drained	1 oz	37	0.0	0.1
drained, approx 6.3 oz	1 can	216	0.0	0.8
drained (A&P)	2 oz	60	<1.0	<1.0
drained (Empress)	2 oz	60	0.0	1.0
solid, drained (Star-Kist)	2 oz	60	<1.0	<1.0
solid 'Prime Catch' drained (Star-Kist)	2 oz	60	<1.0	<1.0
w/o salt, drained	3 oz	111	0.0	0.4
w/o salt, drained	1 oz	37	0.0	0.1
w/o salt, drained, approx 6.3 oz	1 can	216	0.0	0.8

Food Name	Serv. Size	Total Cal.	Carbs GMS	Fat GMS
WHITE				
In oil				
drained	3 oz	158	0.0	6.9
drained, approx 6.3 oz	1 can	331	0.0	14.4
w/o salt, drained	3 oz	158	0.0	6.9
w/o salt, drained, approx 6.3 oz	1 can	331	0.0	14.4
In soybean oil				
chunk, drained	1 oz	53	0.0	2.3
chunk, drained (A&P)	2 oz	150	<1.0	10.0
chunk, drained (Bumble Bee)	2 oz	110	0.0	12.0
chunk, drained (Star-Kist)	2 oz	140	<1.0	10.0
solid, albacore, drained (Bumble Bee)	2 oz	100	0.0	8.0
solid, albacore, drained (Finast)	2 oz	145	<1.0	10.0
solid, albacore, drained (S&W)	2 oz	160	0.0	12.0
solid, albacore, drained (Star-Kist)	2 oz	140	<1.0	10.0
w/o salt, drained	1 oz	53	0.0	2.3
In spring water, solid, fancy albacore (Chicken of the Sea)	2 oz	60	<1.0	1.0
In water				
chunk, diet, drained (Star-Kist)	2 oz	70	<1.0	1.0
chunk, drained (A&P)	2 oz	100	<1.0	5.0
chunk, drained (Bumble Bee)	2 oz	60	0.0	2.0
chunk '60% Less Salt' drained (Star-Kist)	2 oz	70	<1.0	<1.0
drained	3 oz	116	0.0	2.1
drained, approx 6.1 oz	1 can	234	0.0	4.2
solid, albacore, drained (A&P)	2 oz	70	<1.0	<1.0
solid, albacore, drained (Bumble Bee)	2 oz	60	0.0	2.0
solid, albacore, drained (Finast)	2 oz	70	<1.0	1.0
solid, albacore, drained (Pathmark)	2 oz	70	0.0	2.0
solid, albacore, drained (Star-Kist)	2 oz	70	<1.0	1.0
solid, albacore, drained (Weight Watchers)	2 oz	70	<1.0	1.0
w/o salt, drained	3 oz	116	0.0	2.1
w/o salt, drained	1 oz	39	0.0	0.7
w/o salt, drained, approx 6.1 oz	1 can	234	0.0	4.2
TUNA, FROZEN				
(Peter Pan Seafoods) albacore, white, steaks, skinless, boneless, raw	3.5 oz	102	na	4.9
(Peter Pan Seafoods) yellowfin, steaks, skinless, boneless, raw	3.5 oz	131	na	4.1
(SeaPak) steak, w/o seasoning mix	6-oz pkg	180	0.0	2.0
TUNA, SKIPJACK /aku/arctic bonito/katsuo/oceanic bonito. See also BONITO.				
dry-heat cooked	3 oz	112	0.0	1.1
raw	1 lb	468	0.0	4.6
raw	3 oz	88	0.0	0.9

Food Name	Serv. Size	Total Cal.	Carbs GMS	Fat GMS
raw	1 oz	29	0.0	0.3
raw, approx 7 oz	1/2 fillet	204	0.0	2.0
TUNA, YELLOWFIN/ahi				
dry-heat cooked	3 oz	118	0.0	1.0
raw	1 lb	492	0.0	4.3
raw	3 oz	92	0.0	0.8
raw	1 oz	31	0.0	0.3
TUNA ENTRÉE, FROZEN				
noodle casserole *(Stouffer's)*	10 oz	280	33.0	15.0
noodle casserole *(Weight Watchers)*	9 oz	230	27.0	7.0
pie *(Banquet)*	7 oz	540	44.0	33.0
TUNA ENTRÉE, MIX				
au gratin, dry mix *(Tuna Helper)*	1/5 pkg	180	27.0	5.0
buttery rice, dry mix *(Tuna Helper)*	1/5 pkg	160	32.0	2.0
cheesy noodle, dry mix *(Tuna Helper)*	1/5 pkg	160	27.0	4.0
creamy broccoli, dry mix *(Tuna Helper)*	1/5 pkg	200	35.0	4.0
fettuccine Alfredo, dry mix *(Tuna Helper)*	1/5 pkg	160	28.0	3.0
mushroom, creamy, dry mix *(Tuna Helper)*	1/5 pkg	140	28.0	1.0
noodle, creamy, dry mix *(Tuna Helper)*	1/5 pkg	210	29.0	8.0
pot pie, dry mix *(Tuna Helper)*	1/6 pkg	290	31.0	17.0
salad, dry mix *(Tuna Helper)*	1/5 pkg	140	28.0	1.0
tetrazzini, dry mix *(Tuna Helper)*	1/5 pkg	160	26.0	3.0
TUNA LUNCH KIT				
'Charlie's Lunch Kit' w/1 mayo packet *(Star-Kist)*	4.6 oz	290	16.0	15.0
'Charlie's Lunch Kit' w/2 mayo packets *(Star-Kist)*	5 oz	370	16.0	15.0
TUNA MIX				
classic Italian 'Tuna Mix-ins' dry mix *(Bumble Bee)*	1 oz	25	5.0	0.0
garden and herb 'Tuna Mix-ins' dry mix *(Bumble Bee)*	1 oz	25	5.0	0.0
lemon herb 'Tuna Mix-ins' dry mix *(Bumble Bee)*	1 oz	25	6.0	0.0
zesty tomato 'Tuna Mix-ins' dry mix *(Bumble Bee)*	1 oz	25	5.0	0.0
TUNA SALAD				
(Longacre)	1 oz	58	3.0	4.0
(Longacre) 'Saladfest'	1 oz	52	2.0	4.0
TUNA SALAD SPREAD *(Libby's)* 'Spreadables'	1.9 oz	80	5.0	5.0
TUNKA. See GOURD, WHITE.				
TURBOT, DOMESTIC				
raw	1 lb	845	0.0	62.8
raw	1 oz	53	0.0	3.9
raw, approx 7.2 oz	1/2 fillet	380	0.0	28.2
TURBOT, EUROPEAN				
dry-heat cooked	3 oz	104	0.0	3.2
raw	1 lb	432	0.0	13.4
raw	3 oz	81	0.0	2.5

Food Name	Serv. Size	Total Cal.	Carbs GMS	Fat GMS
raw	1 oz	27	0.0	0.8
raw, approx 7.2 oz	1/2 fillet	194	0.0	6.0
TURKEY, ALL CLASSES				
BACK MEAT W/SKIN				
raw	1 lb	896	0.0	59.2
raw	1 oz	56	0.0	3.7
roasted	4 oz	276	0.0	16.3
BREAST MEAT W/SKIN				
raw	1 lb	720	0.0	32.0
raw	1 oz	45	0.0	2.0
roasted	4 oz	214	0.0	8.4
DARK MEAT ONLY				
raw	1 lb	560	0.0	19.2
raw	1 oz	35	0.0	1.2
roasted	1 cup	262	0.0	10.1
roasted	4 oz	212	0.0	8.2
DARK MEAT W/SKIN				
raw	1 lb	720	0.0	40.0
raw	1 oz	45	0.0	2.5
roasted	4 oz	251	0.0	13.1
LEG MEAT W/SKIN				
raw	1 lb	656	0.0	30.4
raw	1 oz	41	0.0	1.9
roasted	4 oz	236	0.0	11.1
LIGHT MEAT ONLY				
raw	1 lb	528	0.0	6.4
raw	1 oz	33	0.0	0.4
roasted	4 oz	178	0.0	3.7
roasted, diced	1 cup	220	0.0	4.5
LIGHT MEAT W/SKIN				
raw	1 lb	72.0	0.0	33.6
raw	1 oz	45	0.0	2.1
roasted	4 oz	223	0.0	9.4
NECK MEAT ONLY				
raw	1 lb	608	0.0	24.0
raw	1 oz	38	0.0	1.5
simmered	4 oz	204	0.0	8.2
SKIN ONLY				
raw	1 lb	1760	0.0	168.0
raw	1 oz	110	0.0	10.5
roasted	1 oz	125	0.0	11.2
WING MEAT W/SKIN				
raw	1 lb	896	0.0	56.0

Food Name	Serv. Size	Total Cal.	Carbs GMS	Fat GMS
raw	1 oz	56	0.0	3.5
roasted	4 oz	260	0.0	14.1
TURKEY, ALTERNATIVE				
(Worthington) roll, smoked, frozen	4 slices	180	5.0	12.0
(Worthington) sliced, smoked, frozen	4 slices	180	5.0	12.0
(Worthington) 'Turkee Slices' canned	2 slices	130	3.0	9.0
(Worthington) '209' canned, drained	2 slices	120	3.0	8.0
TURKEY, BONELESS. See also LUNCHEON MEAT.				
BREAST				
(Butterball) 'Slice 'n Serve'	1 oz	35	<1.0	1.0
(Longacre) 'Gourmet'	1 oz	35	1.0	1.0
(Longacre) 'Gourmet Low Salt'	1 oz	30	1.0	<1.0
(Longacre) 'Premium'	1 oz	30	1.0	1.0
(Longacre) 'Salt Watchers'	1 oz	32	0.0	<1.0
(Mr. Turkey)	1 oz	31	0.3	0.7
Barbecue seasoned *(Butterball)* 'Slice 'n Serve'	1 oz	40	1.0	2.0
Browned				
(Longacre) glazed 'Gourmet'	1 oz	35	1.0	1.0
(Longacre) glazed 'Premium'	1 oz	30	1.0	1.0
(Longacre) roasted 'Gourmet'	1 oz	35	1.0	1.0
(Longacre) roasted 'Premium'	1 oz	30	1.0	1.0
Golden				
(Boar's Head)	1 oz	35	<1.0	1.0
(Boar's Head) skinless	1 oz	30	<1.0	<1.0
Hickory smoked *(Butterball)* 'Slice 'n Serve'	1 oz	35	1.0	1.0
Honey roasted *(Louis Rich)*	1 oz	32	1.2	0.8
Lean, lite				
(Longacre) 'Deli'	1 oz	35	0.0	1.0
(Longacre) skinless 'Deli'	1 oz	35	0.0	<1.0
(Longacre) smoked 'Deli'	1 oz	35	0.0	1.0
Skinless				
(Longacre) 'Catering'	1 oz	35	<1.0	<1.0
(Longacre) 'Gourmet'	1 oz	30	1.0	<1.0
(Longacre) 'Premium'	1 oz	30	1.0	<1.0
(Norbest) 'Blue Label'	1 oz	26	0.4	0.4
(Norbest) 'Norfresh'	1 oz	27	0.5	0.3
(Norbest) 'Norfresh Blue Label'	1 oz	24	0.7	0.3
(Norbest) 'Norfresh Yellow Label'	1 oz	24	0.4	0.5
(Norbest) 'Orange Label'	1 oz	26	0.5	0.2
(Norbest) salt-free 'Blue Label'	1 oz	33	<.1	0.3
(Norbest) 'Tan Label'	1 oz	24	0.5	0.5
(Norbest) 'Yellow Label'	1 oz	26	0.8	0.5

Food Name	Serv. Size	Total Cal.	Carbs GMS	Fat GMS
Smoked				
(Healthy Deli) 'Gourmet'	1 oz	31	0.4	0.5
(Hormel) 'Perma-Fresh'	2 slices	60	0.0	2.0
(Longacre)	1 oz	35	0.0	1.0
(Norbest) 'Gold Label'	1 oz	29	0.1	<.6
(OHSE)	1 oz	30	1.0	1.0
W/skin				
(Norbest) 'Blue Label'	1 oz	28	0.2	0.7
(Norbest) 'Norfresh Orange Label'	1 oz	26	0.1	0.3
(Norbest) 'Norfresh Yellow Label'	1 oz	25	0.1	0.5
(Norbest) 'Orange Label'	1 oz	28	0.1	0.3
(Norbest) prebrowned 'Orange Label'	1 oz	29	0.2	0.8
(Norbest) salt-free 'Blue Label'	1 oz	35	0.2	0.5
(Norbest) smoked 'Orange Label'	1 oz	30	0.9	0.5
(Norbest) 'Yellow Label'	1 oz	26	0.1	0.4
BREAST AND LIGHT MEAT				
(Longacre) browned and roasted	1 oz	40	1.0	2.0
(Longacre) 'Deli Chef'	1 oz	35	1.0	1.0
(Longacre) skinless 'Deli Chef'	1 oz	40	1.0	2.0
BREAST AND THIGH (Norbest) 'Blue Label'	1 oz	31	0.2	0.9
DARK MEAT (Norbest) ham flavor, hickory smoked	1 oz	39	0.1	2.2
OVEN COOKED (OHSE)	1 oz	30	1.0	1.0
ROLL				
(Norbest) white meat 'Orange Label'	1 oz	29	0.5	0.9
(Norbest) white and dark meat 'Orange Label'	1 oz	36	0.3	2.0
SMOKED (Louis Rich)	1 oz	32	0.4	1.0
W/PORK (Healthy Favorites) 'Breakfast Strips'	11 grams	18	0.4	1.0
TURKEY, CANNED				
(Hormel) chunk	6.75 oz	230	0.0	10.0
(Hormel) chunk	2.5 oz	80	1.0	3.0
(Swanson) white	2.5 oz	80	1.0	1.0
(Tyson) 'Wholesale Club Item'	3.5 oz	120	0.0	3.0
TURKEY, FROZEN/REFRIGERATED				
BREAST				
Cooked				
(Land O'Lakes)	3 oz	100	0.0	1.0
(Longacre) 'Cook-N-Bag'	1 oz	38	<1.0	<1.0
(Louis Rich)	1 oz	47	0.1	1.5
(Louis Rich) barbecue	1 oz	33	0.9	1.0
(Louis Rich) hen, w/o wings	1 oz	50	0.1	2.0
(Louis Rich) hickory smoked	1 oz	33	0.8	1.0
(Louis Rich) honey roasted	1 oz	33	1.1	0.8
(Louis Rich) oven roasted	1 oz	31	0.4	0.9

Food Name	Serv. Size	Total Cal.	Carbs GMS	Fa GM
(Louis Rich) roast	1 oz	42	0.2	0.
(Louis Rich) slices	1 oz	39	0.1	0.
(Louis Rich) smoked	1 oz	33	0.2	1.
(Louis Rich) steaks	1 oz	39	0.1	0.
(Louis Rich) tenderloins	1 oz	39	0.2	0.
(Mr. Turkey) barbecue, quarter 'Chub'	1 oz	34	1.0	1.
(Mr. Turkey) oven roasted, quarter 'Chub'	1 oz	34	0.4	1.
(Mr. Turkey) smoked, quarter 'Chub'	1 oz	35	0.3	1.
(Tyson) skinless, boneless 'Wholesale Club Item'	3.5 oz	160	0.0	3.
w/skin, roasted, broth pre-basted	4 oz	143	0.0	3.9
Raw				
(Longacre) 'Cook-N-Bag'	1 oz	27	<1.0	<1.
(Longacre) 'Ready-to-Cook'	1 oz	39	0.0	<1.
(Norbest) steaks, cubed	4 oz	135	<.1	2.
(Norbest) strips and tips 'Tasti-Lean'	4 oz	135	<.1	2.0
(Norbest) tenderloin 'Tasti-Lean Tenders'	4 oz	135	<.1	2.
(Norbest) w/gravy	4 oz	115	1.1	2.
CUTLET *(Norbest)* raw 'Tasti-Lean'	4 oz	135	<.1	2.
DARK MEAT *(Butterball)* w/o skin, roasted, approx 3.5 oz	2 slices	195	na	10.0
DRUMSTICK				
(Land O'Lakes)	3 oz	120	0.0	5.
(Louis Rich) cooked	1 oz	56	0.1	2.
(Louis Rich) cooked 'Fresh Turkey Cuts'	1 oz	55	<1.0	3.0
HINDQUARTER ROAST *(Land O'Lakes)*	3 oz	140	0.0	8.0
LIGHT AND DARK MEAT				
roasted, then seasoned	4 oz	176	3.5	6.8
seasoned raw, then roasted	1 lb	544	29.0	10.0
seasoned raw, then roasted	1 oz	34	1.8	0.6
(Butterball) w/skin, roasted, approx 3.5 oz	2 slices	195	na	10.0
LIGHT MEAT *(Butterball)* w/o skin, roasted, approx 3.5 oz	2 slices	160	na	4.0
THIGH				
w/skin, roasted, pre-basted w/broth	4 oz	178	0.0	9.7
(Land O'Lakes)	3 oz	150	0.0	10.0
(Louis Rich) cooked	1 oz	64	0.1	3.7
(Louis Rich) cooked 'Fresh Turkey Cuts'	1 oz	65	<1.0	4.0
WHOLE				
(Louis Rich) w/o giblets, cooked	1 oz	52	0.1	2.3
(Louis Rich) w/o giblets, cooked 'Fresh Whole Turkey'	1 oz	50	<1.0	2.0
(Norbest) boneless, cooked	1 oz	42	0.3	1.5
(Norbest) boneless, smoked, cooked	1 oz	42	0.3	1.6
WING				
(Land O'Lakes)	3 oz	120	0.0	5.0
(Louis Rich) cooked	1 oz	54	0.1	2.7

Food Name	Serv. Size	Total Cal.	Carbs GMS	Fat GMS
(Louis Rich) cooked 'Drumettes'	1 oz	51	0.1	2.2
(Louis Rich) cooked 'Fresh Turkey Cuts'	1 oz	55	<1.0	3.0
(Louis Rich) drumettes, cooked 'Fresh Turkey Cuts'	1 oz	50	<1.0	2.0
(Louis Rich) portions, cooked	1 oz	54	0.1	2.9
(Louis Rich) portions, cooked 'Fresh Turkey Cuts'	1 oz	55	<1.0	3.0
W/GRAVY (Norbest) raw	4 oz	115	1.1	2.7
YOUNG				
(Land O'Lakes)	3 oz	130	<1.0	7.0
(Land O'Lakes) butter-basted	3 oz	140	<1.0	8.0
(Land O'Lakes) self-basting, w/broth	3 oz	120	<1.0	5.0
TURKEY, FRYER-ROASTER				
BACK MEAT ONLY				
raw	1 lb	544	0.0	16.0
raw	1 oz	34	0.0	1.0
roasted	4 oz	193	0.0	6.4
BACK MEAT W/SKIN				
raw	1 lb	688	0.0	336.0
raw	1 oz	43	0.0	2.1
roasted	4 oz	231	0.0	11.6
BREAST MEAT ONLY				
raw	1 lb	496	0.0	3.2
raw	1 oz	31	0.0	0.2
roasted	4 oz	153	0.0	0.8
BREAST MEAT W/SKIN				
raw	1 lb	560	0.0	12.8
raw	1 oz	35	0.0	0.8
roasted	4 oz	174	0.0	3.6
DARK MEAT ONLY				
raw	1 lb	496	0.0	12.8
raw	1 oz	31	0.0	0.8
roasted	4 oz	184	0.0	4.9
roasted, diced	1 cup	227	0.0	6.0
DARK MEAT W/SKIN				
raw	1 lb	592	0.0	22.4
raw	1 oz	37	0.0	1.4
roasted	4 oz	206	0.0	8.0
LEG MEAT ONLY				
raw	1 lb	496	0.0	11.2
raw	1 oz	31	0.0	0.7
roasted	4 oz	180	0.0	4.3
LEG MEAT W/SKIN				
raw	1 lb	528	0.0	16.0
raw	1 oz	33	0.0	1.0

Food Name	Serv. Size	Total Cal.	Carbs GMS	Fat GMS
roasted	4 oz	193	0.0	6.1
LIGHT MEAT ONLY				
raw	1 lb	496	0.0	1.6
raw	1 oz	31	0.0	0.1
roasted	4 oz	159	0.0	1.3
roasted, diced	1 cup	196	0.0	1.6
LIGHT MEAT W/SKIN				
raw	1 lb	608	0.0	17.6
raw	1 oz	38	0.0	1.1
roasted	4 oz	186	0.0	5.2
SKIN ONLY				
raw	1 lb	1280	0.0	107.2
raw	1 oz	80	0.0	6.7
WING MEAT ONLY				
raw	1 lb	480	0.0	4.8
raw	1 oz	30	0.0	0.3
roasted	4 oz	185	0.0	3.9
WING MEAT W/SKIN				
raw	1 lb	720	0.0	35.2
raw	1 oz	45	0.0	2.2
roasted	4 oz	235	0.0	11.2
TURKEY, GROUND				
Cooked				
	4 oz	260	0.0	15.6
approx 2.9 oz	1 patty	193	0.0	10.8
yield from 1 lb raw	11.6 oz	754	0.0	45.5
(Hudson's)	1 oz	55	0.0	3.7
(Longacre)	1 oz	60	0.0	4.0
(Louis Rich) 85% fat-free	1 oz	60	<1.0	3.0
(Louis Rich) 90% fat-free	1 oz	50	<1.0	3.0
(Louis Rich) 90% fat-free, natural flavorings	1 oz	50	<1.0	2.0
(Mr. Turkey)	1 oz	54	0.0	4.0
Raw				
	1 lb	676	0.0	37.5
	1 oz	40	0.0	2.1
(Norbest)	1 oz	45	0.1	2.6
(Louis Rich) w/natural flavoring	1 oz	50	0.0	2.2
TURKEY, YOUNG HEN				
BACK MEAT W/SKIN				
raw	1 lb	992	0.0	72.0
raw	1 oz	62	0.0	4.5
roasted	4 oz	288	0.0	17.7

Food Name	Serv. Size	Total Cal.	Carbs GMS	Fat GMS
BREAST MEAT W/SKIN				
raw	1 lb	752	0.0	38.4
raw	1 oz	47	0.0	2.4
roasted	4 oz	220	0.0	8.9
DARK MEAT ONLY				
raw	1 lb	592	0.0	22.4
raw	1 oz	37	0.0	1.4
roasted	4 oz	218	0.0	8.8
roasted, diced	1 cup	269	0.0	10.9
DARK MEAT W/SKIN				
raw	1 lb	784	0.0	46.4
raw	1 oz	49	0.0	2.9
roasted	4 oz	263	0.0	14.5
LEG MEAT W/SKIN				
raw	1 lb	688	0.0	33.6
raw	1 oz	43	0.0	2.1
roasted	4 oz	242	0.0	11.9
LIGHT MEAT ONLY				
raw	1 lb	528	0.0	8.0
raw	1 oz	33	0.0	0.5
roasted	4 oz	183	0.0	4.2
roasted, diced	1 cup	225	0.0	5.2
LIGHT MEAT W/SKIN				
raw	1 lb	752	0.0	36.8
raw	1 oz	47	0.0	2.3
roasted	4 oz	235	0.0	10.7
SKIN ONLY				
roasted	1 oz	137	0.0	12.6
WING MEAT W/SKIN				
raw	1 lb	960	0.0	62.4
raw	1 oz	60	0.0	3.9
roasted	4 oz	270	0.0	15.3
TURKEY, YOUNG TOM				
BACK MEAT W/SKIN				
raw	1 lb	81.6	0.0	51.2
raw	1 oz	51	0.0	3.2
roasted	4 oz	270	0.0	15.5
BREAST MEAT W/SKIN				
raw	1 lb	688	0.0	28.8
raw	1 oz	43	0.0	1.8
roasted	4 oz	214	0.0	8.4
DARK MEAT ONLY				
raw	1 lb	560	0.0	19.2

Food Name	Serv. Size	Total Cal.	Carbs GMS	Fat GMS
raw	1 oz	35	0.0	1.2
roasted	4 oz	210	0.0	7.9
roasted, diced	1 cup	259	0.0	9.8
DARK MEAT W/SKIN				
raw	1 lb	688	0.0	35.2
raw	1 oz	43	0.0	2.2
roasted	4 oz	245	0.0	12.3
LEG MEAT W/SKIN				
raw	1 lb	640	0.0	28.8
raw	1 oz	40	0.0	1.8
roasted	4 oz	234	0.0	10.9
LIGHT MEAT ONLY				
raw	1 lb	512	0.0	6.4
raw	1 oz	32	0.0	0.4
roasted	4 oz	175	0.0	3.3
roasted, diced	1 cup	216	0.0	4.1
LIGHT MEAT W/SKIN				
raw	1 lb	704	0.0	32.0
raw	1 oz	44	0.0	2.0
roasted	4 oz	217	0.0	8.7
SKIN ONLY				
raw	1 lb	1664	0.0	157.0
raw	1 oz	104	0.0	9.8
roasted	1 oz	120	0.0	10.6
WING MEAT W/SKIN				
raw	1 lb	848	0.0	51.2
raw	1 oz	53	0.0	3.2
roasted	4 oz	251	0.0	13.0
TURKEY BREAST				
BARBECUED *(Louis Rich)* skinless	1 oz	30	<1.0	<1.0
HONEY ROASTED				
(Louis Rich) 95% fat-free	1-oz slice	35	1.0	1.0
(Louis Rich) skinless	1 oz	30	<1.0	<1.0
OVEN ROASTED				
(Louis Rich) 'Carving Board'	22 grams	21	0.1	0.3
(Louis Rich) 'Fresh Turkey Cuts'	1 oz	45	<1.0	2.0
(Louis Rich) 96% fat-free 'Deli-Thin'	1 slice	10	<1.0	<1.0
(Louis Rich) 97% fat-free	1-oz slice	30	1.0	<1.0
(Louis Rich) 97% fat-free 'Deli-Thin'	1 slice	10	<1.0	<1.0
(Louis Rich) roast 'Fresh Turkey Cuts'	1 oz	40	<1.0	<1.0
(Louis Rich) skinless	1 oz	25	<1.0	<1.0
(Louis Rich) slices 'Fresh Turkey Cuts'	1 oz	40	<1.0	<1.0
(Louis Rich) steaks 'Fresh Turkey Cuts'	1 oz	40	<1.0	<1.0

Food Name	Serv. Size	Total Cal.	Carbs GMS	Fat GMS
(Louis Rich) tenderloins 'Fresh Turkey Cuts'	1 oz	40	<1.0	<1.0
SMOKED				
(Louis Rich) 'Carving Board'	10 grams	9	0.1	0.1
(Louis Rich) 96% fat-free	1 oz	35	<1.0	1.0
(Louis Rich) 97% fat-free 'Deli-Thin'	1 slice	10	<1.0	<1.0
(Louis Rich) 98% fat-free	1-oz slice	20	<1.0	<1.0
(Louis Rich) skinless	1 oz	30	<1.0	<1.0
TURKEY DINNER, FROZEN				
(Banquet)	10.5 oz	390	35.0	20.0
(Banquet) 'Extra Helping'	19 oz	750	68.0	42.0
(Morton)	10 oz	230	28.0	6.0
(Swanson)	11.5 oz	350	42.0	11.0
(Swanson) 'Hungry Man'	17 oz	550	61.0	18.0
BREAST				
(Budget Gourmet) Dijon	11.2 oz	340	37.0	12.0
(Budget Gourmet) sliced	11.1 oz	290	36.0	9.0
(Healthy Choice) medallions, w/vegetables 'Classics'	12.5 oz	350	45.0	6.0
(Le Menu) sliced, w/mushroom gravy	10.5 oz	300	38.0	7.0
(Swanson) w/pasta	11.25 oz	310	36.0	9.0
DIVAN *(Le Menu)* 'LightStyle'	10 oz	260	23.0	7.0
SLICED				
(Freezer Queen)	10 oz	280	36.0	8.0
(Le Menu) 'LightStyle'	10 oz	210	21.0	5.0
TETRAZZINI *(Healthy Choice)*	12.6 oz	340	49.0	6.0
W/DRESSING AND GRAVY				
(Armour) 'Classics'	11.5 oz	320	34.0	12.0
(Banquet) w/dressing and gravy 'Healthy Balance'	11.25 oz	270	41.0	5.0
TURKEY ENTRÉE				
(Dinty Moore) w/dressing and gravy 'American Classics'	10 oz	290	33.0	5.0
(Hormel) and vegetables 'Health Selections' microwave cup	7.25 oz	220	35.0	2.0
(Libby's) w/dressing and gravy 'Diner' microwave cup	7 oz	170	15.0	7.0
(Mountain House) tetrazzini, freeze-dried, prepared	1 cup	200	20.0	8.0
(Turkey by George) hickory barbecue	5 oz	190	8.0	5.0
(Turkey by George) Italian Parmesan	5 oz	170	3.0	5.0
(Turkey by George) lemon pepper	5 oz	160	4.0	4.0
(Turkey by George) mustard tarragon	5 oz	180	3.0	6.0
(Ultra Slim Fast) glazed, w/dressing	10.5 oz	340	49.0	5.0
(Ultra Slim Fast) medallions, in herb sauce	12 oz	280	33.0	6.0
TURKEY ENTRÉE, FROZEN				
À LA KING *(Budget Gourmet)* w/rice	10 oz	390	36.0	18.0
BREAST				
(Healthy Choice) sliced, w/dressing and gravy 'Classics'	10 oz	270	30.0	4.0

Food Name	Serv. Size	Total Cal.	Carbs GMS	Fat GM.
(Lean Cuisine) sliced, w/dressing	7 7/8 oz	200	23.0	5.0
(Lean Cuisine) sliced, w/mushroom sauce and rice	8 oz	230	24.0	7.0
(Stouffer's) roast, w/stuffing and gravy	7 7/8 oz	270	27.0	9.0
(Tyson) 'Gourmet Selections'	11.5 oz	380	51.0	11.0
(Weight Watchers) stuffed	8.5 oz	270	31.0	8.0
CASSEROLE (Pillsbury) 'Microwave Classic'	1 pkg	430	31.0	25.0
CROQUETTES (Freezer Queen) breaded, w/gravy	7 oz	250	19.0	13.0
DIJON (Lean Cuisine)	9.5 oz	210	20.0	6.0
GLAZED (Le Menu) 'LightStyle'	8.25 oz	260	34.0	6.0
HOMESTYLE (Lean Cuisine) w/vegetables and pasta	9 3/8 oz	230	25.0	5.0
MEDALLIONS (Smart Ones) roasted, w/mushroom sauce	8.5 oz	200	35.0	1.0
PIE				
(Banquet)	7 oz	510	39.0	31.0
(Banquet) 'Supreme Microwave'	7 oz	430	30.0	27.0
(Mrs. Paterson's) w/broccoli 'Aussie Pie'	5.5 oz	460	42.0	26.0
(Stouffer's)	10 oz	410	3.0	24.0
(Swanson) 'Hungry Man'	16 oz	650	57.0	36.0
(Swanson) 'Pot Pie'	7 oz	380	36.0	21.0
(Tyson)	9 oz	370	39.0	18.0
ROASTED (Healthy Choice) and mushrooms in gravy	8.5 oz	200	26.0	3.0
SLICED				
(Banquet) w/gravy 'Cookin' Bags'	5 oz	100	5.0	6.0
(Banquet) w/gravy 'Family Entrees'	8 oz	150	8.0	8.0
(Freezer Queen) w/dressing and gravy 'Single Serve'	9 oz	230	32.0	5.0
(Freezer Queen) w/gravy 'Cook-In-Pouch'	5 oz	70	6.0	2.0
(Freezer Queen) w/gravy 'Family Suppers'	7 oz	110	8.0	5.0
(Right Course) in mild curry sauce, w/rice pilaf	8.75 oz	320	40.0	8.0
TETRAZZINI (Stouffer's)	10 oz	400	26.0	23.0
W/DRESSING				
(Freezer Queen) w/dressing and gravy 'Deluxe Family'	7 oz	160	18.0	5.0
(Tyson) 'Looney Tunes Elmer Fudd'	6.55 oz	260	40.0	7.0
W/DRESSING AND POTATOES				
(Swanson) 'Homestyle Recipe'	9 oz	290	30.0	11.0
W/GRAVY (Tyson) 'Gourmet Selections'	9.5 oz	320	34.0	12.0
W/VEGETABLES (Healthy Choice) low fat 'Homestyle'	9.5 oz	230	28.0	3.0
WHITE MEAT (Le Menu) w/stuffing and gravy	8 oz	200	19.0	5.0
TURKEY FAT				
	1 cup	1846	0.0	204.6
	1 oz	255	0.0	28.3
	1 tbsp	115	0.0	12.8
TURKEY GIBLETS				
raw	1 oz	37	0.6	1.2
raw: 1 gizzard, 1 heart, and 1 liver, approx 8.6 oz	1 pkt	315	5.1	10.2

Food Name	Serv. Size	Total Cal.	Carbs GMS	Fat GMS
simmered	4 oz	189	2.4	5.8
simmered, chopped or diced	1 cup	243	3.0	7.4
simmered, w/giblet fat	1 cup	242	3.0	7.4
TURKEY GIZZARD				
raw	1 oz	33	0.2	1.0
raw, approx 4 oz	1 gizzard	132	0.7	4.2
simmered	1 cup	236	0.9	5.6
simmered	4 oz	185	0.7	4.4
TURKEY HAM SALAD				
(Longacre)	1 oz	53	3.0	4.0
(Longacre) 'Saladfest'	1 oz	58	2.0	4.0
TURKEY HEART				
raw	1 oz	41	0.2	2.0
raw, approx 1 oz	1 heart	41	0.2	2.0
simmered	1 cup	257	3.0	8.9
simmered	4 oz	201	2.3	6.9
TURKEY LIVER				
raw	1 oz	39	1.2	1.1
raw, approx 3.6 oz	1 liver	140	4.2	4.1
simmered	1 cup	237	4.8	8.3
simmered	4 oz	192	3.9	6.7
TURKEY NUGGET				
(Louis Rich) 80% fat-free, breaded, cooked	3/4 oz	60	3.0	4.0
TURKEY SALAD				
(Longacre)	1 oz	70	3.0	5.0
(Longacre) 'Saladfest'	1 oz	68	2.0	5.0
TURKEY SEASONING MIX				
(Schilling) roast 'Bag'n Season'	1 pkg	146	20.0	5.0
TURKEY SPREAD				
(Libby's) 'Spreadables'	1.9 oz	100	6.0	6.0
(Underwood) chunky 'Light'	2 1/8 oz	75	2.0	2.0
TURKEY STICK				
(Louis Rich) cooked, breaded, 80% fat-free	.95 oz	80	5.0	5.0
(Louis Rich) cooked, prepared	1 oz	81	4.8	5.0
(The Turkey Store) breast meat, cheese 'Gobble Stix'	1 stick	30	0.5	0.8
(The Turkey Store) breast meat, smoked 'Gobble Stix'	1 stick	25	0.1	0.2
TURMERIC				
ground	1 oz	100	18.4	2.8
ground	1 tbsp	24	4.4	0.7
ground	1 tsp	8	1.4	0.2
ground (Durkee)	1 tsp	9	0.0	tr
ground (Laurel Leaf)	1 tsp	9	0.0	tr
ground (Spice Islands)	1 tsp	7	1.3	0.2

Food Name	Serv. Size	Total Cal.	Carbs GMS	Fat GMS
TURNIP				
boiled, drained	4 oz	20	5.6	0.1
boiled, drained, cubed	1/2 cup	14	3.8	0.1
boiled, drained, mashed	1/2 cup	21	5.6	0.1
raw, cubed	1/2 cup	18	4.1	0.1
raw, trimmed	1 oz	8	1.8	<.1
raw, untrimmed	1 lb	100	22.9	0.4
Canned				
(Allens) diced	1/2 cup	16	2.0	<1.0
(Stokely)	1/2 cup	20	3.0	0.0
Frozen				
boiled, drained	4 oz	26	4.9	0.3
mashed	3 1/3 oz	15	2.8	0.2
(Southern) diced	3.5 oz	17	2.9	0.2
TURNIP GREENS				
boiled, drained	4 oz	23	4.9	0.3
boiled, drained, chopped	1/2 cup	14	3.1	0.2
raw, chopped	1/2 cup	8	1.6	0.1
raw, untrimmed	1 lb	85	18.2	1.0
TURNIP GREENS, CANNED				
Chopped				
(Allens)	1/2 cup	21	3.0	<1.0
(Bush's Best)	1/2 cup	20	3.0	0.0
W/diced turnips				
(Allens) chopped	1/2 cup	19	1.0	<1.0
(Bush's Best)	1/2 cup	25	4.0	0.0
(Stokely)	1/2 cup	20	0.0	0.0
W/liquid	1/2 cup	16	2.8	0.4
TURNIP GREENS, FROZEN				
boiled, drained	10 oz	66	11.0	0.9
boiled, drained	4 oz	34	5.6	0.5
boiled, drained	1/2 cup	25	4.1	0.3
chopped	10 oz	62	10.4	0.9
chopped	1/2 cup	18	3.0	0.3
chopped (Frosty Acres)	3.3 oz	20	4.0	0.0
chopped (Seabrook)	3.3 oz	20	4.0	0.0
chopped (Southern)	3.5 oz	25	3.6	0.3
w/turnips	10 oz	60	9.7	0.5
w/turnips (Seabrook)	3.3 oz	20	3.0	0.0
w/turnips, boiled, drained	4 oz	19	3.3	0.2
TURNIP-ROOTED PARSLEY. See PARSLEY ROOT.				
TURNOVER. See also PASTRY.				
apple, frozen (Pepperidge Farm)	1 turnover	300	34.0	17.0

Food Name	Serv. Size	Total Cal.	Carbs GMS	Fat GMS
apple, refrigerated *(Pillsbury)*	1 turnover	170	23.0	8.0
blueberry, frozen *(Pepperidge Farm)*	1 turnover	310	32.0	19.0
cherry, frozen *(Pepperidge Farm)*	1 turnover	310	32.0	19.0
cherry, refrigerated *(Pillsbury)*	1 turnover	170	23.0	8.0
peach, frozen *(Pepperidge Farm)*	1 turnover	310	34.0	18.0
raspberry, frozen *(Pepperidge Farm)*	1 turnover	310	36.0	17.0

TURTLE, GREEN

Food Name	Serv. Size	Total Cal.	Carbs GMS	Fat GMS
canned	100 gm	106	0.0	0.7
raw	100 gm	89	0.0	0.5

TUSK. See CUSK.

U

Food Name	Serv. Size	Total Cal.	Carbs GMS	Fat GMS

UDON NOODLE. See NOODLE, JAPANESE.
ULTRA SLIM FAST. See DIET DRINK.
UMEBOSHI PLUM. See PLUM, JAPANESE.

V

Food Name	Serv. Size	Total Cal.	Carbs GMS	Fat GMS
VANILLA BAKING CHIPS *(Hershey's)*	1/4 cup	240	25.0	14.0
VANILLA EXTRACT, pure *(Virginia Dare)*	1 tsp	10	0.3	0.0
VANILLA FLAVOR DRINK, CANNED				
(Ensure) liquid nutrition	8 oz	250	34.3	8.8
(Ensure) liquid nutrition 'Plus'	8 oz	355	47.3	12.6
(Ensure) liquid nutrition, w/fiber	8 oz	260	38.3	8.8
(Sego) 'Lite'	10 oz	150	17.0	4.0
(Sego) 'Lite French Vanilla'	10 oz	150	17.0	4.0
(Sego) 'Very Vanilla'	10 oz	225	34.0	5.0
(Sustacal) liquid food, nutritionally complete	8 oz	240	33.0	5.5

VEAL
(NOTE: TRIMMED = Lean; separable fat removed. UNTRIMMED = Separable fat not removed.)
BRAINS

Food Name	Serv. Size	Total Cal.	Carbs GMS	Fat GMS
braised	3 oz	116	0.0	8.2
pan-fried	3 oz	181	0.0	14.2
raw	1 oz	33	0.0	2.3

GROUND

Food Name	Serv. Size	Total Cal.	Carbs GMS	Fat GMS
broiled	1 cup	200	0.0	8.8
broiled	3 oz	146	0.0	6.4
raw	1 cup	325	0.0	15.3

Food Name	Serv. Size	Total Cal.	Carbs GMS	Fat GMS
raw	1 oz	40	0.0	1.9
HEART				
braised	3 oz	158	0.1	5.7
raw	1 oz	31	0.0	1.1
simmered	4 oz	368	0.3	13.4
KIDNEYS				
braised	3 oz	139	0.0	4.8
raw	1 oz	28	0.2	0.9
LEG				
Trimmed				
braised	3 oz	173	0.0	4.3
pan-fried	3 oz	156	0.0	3.9
raw	1 oz	30	0.0	0.5
roasted	3 oz	127	0.0	2.9
Untrimmed				
braised	3 oz	179	0.0	5.4
pan-fried	3 oz	179	0.0	7.1
raw	1 oz	33	0.0	0.9
roasted	3 oz	136	0.0	4.0
LEG AND SHOULDER				
raw, trimmed	1 oz	31	0.0	0.7
trimmed, braised	3 oz	160	0.0	3.7
LIVER				
braised	3 oz	140	2.3	5.9
pan-fried	3 oz	208	3.3	9.7
raw	4 oz	152	5.2	5.0
raw	1 oz	38	1.3	1.2
LOIN				
Trimmed				
braised	3 oz	192	0.0	7.8
raw	1 oz	32	0.0	0.9
roasted	3 oz	149	0.0	5.9
stewed	4 oz	256	0.0	10.4
Untrimmed				
braised	3 oz	241	0.0	14.6
raw	1 oz	46	0.0	2.6
roasted	3 oz	184	0.0	10.5
stewed	4 oz	322	0.0	19.5
LUNGS				
braised	3 oz	88	0.0	2.2
raw	1 oz	25	0.0	0.6
PANCREAS				
braised	3 oz	218	0.0	12.4

od Name	Serv. Size	Total Cal.	Carbs GMS	Fat GMS
raw	1 oz	51	0.0	3.7
B				
Trimmed				
braised	3 oz	185	0.0	6.6
raw	1 lb	544	0.0	17.6
raw	1 oz	34	0.0	1.1
roasted	3 oz	150	0.0	6.3
stewed	4 oz	247	0.0	8.9
Untrimmed				
braised	3 oz	213	0.0	10.6
raw	1 lb	735	0.0	40.9
raw	1 oz	45	0.0	2.5
roasted	3 oz	194	0.0	11.9
stewed	4 oz	285	0.0	14.2
HOULDER, ARM				
Trimmed				
braised	3 oz	171	0.0	4.5
braised, approx 5.6 oz	1 steak	321	0.0	8.5
raw	1 oz	29	0.0	0.6
roasted	3 oz	139	0.0	4.9
roasted, approx 9.6 oz	1 steak	447	0.0	15.8
Untrimmed				
braised	3 oz	201	0.0	8.7
braised, approx 6.1 oz	1 steak	409	0.0	17.7
raw	1 oz	37	0.0	1.5
roasted	3 oz	156	0.0	7.0
HOULDER, BLADE				
Trimmed				
braised	3 oz	168	0.0	5.5
diced, braised	1 cup	277	0.0	9.1
diced, roasted	1 cup	239	0.0	9.6
diced, stewed	1 cup	277	0.0	9.1
raw	1 lb	513	0.0	14.8
raw	1 oz	32	0.0	0.9
roasted	3 oz	145	0.0	5.8
stewed	4 oz	224	0.0	7.3
Untrimmed				
braised	3 oz	191	0.0	8.6
diced, braised	1 cup	315	0.0	14.1
diced, roasted	1 cup	260	0.0	12.1
diced, stewed	1 cup	315	0.0	14.1
raw	1 lb	585	0.0	23.6
raw	1 oz	36	0.0	1.5

Food Name	Serv. Size	Total Cal.	Carbs GMS	F
roasted	3 oz	158	0.0	7
stewed	4 oz	255	0.0	11
SHOULDER, WHOLE				
Trimmed				
braised	3 oz	169	0.0	5
diced, braised	1 cup	279	0.0	8
diced, roasted	1 cup	238	0.0	9
diced, stewed	1 cup	279	0.0	8
raw	1 lb	508	0.0	13
raw	1 oz	31	0.0	0
roasted	3 oz	144	0.0	5
stewed	4 oz	226	0.0	6
Untrimmed				
braised	3 oz	194	0.0	8
diced, braised	1 cup	319	0.0	14
diced, roasted	1 cup	258	0.0	11
diced, stewed	1 cup	319	0.0	14
raw	1 lb	590	0.0	24
raw	1 oz	36	0.0	1
roasted	3 oz	156	0.0	7
stewed	4 oz	259	0.0	11
SIRLOIN				
Trimmed				
braised	3 oz	173	0.0	5
diced, braised	1 cup	286	0.0	9
diced, roasted	1 cup	235	0.0	8
diced, stewed	1 cup	286	0.0	9.
raw	1 lb	499	0.0	11
raw	1 oz	31	0.0	0.
roasted	3 oz	143	0.0	5.
stewed	4 oz	231	0.0	7.
Untrimmed				
braised	3 oz	214	0.0	11.
diced, braised	1 cup	353	0.0	18
diced, roasted	1 cup	283	0.0	14
diced, stewed	1 cup	353	0.0	18.
raw	1 lb	689	0.0	35.
raw	1 oz	43	0.0	2.
roasted	3 oz	172	0.0	8.
stewed	4 oz	286	0.0	14.
SPLEEN				
braised	3 oz	110	0.0	2.
raw	1 oz	27	0.0	0.

od Name	Serv. Size	Total Cal.	Carbs GMS	Fat GMS
HYMUS				
braised	3 oz	148	0.0	3.7
raw	1 oz	28	0.0	0.7
ONGUE				
braised	3 oz	172	0.0	8.6
raw	1 oz	37	0.5	1.5
OP ROUND				
Trimmed				
braised	4 oz	230	0.0	5.8
diced, braised	1 cup	284	0.0	7.1
diced, roasted	1 cup	210	0.0	4.7
diced, stewed	1 cup	284	0.0	7.1
pan-fried in vegetable oil	4 oz	208	0.0	5.2
roasted	4 oz	170	0.0	3.8
stewed	4 oz	230	0.0	5.8
Untrimmed				
diced, roasted	1 cup	224	0.0	6.5
diced, stewed	1 cup	295	0.0	8.9
pan-fried in vegetable oil	4 oz	239	0.0	9.5
roasted	4 oz	181	0.0	5.3
stewed	4 oz	239	0.0	7.2
EAL ENTRÉE, FROZEN				
MARSALA *(Le Menu)* 'LightStyle'	10 oz	230	28.0	3.0
ARMIGIANA				
(Armour) 'Classics'	11.25 oz	400	34.0	22.0
(Le Menu)	11.5 oz	390	36.0	17.0
(Morton)	10 oz	260	35.0	8.0
(Swanson)	12.25 oz	430	42.0	20.0
(Swanson) 'Homestyle Recipe'	10 oz	330	33.0	13.0
(Swanson) 'Hungry Man'	18.25 oz	590	57.0	26.0
(Ultimate 200)	8.2 oz	150	5.0	4.0
Breaded				
(Banquet) 'Cookin' Bags'	4 oz	230	20.0	11.0
(Banquet) 'Family Entrées'	8 oz	370	33.0	18.0
(Freezer Queen)	5 oz	220	17.0	12.0
(Freezer Queen) 'Cook-In-Pouch'	5 oz	220	17.0	12.0
(Freezer Queen) 'Deluxe Family Suppers'	7 oz	300	22.0	15.0
Platter *(Freezer Queen)*	10 oz	400	32.0	20.0
W/pasta Alfredo *(Stouffer's)* homestyle	9.25 oz	350	26.0	15.0
TEAK				
(Hormel)	4 oz	130	2.0	4.0
(Hormel) breaded	4 oz	240	13.0	13.0

VEGETABLE. See individual listings.

Food Name	Serv. Size	Total Cal.	Carbs GMS	
VEGETABLE DISH, CANNED. See also individual listings.				
Corn, beans, and carrots, w/pasta, in tomato sauce				
(Green Giant)	1/2 cup	80	17.0	2
Green beans, potatoes, and mushrooms, in sauce				
(Green Giant)	1/2 cup	50	9.0	2
Snap beans, potatoes, and mushrooms, in sauce				
(Green Giant)	1/2 cup	50	9.0	2
String beans, potatoes, and mushrooms, in sauce				
(Green Giant)	1/2 cup	50	9.0	2
VEGETABLE DISH, FROZEN. See also individual listings.				
Broccoli, cauliflower, carrots				
(Birds Eye) 'Butter Sauce'	3.3 oz	45	6.0	2
(Birds Eye) 'Cheese Sauce'	4.5 oz	110	11.0	5
(Birds Eye) 'Farm Fresh'	4 oz	35	7.0	0
(Green Giant) 'Butter Sauce'	1/2 cup	30	4.0	1
(Green Giant) in cheese sauce	1/2 cup	60	9.0	2
(Green Giant) 'One Serving'	1 pkg	30	7.0	0
(Stokely) 'Singles' w/baby carrots	3 oz	25	5.0	1
(Stokely) w/baby carrots, in cheese sauce	4 oz	70	8.0	3
Broccoli, cauliflower, peppers, w/red peppers 'Farm Fresh'				
(Birds Eye)	4 oz	30	5.0	0
Broccoli, corn, peppers, w/red peppers 'Farm Fresh' (Birds Eye)	4 oz	60	14.0	1
Broccoli, green beans, onions, peppers, w/pearl onions				
and red peppers (Birds Eye)	4 oz	35	7.0	0
Broccoli, peppers, bamboo shoots, mushrooms, w/red				
peppers (Birds Eye)	4 oz	30	5.0	0
Broccoli and carrots, w/rotini, in cheese sauce (Green Giant)	1 pkg	100	17.0	2
Brussels sprouts, cauliflower, carrots (Birds Eye)	4 oz	40	8.0	0
Cauliflower, broccoli, carrots, in cheese sauce				
(Freezer Queen)	5 oz	60	10.0	1
Cauliflower, carrots, snow peas, w/baby carrots and snow				
pea pods (Birds Eye)	4 oz	40	8.0	0
Cauliflower, zucchini, carrots, peppers, w/red peppers				
(Birds Eye)	4 oz	30	6.0	0
Peas, carrots, water chestnuts, w/sugar snap peas and				
baby carrots (Birds Eye)	3.2 oz	50	11.0	0
Zucchini, carrots, onions, mushrooms, w/pearl onions				
(Birds Eye)	4 oz	30	7.0	0
VEGETABLE ENTRÉE				
Chinese style, w/chicken, frozen (Budget Gourmet)	10 oz	280	47.0	7
Country style, w/beef tips (Ultra Slim Fast)	12 oz	230	26.0	5
Italian style, w/chicken, frozen (Budget Gourmet)	10.25 oz	310	50.0	8

Food Name	Serv. Size	Total Cal.	Carbs GMS	Fat GMS
Pot pie, frozen				
(Amy's Kitchen) organic	8 oz	347	45.0	16.0
(Morton) w/beef	7 oz	430	27.0	31.0
(Morton) w/chicken	7 oz	420	27.0	28.0
(Morton) w/turkey	7 oz	420	27.0	28.0
Stir-fry, frozen (Shanghai)	5.1 oz	75	11.0	1.0
VEGETABLE FLAKES (French's) dehydrated	1 tbsp	12	3.0	0.0
VEGETABLE JUICE				
cocktail, canned	6 oz	35	8.3	0.2
cocktail, canned	1/2 cup	23	5.5	0.1
(Biotta) 'Breuss Juice'	6 oz	67	13.2	0.1
(Biotta) 'Cocktail'	6 oz	50	10.1	0.1
(Knudsen & Sons) 'Very Veggie'	8 oz	40	8.0	0.0
(Knudsen & Sons) 'Very Veggie' low sodium	8 oz	40	8.0	0.0
(Knudsen & Sons) 'Very Veggie' organic	8 oz	40	8.0	0.0
(Knudsen & Sons) 'Very Veggie' spicy	8 oz	40	8.0	0.0
(Smucker's) hearty	8 oz	58	13.0	<.1
(Smucker's) hot and spicy	8 oz	58	13.0	<.1
(V•8)	6 oz	35	8.0	0.0
(V•8) 'Light'n Tangy'	6 oz	40	8.0	0.0
(V•8) 'No Salt Added'	6 oz	35	8.0	0.0
(V•8) 'Picante' mild	6 oz	35	8.0	0.0
(V•8) spicy hot	6 oz	35	8.0	0.0
(Veryfine) '100%'	6 oz	32	6.0	0.0
VEGETABLE MARROW SQUASH. See SQUASH, MARROW.				
VEGETABLE OIL. See also individual listings.				
(Crisco)	1 tbsp	120	0.0	14.0
(Finast)	1 tbsp	120	0.0	14.0
(Hain) 'All Blend'	1 tbsp	120	0.0	14.0
(Hain) w/garlic 'Garlic & Oil'	1 tbsp	120	0.0	14.0
(Kroger)	1 tbsp	122	0.0	13.6
(Pathmark)	1 tbsp	120	0.0	14.0
(Pathmark) 'No Frills'	1 tbsp	130	0.0	14.0
(Puritan)	1 tbsp	120	0.0	14.0
(Wesson)	1 tbsp	120	0.0	14.0
VEGETABLE OIL SPRAY. See COOKING SPRAY.				
VEGETABLE OIL SPREAD. See MARGARINE SPREAD.				
VEGETABLE OYSTER. See SALSIFY.				
VEGETABLE SPONGE. See GOURD, DISHCLOTH.				
VEGETABLE STICKS, breaded, frozen (Farm Rich)	4 oz	240	34.0	10.0
VEGETABLES, MIXED, CANNED				
drained	4 oz	53	10.5	0.3
drained	1/2 cup	39	7.6	0.2

Food Name	Serv. Size	Total Cal.	Carbs GMS	F G
w/liquid	4 oz	41	8.1	0
w/liquid	1/2 cup	40	7.0	0
(A&P) 'Eastern'	1/2 cup	45	8.0	<1
(A&P) 'No Salt Added'	1/2 cup	40	9.0	<1
(A&P) 'Western'	1/2 cup	40	9.0	<1
(Bush's Best) 'Mixed Greens'	1/2 cup	20	3.0	0
(Featherweight)	1/2 cup	40	8.0	0
(Finast)	1/2 cup	40	8.0	0
(Finast) 'No Salt Added'	1/2 cup	40	8.0	0
(Freshlike) water packed, w/o salt	1/2 cup	35	8.0	0
(Freshlike) water packed, w/o sugar or salt	1/2 cup	35	8.0	0
(Green Giant) 'Garden Medley'	1/2 cup	35	9.0	0
(Green Giant) 'Pantry Express'	1/2 cup	35	8.0	<1
(LaChoy) 'Chinese'	1/2 cup	12	2.0	0
(LaChoy) 'Chop Suey'	1/2 cup	9	2.0	0
(LaChoy) 'Fancy Mix'	1/2 cup	12	2.0	<1
(P&Q) 'Chunky Eastern'	1/2 cup	40	8.0	<1
(P&Q) 'Chunky Western'	1/2 cup	40	9.0	<1
(Pathmark)	1/2 cup	35	8.0	0
(Pathmark) 'No Salt Added'	1/2 cup	35	7.0	0
(S&W) 'Old Fashioned Harvest'	1/2 cup	35	6.0	0
(Stokely)	1/2 cup	40	8.0	0
(Stokely) 'No Salt or Sugar Added'	1/2 cup	40	8.0	0
(Veg•All) 'Homestyle Large Cut'	1/2 cup	35	9.0	0
(Veg•All) 'Lite'	1/2 cup	35	8.0	0
(Veg•All) 'Original'	1/2 cup	35	8.0	0
VEGETABLES, MIXED, FROZEN				
boiled, drained	10-oz pkg	162	36.0	0.
boiled, drained	4 oz	67	14.8	0
boiled, drained	1/2 cup	54	11.9	0
(A&P)	3.3 oz	65	13.0	<1
(Birds Eye)	3.3 oz	60	13.0	0
(Birds Eye) 'Portion Pack'	3 oz	50	12.0	0
(Freshlike)	3.3 oz	70	13.0	0
(Frosty Acres)	3.3 oz	65	13.0	0
(Green Giant)	1/2 cup	40	9.0	0
(Green Giant) 'Harvest Fresh'	1/2 cup	40	9.0	0
(Green Giant) 'Plain Polybag'	1/2 cup	40	9.0	0
(Health Valley)	1/2 cup	68	14.0	0
(Seabrook)	3.3 oz	65	13.0	0
(Southern)	3.5 oz	69	13.9	0.
(Stokely) 'Singles'	3 oz	60	12.0	1
(Veg•All)	3.3 oz	70	13.0	0.

d Name	Serv. Size	Total Cal.	Carbs GMS	Fat GMS
LIFORNIA STYLE				
(A&P) 'California Blend'	3.3 oz	25	5.0	<1.0
(Freshlike) 'California Blend'	3.3 oz	30	6.0	0.0
(Green Giant) 'American Mixtures'	1/2 cup	25	6.0	0.0
(Veg•All) 'California Blend'	3.3 oz	30	6.0	0.0
NESE STYLE				
(Birds Eye) chow mein, w/Oriental sauce 'Custom Cuisine'	4.6 oz	80	14.0	2.0
(Birds Eye) chow mein, w/seasoned sauce	3.3 oz	90	12.0	4.0
(Birds Eye) 'Stir-Fry'	3.3 oz	35	8.0	0.0
UCKWAGON STYLE				
(Freshlike) 'Chuckwagon Blend'	3.3 oz	70	16.0	1.0
(Veg•All) 'Chuckwagon Blend'	3.3 oz	70	16.0	1.0
UNTRY STYLE				
(Birds Eye) 'International Rice Recipes'	3.3 oz	90	19.0	0.0
(Freshlike) 'Country Blend'	3.3 oz	50	12.0	0.0
(Green Giant) 'American Mixtures Heartland'	1/2 cup	25	6.0	0.0
(Veg•All) 'Country Blend'	3.3 oz	50	12.0	0.0
TCH STYLE (Frosty Acres)	3.2 oz	30	5.0	0.0
R BEEF				
(Birds Eye) Oriental style, w/sauce	4.6 oz	90	11.0	4.0
(Birds Eye) w/cream mushroom 'Custom Cuisine'	4.6 oz	60	9.0	2.0
R CHICKEN				
(Birds Eye) w/tomato basil sauce	4.6 oz	110	17.0	3.0
(Birds Eye) w/wild rice, in white wine sauce	4.6 oz	100	19.0	0.0
R CHICKEN OR FISH (Birds Eye) w/Dijon mustard sauce	4.6 oz	70	9.0	3.0
R CHICKEN OR SHRIMP (Birds Eye) w/delicate herb sauce	4.6 oz	90	8.0	5.0
R SOUP				
(Freshlike)	3.3 oz	50	11.0	0.0
(Veg•All)	3.3 oz	50	11.0	0.0
R STEW				
(A&P)	4 oz	60	13.0	<1.0
(Freshlike) 5-ways	3.3 oz	50	12.0	0.0
(Freshlike) 4-ways	3.3 oz	50	11.0	0.0
(Frosty Acres)	3 oz	42	10.0	0.0
(Kohl's)	3.3 oz	50	10.0	<1.0
(Ore-Ida)	3 oz	60	12.0	<1.0
(Veg•All) 5-ways	3.3 oz	50	12.0	0.0
(Veg•All) 4-ways	3.3 oz	50	11.0	0.0
ENCH STYLE (Birds Eye) 'International Recipes'	3.3 oz	110	23.0	0.0
BUTTER SAUCE				
(Finast)	3.3 oz	70	15.0	4.0
(Green Giant)	1/2 cup	60	11.0	2.0

Food Name	Serv. Size	Total Cal.	Carbs GMS
ITALIAN STYLE			
(A&P) blend	3.3 oz	40	8.0
(Birds Eye) 'International Recipes'	3.3 oz	100	11.0
(Freshlike) 'Italian Blend'	3.3 oz	30	7.0
(Freshlike) 'Italian Blend' food service	3.3 oz	25	5.0
(Veg•All) 'Italian Blend'	3.3 oz	30	7.0
(Veg•All) 'Italian Blend' food service	3.3 oz	25	5.0
JAPANESE STYLE			
(Birds Eye) 'International Recipes'	3.3 oz	90	10.0
(Birds Eye) 'Stir-Fry'	3.3 oz	30	7.0
LE SUEUR STYLE *(Green Giant)* 'Valley Combinations'	1/2 cup	70	12.0
MANHATTAN STYLE *(Green Giant)* 'American Mixtures'	1/2 cup	25	5.0
MIDWESTERN STYLE			
(Freshlike) 'Midwestern Blend'	3.3 oz	40	8.0
(Veg•All) 'Midwestern Blend'	3.3 oz	40	8.0
NEW ENGLAND STYLE			
(Birds Eye) 'International Recipes'	3.3 oz	130	14.0
(Green Giant) 'American Mixtures'	1/2 cup	70	14.0
ORIENTAL STYLE			
(A&P) blend	3.3 oz	25	5.0
(Birds Eye) 'International Recipes'	3.3 oz	70	8.0
(Freshlike) 'Oriental Blend'	3.3 oz	25	5.0
(Frosty Acres)	3.2 oz	25	5.0
(Veg•All) 'Oriental Blend'	3.3 oz	25	5.0
SAN FRANCISCO STYLE			
(Birds Eye) 'International Recipes'	3.3 oz	100	11.0
(Green Giant) 'American Mixtures'	1/2 cup	25	7.0
SANTA FE STYLE *(Green Giant)* 'American Mixtures'	1/2 cup	70	16.0
SCANDINAVIAN STYLE			
(Freshlike) 'Scandinavian Blend'	3.3 oz	45	9.0
(Veg•All) 'Scandinavian Blend'	3.3 oz	45	9.0
SEATTLE STYLE *(Green Giant)* 'American Mixtures'	1/2 cup	25	7.0
SPANISH STYLE *(Birds Eye)* 'International Recipes'	3.3 oz	110	24.0
WESTERN STYLE *(Green Giant)* 'American Mixtures'	1/2 cup	60	12.0
WINTER VEGETABLES			
(A&P) blend	3.3 oz	24	6.0
(Freshlike) 'Winter Blend'	3.3 oz	25	5.0
(Veg•All) 'Winter Blend'	3.3 oz	25	5.0
W/PASTA			
(Birds Eye) cheese tortellini, in tomato sauce 'For One'	5.5 oz	210	31.0
(Birds Eye) in Stroganoff sauce 'Custom Cuisine'	4.6 oz	120	15.0
(Birds Eye) in white cheese sauce 'Custom Cuisine'	4.6 oz	150	19.0
(Birds Eye) primavera style, w/seasoned sauce	3.3 oz	120	14.0

Food Name	Serv. Size	Total Cal.	Carbs GMS	Fat GMS
(Stokely) rotini, in cheddar cheese sauce 'Singles'	4 oz	100	15.0	3.0
(Stokely) shells, in Italian style sauce 'Singles'	4 oz	170	5.0	15.0
w/TERIYAKI SAUCE (Stokely) 'Singles'	4 oz	100	24.0	0.0
w/WHITE AND WILD RICE, pilaf (Stokely) 'Singles'	4 oz	80	17.0	0.0
VEGETABLES, MIXED, MICROWAVE				
(Green Giant) 'Microwave Shelf-Pack'	1/2 cup	35	8.0	<1.0
(Pantry Express) 'Microwave Shelf-Pack'	1/2 cup	35	8.0	<1.0
VEGETARIAN ENTRÉE. See also individual listings.				
(Amy's Kitchen) Salisbury steak, organic, frozen 'Country Dinner'	11 oz	482	48.0	19.0
(Ken & Robert's) patty, frozen 'Truly Amazing'	2.5-oz patty	110	19.0	2.0
(LaChoy) chow mein, w/o meat, canned	3/4 cup	35	6.0	0.4
(Natural Touch) patty, frozen 'Dinner Entree'	3 oz	230	6.0	14.0
(Tofutti) tortellini, meatless, frozen	2 oz	220	38.0	2.0
(Worthington) roast, frozen 'Dinner Roast'	2 oz	120	5.0	8.0
VEGETARIAN ENTRÉE MIX. See also individual listings.				
(Tofu Classics) stroganoff, creamy, prepared w/tofu	1/2 cup	94	11.0	3.0
(Tofu Classics) stroganoff, creamy, prepared w/tofu and salted butter	1/2 cup	127	11.0	7.0

VEGETARIAN FOODS. See BACON, ALTERNATIVE; BEEF, ALTERNATIVE; BEEF JERKY, ALTERNATIVE; BURGER, VEGETARIAN; BURGER MIX, VEGETARIAN; CHICKEN, ALTERNATIVE; CRAB, ALTERNATIVE; FISH FILLET, ALTERNATIVE; HAM, ALTERNATIVE; LUNCHEON MEAT, ALTERNATIVE; MEAT, ALTERNATIVE; MEAT LOAF MIX, ALTERNATIVE; SAUSAGE, ALTERNATIVE; SCALLOP, ALTERNATIVE; SPREAD, VEGETARIAN; TUNA, ALTERNATIVE; TURKEY, ALTERNATIVE; VEGETARIAN ENTRÉE; and individual listings.

VENISON. See ANTELOPE; CARIBOU; DEER; ELK; MOOSE.

	Serv. Size	Total Cal.	Carbs GMS	Fat GMS
VIENNA SAUSAGE, CANNED				
beef and pork	1 oz	79	0.6	7.1
2 inches long, 7/8 inch diam	1 sausage	45	0.3	4.0
(Armour) chicken, in beef stock 'Premium' lite	2 oz	150	1.0	13.0
(Armour) hot and spicy	2.5 oz	190	3.0	17.0
(Armour) in barbecue sauce	2.5 oz	190	4.0	17.0
(Armour) in beef stock	2 oz	180	1.0	17.0
(Armour) in beef stock, lite	2 oz	150	1.0	13.0
(Armour) smoked	2 oz	180	1.0	17.0
(Hormel)	1 oz	69	2.0	7.0
(Hormel) chicken	1 oz	56	1.0	5.0
(Hormel) w/o broth	4 links	200	1.0	18.0
(Libby's) chicken, in beef broth	2 oz	130	3.0	10.0
(Libby's) in barbecue sauce	2.5 oz	180	2.0	15.0
(Libby's) in beef broth	2 oz	160	1.0	15.0
VINE SPINACH/basella				
raw	1 lb	86	15.4	1.4

Food Name	Serv. Size	Total Cal.	Carbs GMS
raw	3.5 oz	19	3.4
VINEGAR			
APPLE CIDER			
	1 cup	34	14.2
	1 tbsp	2	0.9
(Great Impressions)	1 tbsp	7	0.9
(Hain)	1 tbsp	2	4.0
(Heinz)	.51 oz	2	0.0
(Heinz) gourmet 'Decanter'	.51 oz	4	0.0
(Indian Summer)	1 cup	40	14.0 <
(Lucky Leaf)	1 oz	4	2.0
(Musselman's)	1 oz	4	2.0
(Spectrum Naturals) filtered	1 tbsp	7	2.0
(Spectrum Naturals) unfiltered	1 tbsp	7	2.0
(White House)	1 oz	4	2.0
BROWN RICE			
(Spectrum Naturals) organic	1 tbsp	0	0.0
(Spectrum Naturals) organic, seasoned	1 tbsp	10	2.0
WHITE			
	1 cup	29	12.0
	1 tbsp	2	0.8
(Heinz)	1 tbsp	2	0.0
(Indian Summer)	1 cup	30	12.0 <1
(Lucky Leaf)	1 oz	4	2.0
(Musselman's)	1 oz	4	2.0
(Spectrum Naturals) organic	1 tbsp	0	0.0
WINE			
(Great Impressions) basil	1 tbsp	7	0.6
(Great Impressions) paprika, hot	1 tbsp	6	0.6
(Great Impressions) raspberry	1 tbsp	7	1.0
(Heinz) gourmet 'Decanter'	.51 oz	4	0.0
(Heinz) tarragon, gourmet 'Decanter'	.51 oz	2	0.0
(Lucky Leaf) red	1 oz	0	0.0
(Musselman's) red	1 oz	0	0.0
(Regina) all varieties	1 oz	4	0.0
(Spectrum Naturals) garlic, organic	1 tbsp	0	0.0
(Spectrum Naturals) Italian herb, organic	1 tbsp	0	0.0
(Spectrum Naturals) raspberry, organic	1 tbsp	10	0.0
(Spectrum Naturals) red, organic	1 tbsp	0	0.0
(Spectrum Naturals) white, organic	1 tbsp	0	0.0
VITA JUICE (Knudsen & Sons)	8 oz	90	21.0
VODKA. See ALCOHOLIC BEVERAGES.			

W

Food Name	Serv. Size	Total Cal.	Carbs GMS	Fat GMS
WAFFLE, FROZEN				
(Aunt Jemima) 'Original' 2.5 oz	1 waffle	173	27.8	5.6
(Downyflake)	2 waffles	120	20.0	3.0
(Downyflake) 'Crisp & Healthy'	1 waffle	80	16.0	1.0
(Downyflake) 'Hot-N-Buttery'	2 waffles	180	27.0	6.0
(Downyflake) 'Jumbo'	2 waffles	170	30.0	4.0
(Eggo) 'Homestyle'	1 waffle	120	16.0	5.0
(Eggo) 'Nutri-Grain'	1 waffle	130	18.0	5.0
(Roman Meal)	2 waffles	280	33.0	14.0
APPLE (Eggo) 'Fruit Top'	3.1 oz	190	32.0	6.0
APPLE CINNAMON				
(Aunt Jemima) 2.5 oz	1 waffle	176	28.8	5.6
(Downyflake) 'Crisp & Healthy'	1 waffle	80	16.0	1.0
(Eggo)	1 waffle	130	18.0	5.0
(Van's)	1 waffle	75	8.4	2.0
BLUEBERRY				
(Aunt Jemima) 2.5 oz	1 waffle	175	29.2	5.2
(Downyflake)	2 waffles	180	32.0	4.0
(Eggo)	1 waffle	130	18.0	5.0
(Eggo) 'Fruit Top'	3.1 oz	190	32.0	6.0
(Krusteaz) 1.2 oz	1 waffle	110	19.0	3.0
BUTTERMILK				
(Aunt Jemima) 2.5 oz	1 waffle	179	28.7	5.8
(Downyflake)	2 waffles	190	32.0	5.0
(Downyflake) 'Jumbo'	2 waffles	170	30.0	4.0
(Eggo)	1 waffle	120	16.0	5.0
(Krusteaz) 1.2 oz	1 waffle	100	16.0	2.0
GOLDEN (Krusteaz) 1.2 oz	1 waffle	100	16.0	2.0
HONEY ALMOND (Van's)	1 waffle	75	8.4	2.0
MULTIGRAIN				
(Downyflake)	2 waffles	250	28.0	4.0
(Van's)	1 waffle	75	8.4	2.0
OAT BRAN				
(Aunt Jemima)	2.5 oz	154	29.4	2.8
(Downyflake)	2 waffles	260	30.0	13.0
(Eggo) 'Common Sense'	1 waffle	110	16.0	4.0
(Eggo) w/fruit and nut 'Common Sense'	1 waffle	120	17.0	5.0
(Van's) 'Belgian'	1 waffle	89	11.0	2.0
ORIGINAL (Van's) 'Belgian'	1 waffle	86	14.0	2.0
PEACH (Eggo) 'Fruit Top'	3.1 oz	190	30.0	6.0
RAISIN BRAN (Eggo) 'Nutri-Grain'	1 waffle	130	18.0	5.0

Food Name	Serv. Size	Total Cal.	Carbs GMS	
RICE BRAN *(Downyflake)*	2 waffles	210	25.0	1
SEVEN GRAIN *(Van's)* 'Belgian'	1 waffle	88	9.9	
STRAWBERRY				
(Eggo)	1 waffle	130	18.0	
(Eggo) 'Fruit Top'	1 waffle	190	31.0	
WHOLE-GRAIN WHEAT *(Aunt Jemima)*	1 waffle	154	29.4	
WAFFLE BREAKFAST, FROZEN				
(Swanson) Belgian, w/sausage 'Great Starts'	2.85 oz	280	21.0	1
(Swanson) Belgian, w/strawberries and sausage	3.5 oz	210	31.0	
(Swanson) w/bacon 'Great Starts'	2.2 oz	230	19.0	1
WAFFLE MIX. See PANCAKE/WAFFLE MIX.				
WAKAME. See SEAWEED.				
WALNUT, BLACK				
Dried				
	1 oz	172	3.4	16
chopped	1 cup	759	15.1	7
finely ground	1 cup	486	9.7	4
in shell	1 lb	661	13.2	6
Raw *(Planters)*	1 oz	180	3.0	17
Shelled *(Fisher)*	1 oz	170	3.0	16
WALNUT, ENGLISH				
Dried				
	1 lb	1310	37.4	126
halves	1 cup	642	18.3	61
halves, approx 14	1 oz	182	5.2	17
in shell	1 lb	1310	37.4	126
pieces or chips	1 cup	770	22.0	74
(Diamond)	1 oz	192	4.0	19
(Fisher) chopped	1 oz	180	5.0	18
(Fisher) ground	1 oz	180	5.0	18
(Planters) halves	1 oz	190	3.0	20
(Planters) pieces	1 oz	190	3.0	20
(Planters) whole	1 oz	190	3.0	20
Raw *(Fisher)*	1 oz	180	5.0	18
WALNUT, PERSIAN				
Dried, in shell	1 lb	1310	37.4	126
Dried, shelled				
halves	1 cup	642	18.3	61
halves, approx 14	1 oz	182	5.2	17
pieces or chips	1 cup	770	22.0	74
(Diamond)	1 oz	192	4.0	19
(Planters) halves	1 oz	190	3.0	20
(Planters) pieces	1 oz	190	3.0	20

Food Name	Serv. Size	Total Cal.	Carbs GMS	Fat GMS
(Planters) whole	1 oz	190	3.0	20.0
WALNUT OIL				
	1 cup	1927	0.0	218.0
	1 tbsp	120	0.0	13.6
(Hain)	1 tbsp	120	0.0	14.0
(Spectrum Naturals)	1 tbsp	120	0.0	14.0
WASABI	1/4 oz	24	4.9	<.1
WATER, BOTTLED				
(Perrier)	1 cup	0	0.0	0.0
(Perrier)	6.5-oz bottle	0	0.0	0.0
(Poland Spring)	1 cup	0	0.0	0.0
distilled *(Arrowhead)*	1 liter	0	0.0	0.0
drinking *(Arrowhead)*	1 liter	0	0.0	0.0
fluoridated *(Arrowhead)*	1 liter	0	0.0	0.0
mineral *(Perrier)*	1 liter	0	0.0	0.0
sparkling, natural, unflavored *(Clearly Canadian)*	6 oz	0	0.0	0.0
spring *(Arrowhead)*	1 liter	0	0.0	0.0
spring, Arizona Tule *(Arrowhead)*	1 liter	0	0.0	0.0
Vichy *(Schweppes)*	6 oz	0	0.0	0.0
WATER, SPARKLING, FLAVORED. See also SOFT DRINKS AND MIXERS.				
BLACK CHERRY				
'Refresher' *(Quest)*	10 oz	2	0.0	0.0
'Refresher' *(Quest)*	8 oz	2	0.0	0.0
BLACKBERRY, 'Mountain Blackberry' *(Clearly Canadian)*	6 oz	70	16.0	0.0
CHERRY, 'Wild Cherry' *(Clearly Canadian)*	6 oz	70	16.0	0.0
CHERRY-BLACKBERRY, w/juice *(Cascadia)*	6 oz	2	0.0	0.0
CRANBERRY, 'Coastal Cranberry' *(Clearly Canadian)*	6 oz	70	16.0	0.0
GRAPEFRUIT, w/juice *(Cascadia)*	6 oz	2	0.0	0.0
GUAVA-BERRY, w/juice *(Cascadia)*	6 oz	2	0.0	0.0
LEMONAID, w/juice *(Cascadia)*	6 oz	2	0.0	0.0
LEMON-LIME *(H2OH!)*	6 oz	0	0.0	0.0
LOGANBERRY, 'Western Loganberry' *(Clearly Canadian)*	6 oz	70	16.0	0.0
NATURAL BERRY *(H2OH!)*	6 oz	0	0.0	0.0
PEACH, 'Orchard Peach' *(Clearly Canadian)*	6 oz	70	16.0	0.0
PEACH-CITRUS				
'Refresher' *(Quest)*	10 oz	2	0.0	0.0
'Refresher' *(Quest)*	8 oz	2	0.0	0.0
RASPBERRY				
'Country Raspberry' *(Clearly Canadian)*	6 oz	70	16.0	0.0
'Refresher' *(Quest)*	10 oz	2	0.0	0.0
'Refresher' *(Quest)*	8 oz	2	0.0	0.0
RED RASPBERRY				
'Refresher' *(Quest)*	10 oz	2	0.0	0.0

Food Name	Serv. Size	Total Cal.	Carbs GMS	Fat GMS
'Refresher' (Quest)	8 oz	2	0.0	0.0
STRAWBERRY-KIWI				
'Refresher' (Quest)	10 oz	2	0.0	0.0
'Refresher' (Quest)	8 oz	2	0.0	0.0
TANGERINE-LIME				
'Refresher' (Quest)	10 oz	2	0.0	0.0
'Refresher' (Quest)	8 oz	2	0.0	0.0
WATER BUFFALO				
raw	1 lb	449	0.0	6.2
raw	1 oz	28	0.0	0.4
roasted	3 oz	111	0.0	1.5
roasted, diced, approx 4.9 oz	1 cup	183	0.0	2.5
WATER CHESTNUT, CHINESE/matai				
approx 1.7 oz	4 fruits	38	8.6	0.0
slices	1/2 cup	66	14.8	0.1
trimmed	1 oz	30	6.8	<.1
untrimmed	1 lb	369	83.6	0.4
Canned				
sliced, w/liquid	1/2 cup	35	8.7	0.0
w/liquid	4 oz	57	14.1	0.1
w/liquid	4 fruits	14	3.5	0.0
(LaChoy)	1.28 oz	18	4.5	<.1
(LaChoy) chopped	.6349 oz	9	2.2	0.1
(LaChoy) sliced	1/4 cup	18	4.0	<1.0
(LaChoy) sliced	.776 oz	11	2.7	0.1
(LaChoy) whole	4 fruits	14	4.0	<1.0
(LaChoy) whole	.6702 oz	10	2.3	0.1
WATER CONVOLVULUS. See CABBAGE, SKUNK.				
WATERCRESS				
chopped	1/2 cup	2	0.2	0.0
fresh	1 sprig	0	0.0	0.0
trimmed	1 oz	3	0.4	<.1
untrimmed	1 lb	46	5.4	0.4
WATERMELON				
diced	1 cup	51	11.5	0.7
diced	1/2 cup	25	5.7	0.3
sliced, 1/16 of 10-inch-diam fruit	1 slice	154	34.6	2.1
trimmed	1 oz	9	2.0	0.1
untrimmed	1 lb	74	16.9	1.0
WATERMELON SEED, DRIED				
in hard coat	1 lb	935	25.7	79.5
kernels	1 cup	602	16.5	51.2
kernels	1 oz	158	4.3	13.4

Food Name	Serv. Size	Total Cal.	Carbs GMS	Fat GMS
WAX BEAN, CANNED				
(Allens)	1/2 cup	15	3.0	<1.0
(Del Monte) golden, cut	1/2 cup	20	4.0	0.0
(Del Monte) golden, French style	1/2 cup	20	4.0	0.0
(Stokely)	1/2 cup	20	4.0	0.0
(Stokely) 'No Salt or Sugar'	1/2 cup	20	4.0	0.0
WAX BEAN, FROZEN				
(Frosty Acres)	3 oz	25	5.0	0.0
(Seabrook) cut	3 oz	25	5.0	0.0
WAX GOURD. See GOURD, WAX.				
WELSH ONION. See ONION, WELSH.				
WELSH RAREBIT				
(Snow's) canned	1/2 cup	170	10.0	11.0
(Stouffer's) frozen	5 oz	270	9.0	20.0
WESTERN DINNER, FROZEN				
(Banquet)	11 oz	630	40.0	41.0
(Morton)	10 oz	290	29.0	14.0
(Swanson)	11.5 oz	430	43.0	19.0
WHALE, raw	100 gm	156	0.0	7.5
WHEAT, SPROUTED				
	1/3 cup	71	15.3	0.5
	1 oz	56	12.1	0.4
WHEAT, WHOLE GRAIN				
DURUM				
	1 cup	650	136.6	4.7
	1/2 cup	325	68.3	2.4
	1 oz	96	20.2	0.7
HARD RED				
spring	1 cup	631	130.6	3.7
spring	1/2 cup	316	65.3	1.8
spring	1 oz	93	19.3	0.5
spring or winter *(Arrowhead Mills)*	2 oz	190	41.0	1.0
winter	1 cup	628	136.7	3.0
winter	1/2 cup	314	68.3	1.5
winter	1 oz	93	20.2	0.4
HARD WHITE				
	1 cup	656	145.7	3.3
	1/2 cup	328	72.9	1.6
	1 oz	97	21.5	0.5
SOFT RED				
for pastry *(Arrowhead Mills)*	2 oz	190	41.0	1.0
winter	1 cup	556	124.7	2.6
winter	1/2 cup	278	62.4	1.3

Food Name	Serv. Size	Total Cal.	Carbs GMS	Fat GMS
winter	1 oz	94	21.0	0.4
SOFT WHITE				
	1 cup	571	126.6	3.3
	1/2 cup	286	63.3	1.7
	1 oz	96	21.4	0.6
WHEAT BRAN				
crude	1/2 cup	65	19.4	1.3
crude	1 oz	61	18.3	1.2
crude	2 tbsp	15	4.5	0.3
crude *(Arrowhead Mills)*	2 oz	50	30.0	2.0
toasted *(Kretschmer)*	1 oz	57	14.8	2.3
unprocessed *(Quaker)*	2 tbsp	8	3.8	0.2
WHEAT CAKE				
(Quaker) 'Grain Cakes'	1 cake	34	6.7	0.3
(Quaker) lightly salted	1 cake	35	7.0	0.0
WHEAT FLAKES *(Arrowhead Mills)*	2 oz	210	42.0	1.0
WHEAT FLOUR				
RYE				
(Pillsbury's Best) medium-colored	1 cup	400	83.0	2.0
(Pillsbury's Best) w/wheat 'Bohemian Style'	1 cup	400	86.0	1.0
WHITE				
(Drifted Snow)	1 cup	400	87.0	1.0
(Softasilk)	1/4 cup	100	23.0	0.0
(Wondra)	1 cup	400	87.0	1.0
All-purpose				
enriched	1/2 cup	226	47.3	0.6
enriched	1 oz	103	21.6	0.3
enriched, calcium-fortified	1/2 cup	226	47.3	0.6
(Ballard)	1 cup	400	87.0	1.0
(Ceresota)	4 oz	390	82.5	1.0
(Gold Medal)	1 cup	400	87.0	1.0
(Heckers)	4 oz	390	82.5	1.0
(Pillsbury's Best)	1 cup	400	87.0	1.0
(Red Band)	1 cup	390	85.0	1.0
(Robin Hood)	1 cup	400	85.0	1.0
(White Deer)	1 cup	400	87.0	1.0
All-purpose, unbleached				
enriched	1/2 cup	226	47.3	0.6
(Arrowhead Mills)	2 oz	200	53.0	1.0
(Gold Medal)	1 cup	400	87.0	1.0
(Pillsbury's Best)	1 cup	400	86.0	1.0
(Robin Hood)	1 cup	400	85.0	1.0

Food Name	Serv. Size	Total Cal.	Carbs GMS	Fat GMS
Bread				
enriched	1/2 cup	249	50.0	1.1
enriched	1 oz	102	20.6	0.5
(Gold Medal) 'Better for Bread'	1 cup	400	83.0	1.0
(Pillsbury's Best)	1 cup	400	83.0	2.0
Cake				
enriched	1/2 cup	195	42.1	0.5
enriched	1 oz	103	22.1	0.2
Self-rising				
enriched	1/2 cup	219	46.0	0.6
enriched	1 oz	100	21.0	0.3
(Aunt Jemima) enriched	1 oz	109	23.6	0.3
(Ballard)	1 cup	380	84.0	1.0
(Gold Medal)	1 cup	380	83.0	1.0
(Pillsbury's Best)	1 cup	380	84.0	1.0
(Pillsbury's Best) unbleached	1 cup	380	84.0	1.0
(Red Band)	1 cup	380	83.0	1.0
(Robin Hood)	1 cup	380	83.0	1.0
Shake and blend *(Pillsbury's Best)*	2 tbsp	50	11.0	0.0
Tortilla mix				
enriched	1/3 cup	150	24.8	3.9
enriched	1 oz	115	19.0	3.0
WHOLE GRAIN				
	1/2 cup	203	43.5	1.1
	1 oz	96	20.6	0.5
(Arrowhead Mills) pastry	2 oz	180	41.0	1.0
(Arrowhead Mills) stone ground	2 oz	200	40.0	1.0
(Ceresota)	4 oz	400	80.0	2.0
(Gold Medal)	1 cup	350	78.0	2.0
(Gold Medal) blend	1 cup	380	84.0	2.0
(Heckers)	4 oz	400	80.0	2.0
(Krusteaz)	1 cup	450	90.0	2.0
(Pillsbury's Best)	1 cup	400	80.0	2.0
WHEAT GERM				
crude	1/4 cup	104	15.0	2.8
crude	1 oz	102	14.7	2.8
toasted	1 cup	431	56.1	12.1
toasted	1 oz	108	14.1	3.0
(Arrowhead Mills) raw	2 oz	210	26.0	6.0
(Kretschmer)	1 oz	103	12.3	3.4
(Kretschmer) honey crunch	1 oz	105	15.2	2.8
WHEAT GERM OIL				
	1 cup	1927	0.0	218.0

Food Name	Serv. Size	Total Cal.	Carbs GMS	Fat GMS
. . . .	1 tbsp	120	0.0	13.6
(Spectrum Naturals) unrefined	1 tbsp	120	0.0	14.0
WHEAT GLUTEN *(Arrowhead Mills)* 'Vita 1' toasted	1 oz	100	9.0	1.0
WHEAT NUTS				
macadamia flavor, w/o salt	1 oz	176	7.9	16.0
other flavors, w/o salt	1 oz	184	5.9	17.7
unflavored, w/salt added	1 oz	177	6.7	16.4
WHEAT PILAF MIX, dry mix *(Casbah)*	1 oz	100	20.0	0.0
WHELK				
moist-heat cooked	3 oz	234	13.2	0.7
raw	1 lb	623	35.2	1.8
raw	3 oz	116	6.6	0.3
raw	1 oz	39	2.2	0.1
WHEY				
Acid				
dry	1 cup	193	41.9	0.3
dry	1 oz	96	20.8	0.2
dry	1 tbsp	10	2.1	0.0
fluid	1 quart	235	50.4	0.9
fluid	1 cup	59	12.6	0.2
fluid	1 oz	7	1.5	<.1
Sweet				
dry	1 cup	512	108.0	1.5
dry	1 oz	100	21.1	0.3
dry	1 tbsp	26	5.6	0.1
fluid	1 quart	263	50.6	3.5
fluid	1 cup	66	12.6	0.9
fluid	1 oz	8	1.5	0.1
WHIPPED TOPPING. See CREAM TOPPING.				
WHISKEY. See ALCOHOLIC BEVERAGES.				
WHISKEY SOUR. See ALCOHOLIC BEVERAGES.				
WHITE BEAN				
boiled	4 oz	158	28.5	0.4
boiled	1/2 cup	125	22.6	0.3
raw	1/2 cup	336	60.9	0.9
raw	1 oz	94	17.1	0.2
small, boiled	4 oz	161	29.3	0.7
small, boiled	1/2 cup	128	23.2	0.6
small, raw	1/2 cup	363	67.2	1.3
small, raw	1 oz	95	17.6	0.3
WHITE BEAN, CANNED				
. . . .	1/2 cup	153	28.7	0.4
w/liquid	4 oz	133	24.9	0.3

Food Name	Serv. Size	Total Cal.	Carbs GMS	Fat GMS

WHITE-FLOWERED GOURD. See GOURD, BOTTLE.

WHITE GOURD. See GOURD, WHITE.

WHITEFISH

dry-heat cooked	3 oz	146	0.0	6.4
dry-heat cooked, approx 7 oz	1 fillet	265	0.0	11.6
raw	1 lb	610	0.0	26.6
raw	3 oz	114	0.0	5.0
raw	1 oz	38	0.0	1.7
raw, approx 7 oz	1 fillet	265	0.0	11.6
smoked	4 oz	122	0.0	1.1
smoked	3 oz	92	0.0	0.8
smoked	1 oz	30	0.0	0.3

WHITING, MIXED SPECIES/silver hake

dry-heat cooked	4 oz	130	0.0	1.9
dry-heat cooked	3 oz	98	0.0	1.4
raw	1 lb	408	0.0	6.0
raw	3 oz	77	0.0	1.1
raw	1 oz	26	0.0	0.4

WHITING, MIXED SPECIES, FROZEN

(Booth)	4 oz	100	0.0	1.0
(Booth) 'Individually Wrapped'	4 oz	80	0.0	1.0

WILD BERRY DRINK

(Hi-C)	6 oz	92	22.5	0.1
(Hi-C) aseptic box or chilled	6 oz	90	22.0	0.0
(Hi-C) boxed	8.45 oz	129	31.7	0.1
(Hi-C) chilled	6 oz	90	22.0	0.0
(Tropicana) 'Juice Sparkler'	8 oz	110	27.0	0.0

WINE. See ALCOHOLIC BEVERAGES.

WINE, COOKING. See also ALCOHOLIC BEVERAGES.

Burgundy (Regina)	1/4 cup	2	<1.0	<1.0
Marsala (Holland House)	1 oz	9	2.3	0.0
red (Holland House)	1 oz	6	1.5	0.0
Sauternes (Regina)	1/4 cup	2	<1.0	<1.0
sherry (Holland House)	1 oz	5	1.2	0.0
sherry (Regina)	1/4 cup	20	5.0	<1.0
vermouth (Holland House)	1 oz	2	<1.0	0.0
white (Holland House)	1 oz	2	<1.0	0.0

WINGED BEAN/goa bean

boiled, drained	4 oz	43	3.6	0.7
immature seeds, boiled, drained	1/2 cup	12	1.0	0.2
immature seeds, raw, approx .6 oz	1 pod	8	0.7	0.1
immature seeds, slices, raw	1 cup	22	1.9	0.4
mature seeds, boiled, drained	1/2 cup	126	12.8	5.0

Food Name	Serv. Size	Total Cal.	Carbs GMS	Fat GMS
mature seeds, raw	1/2 cup	372	38.0	14.9
trimmed, raw	1 oz	14	1.2	0.2
untrimmed, raw	1 lb	218	19.2	3.9
WINGED BEAN, DRIED				
boiled	4 oz	167	16.9	6.6
boiled	1/2 cup	126	12.8	5.0
raw	1/2 cup	372	38.0	14.9
raw	1 oz	116	11.8	4.6
WINGED BEAN LEAVES				
trimmed	1 lb	336	64.0	5.0
trimmed	1 oz	21	4.0	0.3
WOLF FISH/ocean catfish				
dry-heat cooked	3 oz	105	0.0	2.6
frozen (Booth)	4 oz	115	0.0	20.0
raw	1 lb	437	0.0	10.8
raw	3 oz	82	0.0	2.0
raw	1 oz	27	0.0	0.7
raw, approx 5.4 oz	1/2 fillet	147	0.0	3.7
WON TON SKIN				
	1 oz	83	16.4	0.4
	1 wrapper	23	4.6	0.1
(Nasoya)	1 wrapper	23	4.5	0.0
WON TON SOUP. See SOUP.				

Y

Food Name	Serv. Size	Total Cal.	Carbs GMS	Fat GMS
YAKIDOFU. See TOFU.				
YAM				
boiled and drained, or baked	4 oz	132	31.2	0.2
boiled and drained, or baked, cubed	1/2 cup	79	18.8	0.1
raw, cubed	1/2 cup	89	20.9	0.1
raw, trimmed	1 oz	33	7.9	<.1
raw, untrimmed	1 lb	460	108.8	0.7
Mountain/Hawaiian				
raw, approx 8.25 inches long	1 yam	281	68.5	0.4
raw, cubed	1/2 cup	46	11.1	0.1
raw, trimmed	1 oz	19	4.6	<.1
raw, untrimmed	1 lb	253	61.4	0.4
steamed	4 oz	93	22.7	0.1
steamed, cubed	1/2 cup	59	14.4	0.1
YAM, CANNED (Bush's Best)	1/2 cup	120	28.0	0.0

Food Name	Serv. Size	Total Cal.	Carbs GMS	Fat GMS
YAM BEAN TUBER. See JICAMA.				
YARDLONG BEAN/asparagus bean				
boiled, drained	4 oz	53	10.4	0.1
boiled, drained, approx 13.25 inches long	1 pod	7	1.3	0.0
boiled, drained, sliced	1 cup	49	9.6	0.1
boiled, drained, sliced	1/2 cup	25	4.8	0.1
mature, boiled	1/2 cup	101	18.1	0.4
mature, raw	1/2 cup	291	52.0	1.1
raw, approx 13.25 inches long	1 pod	6	1.0	0.1
raw, sliced	1 cup	43	7.6	0.4
raw, sliced	1/2 cup	22	3.8	0.2
raw, trimmed	1 oz	13	2.4	0.1
raw, untrimmed	1 lb	203	36.0	1.7
Dried				
boiled	4 oz	134	23.9	0.5
boiled	1/2 cup	102	18.1	0.4
raw	1/2 cup	292	52.0	1.1
raw	1 oz	98	17.6	0.4
YEAST, BAKER'S				
active dry	1 oz	79	10.9	0.5
active dry	1 tbsp	35	4.6	0.6
active dry	.25-oz pkg	21	2.7	0.3
compressed	100 gm	105	18.1	1.9
compressed	.6-oz cake	18	3.1	0.3
compressed, fortified	1 oz	24	3.1	0.1
compressed, not fortified	1 oz	24	3.1	0.1
YEAST, BREWER'S				
debittered	1 oz	79	10.8	0.3
debittered	1 tbsp	23	3.1	0.1
(Fleischmann's) 'Active Dry/RapidRise'	1/4 oz	20	3.0	0.0
(Red Star) 'Active Dry'	1/4 oz	15	2.0	0.0
YEAST, TORULA	1 oz	78	10.4	0.3
YELLOW BEAN				
mature, boiled	1/2 cup	127	22.2	1.0
mature, raw	1/2 cup	338	59.5	2.5
Dried				
boiled	4 oz	163	28.7	1.2
boiled	1/2 cup	126	22.2	1.0
raw	1/2 cup	338	59.5	2.6
raw	1 oz	98	17.2	0.7
YELLOW MOMBIN. See JOBO.				
YELLOWEYE BEAN *(B&M)* canned, baked style	8 oz	326	50.0	7.0
YELLOW-EYED PEAS. See BLACK-EYED PEAS.				

Food Name	Serv. Size	Total Cal.	Carbs GMS	Fat GMS
YELLOWTAIL, MIXED SPECIES				
dry-heat cooked	3 oz	159	0.0	5.7
raw	1 lb	662	0.0	23.8
raw	3 oz	124	0.0	4.4
raw	1 oz	41	0.0	1.5
YOGURT				
(Colombo) 'Fruit on the Bottom' all flavors	8 oz	230	36.0	6.0
(Colombo) 'Nonfat Fruit on the Bottom' all flavors	8 oz	190	38.0	<1.0
(Colombo) 'Nonfat Lite Minipack' all flavors	4.4 oz	100	20.0	0.0
(Crowley) 'Sundae Style' all flavors	8 oz	250	47.0	2.0
(Crowley) 'Swiss Style' all flavors	8 oz	240	48.0	2.0
(Dannon) 'Extra Smooth' all flavors	4.4 oz	130	24.0	2.0
(Dannon) 'Hearty Nuts & Raisins' all flavors except vanilla	8 oz	260	48.0	3.0
(Knudsen) 'Lowfat' all flavors except strawberry	8 oz	240	43.0	4.0
(Light n' Lively) 'Free' all flavors except strawberry	4.4 oz	50	8.0	0.0
(Ripple) '70' fat-free, all flavors	6 oz	70	13.0	0.0
(Yoplait) 'Fat-free' all flavors	6 oz	150	31.0	0.0
(Yoplait) 'Light' all flavors	6 oz	90	14.0	0.0
(Yoplait) 'Light' all flavors	4 oz	60	9.0	0.0
APPLE CRISP (New Country) 'Lowfat'	6 oz	150	30.0	2.0
BANANA				
(Dannon) 'Sprinkl'ins' lowfat	4.1 oz	140	24.0	2.0
(Yoplait) 'Custard Style'	6 oz	180	30.0	3.0
BANANA BERRY				
(Light n' Lively) lowfat, 1% milkfat, cultured	4.4 oz	130	24.0	1.0
BERRIES (Yoplait) 'Breakfast' w/wheat, raisins, and walnuts	6 oz	200	39.0	2.0
BLACK CHERRY				
(Alta•Dena) 'Blended European Style'	8 oz	190	38.0	<1.0
(Alta•Dena) 'Naja' fruit-on-the-bottom	8 oz	240	40.0	4.0
(Breyers) 'Lowfat'	8 oz	260	49.0	3.0
(Knudsen) 'Cal 70'	6 oz	70	12.0	0.0
(Light n' Lively)	8 oz	230	44.0	2.0
(Light n' Lively) '100'	8 oz	100	17.0	0.0
(Mountain High) 'Honey Light' natural	8 oz	190	35.0	1.0
(TCBY) 'Light'	8 oz	100	17.0	0.0
BLUEBERRY				
(Alta•Dena) 'Maya' fruit-on-the-bottom	8 oz	280	39.0	9.0
(Breyers) 'Lowfat'	8 oz	250	48.0	2.0
(Dannon) 'Blended' fat-free	6 oz	160	33.0	0.0
(Dannon) 'Light' nonfat	8 oz	100	19.0	0.0
(Knudsen) 'Cal 70'	6 oz	70	11.0	0.0
(Light n' Lively)	8 oz	240	46.0	2.0
(Light n' Lively)	4.4 oz	130	26.0	1.0

Food Name	Serv. Size	Total Cal.	Carbs GMS	Fat GMS
(Light n' Lively) 'Free' nonfat	4.4 oz	50	8.0	0.0
(Light n' Lively) '100'	8 oz	90	15.0	0.0
(Mountain High) 'Honey Light' natural	8 oz	190	35.0	<1.0
(Mountain High) w/other natural flavors	8 oz	220	31.0	6.0
(New Country) 'Supreme'	6 oz	150	31.0	2.0
(TCBY)	8 oz	220	42.0	2.0
(TCBY) 'Light' nonfat, w/aspartame	8 oz	100	17.0	0.0
(Weight Watchers) 'Ultimate 90'	8 oz	90	13.0	0.0
(Yogi) 'Sundae' cheesecake, w/gelatin	5.6 oz	50	14.0	<1.0
(Yoplait) 'Fruit-on-the-Bottom'	6 oz	170	35.0	0.0
(Yoplait) 'Light' fat-free	6 oz	90	16.0	0.0
(Yoplait) 'Original' 99% fat-free	6 oz	180	32.0	2.0
(Yoplait) 'Parfait Style' blueberry and vanilla	6 oz	200	34.0	3.0
BOYSENBERRY *(Yoplait)* 'Original' 99% fat-free	6 oz	180	32.0	2.0
CAPPUCCINO *(Dannon)* 'Light' nonfat	8 oz	100	16.0	0.0
CHERRIES JUBILEE *(Weight Watchers)* 'Ultimate 90'	8 oz	90	13.0	0.0
CHERRY				
(Dannon) 'Sprinkl'ins' lowfat	4.1 oz	140	24.0	2.0
(Light n' Lively)	4.4 oz	140	27.0	1.0
(New Country) 'Supreme'	6 oz	150	32.0	2.0
(Yoplait) 'Breakfast Yogurt' w/almonds	6 oz	200	38.0	3.0
(Yoplait) 'Custard Style'	6 oz	180	30.0	4.0
(Yoplait) 'Light' fat-free	6 oz	90	16.0	0.0
(Yoplait) 'Original' 99% fat-free	6 oz	180	32.0	2.0
(Yoplait) 'Parfait Style' cherry and vanilla	6 oz	200	34.0	3.0
CHERRY-VANILLA				
(Dannon) 'Light' nonfat	8 oz	100	18.0	0.0
(Dannon) 'Sprinkl'ins' lowfat	4.1 oz	140	24.0	2.0
(Lite-Line) 'Swiss Style 1%'	8 oz	240	45.0	2.0
(TCBY)	8 oz	220	42.0	2.0
(Yogi) w/gelatin 'Sundae'	5.6 oz	50	14.0	<1.0
(Yoplait) fat-free 'Light Custard Style'	6 oz	90	17.0	0.0
COFFEE				
(Bison) 'Lowfat'	8 oz	210	33.0	4.0
(Dannon) 'Fresh Flavors'	8 oz	200	34.0	3.0
(Friendship) 'Lowfat'	8 oz	210	35.0	3.0
CRANBERRY-RASPBERRY *(Weight Watchers)* 'Ultimate 90'	8 oz	90	13.0	0.0
FRUIT CRUNCH *(New Country)* 'Lowfat'	6 oz	150	30.0	2.0
GRAPE				
(Dannon) lowfat 'Sprinkl'ins'	4.1 oz	140	24.0	2.0
(Light n' Lively)	4.4 oz	130	24.0	1.0
HAWAIIAN SALAD *(New Country)* 'Lowfat'	6 oz	150	31.0	2.0

Food Name	Serv. Size	Total Cal.	Carbs GMS	Fat GMS
LEMON				
(Alta•Dena) 'Naja' fruit-on-the-bottom	8 oz	240	40.0	4.0
(Bison) 'Lowfat'	8 oz	210	33.0	4.0
(Dannon) 'Fresh Flavors'	8 oz	200	34.0	3.0
(Knudsen) 'Cal 70'	6 oz	70	12.0	0.0
(Light n' Lively) '100'	8 oz	100	16.0	0.0
(Mountain High) 'Natural'	8 oz	220	31.0	6.0
(New Country) 'Supreme'	6 oz	150	31.0	2.0
(Weight Watchers) 'Ultimate 90'	1 cup	90	13.0	0.0
(Yoplait) 'Original' 99% fat-free	6 oz	180	32.0	2.0
LEMON CHIFFON				
(Dannon) 'Blended' fat-free	6 oz	150	30.0	0.0
(Dannon) 'Light' non-fat	8 oz	100	15.0	0.0
(Yogi) 'Sundae' w/gelatin	5.6 oz	50	14.0	<1.0
MIXED BERRIES				
(Alta•Dena) 'Blended European Style'	8 oz	190	39.0	<1.0
(Breyers) 'Lowfat'	8 oz	250	48.0	2.0
(New Country) 'Lowfat'	6 oz	150	31.0	2.0
(Yoplait) 'Custard Style'	6 oz	180	30.0	4.0
(Yoplait) 'Original' 99% fat-free	6 oz	180	32.0	2.0
ORANGE				
(Dannon) 'Fruit-on-the-Bottom'	8 oz	230	44.0	3.0
(New Country) 'Supreme'	6 oz	150	31.0	2.0
ORANGE-PINEAPPLE (Yogi) 'Sundae' w/gelatin	5.6 oz	50	14.0	<1.0
PEACH				
(Alta•Dena) 'Naja' fruit-on-the-bottom	8 oz	240	40.0	4.0
(Alta•Dena) nonfat, fruit-on-the-bottom	8 oz	190	36.0	<1.0
(Breyers) 'Lowfat'	8 oz	250	48.0	2.0
(Carnation) 'Smooth'n Creamy' fruit on the bottom	8 oz	250	47.0	3.0
(Dannon) 'Fruit-on-the-Bottom'	8 oz	230	44.0	3.0
(Dannon) 'Light' nonfat	8 oz	100	17.0	0.0
(Knudsen) 'Cal 70'	6 oz	70	11.0	0.0
(Light n' Lively)	8 oz	240	46.0	2.0
(Light n' Lively)	4.4 oz	130	26.0	1.0
(Light n' Lively) '100'	8 oz	100	16.0	0.0
(Lite-Line) 'Swiss Style 1%'	8 oz	230	42.0	2.0
(Mountain High) 'Natural'	8 oz	220	31.0	6.0
(New Country) 'Lowfat' 'n cream	6 oz	150	31.0	2.0
(TCBY)	8 oz	220	36.0	2.0
(Weight Watchers) 'Ultimate 90'	8 oz	90	13.0	0.0
(Yogi) 'Sundae' peachy peach, w/gelatin	5.6 oz	50	14.0	<1.0
(Yoplait) 'Crunch 'N Yogurt' nonfat, w/granola	7 oz	220	43.0	2.0
(Yoplait) 'Fruit-on-the-Bottom'	6 oz	170	35.0	0.0

Food Name	Serv. Size	Total Cal.	Carbs GMS	Fat GMS
(Yoplait) 'Light' fat-free	6 oz	90	16.0	0.0
(Yoplait) 'Light Custard Style' fat-free	6 oz	90	17.0	0.0
(Yoplait) 'Original' 99% fat-free	6 oz	180	32.0	2.0
(Yoplait) 'Parfait Style' peach and vanilla	6 oz	200	34.0	3.0
PIÑA COLADA				
(Yoplait)	6 oz	190	32.0	3.0
(Yoplait) 'Original' 99% fat-free	6 oz	180	32.0	2.0
PINEAPPLE				
(Breyers) 'Lowfat'	8 oz	250	50.0	2.0
(Knudsen) 'Cal 70'	6 oz	70	12.0	0.0
(Light n' Lively)	8 oz	230	47.0	2.0
(Light n' Lively)	4.4 oz	130	26.0	1.0
(Yoplait) 'Original' 99% fat-free	6 oz	180	32.0	2.0
PLAIN				
(Alta•Dena) nonfat	8 oz	100	13.0	<1.0
(Bison) 'Lowfat'	8 oz	150	17.0	4.0
(Bison) 'Nonfat'	8 oz	120	16.0	0.0
(Breyers) 'Lowfat'	8 oz	140	16.0	3.0
(Colombo)	8 oz	160	13.0	8.0
(Colombo) 'Nonfat Lite'	8 oz	110	17.0	<1.0
(Crowley)	8 oz	160	14.0	8.0
(Crowley) 'Lowfat'	8 oz	140	17.0	2.0
(Crowley) 'Nonfat'	8 oz	120	17.0	<1.0
(Dannon) 'Lowfat'	8 oz	140	16.0	4.0
(Dannon) 'Nonfat'	8 oz	110	16.0	0.0
(Friendship) 'Lowfat 1.5%'	8 oz	150	17.0	3.0
(Knudsen)	8 oz	200	16.0	9.0
(Knudsen) 'Lowfat'	8 oz	160	17.0	5.0
(Lite-Line) 'Swiss Style 1.5%'	8 oz	140	18.0	2.0
(Meadow Gold) lowfat, 2% milkfat	8 oz	160	16.0	5.0
(Mountain High)	8 oz	200	16.0	9.0
(Weight Watchers) 'Nonfat'	8 oz	90	13.0	<1.0
(Yoplait)	6 oz	130	15.0	3.0
(Yoplait) fat-free	8 oz	120	17.0	0.0
(Yoplait) 'Nonfat'	8 oz	120	18.0	0.0
(Yoplait) 'Original' 98% fat-free	6 oz	120	15.0	2.0
RAINBOW PUNCH *(Yoplait)* 'Trix'	6 oz	190	31.0	3.0
RASPBERRY				
(Alta•Dena) 'Blended European Style'	8 oz	180	37.0	<1.0
(Dannon) 'Blended' fat-free	6 oz	150	30.0	0.0
(Dannon) 'Fruit-on-the-Bottom'	8 oz	240	45.0	3.0
(Dannon) 'Light' nonfat	8 oz	100	18.0	0.0
(Meadow Gold) 'Sundae Style' lowfat, natural	8 oz	250	42.0	4.0

Food Name	Serv. Size	Total Cal.	Carbs GMS	Fat GMS
(Mountain High) 'Honey Light' natural	8 oz	190	35.0	<1.0
(TCBY)	8 oz	220	42.0	2.0
(Weight Watchers) 'Ultimate 90'	8 oz	90	13.0	0.0
(Yoplait) fat-free 'Light'	6 oz	90	16.0	0.0
(Yoplait) 'Fruit-on-the-Bottom'	6 oz	170	35.0	0.0
(Yoplait) 'Original' 99% fat-free	6 oz	180	32.0	2.0
RED RASPBERRY				
(Alta•Dena) 'Naja' fruit-on-the-bottom	8 oz	240	40.0	4.0
(Breyers) 'Lowfat'	8 oz	250	48.0	2.0
(Carnation) 'Smooth'n Creamy' fruit on the bottom	8 oz	250	47.0	3.0
(Knudsen) 'Cal 70'	6 oz	70	11.0	0.0
(Light n' Lively)	8 oz	230	43.0	2.0
(Light n' Lively)	4.4 oz	130	24.0	1.0
(Light n' Lively) 'Free' nonfat	4.4 oz	50	8.0	0.0
(Light n' Lively) '100'	8 oz	90	15.0	0.0
(Meadow Gold) lowfat, 1.5% milkfat	8 oz	250	42.0	4.0
(New Country) 'Supreme'	6 oz	150	31.0	2.0
STRAWBERRY				
(Alta•Dena) 'Blended European Style'	8 oz	180	37.0	<1.0
(Alta•Dena) 'Maya' fruit-on-the-bottom	8 oz	280	39.0	9.0
(Alta•Dena) 'Naja' fruit-on-the-bottom	8 oz	240	40.0	4.0
(Breyers) 'Lowfat'	8 oz	250	48.0	2.0
(Carnation) 'Smooth'n Creamy' fruit on the bottom	8 oz	230	44.0	3.0
(Colombo)	8 oz	210	29.0	7.0
(Crowley) 'Nonfat'	8 oz	190	35.0	<1.0
(Dannon) 'Blended' fat-free	6 oz	150	30.0	0.0
(Dannon) 'Fruit-on-the-Bottom'	8 oz	230	45.0	3.0
(Dannon) 'Light' nonfat	8 oz	100	17.0	0.0
(Dannon) 'Sprinkl'ins' lowfat	4.1 oz	140	24.0	2.0
(Knudsen) 'Cal 70'	6 oz	70	11.0	0.0
(Knudsen) 'Lowfat'	8 oz	250	45.0	4.0
(Light n' Lively)	8 oz	240	45.0	2.0
(Light n' Lively)	4.4 oz	130	25.0	1.0
(Light n' Lively) 'Free'	4.4 oz	50	8.0	0.0
(Light n' Lively) '100'	8 oz	90	15.0	0.0
(Lite-Line) 'Lowfat 1%'	8 oz	240	46.0	2.0
(Mountain High) 'Honey Light' natural	8 oz	190	35.0	<1.0
(New Country) 'Supreme'	6 oz	150	30.0	2.0
(TCBY)	8 oz	220	43.0	2.0
(Weight Watchers) 'Ultimate 90'	8 oz	90	13.0	0.0
(Yoplait) 'Custard Style'	6 oz	180	30.0	3.0
(Yoplait) 'Fruit-on-the-Bottom'	6 oz	170	35.0	0.0
(Yoplait) 'Light' fat-free	6 oz	90	16.0	0.0

Food Name	Serv. Size	Total Cal.	Carbs GMS	Fat GMS
(Yoplait) 'Light Custard Style' fat-free	6 oz	90	17.0	0.0
(Yoplait) 'Original' 99% fat-free	6 oz	180	32.0	2.0
(Yoplait) 'Parfait Style' strawberry and vanilla	6 oz	200	34.0	3.0
STRAWBERRY CHEESECAKE *(Yogi)* 'Sundae' w/gelatin	5.6 oz	50	14.0	<1.0
STRAWBERRY FRUIT BASKET *(Knudsen)* 'Cal 70'	6 oz	70	11.0	0.0
STRAWBERRY FRUIT CUP				
(Dannon) 'Light' nonfat	8 oz	100	17.0	0.0
(Light n' Lively)	8 oz	240	47.0	2.0
(Light n' Lively)	4.4 oz	130	26.0	1.0
(Light n' Lively) 'Free' nonfat	4.4 oz	50	8.0	0.0
(Light n' Lively) '100'	8 oz	90	15.0	0.0
(New Country) 'Lowfat'	6 oz	150	30.0	2.0
STRAWBERRY-ALMOND *(Yoplait)* 'Breakfast Yogurt'	6 oz	200	38.0	3.0
STRAWBERRY-BANANA				
(Alta•Dena) nonfat, fruit-on-the-bottom	8 oz	180	35.0	<1.0
(Breyers) 'Lowfat'	8 oz	250	50.0	2.0
(Carnation) 'Smooth'n Creamy' fruit on the bottom	8 oz	240	42.0	4.0
(Dannon) 'Fruit-on-the-Bottom'	8 oz	230	44.0	3.0
(Dannon) 'Light' nonfat	8 oz	100	17.0	0.0
(Dannon) lowfat 'Sprinkl'ins'	4.1 oz	140	24.0	2.0
(Knudsen) 'Cal 70'	6 oz	70	12.0	0.0
(Light n' Lively)	8 oz	260	52.0	2.0
(Light n' Lively)	4.4 oz	140	29.0	1.0
(Light n' Lively) 'Free' nonfat	4.4 oz	50	8.0	0.0
(Mountain High) 'Honey Light' natural	8 oz	190	35.0	<1.0
(New Country)	6 oz	150	31.0	2.0
(TCBY)	8 oz	220	43.0	2.0
(Weight Watchers) 'Ultimate 90'	8 oz	90	13.0	0.0
(Yoplait) 'Breakfast' w/wheat and walnuts	6 oz	200	40.0	2.0
(Yoplait) 'Fruit-on-the-Bottom'	6 oz	170	35.0	0.0
(Yoplait) 'Light' fat-free	6 oz	90	16.0	0.0
(Yoplait) 'Original' 99% fat-free	6 oz	180	32.0	2.0
(Yoplait) 'Trix' bash	6 oz	190	31.0	3.0
STRAWBERRY-RHUBARB *(Yoplait)*	6 oz	190	32.0	3.0
TRIPLE CHERRY *(Yoplait)* 'Trix'	6 oz	190	31.0	3.0
TROPICAL FRUIT				
(Dannon) 'Light' nonfat	8 oz	100	18.0	0.0
(Ripple) '70'	6 oz	70	13.0	0.0
(Weight Watchers) 'Ultimate 90'	8 oz	90	13.0	0.0
(Yoplait) 'Breakfast' w/wheat, raisins, and nuts	6 oz	200	41.0	3.0
VANILLA				
(Bison) 'Lowfat'	8 oz	210	33.0	4.0
(Breyers) 'Lowfat' vanilla bean	8 oz	230	41.0	3.0

Food Name	Serv. Size	Total Cal.	Carbs GMS	Fat GMS
(Colombo) French	8 oz	215	30.0	7.0
(Colombo) 'Nonfat Lite'	8 oz	160	30.0	<1.0
(Crowley) 'Lowfat'	8 oz	200	33.0	2.0
(Dannon) 'Blended' French, fat-free	6 oz	150	31.0	0.0
(Dannon) 'Fresh Flavors'	8 oz	200	34.0	3.0
(Dannon) 'Fresh Flavors'	4.4 oz	110	20.0	2.0
(Dannon) 'Hearty Nuts & Raisins' w/wheat	8 oz	270	48.0	5.0
(Dannon) 'Light' nonfat	8 oz	100	16.0	0.0
(Friendship) 'Lowfat'	8 oz	210	35.0	3.0
(Knudsen) 'Cal 70'	6 oz	70	11.0	0.0
(Knudsen) 'Lowfat'	8 oz	240	43.0	4.0
(New Country) 'Lowfat' French	6 oz	150	31.0	2.0
(Weight Watchers) 'Ultimate 90'	1 cup	90	13.0	0.0
(Yoplait)	6 oz	180	29.0	3.0
(Yoplait) 'Crunch 'N Yogurt' w/granola, nonfat	7 oz	220	43.0	2.0
(Yoplait) 'Custard Style'	6 oz	180	30.0	4.0
(Yoplait) 'Custard Style'	4 oz	130	20.0	3.0
(Yoplait) 'Fat-free'	6 oz	150	28.0	0.0
(Yoplait) 'Light Custard Style' fat-free	6 oz	90	17.0	0.0
(Yoplait) 'Nonfat'	8 oz	180	35.0	0.0
WILD BERRY *(Light n' Lively)* lowfat, 1% milkfat, cultured	4.4 oz	140	28.0	1.0
YOGURT, FROZEN				
(Alta•Dena) apricot mango, nonfat	4 oz	90	20.0	0.0
(Ben & Jerry's)				
apple pie	1/2 cup	170	32.0	3.0
banana strawberry	1/2 cup	160	32.0	2.0
blueberry	1/2 cup	160	32.0	2.0
cherry Garcia	1/2 cup	170	31.0	3.0
chocolate fudge brownie	1/2 cup	190	35.0	4.0
chocolate raspberry swirl	1/2 cup	200	40.0	2.5
coffee almond fudge	1/2 cup	200	30.0	7.0
English toffee crunch	1/2 cup	190	32.0	6.0
(Bison) chocolate	3.5 oz	94	18.0	2.0
(Breyers)				
black cherry	1/2 cup	120	24.0	1.0
chocolate	1/2 cup	120	24.0	1.0
peach	1/2 cup	110	22.0	1.0
red raspberry	1/2 cup	120	23.0	1.0
strawberry	1/2 cup	110	22.0	1.0
strawberry-banana	1/2 cup	110	22.0	1.0
vanilla	1/2 cup	120	23.0	1.0
(Colombo)				
banana split, lowfat, 'Sundae Style'	3 oz	100	20.0	1.0

Food Name	Serv. Size	Total Cal.	Carbs GMS	Fat GMS
Bavarian chocolate chunk, 'Gourmet'	3 oz	120	18.0	4.0
caramel fudge sundae, lowfat, 'Sundae Style'	3 oz	100	21.0	1.0
caramel-pecan chunk, 'Gourmet'	3 oz	120	19.0	3.0
chocolate peanut butter twist, 'Sundae Style'	3 oz	110	18.0	3.0
dream, 'Gourmet'	3 oz	90	16.0	2.0
Heath bar crunch, 'Gourmet'	3 oz	130	19.0	5.0
mocha Swiss almond, 'Gourmet'	3 oz	120	17.0	5.0
nonfat, lite	4 oz	95	21.0	0.0
peanut butter cup, 'Gourmet'	3 oz	140	16.0	7.0
plain, lowfat	4 oz	99	18.0	2.0
plain, 'Nonfat Lite'	4 oz	95	21.0	0.0
strawberry passion, 'Gourmet'	3 oz	100	18.0	2.0
wild raspberry cheesecake, 'Gourmet'	3 oz	100	18.0	2.0
(Crowley)				
cherry	3 oz	80	16.0	1.0
chocolate	3 oz	80	15.0	2.0
peach	3 oz	80	16.0	1.0
raspberry	3 oz	80	16.0	1.0
strawberry	3 oz	80	16.0	1.0
vanilla	3 oz	80	15.0	2.0
(Dannon)				
cappuccino, nonfat, 'Light'	4 oz	80	19.0	0.0
caramel pecan, 'Pure Indulgence'	4 oz	180	22.0	8.0
cherry vanilla swirl, nonfat, 'Light'	4 oz	90	21.0	0.0
chocolate, nonfat, 'Light'	4 oz	80	19.0	<1.0
chocolate, 'Pure Indulgence'	3 oz	130	24.0	3.0
chocolate nut, chunky, 'Pure Indulgence'	4 oz	190	24.0	9.0
chunky chocolate nut, 'Pure Indulgence'	4 oz	190	24.0	9.0
cookies and cream, 'Pure Indulgence'	4 oz	180	18.0	7.0
Heath bar crunch, 'Pure Indulgence'	4 oz	170	25.0	7.0
peach, nonfat, 'Light'	4 oz	80	19.0	0.0
red raspberry, nonfat, 'Light'	4 oz	90	21.0	0.0
strawberry, nonfat, 'Light'	4 oz	80	19.0	0.0
vanilla, nonfat, 'Light'	4 oz	80	20.0	0.0
vanilla, 'Pure Indulgence'	3 oz	130	25.0	3.0
(Dreyer's)				
black cherry vanilla, nonfat, 'Inspirations'	4 oz	90	19.0	0.0
blueberry, 'Inspirations'	3 oz	80	15.0	1.0
cherry, 'Inspirations'	3 oz	80	15.0	1.0
chocolate, 'Inspirations'	3 oz	80	15.0	1.0
peach, 'Inspirations Perfectly Peach'	3 oz	80	15.0	1.0
raspberry, 'Inspirations'	3 oz	80	15.0	1.0
strawberry, 'Inspirations'	3 oz	80	15.0	1.0

Food Name	Serv. Size	Total Cal.	Carbs GMS	Fat GMS
strawberry-banana, 'Inspirations'	3 oz	80	15.0	1.0
vanilla chocolate swirl, nonfat, 'Inspirations'	4 oz	90	19.0	0.0
vanilla-raspberry swirl, 'Inspirations'	3 oz	80	15.0	1.0
(Elan) chocolate almond	1/2 cup	160	23.0	7.0
(Häagen-Dazs)				
chocolate	3 oz	130	21.0	3.0
peach	3 oz	120	20.0	3.0
praline pandemonium, 'Exträas'	4 oz	240	33.0	9.0
strawberry	3 oz	120	21.0	3.0
strawberry cheesecake craze, 'Exträas'	4 oz	210	31.0	7.0
vanilla almond crunch	3 oz	150	22.0	5.0
(Natural Nectar) chocolate, 'Fi-Bar Lite'	2.5 oz	190	29.0	6.0
(Sealtest)				
black cherry, nonfat, 'Free'	1/2 cup	110	24.0	0.0
chocolate, nonfat, 'Free'	1/2 cup	110	24.0	0.0
peach, nonfat, 'Free'	1/2 cup	100	23.0	0.0
red raspberry, nonfat, 'Free'	1/2 cup	100	23.0	0.0
strawberry, nonfat, 'Free'	1/2 cup	100	22.0	0.0

YOGURT, FROZEN, SOFT-SERVE

Food Name	Serv. Size	Total Cal.	Carbs GMS	Fat GMS
(Bresler's)				
'Gourmet' all flavors, 1 oz	1/2 cup	29	5.5	0.5
'Lite' all flavors, 1 oz	1/2 cup	27	6.0	0.0
(Crowley)				
banana, 'Peaks of Perfection,' 3.5 oz	1/2 cup	100	19.0	2.0
chocolate, 'Peaks of Perfection,' 3.5 oz	1/2 cup	100	19.0	2.0
lemon, 'Peaks of Perfection,' 3.5 oz	1/2 cup	100	19.0	2.0
plain, 'Peaks of Perfection,' 3.5 oz	1/2 cup	90	20.0	1.0
raspberry, 'Peaks of Perfection,' 3.5 oz	1/2 cup	100	19.0	2.0
strawberry, 'Peaks of Perfection,' 3.5 oz	1/2 cup	100	19.0	2.0
vanilla, 'Peaks of Perfection,' 3.5 oz	1/2 cup	100	19.0	2.0
(Dannon)				
blueberry	1/2 cup	100	18.0	2.0
butter pecan	1/2 cup	100	18.0	2.0
cappuccino	1/2 cup	100	18.0	2.0
cheesecake	1/2 cup	100	18.0	2.0
chocolate	1/2 cup	120	23.0	2.0
lemon meringue	1/2 cup	100	18.0	2.0
peach	1/2 cup	100	18.0	2.0
piña colada	1/2 cup	100	18.0	2.0
raspberry	1/2 cup	100	18.0	2.0
red raspberry, 'Nonfat'	1/2 cup	90	21.0	0.0
strawberry	1/2 cup	100	18.0	2.0
strawberry-banana	1/2 cup	100	18.0	2.0

Food Name	Serv. Size	Total Cal.	Carbs GMS	Fat GMS
(Häagen-Dazs)				
banana, nonfat	1 oz	25	5.0	0.0
chocolate	1 oz	30	4.0	1.0
chocolate, nonfat	1 oz	30	6.0	0.0
coffee	1 oz	28	4.0	1.0
raspberry	1 oz	30	5.0	1.0
strawberry, nonfat	1 oz	25	5.0	0.0
vanilla	1 oz	28	4.0	1.0
YOGURT BAR, FROZEN				
(Dole)				
cherry 'Fruit & Yogurt'	1 bar	80	17.0	<1.0
raspberry 'Fruit & Yogurt'	1 bar	70	17.0	<1.0
strawberry 'Fruit & Yogurt'	1 bar	70	17.0	<1.0
(Häagen-Dazs)				
cherry chocolate fudge	1 bar	230	28.0	12.0
peach	1 bar	100	18.0	1.0
piña colada	1 bar	100	21.0	1.0
raspberry and vanilla	1 bar	100	19.0	1.0
strawberry daiquiri	1 bar	100	20.0	1.0
tropical orange passion	1 bar	100	21.0	1.0
YOGURT DESSERT *(Sara Lee)* 'Free & Light'	1/10 pkg	120	26.0	1.0
YOGURT FLAVORED DRINK				
(Dannon) all flavors	8 oz	190	32.0	4.0
(Yogloo) fruit basket	10 oz	170	40.0	0.0
(Yogloo) original	10 oz	170	40.0	0.0
(Yogloo) peach	10 oz	170	40.0	0.0
(Yogloo) strawberry	10 oz	170	40.0	0.0
YOKAN	1 oz	74	17.2	(tr)
YUCA. See CASSAVA.				

Z

Food Name	Serv. Size	Total Cal.	Carbs GMS	Fat GMS
ZITI ENTRÉE, FROZEN				
(Budget Gourmet) 'Side Dish' in marinara sauce	6.25 oz	220	25.0	9.0
ZUCCHINI. See also SQUASH, SUMMER.				
baby, raw	1 large	3	0.5	0.1
baby, raw	1 med	2	0.3	0.0
boiled, drained	4 oz	18	4.5	0.1
raw	1 lb	62	12.5	0.6
raw, trimmed	1 oz	4	0.8	<.1
w/skin, boiled, drained, mashed	1/2 cup	19	4.7	0.1

Food Name	Serv. Size	Total Cal.	Carbs GMS	Fat GMS
w/skin, boiled, drained, sliced	1/2 cup	14	3.5	0.0
w/skin, raw, sliced	1/2 cup	9	1.9	0.1
Canned				
in tomato juice	1/2 cup	33	7.8	0.1
Italian style	1/2 cup	33	7.8	0.1
(Del Monte) in tomato sauce	1/2 cup	30	8.0	0.0
(Progresso) Italian style	1/2 cup	50	8.0	2.0
Frozen				
w/skin, unprepared	10-oz pkg	48	10.2	0.4
(Seabrook)	3.3 oz	16	3.0	0.0
(Southern)	3.5 oz	18	3.6	0.1
(Stilwell) 'Quick Krisp' breaded	3.3 oz	200	24.0	10.0

Free Software Version of this Book!

Query - *Instantly* locate all foods that meet *all* the criteria you specify. For instance, display all hamburgers and cheeseburgers from ten selected restaurants that contain less than 35 gm of *Carbohydrate* and sort them from low-to-high (or high-to-low) based on *Calories from Fat*.

Collect Avery Publishing Group's entire NutriBase Series of books and receive the entire NutriBase software library free!

How to Get Your Free Software
NutriBase Guide to Carbohydrates, Calories, & Fat in Your Food

1. Fill out this order form (photocopy acceptable).

2. Attach the original register receipt for the <u>NutriBase Guide to Carbohydrates, Calories, and Fat in Your Food</u>.

3. Include a $5.00 check or money order (payable to CyberSoft, Inc.) per copy to cover shipping and handling.

4. Send the three items listed above to:

    CyberSoft, Incorporated
    3646 E. Ray Rd., # B16-8
    Phoenix AZ 85044-7116

Name: _____

Address: _____

Address: _____

City: _____ State: _____ ZIP: _____

Telephone Number: _____

Software Format Preference: Windows _____ DOS _____

Note: *This free software offer is valid only for the book title purchased. Additional free software titles require the purchase of the corresponding NutriBase Series book titles. NutriBase Series software titles are not available for sale—they are available only as free complements to their hard copy book versions. This offer is subject to expiration without notice after January 1, 1997.*

Free Software Version of this Book!

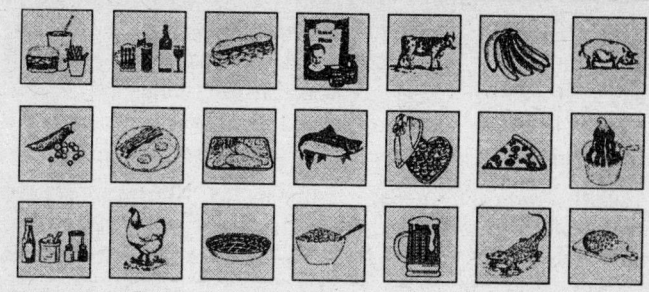

The NutriBase Guide to Carbohydrates, Calories, and Fat in Your Food

Congratulations! Your purchase of this book entitles you to a free copy of the software edition of the <u>NutriBase Guide to Carbohydrates, Calories, and Fat in Your Food</u>. Get the best of both worlds–the portability and convenience of hard copy, plus the analytical capabilities of the NutriBase Series software.

Your free software will provide you with instant access to all of the information in this book including *Food Names, Comments, Brand Names, Serving Sizes, Total Calories, Carbohydrate Grams, Fat Grams* and *Calories from Fat*. Harness the power of your DOS or Windows PC and tap into a wide range of capabilities:

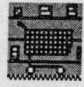 **Comprehensive Data** - NutriBase software will provide you with information for every food item in this book–a total of 47,547 food items. The software features over 31,000 brand name foods and thousands of generic food entries.

 View - Click on this software icon to instantly display an alphabetized view of food items in a conventional "spreadsheet view." Your NutriBase software also features over 3,100 menu items from more than 70 restaurants.

 Rank - Instantly rank foods based on their values for any nutrient. For instance, rank all of the Frozen Entrees from low-to-high or high-to-low based on *Calories, Carbohydrates, Fat Grams,* or *Calories from Fat*.